Encyclopedia of

MEDICAL DECISION MAKING

Editorial Board

Encyclopedia of

MEDICAL DECISION MAKING

MICHAEL W. KATTAN, EDITOR

Cleveland Clinic

MARK E. COWEN, ASSOCIATE EDITOR

St. Joseph Mercy Health System, Michigan

Volume 1

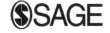

Los Angeles | London | New Delhi
Singapore | Washington DC

A SAGE Reference Publication

For information:

SAGE Publications, Inc.
2455 Teller Road
Thousand Oaks, California 91320
E-mail: order@sagepub.com

SAGE Publications Ltd.
1 Oliver's Yard
55 City Road
London, EC1Y 1SP
United Kingdom

SAGE Publications India Pvt. Ltd.
B 1/I 1 Mohan Cooperative Industrial Area
Mathura Road, New Delhi 110 044
India

SAGE Publications Asia-Pacific Pte. Ltd.
33 Pekin Street #02-01
Far East Square
Singapore 048763

Library of Congress Cataloging-in-Publication Data

Encyclopedia of medical decision making/editor, Michael W. Kattan ; associate editor, Mark E. Cowen.
    p. ; cm.
Includes bibliographical references and index.
ISBN 978-1-4129-5372-6 (cloth)

  1. Medicine—Decision making—Encyclopedias. 2. Clinical medicine—Decision making—Encyclopedias.
3. Diagnosis—Decision making—Encyclopedias. I. Kattan, Michael W. II. Cowen, Mark E.
[DNLM: 1. Clinical Medicine—Encyclopedias—English. 2. Decision Making—Encyclopedias—English. 3. Costs and Cost Analysis—Encyclopedias—English. 4. Decision Support Techniques—Encyclopedias—English. 5. Patient Participation—Encyclopedias—English. 6. Quality of Health Care—Encyclopedias—English. WB 13 E56289 2009]

R723.5.E53 2009
610.3—dc22   2009004379

09 10 11 12 13 10 9 8 7 6 5 4 3 2 1

Publisher:	Rolf A. Janke
Assistant to the Publisher:	Michele Thompson
Acquisitions Editor:	Jim Brace-Thompson
Developmental Editor:	Carole Maurer
Reference Systems Manager:	Leticia Gutierrez
Reference Systems Coordinator:	Laura Notton
Production Editor:	Tracy Buyan
Copy Editor:	QuADS Prepress (P) Ltd.
Typesetter:	C&M Digitals (P) Ltd.
Proofreaders:	Jenifer Kooiman, Scott Oney
Indexer:	Virgil Diodato
Cover Designer:	Gail Buschman
Marketing Manager:	Amberlyn McKay

Contents

List of Entries

Reader's Guide

The alphabetical organization of an encyclopedia facilitates access to information when the reader can identify the topic of interest. Some readers, on the other hand, may prefer to use the encyclopedia as a source for topical study and to sample key concepts of an academic discipline sequentially. This Reader's Guide is an attempt to catalog essays to mirror the components of the decision-making process. Many essays could be grouped under more than one category, and some titles might have more than one connotation. The following organization is offered as one of many possible ways to guide topical reading:

Basis for Making the Decision. These essays examine criteria by which the optimal choice among available alternatives can be identified. Some methods, particularly those drawn from the field of health economics or used by decision analysts, are quantitative and permit the rank ordering of potential decision strategies. However, there are also other considerations used in making a final decision, sometimes on philosophical or ethical grounds.

Biostatistics and Clinical Epidemiology: The Assessment of the Likelihood of Possible Consequences or Outcomes. These entries present some of the techniques used to determine the probabilities of health outcomes, to determine if the results of a clinical study are due to chance or some alternate explanation, and to assess the accuracy of diagnostic tests and prognostic algorithms. These concepts often underlie the approaches described in essays throughout the Encyclopedia, and provide background for understanding the Methods sections of scientific publications.

Decision Analysis and Related Mathematical Models. These essays present techniques for a rational or prescriptive decision-making process for an individual or population. The choice to be made, the possible consequences, their value or cost, and their likelihood of occurring are combined to identify the optimal decision.

Health Outcomes and Measurement. These essays discuss some of the possible health outcomes that follow a medical or health policy decision and how they can be measured or quantified. Some of these essays provide a foundation for understanding health-related surveys and evaluations of the quality of care provided by health professionals or health systems.

Impact or Weight or Utility of the Possible Outcomes. These essays examine the value or "utility" placed on certain health outcomes to indicate their relative level of desirability or preference in the eyes of patients or the general population. Some essays describe the methods for determining this value, whereas others describe how utilities can be combined and aggregated in decision analyses or economic analyses.

Other Techniques, Theories, and Tools to Understand and to Assist Decision Making. Although the following essays do not fit neatly into the other categories, they represent a valuable array for understanding patients and healthcare delivery systems, and provide potential resources for guiding clinicians and patients in making sound decisions.

Perspective of the Decision Maker. The relevant components of decision making and the considerations used to determine a course of action may differ according to the point of view or perspective of the person or entity empowered to choose. The following essays include examples of health-related scenarios for decision making by individuals, clinicians, health systems, governments, and other entities.

The Psychology Underlying Decision Making. These essays represent scholarly work to understand how humans appropriate, use, and process information when they make their choices. Influences on, vulnerabilities associated with, and strategies developed to improve decision making are discussed.

Basis for Making the Decision

Biostatistics and Clinical Epidemiology

About the Editors

General Editor

Michael W. Kattan is Chairman of the Department of Quantitative Health Sciences at Cleveland Clinic. He is also Professor of Medicine, Epidemiology, and Biostatistics at Cleveland Clinic Lerner College of Medicine of Case Western Reserve University. Prior to joining Cleveland Clinic, he was Associate Attending Outcomes Research Scientist at Memorial Sloan-Kettering Cancer Center and Associate Professor of Biostatistics in Urology at Cornell University in New York City. He began his academic career as an assistant professor of urology and medical informatics at Baylor College of Medicine in Houston, Texas, where he also obtained his postdoctorate in medical informatics.

His primary research interest lies in prescriptive medical decision making—how physicians and patients should make decisions. Specifically, he is most interested in medical prediction: how, why, and when. He has received multiple patents for his work in this area and coauthored about 300 articles in peer-reviewed journals. In 2008, he received the Eugene Saenger Distinguished Service Award from the Society for Medical Decision Making. He serves or has served on the editorial boards for several journals, including *Cancer Investigation, Nature Clinical Practice Urology, Medical Decision Making, Clinical Genitourinary Cancer, Urologic Oncology, Journal of Urology,* and *Urologic Oncology: Seminars and Original Investigation.* His PhD is in management information systems, with a minor in statistics, from the University of Houston. He also has a master's of business administration, with concentration in computer information systems and quantitative analysis, from the University of Arkansas. His undergraduate degree is in food science, also from the University of Arkansas.

Associate Editor

Mark E. Cowen, MD, is Chief of Clinical Decision Services at the St. Joseph Mercy Health System, Ann Arbor, Michigan. He was founder and president of a private group practice in internal medicine and served as a clinical instructor for the University of Michigan Medical School for a number of years. After receiving a master of science degree in epidemiology from the Harvard School of Public Health, he was Vice President, Performance Improvement, of Allegiance LLC, a physician-hospital organization for managed care. He is currently on the editorial board of the *American Journal of Managed Care.* His research has been largely driven by questions arising from daily responsibilities with managed care or hospitalized patient populations. A concurrent interest in prostate cancer screening and treatment decisions led to the development of a Markov model and collaborations with Dr. Kattan to study various components of decision making regarding this disease. He has been a member of the prostate cancer outcomes task force of the American Urological Association. He received his undergraduate and medical degrees from the University of Michigan.

Contributors

A E Ades
University of Bristol

Arpita Aggarwal
*Virginia Commonwealth
University*

Laith Alattar
University of Michigan

Daniel Almirall
*Duke University School of
Medicine*

Allen Andrew Alvarez
*University of the
Philippines*

Andrea Angott
University of Michigan

Noriaki Aoki
University of Texas–Houston

Arlene S. Ash
*Boston University School of
Medicine*

Koula Asimakopoulou
King's College London

Carla Bann
RTI International

Paul G. Barnett
*U.S. Department of Veterans
Affairs*

Barbara A. Bartman
*Agency for Healthcare Research
and Quality*

Daniel Beavers
Baylor University

J. Robert Beck
Fox Chase Cancer Center

James F. Bena
Cleveland Clinic

George Bergus
University of Iowa

Whitney Berta
University of Toronto

Harald Binder
University Medical Center

Jakob B. Bjorner
QualityMetric Inc.

Eugene H. Blackstone
Cleveland Clinic

Gerhard Blasche
Medical University of Vienna

Han Bleichrodt
Erasmus University

Donald Bordley
*University of Rochester Medical
Center*

Emanuele Borgonovo
Bocconi University

Brian H. Bornstein
University of Nebraska–Lincoln

Mari Botti
Deakin University

Dave Bouckenooghe
*Vlerick Leuven Gent
Management School*

Aziz A. Boxwala
Harvard Medical School

Eduard Brandstätter
*Johannes Kepler University
of Linz*

John E. Brazier
University of Sheffield

Karen E. Bremner
University Health Network

Frank Brennan
Calvary Hospital

Andrew H. Briggs
University of Glasgow

Arndt Bröder
University of Bonn

Werner Brouwer
Erasmus MC Rotterdam

Tracey Bucknall
Deakin University

Marc Buelens
*Vlerick Leuven Gent
Management School*

Robert S. Butler
Cleveland Clinic

Scott B. Cantor
University of Texas M. D.
Anderson Cancer Center

Linda Jean Carroll
University of Alberta

Lydia L. Chen
University of Michigan

Ying Qing Chen
Fred Hutchinson Cancer
Research Center

Karis K. F. Cheng
Chinese University of Hong
Kong

V. K. Chetty
Boston University

Ling-Hsiang Chuang
Centre for Health Economics

Felix K.-H. Chun
University of Hamburg

Leslie Citrome
New York University Medical
Center

Nancy S. Clark
University of Rochester Medical
Center

Karl Claxton
University of York

Phaedra Corso
University of Georgia

Michael Cousins
University of Sydney Pain
Management Research
Institute

William Dale
University of Chicago

Jarrod E. Dalton
Cleveland Clinic

Laura J. Damschroder
Ann Arbor VA HSR&D Center
of Excellence

Raisa Deber
University of Toronto

Richard A. Demme
University of Rochester Medical
Center

Francisco J. Díez
UNED (Spain)

Peter H. Ditto
University of California, Irvine

Robert S. Dittus
Vanderbilt University

Jason N. Doctor
University of Southern
California

Ray Dolan
University College London

Michael R. Dougherty
University of Maryland

Stephan Dreiseitl
Upper Austria University of
Applied Sciences

Marek J. Druzdzel
University of Pittsburgh

Michael Dunn
University of Oxford

Mette Ebbesen
University of Aarhus

Mark H. Eckman
University of Cincinnati

Heather Edelblute
University of North Carolina at
Chapel Hill

Eric L. Eisenstein
Duke University Medical Center

A. Christine Emler
Veterans Administration

David Epstein
University of York

Ronald Epstein
University of Rochester Medical
Center

Steven Estrada
Cornell University

Margot M. Eves
Cleveland Clinic

Zhaozhi Fan
Memorial University of
Newfoundland

Deb Feldman-Stewart
Queen's University

Elisabeth Fenwick
University of Glasgow

Paul J. Ford
Cleveland Clinic

Liana Fraenkel
Yale University

Daniel J. France
Vanderbilt University Medical
Center

Jenny V. Freeman
University of Sheffield

Alex Z. Fu
Cleveland Clinic

Amiram Gafni
McMaster University

Wolfgang Gaissmaier
Max Planck Institute for
Human Development

Mirta Galesic
Max Planck Institute for
Human Development

Rocio Garcia-Retamero
University of Granada

Jason Gatliff
Cleveland Clinic

Constantine Gatsonis
Brown University

R. Brian Giesler
Butler University

Gerd Gigerenzer
*Max Planck Institute for
Human Development*

John Gilmour
*Gilmour and Associates
Physiotherapy*

Alan Girling
University of Birmingham

Julie Goldberg
University of Illinois at Chicago

Morton P. Goldman
Cleveland Clinic

Mithat Gönen
*Memorial Sloan-Kettering
Cancer Center*

Banu Gopalan
Cleveland Clinic

Carolyn C. Gotay
University of British Columbia

Markus Graefen
University of Hamburg

Erika Graf
University Medical Center

Dan Greenberg
*Ben Gurion University of the
Negev*

Kalle Grill
Royal Institute of Technology

Erik J. Groessl
*VA San Diego/University of
California, San Diego*

Scott D. Grosse
Centers for Disease Control

Enzo Grossi
Bracco

Frank M. Guess
University of Tennessee

Alexander Haese
University of Hamburg

C. Gregory Hagerty
*Robert Wood Johnson Medical
School*

Susan Halabi
Duke University

Bruce P. Hallbert
Idaho National Laboratory

Robert M. Hamm
*University of Oklahoma Health
Sciences Center*

Seunghee Han
Carnegie Mellon

Ronald B. Harrist
*University of Texas, Austin
Regional Campus*

Kate Haswell
*Auckland University of
Technology*

Katherine Hauser
Cleveland Clinic

Daniel Hausmann
University of Zurich

Ron D. Hays
*University of California, Los
Angeles*

Christopher Hebert
Cleveland Clinic

Glenn Heller
*Memorial Sloan-Kettering
Cancer Center*

Joshua Hemmerich
University of Chicago

Lidewij Henneman
*VU University (Amsterdam)
Medical Center*

Adrian V. Hernandez
Cleveland Clinic

Jørgen Hilden
University of Copenhagen

Richard A. Hirth
*University of Michigan School
of Public Health*

Jeffrey S. Hoch
St. Michael's Hospital

Eduard Hofer
Retired Mathematician

Søren Holm
Cardiff University

Kirsten Howard
University of Sydney

Xuelin Huang
*University of Texas M. D.
Anderson Cancer Center*

Yunchen Huang
Mississippi State University

M. G. Myriam Hunink
*Erasmus University Medical
Center*

Jordan Hupert
*University of Illinois College of
Medicine*

Don Husereau
*Health Technology Assessment
Council*

Lisa I. Iezzoni
*Harvard Medical School/
Institute for Health Policy,
Massachusetts General Hospital*

Lee H. Igel
New York University

Peter B. Imrey
Cleveland Clinic

Hemant Ishwaran
Cleveland Clinic

John L. Jackson Jr.
University of Pennsylvania

Philip Jacobs
University of Alberta

Eric W. Jamoom
University of Florida

Stephen Jan
*George Institute for
    International Health*

Naveed Zafar Janjua
*Aga Khan University, Karachi,
    Pakistan*

Ruth Jepson
University of Stirling

Ava John-Baptiste
University of Toronto

Michael L. Johnson
University of Houston

Robert M. Kaplan
*University of California, Los
    Angeles*

Matthew Karafa
Cleveland Clinic

Pierre I. Karakiewicz
University of Montreal

Jonathan Karnon
University of Adelaide

Catherine Kastanioti
*Technological Educational
    Institution of Kalamata*

David A. Katz
*University of Iowa Carver
    College of Medicine*

H. J. Keselman
University of Manitoba

J. Kievit
*Leiden University Medical
    Center*

Sunghan Kim
University of Toronto

Sara J. Knight
*University of California, San
    Francisco*

Spassena Koleva
University of California, Irvine

Charles Kooperberg
*Fred Hutchinson Cancer
    Research Center*

Wendy Kornbluth
Cleveland Clinic

Olga Kostopoulou
University of Birmingham

Murray Krahn
THETA Collaborative

Ronilda Lacson
Harvard Medical School

Elizabeth B. Lamont
Harvard Medical School

Audrey Laporte
University of Toronto

Franklin N. Laufer
*New York State Department
    of Health*

France Légaré
Université Laval

Allen J. Lehman
*Arthritis Research Centre
    of Canada*

Harold Lehmann
*Johns Hopkins Medical
    Institutions*

Jennifer S. Lerner
Harvard University

Scott R. Levin
Johns Hopkins University

Liang Li
Cleveland Clinic

Matthew H. Liang
Harvard University

Richard Lilford
University of Birmingham, UK

Carol L. Link
*New England Research
    Institutes*

Joseph Lipscomb
*Rollins School of Public Health,
    Emory University*

Benjamin Littenberg
University of Vermont

Lisa M. Lix
University of Saskatchewan

Hilary A. Llewellyn-Thomas
Dartmouth Medical School

Karen E. Lutfey
*New England Research
    Institutes*

Sílvia Mamede
Erasmus University Rotterdam

Edward C. Mansley
Merck & Co., Inc.

P. J. Marang-van de Mheen
Leiden University Medical Centre

Lisa D. Marceau
New England Research Institutes

Kathryn Markakis
University of Rochester Medical Center

Ed Mascha
Cleveland Clinic

Josephine Mauskopf
RTI Health Solutions

Madhu Mazumdar
Weill Cornell Medical College

Dennis J. Mazur
Department of Veterans Affairs Medical Center

Christine M. McDonough
Dartmouth Institute for Health

Craig R. M. McKenzie
Rady School of Management and Psychology Department

John B. McKinlay
New England Research Institutes

Michael McMillan
Cleveland Clinic

Katherine Mead
George Washington University

Alan Meisel
University of Pittsburgh

J. Michael Menke
University of Arizona

Lesley-Ann N. Miller
University of Texas M. D. Anderson Cancer Center

Wilhelmine Miller
GWU School of Public Health and Health Services

Britain Mills
Cornell University

Alex J Mitchell
Consultant and Honorary Senior Lecturer

Nandita Mitra
University of Pennsylvania

Liz Moliski
University of Chicago

Barbara Moore
Gilmour and Associates Physiotherapy

Chaya S. Moskowitz
Memorial Sloan-Kettering Cancer Center

Stephanie Müller
University of Granada

Susan A. Murphy
University of Michigan

Jonathan D. Nelson
University of California, San Diego

Peter J. Neumann
Tufts–New England Medical Center

Angela Neumeyer-Gromen
Max Planck Institute for Human Development

J. Tim Newton
King's College London

Jerry Niederman
Rush University College of Medicine

Annette O'Connor
Ottawa Health Research Institute

Lucila Ohno-Machado
Brigham and Women's Hospital, Harvard Medical School

Sachiko Ohta
Center for Health Service, Outcomes Research and Development–Japan (CHORD-J)

Stephen Olejnik
University of Georgia

Christopher Y. Olivola
Princeton University

Obinna Onwujekwe
College of Medicine, University of Nigeria Enugu

Daniel M. Oppenheimer
Princeton University

Monica Ortendahl
Royal Institute of Technology

Katherine S. Panageas
Memorial Sloan-Kettering Cancer Center

Robert Panzer
University of Rochester Medical Center

Robert Patrick
Cleveland Clinic

Katherine Payne
University of Manchester

Niels Peck
*Academic Medical Center
(Amsterdam)*

Alleene M. Ferguson Pingenot
*California State University,
Stanislaus*

Petra Platzer
Cleveland Clinic

Harold A. Pollack
University of Chicago

Maarten J. Postma
University of Groningen

Georges Potworowski
University of Michigan

Robert K. Pretzlaff
*University of California, Davis
Medical Center*

Lisa Prosser
*University of Michigan Health
System*

Timothy E. Quill
*University of Rochester Medical
Center*

Rob Ranyard
University of Bolton

J. Sunil Rao
*Case Western Reserve
University*

Thomas C. Redman
Navesink Consulting Group

Valerie F. Reyna
Cornell University

Remy Rikers
Erasmus University Rotterdam

Stephen D. Roberts
North Carolina State University

Virginie Rondeau
*Bordeaux School of Public
Health*

Aubri S. Rose
Dartmouth College

Geoffrey L. Rosenthal
*Childrens Hospital, Pediatric
Institute, Cleveland Clinic*

Ingo Ruczinski
Johns Hopkins University

Tracey H. Sach
University of East Anglia

Michi Sakai
*Center for Health Service,
Outcomes Research and
Development–Japan
(CHORD-J)*

Arash Salehi
Mississippi State University

Lacey Schaefer
Mississippi State University

Marilyn M. Schapira
Medical College of Wisconsin

Michael Schlander
*University of Heidelberg,
Mannheim Medical Faculty*

Henk G. Schmidt
Rotterdam

Jesse D. Schold
University of Florida

Alan Schwartz
University of Illinois at Chicago

Mark Sculpher
Centre for Health Economics

John W. Seaman Jr.
Baylor University

Karen R. Sepucha
Massachusetts General Hospital

Anuj K. Shah
Princeton University

James Shanteau
Kansas State University

Ya-Chen Tina Shih
*University of Texas M. D.
Anderson Cancer Center*

Michael Shwartz
Boston University

Uwe Siebert
*UMIT–University for Health
Sciences (Austria)*

Bruce Siegel
George Washington University

Mahender P. Singh
*Massachusetts Institute of
Technology*

Grant H. Skrepnek
University of Arizona

Dean G. Smith
University of Michigan

Kenneth J. Smith
University of Pittsburgh

Martin L. Smith
Cleveland Clinic

Richard D. Smith
*London School of Hygiene and
Tropical Medicine*

Claire F. Snyder
*Johns Hopkins School of
Medicine*

Frank A. Sonnenberg
*UMDNJ–Robert Wood Johnson
Medical School*

Chenni Sriram
Cleveland Clinic

James Stahl
Massachusetts General Hospital

James D. Stamey
Baylor University

Thomas R. Stewart
University at Albany, State University of New York

Ewout W. Steyerberg
Erasmus Medical Center

Anne M. Stiggelbout
Leiden University Medical Center

Theo Stijnen
Leiden University Medical Center

Lesley Strawderman
Mississippi State University

J. Shannon Swan
MGH Institute for Technology Assessment

Carmen Tanner
University of Zurich

Curtis Tatsuoka
Cleveland Clinic

Rick P. Thomas
Oklahoma University

Danielle R. M. Timmermans
EMGO Institute, VU University (Amsterdam) Medical Center

Richard J. Tunney
University of Nottingham

Diane M. Turner-Bowker
QualityMetric Inc.

M. Dolores Ugarte
Universidad Publica de Navarra

Erin Winters Ulloa
VA Boston Healthcare System

Wilbert van den Hout
Leiden University Medical Center

Ben Vandermeer
University of Alberta

Tyler J. VanderWeele
University of Chicago

René (M) van Hulst
University of Groningen

Elisabeth van Rijen
Erasmus University Rotterdam

Marion Verduijn
Leiden University Medical Center

Andrew J. Vickers
Memorial Sloan-Kettering Cancer Center

Ivo Vlaev
University College London

Esteban Walker
Cleveland Clinic

David A. Walsh
University of Southern California

Declan Walsh
Cleveland Clinic

Jochen Walz
Institut Paoli-Calmettes

Bin Wang
University of South Alabama

Xiao-Feng Wang
Cleveland Clinic

Elke U. Weber
Columbia University

Noah J. Webster
Case Western Reserve University

Douglas H. Wedell
University of South Carolina

Saul J. Weiner
VA Center for the Management of Complex Chronic Care/ University of Illinois at Chicago

Kevin Weinfurt
Duke Clinical Research Institute

Brian J. Wells
Cleveland Clinic

Robert L. Winkler
Duke University

Eve Wittenberg
Brandeis University

Sarah E. Worley
Cleveland Clinic

J. Frank Yates
University of Michigan

Jun-Yen Yeh
Cleveland Clinic

Andrew Peng Yu
Analysis Group, Inc.

Changhong Yu
Cleveland Clinic

Marcel Zeelenberg
Tilburg University

Han Zhang
Mississippi State University

Li Zhang
Cleveland Clinic

Sue Ziebland
University of Oxford

Armineh Zohrabian
Centers for Disease Control

Foreword

As the chief academic officer in a cancer research institution, Fox Chase Cancer Center, I meet with each of the new faculty members shortly after their arrival. Recently, a young radiation oncologist came to my office, where we discussed the usual junior faculty issues: adjustment to the center, mentoring, the promotion and tenure process. When I asked him about his research interests, he startled me by expressing a desire to conduct "willingness to pay" studies of new modalities in the radiation therapy of prostate cancer. Then he asked me if I knew anything about this type of research. I admitted I did know a little about it, and offered to refer him to various texts on cost-effectiveness and cost-utility analysis. I could also have sent him to Becker, DeGroot, and Marschak's 1964 paper in *Behavioral Science*, "Measuring Utility by a Single-Response Sequential Method," a foundational article in willingness-to-pay studies, and encouraged him to perform a forward citation search using a tool such as the Web of Science.

Becker et al. (1964) have been cited 255 times since its publication, and the citing articles cover a broad range from econometrics to neuroscience. This might not be the easiest way to learn about a technical topic in valuing health outcomes. Another approach might be a keyword search, focusing on the biomedical literature. PubMed, the Web-based search engine to the comprehensive holdings in the U.S. National Library of Medicine, matches more than 1,100 articles to the text phrase "willingness to pay." Browsing the most recent 50 or so citations turns up a familiar name, Joel Tsevat, a friend who trained with my mentor, Steve Pauker. Downloading a recent paper of Joel's from *Medical Decision Making*, I find in the reference list a few contemporary methods papers on willingness to pay. If these papers suffice for Joel and his team, they are likely good enough for my young colleague.

Such is a typical approach to exploring a specific research topic in biomedical research. I confess to adding Wikipedia to my routine search strategy, as well as Google Scholar. Admittedly, the thrill of the hunt motivates some of my exploration, but the field of medical decision making could use a comprehensive reference. A field that draws from economics, mathematics, medicine, philosophy, psychology, and sociology (and occasionally from many others) is particularly in need of a compendium of ideas and techniques.

This encyclopedia aims to address this need. Didactic articles on more than 300 headwords have been prepared by well over 200 contributors from around the world. Joel Tsevat is on the advisory board for the encyclopedia, along with a number of other leaders who span the disciplines within the field of medical decision making. The article on willingness to pay is written by Obinna Onwujekwe, a health economist and clinician from the London School of Tropical Medicine and Hygiene, based at the University of Nigeria in Enugu, and funded through the Gates Malaria Partnership. I don't know Dr. Onwujekwe, but through this contact, I have discovered more resources on the Internet that can support my research and build my professional network. A well-researched encyclopedia can contribute much to the furthering of knowledge and the application of appropriate techniques to current problems. I look forward to having this reference for our current and future trainees.

At the publication of this encyclopedia, the field is 50 years old if one dates from the publication of Ledley and Lusted's seminal "Reasoning Foundations of Medical Diagnosis" (*Science*, 1959). Table 1 lists frequently cited articles in the field from that point forward, using title words and search terms from MEDLINE and Web of Science. A number of important technical manuscripts are included in this list, as well as "first papers" in several disciplines. Of course, this list is subject to the vagaries of article indexing; papers that focus on "risk" are relatively underrepresented in this set.

Table I Highly cited articles in the field of medical decision making, beginning with Ledley and Lusted's 1959 Science paper

First Author	Short Title	Journal	Year	Cited
Ledley, R. S.	Reasoning foundations of medical diagnosis	Science	1959	312
Wennberg, J. E.	Small area variations in health care delivery	Science	1973	751
Schwartz, W. B.	Decision analysis and clinical judgment	American Journal of Medicine	1973	193
McNeil, B. J.	Primer on certain elements of medical decision making	New England Journal of Medicine	1975	974
Pauker, S. G.	Therapeutic decision-making—cost-benefit analysis	New England Journal of Medicine	1975	223
Pauker, S. G.	Coronary artery surgery—use of decision analysis	Annals of Internal Medicine	1976	107
Kassirer, J. P.	Principles of clinical decision-making—introduction to decision analysis	Yale Journal of Biology and Medicine	1976	102
Weinstein, M. C.	Foundations of cost-effectiveness analysis . . .	New England Journal of Medicine	1977	1,043
Eisenberg, J. M.	Sociologic influences on decision-making by clinicians	Annals of Internal Medicine	1979	225
Shortliffe, E. H.	Knowledge engineering for medical decision making	Proceedings of the IEEE	1979	145
Pauker, S. G.	The threshold approach to clinical decision making	New England Journal of Medicine	1980	480
Griner, P. F.	Selection and interpretation of diagnostic tests . . .	Annals of Internal Medicine	1981	600
McNeil, B. J.	On the elicitation of preferences for alternative therapies	New England Journal of Medicine	1982	604
Beck, J. R.	A convenient approximation of life expectancy (the DEALE) 2 . . .	American Journal of Medicine	1982	256
Beck, J. R.	A convenient approximation of life expectancy (the DEALE) 1 . . .	American Journal of Medicine	1982	253
Beck, J. R.	Markov process in medical prognosis	Medical Decision Making	1983	473
Spiegelhalter, D. J.	Statistical and knowledge-based approaches to CDSS	Journal of the Royal Statistical Society: Series A (General)	1984	156
Greenfield, S.	Expanding patient involvement in care: Effect on health outcomes	Annals of Internal Medicine	1985	635

First Author	Short Title	Journal	Year	Cited
Sox, H. C.	Probability-theory in the use of diagnostic tests	Annals of Internal Medicine	1986	274
Pauker, S. G.	Decision-analysis	New England Journal of Medicine	1987	426
Kassirer, J. P.	Decision-analysis—a progress report	Annals of Internal Medicine	1987	190
Shortliffe, E. H.	Computer programs to support clinical decision making	Journal of the American Medical Association	1987	125
Swets, J. A.	Measuring the accuracy of diagnostic systems	Science	1988	1,339
Detsky, A. S.	Clinician guide to cost-effectiveness analysis	Annals of Internal Medicine	1990	435
Boyd, N. F.	Whose utilities for decision analysis	Medical Decision Making	1990	191
Fryback, D. G.	The efficacy of diagnostic-imaging	Medical Decision Making	1991	303
Hillner, B. E.	Efficacy and cost-effectiveness of adjuvant chemotherapy . . .	New England Journal of Medicine	1991	152
Sonnenberg, F. A.	Markov models in medical decision making . . .	Medical Decision Making	1993	773
Fleming, C.	A decision analysis . . . clinically localized prostate cancer	Journal of the American Medical Association	1993	448
Wu, Y. Z.	Artificial neural networks in mammography	Radiology	1993	250
Smith, T. J.	Efficacy and cost-effectiveness of cancer treatment	Journal of the National Cancer Institute	1993	157
Jaeschke, R.	Users' guides to the med. lit. 3. How to use an article about a diagnostic test B. What are the results?	Journal of the American Medical Association	1994	936
Krahn, M. D.	Screening for prostate cancer—a decision analytic view	Journal of the American Medical Association	1994	256
Omeara, J. J.	A decision analysis . . . for deep vein thrombosis	New England Journal of Medicine	1994	105
Davis, D. A.	Changing physician performance—A review of CME strategies	Journal of the American Medical Association	1995	1,298

(Continued)

Table I   Continued

First Author	Short Title	Journal	Year	Cited
Wilson, I. B.	Linking clinical variables with HRQOL	*Journal of the American Medical Association*	1995	763
Weinstein, M. C.	Recommendations of the panel on CE in health and medicine	*Journal of the American Medical Association*	1996	829
Russell, L. B.	The role of cost-effectiveness analysis in health and medicine	*Journal of the American Medical Association*	1996	502
Pestotnik, S. L.	Implementing antibiotic practice guidelines through CDSS	*Annals of Internal Medicine*	1996	325
Gambhir, S. S.	Decision tree sensitivity analysis for cost-effectiveness of FDG-PET	*Journal of Nuclear Medicine*	1996	170
Partin, A. W.	Combination of PSA, clinical stage, and Gleason score . . .	*Journal of the American Medical Association*	1997	895
Schrag, D.	Decision analysis—effects of prophylactic mastectomy and oophorectomy	*New England Journal of Medicine*	1997	239
Fine, M. J.	A prediction rule . . . low-risk patients with community-acquired pneumonia	*New England Journal of Medicine*	1997	1,141
Bates, D. W.	Effect of CPOE . . . on prevention of serious medication errors	*Journal of the American Medical Association*	1998	631
Hunt, D. L.	Effects of CDSS on physician performance . . .	*Journal of the American Medical Association*	1998	506
Briggs, A.	An introduction to Markov modelling for economic evaluation	*PharmacoEconomics*	1998	143
Gambhir, S. S.	Analytical decision model for . . . solitary pulmonary nodules	*Journal of Clinical Oncology*	1998	116
Grann, V. R.	DA of prophylactic mastectomy/oophorectomy in BRCA-1 positive . . .	*Journal of Clinical Oncology*	1998	115
Schulman, K. A.	The effect of race and sex on physicians' recommendations for cardiac catheterization	*New England Journal of Medicine*	1999	665
Braddock, C. H.	Informed decision making in outpatient practice	*Journal of the American Medical Association*	1999	285
Claxton, K.	A rational framework for decision making by the NICE	*Lancet*	2002	116
Weinstein, M. C.	Principles of good practice for DA modeling in health care evaluation	*Value Health Care*	2003	170

A recently proposed measure of scientific prominence, the h-index, ranks articles in order of times cited since publication. A scholar's or institution's h-index is represented by that article whose rank in terms of times cited is nearest to the actual number of citations. For example, the editor of this encyclopedia, Michael Kattan, has an h-index of 56: His 56th most cited paper has been cited 56 times through this writing. Taking this idea to a search, the topic and title phrase "medical decision making" in the Web of Science (which, unsurprisingly, incorporates more types of articles than covered in this encyclopedia) has an h-index of 131. By comparison, "bioinformatics" has an h-index of 122 and "medical informatics," 40, whereas the comprehensive biomedical topic, "chemotherapy," has an h-index of 239. This suggests to me that the field has attained a level of maturity where comprehensive reference works such as this encyclopedia will add value to teachers and learners. I look forward to browsing this reference and to following the scholarly output of its distinguished board of editors and contributors.

J. Robert Beck, MD
Fox Chase Cancer Center

Introduction

Healthcare decisions affect all of us, whether on a personal, professional, or societal level. We are human, as are all decision makers, and so are blessed and bound by the resources and limitations of the human mind. We cannot predict the future perfectly; we cannot arrange all positive and negative events to our liking; and we may not always understand the available choices. Moreover, even if effective treatments are recognized, financial constraints may force the selection of one option to the exclusion of others. This encyclopedia provides an introduction to some of the pitfalls and potential solutions our species has developed in the quest for achieving better decisions with less regret.

The audience for this encyclopedia is broad, and the need for a compilation of short essays over an equally expansive range of topics is great. There are a number of examples. Patients may wish to understand their vulnerability in interpreting the level of risks and benefits of treatment options, how their decisions are shaped by culture and emotions, or how physicians assess evidence and make diagnoses. Policy makers may seek firsthand knowledge on the basics of economic analyses, health measurement, and bioethics. Clinicians may desire deeper insights into the influences on their own processes of making diagnoses or choosing treatments or understanding the steps by which decision algorithms found in the literature are constructed and evaluated. Ironically, many participating in medical decision making have not accessed the impressive and exciting body of study and scholarship available. The anticipated time commitment and availability of formal courses may have prevented some from exploring the contributions of cognitive psychology, decision analysis, ethics, health economics, health outcomes, biostatistics, and clinical epidemiology. Others may have tried some self-study but become frustrated when confronted with new vocabulary or advanced mathematics. Some potential readers may have had lectures or training in the past but struggle now to retrieve particular points quickly and apply them to their current practices. And many in the target audience may be experts in one aspect of medical decision making but wish to enhance or energize their work by understanding a different perspective.

Satisfying the interests, needs, and time constraints of a diverse audience is challenging. We have attempted to address these, first, by making the encyclopedia instructional, not simply informational. The authors have written clearly, explained carefully the general sense of the mathematical formulae when presented, and provided generously the many and varied examples so that a wide range of readers can understand and appreciate the material. Certainly no encyclopedia can substitute for a textbook or formal course on a particular topic; this encyclopedia provides a quick and comprehensible introduction. Next, we wanted each essay to be understandable on its own account, not critically dependent on previous readings or coursework. Nevertheless, the authors have also suggested related topics and further readings at the ends of the articles. A third consideration guiding the development of this work was that it should reflect international scholarship. The authors represent nearly every continent. Many have contributed to the primary foundations of medical decision making; to have their work represented here together may eventually be viewed as historical.

Given the universality of medical decision making, the list of potential topics to include can quickly grow to an unmanageable length. A conceptual framework is needed to identify the key ideas and organize their elaboration. One approach is to classify studies of medical decision making as either prescriptive (also called normative) or descriptive. Work in the prescriptive area investigates the processes and technology by which optimal medical decisions should be determined. In contrast, descriptive studies examine how decisions actually are made. Perhaps not surprisingly, these two strategies are often in disagreement. Prescriptive decision making often employs formal analyses and algorithms, often via a computer, to calculate the best choice under the circumstances, for instance, maximizing benefit relative to the costs. These algorithms may be complicated, inaccessible, not trusted, and thus not used. In their absence, patients, physicians, or policy makers might use less formal methods to make decisions yet may do as well or better than the more sophisticated approach.

Our encyclopedia addresses both categories—prescriptive and descriptive—through a conceptual structure consisting of six components of classical decision analysis. The first component concerns identification of the decision maker—in other words, who must choose. In general, there are three levels of decision makers, each with a particular perspective: the individual patient or surrogate, the clinician, and society. The second component is the identification of the decision to be made, for instance, the selection of the most likely diagnosis or the therapy with the best chance of cure. The essays pertaining to these first two components generally fall into the descriptive category: how decisions are influenced, finalized, and reviewed afterwards. Generally speaking, these draw heavily from the field of cognitive psychology. The third component concerns the consequences or outcomes of decisions and how these are defined and measured. The corresponding entries generally concern health econometrics and health-related quality-of-life measurement. The fourth category is related, and examines the value of the potential outcomes, often expressed as a monetary sum or a level of desirability termed *utility*. The fifth component in the conceptual framework involves the likelihood or probability of the possible consequences through essays on statistical concepts and clinical epidemiology. The sixth category concerns the mechanism by which individuals, clinicians, and society determine the best

decision. This involves ethics, cultural considerations informed by sociology and anthropology, and prescriptive approaches such as utility maximization as well as descriptive approaches related to cognitive psychology. We have also included a seventh category for the encyclopedia, broadly characterized as pertaining to methods and techniques used to predict outcomes and analyze decisions, whether at the individual patient, cohort, or societal level. The pertinent essays cover mathematical models of disease progression, diagnosis, and prognosis as well as economic evaluations.

The encyclopedia was developed in five basic steps.

Step 1: Leading medical decision-making experts around the world were invited to serve on the editorial board.

Step 2: The senior editorial board editor and the associate editor created a master list of topics corresponding to the conceptual framework presented.

Step 3: The editorial board was asked to nominate individuals to author the list of entries. We also searched PubMed and the Web sites of universities to find people publishing on certain topics, and we consulted with our colleagues for additional suggestions.

Step 4: Contributors were given basic guidelines and instructions regarding the writing of their entries. As previously mentioned, we encouraged them to be thorough in describing the entire topic area and to write in nontechnical, accessible language.

Step 5: The editor and associate editor then reviewed all the entries and asked authors for revisions as necessary.

As with the subject matter, this encyclopedia has its own limitations and imperfections. The first concerns the selection of topics. We anticipate surprise with the selection of some included and chagrin with those not found. Our generic response to those questioning an inclusion is that many of the techniques and tools used in medical decision making are based on methodology developed in a related discipline such as statistics or psychometrics. We wanted to provide interested readers with the opportunity to obtain background in these supporting topics to enhance their enjoyment of the other essays. For those disappointed in the lack of a particular topic, we beg your understanding and trust that your curiosity will lead you to the appropriate reference. The second limitation concerns our attempt to make each essay understandable as a single entity. An inevitable consequence of this editorial approach is some redundancy of content among related essays. We do not foresee this being too problematic with the encyclopedia format. The third limitation concerns the difference between empirical evidence and hypothetical examples for teaching purposes. The field of medical decision making continually develops and includes concepts supported with various levels of evidence. Many of the examples within the essays summarize formal studies referenced at the end of the article. However, other examples are provided as relevant illustrations of the underlying concepts. These should not be taken as firm evidence of the decision practices of a particular culture, profession, or specialty, much less a judgment on the decisions or actions of a given individual.

We conclude with some practical advice for those still reading this Introduction. Start wherever your curiosity is most urgent. If your reading halts due to unfamiliar mathematical notation, consult the essay on "Statistical Notation." If you finish an essay without understanding its major points, read a few entries on the related topics, then return to the original essay. This encyclopedia is a treasure. In the course of its compilation, we have reexperienced the initial joy of discovering concepts and techniques that ultimately changed the directions of our careers.

Michael W. Kattan and Mark E. Cowen

Acknowledgments

I am now severely further indebted to my great and longtime friend, Associate Editor Mark Cowen. He has put an enormous amount of effort into this encyclopedia. Its positive attributes largely belong to him, while the shortcomings rest with me. I picked Mark immediately in the development process because I knew how thoughtful he was. It clearly shows in this encyclopedia.

The SAGE team has been great. Carole Maurer and Laura Notton, most prominently, have really held my hand during this entire project. The SAGE group has put a lot of thought into the encyclopedia process, and it is very good. I thank Neil Salkind at Studio B for identifying me to spearhead this project.

I also thank my star-studded advisory board. I was very pleasantly surprised with how willing these very accomplished folks were to volunteer for this project, given their many time commitments on their time. Their diversity was of tremendous value in identifying the broad listing of topics necessary for a comprehensive text like this.

Furthermore, they helped me identify excellent authors for many of the entries.

On a personal level, many people have taken it on themselves to position me to be able to edit this encyclopedia. The individual who has done the most is, without question, Peter T. Scardino, Chief of Surgery at Memorial Sloan-Kettering Cancer Center. For over a decade, Peter single-handedly sponsored and promoted my career. Whatever success I have had can easily be traced to him, an unmatched combination of brilliance, kindness, and humility. More thanks go to Bob Beck and Scott Cantor, who initiated and propelled, respectively, my medical-decision-making exposure. Along those lines, I thank my many colleagues in the Society for Medical Decision Making for their relentless thirst for new knowledge. I must also thank the leadership at Cleveland Clinic for protecting my time so that I might devote it to this project. And finally, I thank my family (Grace, Madeleine, and Lily), who put up with a lot of unattractive behavior on my part.

Michael W. Kattan

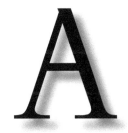

ACCEPTABILITY CURVES AND CONFIDENCE ELLIPSES

Acceptability curves and confidence ellipses are both methods for graphically presenting the uncertainty surrounding the estimate of cost-effectiveness. A confidence ellipse provides a visual representation of the region containing $x\%$ (where x is usually 95) of the uncertainty. An acceptability curve provides a graphical representation of the probability that an intervention is cost-effective compared with the alternative(s), given the data. Confidence ellipses can only be used for comparisons between two interventions, whereas acceptability curves can be produced for decisions involving multiple interventions. Confidence ellipses are determined parametrically from information about the distribution of costs and effects (mean, variance, and covariance). The acceptability curve can be determined from the confidence ellipse or direct from the data following an assessment of uncertainty through bootstrapping (for trial data) or probabilistic sensitivity analysis (of modeling analyses). Both are specified as appropriate methods for presenting uncertainty in cost-effectiveness in the *Guide to the Methods of Technology Appraisal* produced by the National Institute for Clinical Excellence (NICE) in the United Kingdom. This entry reviews the concepts of confidence ellipses and cost-effectiveness acceptability curves (CEACs) for the presentation of uncertainty surrounding the cost-effectiveness, detailing their construction, use, and interpretation.

The concept of the cost-effectiveness acceptability frontier (CEAF) is also introduced.

Confidence Ellipse

A confidence ellipse provides a visual representation of the uncertainty surrounding costs and effects (or indeed any two variables). The ellipse provides a region on the cost-effectiveness plane that should contain $x\%$ (e.g., 95%) of the uncertainty. By varying x, a series of contour lines can be plotted on the cost-effectiveness plane, each containing the relevant proportion of the cost and effect pairs. Figure 1 illustrates 95%, 50%, and 5% confidence ellipses.

Construction of the confidence ellipse requires the assumption that the costs and effects follow a bivariate normal distribution, that is, for each value of cost, the corresponding values of effect are normally distributed (and vice versa).

The drawback with the confidence ellipse is that while it presents the uncertainty around the costs and effects, it does not deal with the uncertainty surrounding the incremental cost-effectiveness ratio (ICER). One solution to this is to use the boundaries of the relevant confidence ellipse to approximate confidence intervals (e.g., 95%) for the ICER. This interval is given by the slopes of the rays from the origin, which are just tangential to the relevant ellipse (identified in Figure 2). Note that these will be overestimates of the confidence interval.

The particular shape and orientation of the confidence ellipse will be determined by the covariance

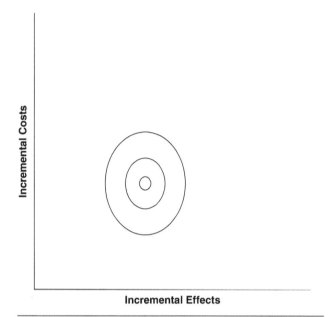

Figure 1   Confidence ellipses on the cost-effectiveness plane

of the costs and effects. This will in turn affect the confidence intervals estimated from the ellipse. Figure 3 illustrates the influence of the covariance on the confidence ellipse and the confidence limits.

Cost-Effectiveness Acceptability Curves

In contrast, the acceptability curve (or cost-effectiveness acceptability curve [CEAC]) focuses on the uncertainty surrounding the cost-effectiveness. An acceptability curve provides a graphical presentation of the probability that the intervention is cost-effective (has an ICER below the cost-effectiveness threshold) compared with the alternative intervention(s), given the data, for a range of values for the cost-effectiveness threshold. It should be noted that this is essentially a Bayesian view of probability (probability that the hypothesis is true given the data) rather than a frequentist/classical view of probability (probability of getting the data, or data more extreme, given that the hypothesis is true). It has been argued that this is more appropriate to the decision maker, who is concerned with the probability that the intervention is cost-effective (hypothesis is correct) given the cost-effectiveness results. However, a frequentist interpretation of the acceptability curve has been suggested, as the $1 - p$ value of a one-sided test of significance.

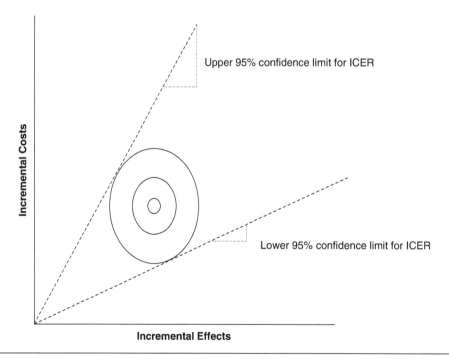

Figure 2   Estimation of the confidence interval from the confidence ellipse

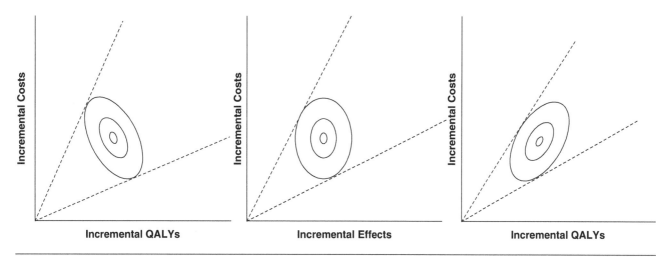

Figure 3 Covariance and the confidence ellipse: (a) negative covariance between cost and effect, (b) independent cost and effect (0 covariance), and (c) positive covariance between cost and effect

Acceptability curves were originally introduced as an alternative to presentation of confidence intervals around the ICER, given the methodological difficulties involved with determining confidence intervals for ratio statistics, including the nonnegligible probability of a small or nonexistent effect difference that would cause the ICER to be undefined and make the variance intractable. Figure 4 presents a CEAC for an intervention.

Constructing a CEAC

The CEAC is derived from the joint distribution of incremental costs and incremental effects. When cost and effect data originate from a clinical trial, the joint distribution is generally determined through nonparametric bootstrapping. When a model has been used, probabilistic sensitivity analysis (Monte Carlo simulation) can be used to translate the uncertainty surrounding the model parameters into uncertainty in costs and effects. As such, the construction of the acceptability curve has no requirement for parametric assumptions regarding the joint distribution of costs and effects.

For any specified cost-effectiveness threshold, the probability that the intervention is cost-effective is calculated simply as the proportion of the cost and effect pairs (plotted on the cost-effectiveness plane) lying below a ray with slope equal to the specific threshold. Since the cost-effectiveness threshold is generally not explicitly defined, this calculation is repeated for different values of the cost-effectiveness threshold. The process usually starts with the threshold = 0 (indicating that society cares only for reduced costs) and ends with the threshold = ∞ (indicating that society cares only for increased effects). The acceptability curve is constructed by plotting probabilities (y-axis) against the cost-effectiveness threshold (x-axis). Figure 5 illustrates the process of constructing the acceptability curve illustrated in Figure 4.

Rules for the CEAC

1. The value at which the acceptability curve cuts the y-axis (i.e., when cost-effectiveness threshold = 0) is determined by the extent of the joint distribution that falls below the x-axis on the cost-effectiveness plane (i.e., involves cost savings). If any of the joint distribution involves cost savings, the curve will not start at 0.

2. The value to which the acceptability curve asymptotes (as the cost-effectiveness threshold approaches infinity) is determined by the extent of the joint distribution falling to the right of the y-axis (i.e., involving increased effects). If any of the joint distribution involves negative effects, the curve will not asymptote to 1.

3. The shape of the acceptability curve will depend solely on the location of the joint distribution within the incremental cost-effectiveness plane.

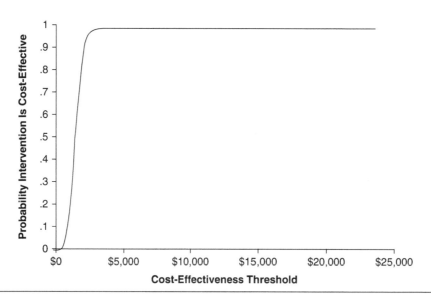

Figure 4   Cost-effectiveness acceptability curve

Incremental cost-effect pairs that fall in the northwest quadrant are never considered cost-effective and, therefore, are never counted in the numerator of the estimate. Incremental cost-effect pairs that fall in the southeast quadrant are always considered cost-effective and, therefore, are always counted in the numerator of the estimate. As the threshold increases from zero to infinity, incremental cost-effect pairs in the northeast and southwest quadrants may or may not be considered cost-effective (and therefore included in the numerator) depending on the value of the threshold. As such, the acceptability curve is not necessarily monotonically increasing with the cost-effectiveness threshold, and therefore, it does not represent a cumulative distribution function.

Interpreting and Misinterpreting the CEAC

For a specific cost-effectiveness threshold (x-axis), the acceptability curve presents the probability (read off on the y-axis) that the data are consistent with a true cost-effectiveness ratio falling below that value. It presents a summary measure of the joint uncertainty in the estimate of incremental cost-effectiveness, thus providing the decision maker with a measure of the uncertainty associated with the selection of a particular intervention as cost-effective.

Note that the acceptability curve *should not* be read in the opposite direction (i.e., from the y-axis to the x-axis) as this would imply that the cost-effectiveness threshold is flexible and determined by the required probability level (confidence) rather than externally set and based on society's willingness to pay for health effects. For example, the curve should not be read to determine the cost-effectiveness threshold (x-axis) required to provide at least a .95 probability that the intervention is cost-effective ($p < .05$).

Statements concerning the acceptability curve should be restricted to those regarding the uncertainty of the estimate of cost-effectiveness. An acceptability curve *should not*, in general, be used to make statements about whether the intervention is actually cost-effective compared with the alternative(s).

Presenting Multiple Acceptability Curves

There are two situations in which it may be useful and/or necessary to present multiple acceptability curves: (1) where there are different patient subgroups and (2) where there are multiple interventions to be compared. The methods for handling and displaying these two situations are very different.

Multiple Patient Subgroups

With analyses involving different patient subgroups, the cost-effectiveness of the intervention for each subgroup is entirely independent from that for other subgroups. Each acceptability curve presents the probability that the intervention is cost-effective compared with the comparator(s), given the data, for a particular subgroup. As such,

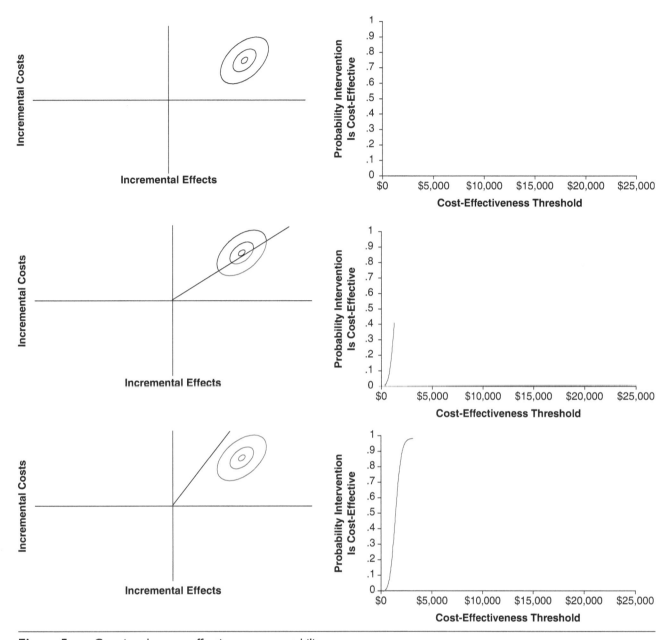

Figure 5   Creating the cost-effectiveness acceptability curve

each acceptability curve should be read and interpreted independently. Such curves can be plotted separately or, to save space, together, but the interpretation remains the same.

Multiple Interventions

With analyses involving multiple (mutually exclusive) interventions, the cost-effectiveness of each intervention must be compared with the available alternatives and assessed simultaneously. The same is true of the probability that each intervention is

cost-effective compared with the available alternatives, given the data. With mutually exclusive, collectively exhaustive interventions, the vertical sum of the probabilities must equal 1 for every value of the cost-effectiveness threshold (i.e., one of the interventions must be cost-effective). Therefore, in contrast to the multiple subgroup case, when presenting acceptability curves for multiple (mutually exclusive) interventions, the curves should be read and interpreted together. However, this presentation of multiple acceptability curves can cause confusion with interpretation and lead to a temptation to identify the cost-effective intervention from the acceptability curves, as that with the highest probability for each cost-effectiveness threshold. As stated above, the acceptability curves present only the probability that the intervention is cost-effective compared with the alternative(s), given the data. They do not identify whether the intervention, or which intervention, is cost-effective. This is identified through comparison of the ICER with the cost-effectiveness threshold, with the cost-effective intervention identified as that with the largest ICER falling below the cost-effectiveness threshold.

Acceptability Frontier

One method suggested to avoid the problem of misinterpretation associated with multiple acceptability curves is the presentation of a CEAF. The CEAF is created by graphing the probability that the intervention is cost-effective only over the range at which it is identified as such on the basis of the ICER. As the name suggests, this provides a frontier produced from the relevant sections of the individual acceptability curves. It should be noted that the appropriate construction of the CEAF requires that the cost-effective intervention is identified for each value of the threshold and then the probability is plotted for this intervention for this threshold. Breaks in the acceptability frontier may occur at the point where the cost-effective intervention changes (i.e., where the cost-effectiveness threshold equals the ICER between the two interventions). Note that the acceptability frontier, created in this way, is not necessarily the same as that created from the outermost boundary of the individual acceptability curves. Figure 6 presents multiple acceptability curves and the associated CEAF.

Elisabeth Fenwick

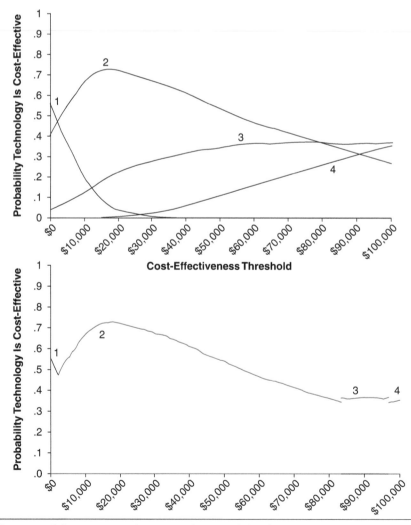

Figure 6   Multiple acceptability curves and associated acceptability frontier

See also Confidence Intervals; Cost-Effectiveness Analysis; Decision Trees: Sensitivity Analysis, Basic and Probabilistic; Managing Variability and Uncertainty; Marginal or Incremental Analysis, Cost-Effectiveness Ratio

Further Readings

Briggs, A. H., & Fenn, P. (1998). Confidence intervals or surfaces? Uncertainty on the cost-effectiveness plane. *Health Economics, 7,* 723–740.

Fenwick, E., Claxton, K., & Sculpher, M. (2001). Representing uncertainty: The role of cost-effectiveness acceptability curves. *Health Economics, 10,* 779–787.

Fenwick, E., O'Brien, B., & Briggs, A. (2004). Cost-effectiveness acceptability curves: Facts, fallacies and frequently asked questions. *Health Economics, 13,* 405–415.

Van Hout, B. A., Al, M. J., Gordon, G. S., & Rutten, F. F. H. (1994). Costs, effects and c/e-ratios alongside a clinical trial. *Health Economics, 3,* 309–319.

ACCOUNTABILITY

Accountability refers to the implicit or explicit expectation that one may be called on to justify one's beliefs, feelings, and actions to others. Although most theories of decision making have conveniently assumed that decision makers act as isolated individuals, decision makers, including those in the field of medicine, seldom think and act free from social influences.

Decision making in the field of medicine is fraught with complex, conflicting pressures from various parties, including patients, physicians, hospitals, health policy makers, and insurers, that promote distinct and often competing objectives, such as maximizing life expectancy versus optimizing quality of life, or weighing quality of treatment against economic constraints. Therefore, to best structure accountability relationships and ultimately to improve the quality of decisions in the medical setting, careful analysis of accountability is warranted.

This entry reviews findings from empirical research that addresses the impact of many types of accountability on decision making and attempts to identify the conditions under which accountability will improve decision making.

Many Kinds of Accountability

It is intuitive to think that accountability will breed hard thinking and that thinking harder will translate to thinking better. But according to reviews of the accountability literature, accountability promotes self-critical and effortful thinking only under certain conditions.

Different types of accountability can be distinguished based on the specific nature of justification an individual is expected to provide for his or her decisions: To whom is he or she accountable, for what, and according to what ground rules must he or she justify his or her decisions? For example, a decision maker may be accountable to an audience with known versus unknown views, to authority figures whom the decision maker may perceive as legitimate or illegitimate, and for either the outcome or the process of the decision.

Based on their review of the accountability literature, Jennifer Lerner and Phillip Tetlock reported that decision makers engage in more careful thinking only when they learn prior to forming any opinions about the decision that they will be accountable to an audience (a) whose views are unknown, (b) who is interested in accuracy, (c) who is more interested in processes rather than outcomes, (d) who is reasonably well informed, and (e) who has a legitimate reason for probing the reasons behind decisions. Therefore, simply leading decision makers to expect to justify their decisions to others is insufficient to promote thorough decision making. Instead, organizations and authorities must methodically tailor accountability structures to promote more careful thought processes.

Will Accountability Improve Decision Making?

Although making a decision maker accountable to an unknown audience before the decision is made promotes more careful thought processes, employing this specific kind of accountability by no means ensures improved decision making. Rather, the effects of accountability depend on the types of decisions and the cognitive processes involved, resulting in some improved decisions, some unchanged decisions, and some degraded decisions.

When Accountability Improves Decision Making

Predecisional accountability to an unknown audience improves decision making to the extent that suboptimal decisions would—under default conditions—result from lack of effort and self-critical attention to the decision process. In other words, as long as improvements in decision making require only greater attention to the information provided, and not acquisition of special skills or training in formal decision rules, the concentrated thinking motivated by accountability pressure will result in thinking better. For example, research has shown that accountable decision makers with a heightened awareness of decision processes made better decisions, specifically, by reducing the tendency for happiness from an unrelated event to elicit heuristic, stereotypic judgments; by reducing blind commitment to a prior course of action in an effort to recoup sunk costs; and by decreasing the likelihood of mindlessly rating a conjunctive event (e.g., shy librarian) as more likely than a simple event (e.g., librarian).

When Accountability Has No Effect on Decision Making

Predecisional accountability to an unknown audience has no effect on decision making if knowledge of formal decision rules (e.g., Bayes's theorem, expected utility theory) that cannot be acquired through increased attention to the decision process is critical for improvements on decision tasks. For instance, accountability had no effect on insensitivity to base rate information; even with increased awareness of their decision process, decision makers often failed to adjust their probability estimates for the frequency of a specific event in some relevant population. As an example, when asked to estimate the probability of a woman having breast cancer given a positive mammogram with 90% sensitivity and 93% specificity, most participants failed to take the base rate of breast cancer in the woman's age group (.8%) into account even when it was clearly provided to them, no matter how hard they were pressured to think.

When Accountability Degrades Decision Making

Predecisional accountability to an unknown audience can actually degrade decision making when certain decision-making biases result from using normatively proscribed information or when the option that appears easiest to justify also happens to be a biased option. For example, increased effort in accountable decision makers led them to increase integration of nondiagnostic information into predictions and resulted in dilution of critical diagnostic information.

Decomposing Accountability

To fully understand how accountability influences a given decision context, it is worth recognizing that even the simplest form of accountability necessarily implicates several empirically distinguishable subphenomena: (a) *the mere presence of another person* (decision makers expect that another person will observe their performance), (b) *identifiability* (decision makers expect that what they say or do will be linked to them personally), (c) *evaluation* (decision makers expect that their performance will be assessed by another person according to some normative ground rules and with some implied consequences), and (d) *reason giving* (decision makers expect that they must give reasons for what they say or do). More research is needed to clarify how these phenomena might affect the impact of accountability.

Accountability and Medical Decision Making

Assuming that accountability is a social panacea, people propose accountability as a solution to all sorts of problems. However, research has documented that accountability is not a singular phenomenon that solves every problem. Only highly specialized forms of accountability will elicit increased cognitive effort in decision makers. More cognitive effort is not always beneficial and sometimes makes matters even worse. Moreover, accountability inherently implicates empirically distinguishable subphenomena, which may or may not influence decision makers in a consistent direction. Accountability as a whole is a complex construct that interacts with individual characteristics of the decision maker and properties of the decision-making environment to produce an array of effects. Decision makers and their superiors should carefully research the decision environment and decision task to use accountability pressure to advantage in medical decision making.

Seunghee Han and Jennifer S. Lerner

See also Bias; Cognitive Psychology and Processes; Decision Quality; Judgment; Social Factors

Further Readings

Lerner, J. S., & Tetlock, P. E. (1999). Accounting for the effects of accountability. *Psychological Bulletin, 125,* 255–275.

Lerner, J. S., & Tetlock, P. E. (2003). Bridging individual, interpersonal, and institutional approaches to judgment and choice: The impact of accountability on cognitive bias. In S. Schneider & J. Shanteau (Eds.), *Emerging perspectives on judgment and decision making* (pp. 431–457). Cambridge, UK: Cambridge University Press.

Tetlock, P. E. (1999). Accountability theory: Mixing properties of human agents with properties of social systems. In J. Levine, L. Thompson, & D. Messick (Eds.), *Shared cognition in organizations: The management of knowledge* (pp. 117–137). Hillsdale, NJ: Erlbaum.

ADVANCE DIRECTIVES AND END-OF-LIFE DECISION MAKING

Advance directives are oral or written statements given by competent individuals regarding the medical treatment they would like to receive should an incapacitating injury or illness preclude their ability to make or express their own decisions. They are most often used to make decisions when a person is near the end of life, and difficult choices must be made about the use or withdrawal of life-sustaining medical treatment.

Rapid advances in medical technology over the past several decades have made end-of-life decision making an increasingly important and complex challenge for patients, their families, and healthcare professionals. Advance directives play a role in many end-of-life decisions, and their use is encouraged by medical professionals and supported by state and federal law. This entry describes the main types of advance directives, their social and legal history, some of their limitations as aids to effective end-of-life decision making, and some strategies suggested for addressing these limitations.

Types of Advance Directives

There are two primary types of advance directives. *Instructional advance directives*, also known as living wills, contain instructions about the type of life-sustaining treatment an individual would like to receive should he or she become incapacitated. Such instructions can range from legal documents prepared with the help of an attorney to verbal statements made to a family member or a physician. They can be general and express values and goals that the individual feels should guide medical care (e.g., emphasize quality over quantity of life) or relevant religious values. Or they can be specific and carefully delineate particular medical treatments to be used or withheld in particular medical conditions. Most often, instructional directives express a desire to withhold aggressive life-sustaining treatments, but they can also be used to request such treatments. In addition, they can specify preferences regarding pain management, organ donation, or dying at home as opposed to in a hospital.

Proxy advance directives designate another person as a surrogate decision maker, or a proxy, for the patient should he or she become incapacitated. Proxy directives are also known as *durable powers of attorney for healthcare* and *surrogate appointments*. The surrogate decision maker is usually a spouse or another close family member. Proxy directives convey the legal right to make treatment decisions but do not necessarily contain explicit guidance regarding what those treatments should be.

Advance directives can be created without using any prepared forms, but the majority of U.S. states provide standard forms that follow specific state statutes. Verbal statements are also considered legal advance directives, especially if recorded by a medical professional in a patient's chart.

Another common kind of instructional advance directive is a *Do Not Resuscitate* (DNR) order, which is recorded in a medical chart and indicates a desire to not receive cardiopulmonary resuscitation (CPR). Because resuscitating treatments often fail, such orders are also sometimes called *Do Not Attempt Resuscitation* (DNAR) orders. Also, because decisions besides those involving resuscitation must often be made, a more comprehensive type of medical order form called *Physician Orders for Life-Sustaining Treatment* (POLST) has recently been developed and adopted for use in several states. POLST forms record a patient's wishes for a number of different life-sustaining treatments and require both patients and physicians to sign, indicating that they have discussed these preferences.

Advance Directives Versus Physician-Assisted Suicide

Advance directives should not be confused with the more controversial issue of physician-assisted suicide. Advance directives involve choices about whether to accept or refuse particular kinds of life-sustaining medical treatment in the event of incapacitation. Physician-assisted suicide involves a competent, terminally ill person asking a physician to knowingly and intentionally provide the means to end his or her life. The use of advance directives to refuse unwanted medical treatment near the end of life is endorsed widely by medical associations and supported by U.S. state and federal law. Advance directives have achieved similar levels of acceptance in a number of European countries. In contrast, physician-assisted suicide is much more controversial and, at this time, is legal only in the state of Oregon and a few European countries (e.g., the Netherlands) under very narrow sets of conditions.

The Social and Legal History of Advance Directives

The concept of advance directives emerged in the late 1960s as medical technology made it increasingly possible to prolong the lives of seriously ill individuals, especially individuals with minimal cognitive functioning or severe and chronic pain, who have little or no hope for ultimate recovery. Many people view the use of life-sustaining medical treatment in such situations as not so much extending life as extending the process of dying. This created a challenge to the "technological imperative" that physicians should use all means at their disposal to prolong life. The concept of advance directives was thus created to allow people to exert some control over the medical treatment they receive at the end of their lives.

Advance directives were a response to a practical problem. At the time difficult medical decisions must be made about the use of life-sustaining treatments, many patients are already too sick to decide for themselves. In 1969, attorney Luis Kutner suggested that individuals too ill to make decisions for themselves could maintain their ability to influence the use of life-sustaining medical treatments by documenting treatment wishes prior to incapacitation in what he termed a "living will."

The issues of advance directives and end-of-life decision making did not enter public consciousness, however, until the controversial 1976 court case of *In re Quinlan*. In that case, the New Jersey Supreme Court considered the dilemma of Karen Ann Quinlan, a young woman who suffered severe brain damage after mixing alcohol and tranquilizers at a party and was left in a persistent vegetative state. Her parents sought to remove her from the respirator that was maintaining her life, but hospital administrators asked for a court ruling on the matter because of concerns about legal liabilities. The court granted her parents' request for removal of the respirator, finding that it infringed on Quinlan's right to privacy protected under the Constitution. The decision was important because it concluded that not only did a competent person have a constitutionally protected right to refuse life-sustaining treatment but that this right was not diminished by Quinlan's incapacitation. The court went on to say that while Quinlan could obviously not exercise this right herself, her parents could on her behalf, using their "best judgment" on how she would decide for herself.

An even more crucial legal decision supporting the use of instructional advance directives was *Cruzan v. Director, Missouri Department of Health*, decided by the U.S. Supreme Court in 1990. The case involved 24-year-old Nancy Cruzan, who suffered a car accident that left her in a persistent vegetative state with no hope for recovery. Cruzan's parents sought legal action to remove her from life support but were opposed by Missouri state officials. The U.S. Supreme Court confirmed not only Cruzan's constitutionally protected right to refuse medical treatment but also a state's right to set its own standard for determining sufficient evidence of an incompetent person's wishes. In this case, Missouri's standard required "clear and convincing evidence" of an incompetent patient's prior wishes, and an instructional advance directive is often seen as the best method of meeting this strict evidentiary standard.

The controversy surrounding the Cruzan case helped spur important legislation, and in 1990, the U.S. Congress passed the Patient Self-Determination Act. The act stipulates that all hospitals receiving Medicaid or Medicare reimbursement must inform patients of (a) their right to accept or refuse treatment, (b) their rights under existing state laws regarding advance directives, and (c) any policies the institution has regarding the withholding or withdrawing of life-sustaining treatments. Institutions are also required to engage in ongoing educational activities for both their employees and the general public regarding the right to accept or refuse treatment and the opportunity for drafting or signing advance directives. Moreover, state legislation has been passed over the past two decades making some form of advance directives (instructional, proxy, or both) legal in all 50 states and the District of Columbia.

More recently, the case of Theresa Marie (Terri) Schiavo brought intense worldwide media attention to the issue of end-of-life decision making. Schiavo was a 26-year-old Florida housewife when her heart unexpectedly stopped in 1990, leaving her immobile and uncommunicative for the next 15 years. Schiavo left no advance directive and members of her immediate family disagreed vehemently about whether or not she should be removed from the machines that were supplying her with food and fluids. Although a series of court decisions had sided with the arguments of Schiavo's husband, Michael, that she should be removed from life support, her parents and siblings continued to battle, both in legal court and in the court of public opinion, arguing that she would want to be kept alive in her current condition, and even that she was currently responsive to external stimulation. Schiavo died on March 31, 2005, 13 days after her feeding and fluid tubes were ordered disconnected by a Florida trial judge. The case raised public awareness of advance directives and the complex and emotionally charged nature of end-of-life decision making.

Limitations of Advance Directives

A number of researchers and ethicists now express skepticism regarding the effectiveness of advance directives to improve end-of-life medical decision making. The challenges of making decisions for incapacitated individuals are complex and multifaceted. End-of-life decisions involve multiple individuals, including the patient, his or her loved ones, and physicians. Information must be passed from one individual to another, and each individual has motivations that may conflict and decision-making limitations that must be overcome. Of particular concern are low completion rates of advance directives (particularly among some ethnic groups), the stability of preferences for life-sustaining treatment across changes in an individual's psychological and medical condition, and the effectiveness and accuracy of surrogate decision making.

The first challenge facing the use of advance directives is that most people do not have one. Estimates suggest that fewer than 25% of U.S. adults have an advance directive. Completion rates are not substantially higher for individuals with serious chronic diseases, and interventions designed to increase the rate of advance directive completion have shown limited effectiveness. Completion rates are particularly low for some ethnic groups, including African Americans, Latinos, and Native Americans. One source of cultural differences may be differential value placed on autonomy. In Western philosophy, family members are generally viewed as a source of emotional support, not active participants in the decision-making process. In many East Asian and other cultures, however, the importance of filial duty or protecting the elderly may lead a family to make decisions for a fully competent adult and withhold information about prognosis. In addition, in traditional Hawaiian, Chinese, and Japanese cultures, it is commonly believed that talking about death may bring on death or spiritual pollution. Planning ahead via advance directives is often resisted by individuals with these cultural backgrounds because it is seen as interfering with deeply held cultural traditions and the natural course of life and death.

A second problem with instructional advance directives in particular concerns the appropriateness of projecting treatment wishes of competent individuals onto future states of incompetence. Preferences for life-sustaining treatment have been found to be highly context dependent and can be altered by an individual's current psychological and physical state, as well as the way questions soliciting treatment preferences are framed. People may have difficulty imagining what life would be like in severely impaired health states. Research suggests that almost one third of individuals change their preferences about any given life-sustaining medical treatment over a period of 1 to 2 years. Moreover, the majority of individuals whose life-sustaining treatment preferences change over time are unaware of these changes and, thus, are unlikely to revise their advance directives. These issues raise concerns about whether an instructional directive completed years before an incapacitating illness can be taken as an accurate representation of a patient's current treatment wishes.

A parallel concern exists for the usefulness of proxy directives. Researchers have examined the ability of potential surrogate decision makers to predict a close relative's life-sustaining treatment wishes. In these studies, an individual records his or her treatment preferences for various end-of-life scenarios (e.g., irreversible coma, end-stage cancer, debilitating stroke), and a surrogate decision maker (e.g., a loved one or physician) is asked to predict those preferences. Research has consistently shown that surrogate accuracy in predicting a patient's life-sustaining treatment wishes rarely exceed chance levels. Surrogate decision makers have been found to show at least two types of prediction biases. The first is an overtreatment bias, that is, predicting that family members will want life-sustaining treatment

more often than they really do, thus choosing to "err on the side of life." This bias is weaker in predictions made by physicians, who have sometimes been found to show an undertreatment bias. The second is a projection bias in which surrogates (both family members and physicians) have been found to err by assuming that individuals will have wishes for life-sustaining treatment that are similar to their own.

Last, it should be noted that decisions about treatment for a loved are not purely rational ones. Individuals who are placed in the position of being directly responsible for taking the action that ends the life of a loved one may experience strong emotional conflict. Thus, even if a surrogate knows full well that a loved one does not want to receive life-sustaining treatment, the surrogate may find it difficult to honor that wish. Another point of conflict may occur if the patient's known wishes conflict with religious or other deeply held values of the surrogate, as well as if different family members disagree about what the patient would have wanted.

Improving End-of-Life Decision Making

Although research has uncovered a number of important limitations of advance directives, several strategies have been advocated that may improve their effectiveness.

Studies show that when asked about their personal wishes, most individuals express generally positive attitudes about planning for the end-of-life, but many express ambivalence toward completing specific instructional directives and, instead, seem more positively inclined toward informal discussion that focuses on general values and goals. Many individuals are comfortable leaving end-of-life medical decisions to their families and indicate that in the event of a disagreement between their own documented preferences and the opinions of their loved ones, their family's rather than their own directions should be followed. As noted above, such attitudes are particularly pronounced in some cultural groups. Therefore, broad-based attempts to encourage healthy people to document increasingly specific instructional advance directives may be misguided. Instead, some scholars have argued that it is better to focus on encouraging the completion of proxy advance directives, and virtually all agree that people should be encouraged to view completion of an advance directive document as only one part of a broader strategy of advance care planning that includes maintaining an ongoing discussion about end-of-life treatment wishes with loved ones and physicians.

Another approach that attempts to overcome the hypothetical nature of general advance directives is the use of disease-specific advance directives. These are directives developed for patients with a particular medical condition (e.g., AIDS) and allow them to document their wishes for the specific decisions that individuals with their condition are most likely to face. Proponents of this approach argue that because the patient already has some experience with the illness, treatment choices are less hypothetical and, thus, more durable and authentic.

Finally, some shortcomings of standard advance directives may be overcome by the use of medical orders for life-sustaining treatment. Like disease-specific advance directives, medical orders can be written based on the individual's current medical condition and, thus, may be more accurate and up-to-date expressions of end-of-life wishes than generic directives completed months or years prior to hospitalization. Advocates of the POLST program argue that in contrast to standard instructional advance directives that are typically more philosophical reflections of an individual's preferences about an unknown future, the POLST is immediately actionable and can be followed by licensed medical staff such as nursing facility nurses and emergency medical technicians. Some recent research supports the effectiveness of the POLST program in ensuring that patients' treatment preferences are honored.

Peter H. Ditto and Spassena Koleva

See also Biases in Human Prediction; Bioethics; Context Effects; Cultural Issues; Decision Making in Advanced Disease; Surrogate Decision Making

Further Readings

Brett, A. S. (1991). Limitations of listing specific medical interventions in advance directives. *Journal of the American Medical Association, 266,* 825–828.

Buchanan, A. E., & Brock, D. W. (1990). *Deciding for others: The ethics of surrogate decision making.* Cambridge, UK: Cambridge University Press.

Cicirelli, V. G. (1997). Relationship of psychosocial and background variables to older adults' end-of-life decisions. *Psychology and Aging, 12,* 72–83.

Ditto, P. H., Danks, J. H., Smucker, W. D., Bookwala, J., Coppola, K. M., Dresser, R., et al. (2001). Advance directives as acts of communication: A randomized controlled trial. *Archives of Internal Medicine, 161,* 421–430.

Ditto, P. H., Hawkins, N. A., & Pizarro, D. A. (2005). Imagining the end of life: On the psychology of advance medical decision making. *Motivation and Emotion, 29,* 475–496.

Emanuel, L. L., Danis, M., Pearlman, R. A., & Singer, P. A. (1995). Advance care planning as a process: Structuring the discussions in practice. *Journal of the American Geriatrics Society, 43,* 440–446.

Fagerlin, A., Ditto, P. H., Danks, J. H., Houts, R., & Smucker, W. D. (2001). Projection in surrogate decisions about life-sustaining medical treatment. *Health Psychology, 20,* 166–175.

Hickman, S. E., Hammes, B. J, Moss, A. H., & Tolle, S. W. (2005). Hope for the future: Achieving the original intent of advance directives. *Hastings Center Report Special Report, 35*(6), S26–S30.

Kwak, J., & Haley, W. E. (2005). Current research findings on end-of-life decision making among racially or ethnically diverse groups. *The Gerontologist, 45,* 634–641.

The President's Council on Bioethics. (2007). *Taking care: Ethical caregiving in our aging society.* Washington, DC: Government Printing Office.

ALLAIS PARADOX

The *independence axiom* of expected utility theory offers a compelling reason for making a decision. According to this axiom, a choice between two alternatives should depend only on features in which alternatives differ but not on features in which the alternatives are equal. Any feature that is the same for both alternatives, therefore, should not influence the choice a rational person makes. For instance, when choosing between two therapies with exactly the same side effects, a rational doctor would ignore these side effects. That is, rational choice is *independent* of the alternatives' shared features.

This axiom seems very intuitive; if two therapies have the same side effects, it does not matter whether they are small or severe. Hence, rational decision makers base their choices on the distinctive rather than the shared features of the choice alternatives. In the early 1950s, however, French economist Maurice Allais proposed choice problems that challenged the independence axiom as a descriptive principle for risky choice. To illustrate this paradox, known as the Allais paradox, consider the following Allais-type choice problems presented by Adam Oliver: Which of the following would you prefer?

A: Living for 12 years in full health then death, with a chance of 100%

B: Living for 18 years in full health then death, with a chance of 10%

Living for 12 years in full health then death, with a chance of 89%

Immediate death, with a chance of 1%

The majority of people selected Alternative A over B.

C: Living for 12 years in full health then death, with a chance of 11%

Immediate death, with a chance of 89%

D: Living for 18 years in full health then death, with a chance of 10%

Immediate death, with a chance of 90%

In the second problem, most people chose Alternative D, which constitutes a violation of the independence axiom. Table 1 shows why.

Alternatives A and B share an 89% chance of living for 12 years. Because this shared feature should not influence the choice, it can be cancelled out. Similarly, Alternatives C and D share an 89% chance of immediate death, which can be cancelled out again. Importantly, after the shared features in each problem (i.e., the bold column in Table 1) have been cancelled out, both problems become identical. A rational decision maker, thus, should choose A and C or B and D, but not A and D.

Explaining the Allais Paradox

To account for the Allais paradox, two prominent explanations have surfaced: prospect theory and

Table 1   Illustration of the Allais paradox

Alternative	10 Blue	89 Red	1 Green
A	12	**12**	12
B	18	**12**	0
C	12	**0**	12
D	18	**0**	0

Note: The chances in the Allais paradox are symbolized by an urn containing 10 blue balls, 89 red balls, and 1 green ball. Cell entries represent numbers in years living in full health for each alternative in the Allais paradox.

the priority heuristic. Prospect theory by Daniel Kahneman and Amos Tversky explains the Allais paradox by adding complex nonlinear transformations of utilities and probabilities on top of the expected utility framework. The priority heuristic by Eduard Brandstätter, Gerd Gigerenzer, and Ralph Hertwig is motivated by first principles, so as to avoid ending up with the worst of two minimum consequences. The heuristic consists of three steps (assuming nonnegative consequences). In the first step, people compare the alternatives' *minimum consequences*. They select the alternative with the higher minimum consequence, if this difference is large (i.e., equal to or larger than 10% of the problem's best consequence). Otherwise, they compare the *chances* of the minimum consequences. They select the alternative with the smaller chance of the minimum consequence, if this difference is large (i.e., equal or larger than 10%). Otherwise, they compare the *maximum consequences* and select the alternative with the higher maximum consequence.

In the choice between A and B, 12 and 0 years represent the minimum consequences. Because this difference is large (i.e., 12 years exceeds 10% of 18 years), people are predicted to select the alternative with the higher minimum consequence, which is A. That is, the heuristic predicts the majority choice correctly.

In the second choice problem, the minimum consequences (0 and 0) do not differ. In the second step, the chances of the minimum consequences, 89% and 90%, are compared, and this difference is small (i.e., less than 10 percentage points). The higher maximum consequence, 18 versus 12 years, thus, decides choice, and people are predicted to select Alternative *D*, which is the majority choice. Together, the pair of predictions makes the Allais paradox.

Oliver asked participants to think aloud while making both decisions. In the first problem, living for 12 years with certainty was often a decisive reason for choosing Alternative *A*. In the second problem, participants most often stated that the difference between a chance of 10% and 11% (i.e., the logical complements to 90% and 89%) was negligible and that the maximum consequence determined their choice. The latter protocol conforms with the priority heuristic, which assumes comparisons across alternatives, but not with prospect theory, which assumes utility calculations within alternatives.

Adhering to the independence axiom, as implied by expected utility theory, is one criterion for rational choice. Avoiding the worst consequence, as implied by the priority heuristic, is another compelling reason. In conclusion, the Allais paradox makes clear that people do not always follow one principle only.

Eduard Brandstätter

See also Bounded Rationality and Emotions; Certainty Effect; Expected Utility Theory; Prospect Theory

Further Readings

Allais, M. (1979). Criticism of the neo-Bernoullian formulation as a behavioural rule for rational man. In M. Allais & O. Hagen (Eds.), *Expected utility hypotheses and the Allais paradox* (pp. 74–106). Dordrecht, the Netherlands: Reidel.

Brandstätter, E., Gigerenzer, G., & Hertwig, R. (2006). The priority heuristic: Making choices without trade-offs. *Psychological Review, 113,* 409–432.

Oliver, A. J. (2003). A quantitative and qualitative test of the Allais paradox using health outcomes. *Journal of Economic Psychology, 24,* 35–48.

ANALYSIS OF COVARIANCE (ANCOVA)

Analysis of covariance (ANCOVA) is a statistical model introduced by Sir Ronald Fisher that combines features of analysis of variance (ANOVA) with those of regression analysis. The purpose of ANCOVA is to examine differences between levels of one or more grouping variables on an outcome measure after controlling for variation or differences between populations on one or more nuisance variables. The grouping variable often represents different treatments, the outcome measure is the consequence of those treatments, and the nuisance variable either obscures true treatment differences or is a confounding variable that offers an alternative explanation for differences on the outcome other than the treatments.

The ANCOVA model is often underused in experimental research and misinterpreted in quasi-experimental studies. Researchers may not recognize the benefit of using a covariate to reduce unexplained variation among units to increase statistical power in experimental studies. The inclusion of the covariate can substantially increase the sensitivity of group comparisons or reduce the necessary sample size to detect meaningful population differences. In quasi-experiments, researchers may fail to recognize the limitations of the ANCOVA model and overinterpret the results of the analyses. Because of specification and measurement errors, the statistical model cannot totally compensate for a lack of random assignment and equate the populations being compared. However, when used properly, the ANCOVA model can be an essential statistical tool to identify differences among populations on outcomes of interest.

Research Design

The simplest application of this model involves one grouping variable (*G*) having two levels (e.g., a herbal supplement treatment vs. a placebo), a single outcome variable (*Y*) (e.g., blood pressure) and a single nuisance variable, referred to as a covariate (*X*) (e.g., body mass index [BMI]) measured before the formation of the groups or before the start of the treatments. While the application of the model is identical when groups are formed using a random or nonrandom process, the primary purpose and the interpretation of the results are substantially different. When the formation of the groups is based on a random process (e.g., use of random numbers matched with participant identification numbers to assign individuals to treatment levels), the research design is referred to as an *experiment* and is often represented as follows:

$$R \ X \ G_1 \ Y,$$

$$R \ X \ G_2 \ Y,$$

where R represents the random assignment of units to the treatment groups; X is a covariate; G_1 and G_2 represent intervention and placebo groups, respectively; and Y is the outcome of interest. When group formation is based on a nonrandom process (e.g., self-selection) the research design is referred to as a *quasi-experiment* and is often represented as follows:

$$X \ G_1 \ Y,$$

$$X \ G_2 \ Y,$$

where terms are defined as above.

Data Example

Suppose a sample of 12 overweight patients having high systolic blood pressure volunteered to investigate the usefulness of a herbal supplement over a 2-month trial period. Half of the volunteers are randomly assigned to receive the herbal supplement, while the other half are given a placebo. Before beginning the investigation, each individual's BMI is computed. When the treatment period ends, systolic blood pressure is assessed. Table 1 presents hypothetical data along with means and standard deviations (*SD*s). These data will be used to demonstrate the use and interpretation of the ANCOVA model.

Structural Model

The ANCOVA model that can represent data from both designs can be written as follows:

$$Y_{ij} = \mu + \alpha_j + \beta_{Y|X}(X_{ij} - \bar{X}) + \varepsilon_{ij},$$

where Y_{ij} is the outcome score for individual i in Group j ($i = 1, \ldots, n_j$; $j = 1, \ldots, J$), μ the grand mean on the outcome measure, α_j the deviation of the mean of population j on the outcome measure from the grand mean, $\beta_{y|x}$ the common regression slope of the outcome on the covariate, X_{ij} the covariate (e.g., pretest) score for individual i in Group j, $\bar{X}$ the observed grand mean on the covariate measure, and ε_{ij} the model error, a measure of individual differences.

Table 1   Body mass index and systolic blood pressure scores (post) for volunteers receiving an herbal diet supplement or placebo

	Herbal Supplement		Placebo	
	BMI	*Post*	*BMI*	*Post*
	50	150	45	147
	40	142	26	135
	7	120	40	152
	32	129	30	128
	45	132	52	165
	36	138	37	140
Mean	38.3	135.2	38.3	144.5
SD	8.45	10.51	9.56	13.16

Before discussing the hypotheses that can be tested with this model, it is very important to note that a common regression slope, β, of Y on X is assumed for this model. That is, the regression slope of Y on X is assumed to be identical for all populations being compared. This assumption is important for two reasons. First, if the slopes are not equal, the statistical model is incorrect and the subsequent ANCOVA hypothesis tests may be statistically invalid. Second, unequal regression slopes indicate that there is an interaction between the grouping variable and the covariate. That is, differences between the populations vary depending on the value of the covariate. For example, the difference in blood pressure between a population receiving an herbal supplement and the placebo may only occur for individuals having high BMI scores. In this context, testing for average differences between populations can be inappropriate or misleading. When an interaction is present, alternative analyses (e.g., Johnson-Neyman procedure) may be recommended.

Hypotheses

To determine whether the assumption of a common regression slope is tenable, a statistical test for the equality of the separate regression slopes should be conducted (i.e., H_0: $\beta_{y|x1} = \beta_{y|x2}$) with the criterion for statistical significance set at a slightly elevated level (e.g., $\alpha = .10$ or $.15$) to reduce the risk of concluding equal slopes when in fact they differ.

For the data in Table 1, the regression slopes of post on BMI are 1.03 and 1.25, respectively. The observed difference between sample estimates is not statistically significant ($F(1, 8) = .230$, $p = .644$). The ANCOVA model is therefore judged appropriate for these data.

If the ANCOVA model is appropriate, two hypotheses can be tested. One hypothesis examines the relationship between the covariate and the outcome measure: H_0: $\beta_{y|x} = 0$. From a substantive perspective, this hypothesis is generally of little interest. Often the covariate and the outcome measures are obtained from the same test administered twice, so a relationship is to be expected. If there is no relationship between the covariate and the outcome measure, then X and Y are independent and knowledge of X is of little statistical value. For the

current data set, the pooled or average regression slope is 1.15. The relationship between BMI and postsystolic blood pressure is statistically significant at $\alpha = .05$ ($F(1, 9) = 28.64$, $p = .000$).

A second hypothesis, and the primary hypothesis of interest, that can be tested with the ANCOVA model can be written as: H_0: $\alpha_j = 0$ for all j, or equivalently as H_0: $_{adj} \mu_1 = {}_{adj} \mu_2 = \cdots = {}_{adj} \mu_j$. The exact meaning of this hypothesis depends on whether the research design is experimental or quasi-experimental. An adjusted mean for population j is defined as

$$_{adj}\mu_j = \mu_{Y_j} - \beta_{Y|X}(\mu_{\bar{X}_j} - \mu_{\bar{X}}),$$

where μ_{Y_j} and μ_{X_j} are the means for population j on the outcome and covariate measures, respectively, and $\mu_{X_.}$ is the grand mean across all populations on the covariate.

If two populations are compared, the hypothesis may be written as

$$H_0 : {}_{adj}\mu_1 - {}_{adj}\mu_2 = 0,$$

or

$$H_0 : (\mu_{Y_1} - \mu_{Y_2}) - \beta_{Y|X}(\mu_{X_1} - \mu_{X_2}) = 0.$$

The hypothesis on difference between the adjusted population means can be seen as a hypothesis on the difference between the population means on the outcome measure minus the product of the difference between the population covariate means and $\beta_{Y/X}$. Where $\beta_{Y/X}$ is a measure of the degree to which the covariate can predict the outcome measure. An estimate of the difference between adjusted population means is provided by substituting sample estimates for the parameters in the hypothesis:

$$(\bar{Y}_1 - \bar{Y}_2) - b_{Y|X}(\bar{X}_1 - \bar{X}_2).$$

Experimental Design

When units are randomly assigned to the groups, there would be no difference between the populations on the covariate measure, $\mu_{x1} - \mu_{x2} = 0$, and no true adjustment is made nor is one necessary. In an experiment, the hypothesis on the adjusted population means is identical to the hypothesis tested in a posttest-only design using analysis of variance. The equality of means on the covariate measure refers to only the populations, not the sample means. Sample means typically differ slightly and small differences between adjusted and unadjusted sample outcome means are generally observed. But hypotheses are statements regarding populations, not samples, so the small differences in sample means can be safely ignored. In the present example, sample BMI means are identical (i.e., $\bar{X}_1 = \bar{X}_2 = 38.3$).

Quasi-Experimental Design

In quasi-experimental studies, populations being compared typically differ on the covariate measure $\mu_{x1} - \mu_{x2} \neq 0$. For example, individuals who choose to take herbal supplements may also exercise more than individuals who do not take the supplements. The difference in blood pressure between the two populations may be related to the amount of exercise rather than the herbal supplement. With the ANCOVA model, differences on the outcome measure can to some extent be adjusted for the difference on the covariate. The question, however, is whether this adjustment is sufficient. The answer is generally no. There are two problems when the populations being compared are not equivalent on all relevant variables that could explain differences on the outcome variable other than the treatments. First, if populations differ on one variable, X, they are likely to differ on other variables as well, and these additional variables might also provide an alternative explanation for population differences on the outcome. It is possible to extend the ANCOVA model to include multiple covariates, but it is impossible to know and to specify all the other relevant confounding variables. This is known as the specification error problem. Second, even if the populations differed on only one variable, X, the adequacy of the adjustment would depend on the estimation of the population slope $\beta_{y|x}$. The reliability (i.e., consistency) with which the covariate is measured affects the estimate of $\beta_{y|x}$. The relationship between $\beta_{Y|X}$ and the sample estimate $b_{Y|X}$ is $b_{Y|X} = \beta_{Y|X} \rho_{XX}$, where ρ_{xx} is the reliability of the covariate measure (e.g., BMI). Because the covariate is never perfectly reliable, measurement error leads to an underestimation of the relationship between X and Y, and the pooled regression

slope, $b_{Y|X}$, is too small and the difference in outcome means is underadjusted. This is known as the measurement error problem. In our example, the pooled slope was computed as $b_{Y|X} = 1.15$. If the BMI is measured with .70 reliability, the correct adjustment should have been 1.64. Consequently, the adjustment is insufficient, and it is not possible to attribute differences in the outcome variable solely to the treatment. In the current example, the mean BMI score for both groups was identical, so the underestimation of the relationship is irrelevant. No adjustment to postsystolic blood pressure is needed.

The hypothesis regarding the grouping variable tested with the ANCOVA model is therefore different when the research design is experimental or quasi-experimental. In an experimental design, the hypothesis tested is unambiguous. Differences in the outcome variable can be attributed to differences in the grouping variable. But in a quasi-experimental study, because of measurement error with the covariate and the inability to specify and measure all relevant confounding variables, differences between populations on the outcome measure cannot be attributed solely to differences in the grouping variable. The ANCOVA model cannot be used to completely compensate for a lack of random assignment, and the results of the analysis must be interpreted cautiously.

Statistical Power

As discussed above in an experimental study, the ANCOVA and ANOVA models test the hypothesis that the population means on the outcome variable are identical. It might then be asked, why go to the trouble and expense of collecting additional data prior to the formation of the groups? The answer is greater sensitivity (i.e., statistical power) to detect a difference between populations. Both ANOVA and ANCOVA models compute a test statistic, F, by taking the ratio of the variation among group means multiplied by n, the common group size (e.g., $n = 6$) to the unexplained variation of units within the groups. Because in an experiment adjusted and unadjusted means are, within sampling error, equivalent, the two statistics differ only in terms of the unexplained variation among the units. The unexplained variation is individual differences attributable to multiple causes (e.g., initial blood pressure, BMI, activity levels). With the ANOVA model, the unexplained variation of the units in the populations being compared on the outcome measure can be represented as $\sigma^2_{Y|G}$. If a covariate is available and is used, it can explain some of the unexplained variation in the outcome measure, and the remaining variation for the ANCOVA model can be written as $\sigma^2_{Y|GX} = \sigma^2_{Y|G}(1 - \rho^2)$, where ρ^2 is the population correlation between the covariate and the outcome measure. The greater the correlation between the two measures, the smaller the unexplained variation in the ANCOVA model relative to the ANOVA model, $\sigma^2_{Y|GX} < \sigma^2_{Y|G}$. The smaller the unexplained variation, the more sensitive the analysis to a true population difference between the intervention and the placebo. This sensitivity is manifested in a larger computed F statistic.

In the current data set, if the BMI is ignored, $\sigma^2_{Y|G}$ is estimated using the average within-group variance on postsystolic blood pressure,

$$141.8 = \frac{(10.51)^2 + (13.16)^2}{2}.$$

Including BMI scores as a covariate, $\sigma^2_{Y|GX}$ is estimated as 37.7. Ignoring the BMI scores, the observed difference between posttreatment means (135.2 vs. 144.5) is not statistically significant ($F(1, 10) = 1.843$, $p = .204$). But after considering individual differences in the BMI scores, the difference between means on the postsystolic blood pressure is statistically significant ($F(1, 9) = 6.936$, $p = .027$).

Effect Size

The statistical evaluation of α_j in the ANCOVA model is useful in determining whether observed difference in the adjusted sample means represent a true difference in population means or is an artifact of sampling error (i.e., chance differences between units in the samples studied). But this analysis provides no information on the magnitude of the true difference. Two useful indices of effect size are the standardized mean difference and η^2.

The standardized mean difference (δ) is useful when comparing two populations, and it defines the difference in population means in terms of the

population standard deviation on the outcome measure:

$$\delta = \frac{\text{adj}\,\mu_{G_1} - \text{adj}\,\mu_{G_2}}{\sigma_{Y|G}}.$$

A sample estimate of δ is provided by using sample estimates of the parameters:

$$d = \frac{\text{adj}\,\bar{Y}_{G_1} - \text{adj}\,\bar{Y}_{G_2}}{S_{Y|G}},$$

where $S_{Y|G}$ equals the pooled within-group standard deviation on the outcome measure. Note that when computing the standardized-mean difference, the denominator includes the variation associated with the covariate. For the current data, d is computed to equal $-.78$ [$(135.2-144.5)/\sqrt{141.8}$]. The herbal supplement reduced systolic blood pressure .78 standard deviation units compared with the placebo.

Eta-square is useful when it is desirable to define the effect as the proportion of the total variation that is associated with the grouping variable:

$$\eta^2 = \frac{\sigma^2_G}{\sigma^2_G + \sigma^2_{ID}},$$

where σ^2_G is the variation associated with the grouping variable and σ^2_{ID} the unexplained variation due to individual differences.

A sample estimate of η^2 is provided using sample estimates of the parameters:

$$\hat{\eta}^2 = \frac{SS_G}{SS_G + SS_{ID}},$$

where SS_G is the sum of squares for the grouping variable and SS_{ID} the sum of squares for individual differences.

Individual differences include unexplained variation and variation associated with the covariate, that is, $SS_{ID} = SS_X + SS_{Y|GX}$. Both the results of the statistical test for population mean differences and effect size should be reported when summarizing the results of the ANCOVA model. For the current data,

$$\hat{\eta}^2 = 0.156 \left(= \frac{261.333}{261.333 + 1079.237 + 339.096} \right).$$

Contrast Analysis

If more than two populations are compared simultaneously (e.g., herbal supplement vs. yoga vs. placebo) the omnibus hypothesis test $H_0: \alpha_j = 0$ for all j does not identify which populations differ. To identify specific differences between and among populations, contrasts must be examined and tested. A contrast is a linear composite of means: $\psi = \Sigma c_j\, \mu_j$, with $\Sigma c_j = 0$, where c_j is the contrast coefficient for population j. The hypothesis tested is $H_0\colon \psi = 0$, (e.g., $H_{0(1)}\colon \psi = \mu_1 - \mu_2 = 0$, or $H_{0(2)}\colon \psi = .5\mu_1 + .5\mu_2 - \mu_3, = 0$). A sample estimate, $\hat{\psi}$, is provided using sample estimates of the parameters, for example, $\hat{\psi} = {}_{\text{adj}}\bar{Y}_1 - {}_{\text{adj}}\bar{Y}_2$. To test the hypothesis, a t test statistic is formed by taking the ratio of the sample estimate of the contrast to the standard error of the contrast,

$$t = \frac{\hat{\psi}}{S_{\hat{\psi}}}.$$

Because multiple contrasts are generally tested in a single study, several strategies have been suggested for evaluating the t statistic depending on what is judged to be an acceptable risk of a Type I error and statistical power.

Data Assumptions

The statistical validity of the hypotheses tested using the ANCOVA model depends on whether several assumptions regarding the units in the populations being compared are met. In addition to the assumption that the separate regression slopes of the outcome on the covariate are the same for all populations, which was discussed earlier, the ANCOVA model also assumes that the relationship between covariate and the outcome is linear and that the model errors, ε_{ij}, are (a) independent of each other, (b) normally distributed at each level of the covariate, and (c) have equal variance at each level of the covariate both within each population and between the populations being compared.

The assumption of linearity can be examined by testing within each group the statistical significance of the Pearson correlation between the covariate and the outcome. For the current data, the separate correlations between BMI and postsystolic blood pressure are .827 and .906 for the herbal and placebo groups, respectively. Both correlations are statistically significant at the .05 level. Further examining a scatter plot of the data shows a consistent increase in postsystolic blood pressure with increasing BMI scores for each group. A linear relationship is reasonable to assume.

Model errors refer to the difference between actual postsystolic pressure and predicted postsystolic blood pressure from BMI, $Y_{ig} - \hat{Y}_{ig}$. These errors are sometimes referred to as residuals. The independence assumption implies that individuals do not influence each other with respect to the outcome under investigation. Determination of whether this assumption is tenable is best judged based on how data were collected. If there is little interaction among the units between and within each group, the assumption is likely met.

The assumptions regarding the distributions of model errors (normality and equal variance) are best examined by plotting the errors (residuals) for each group around the separate regression lines using the common slope. The homogeneity of error variance assumption can also be examined by comparing mean square error estimates, $S^2_{Y|X_j}$ from the regression lines in each group. For the current study, $S^2_{Y|X_1} = 43.6$ and $S^2_{Y|X_2} = 38.8$, so the variance of errors between the groups appear similar.

The ANCOVA model is generally robust to moderate violations of these data assumptions, particularly when the number of units per group is equal.

Stephen Olejnik and H. J. Keselman

See also Analysis of Variance (ANOVA); Hypothesis Testing

Further Readings

Harwell, M. (2003). Summarizing Monte Carlo results in methodological research: The single-factor fixed-effect ANCOVA case. *Journal of Educational and Behavioral Statistics, 28,* 45–70.

Huitema, B. E. (1980). *The analysis of covariance and alternatives.* New York: Wiley.

Kirk, R. E. (1995). *Experimental design procedures for the behavioral sciences* (3rd ed.). Pacific Grove, CA: Brooks/Cole.

Olejnik, S., & Algina, J. (2000). Measures of effect size for comparative studies: Applications, interpretations, and limitations. *Contemporary Educational Psychology, 25,* 242–286.

Olejnik, S., & Algina, J. (2003). Generalized eta and omega squared statistics: Measures of effect size for some common research designs. *Psychological Methods, 8,* 434–447.

Pedhazur, E. J. (1997). *Multiple regression in behavioral research: Explanation and prediction* (3rd ed.). Fort Worth, TX: Harcourt Brace.

Pedhazur, E.J., & Schmelkin, L. P. (1991). *Measurement, design, and analysis: An integrated approach.* Hillsdale, NJ: Lawrence Erlbaum.

Porter, A. C., & Raudenbush, S. W. (1987). Analysis of covariance: Its model and use in psychological research. *Journal of Counseling Psychology, 34,* 383–392.

Shaffer, J. P. (1995). Multiple hypothesis testing. *Annual Review of Psychology, 46,* 561–584.

Toothaker, L. E. (1991). *Multiple comparisons for researchers.* Newbury Park, CA: Sage.

ANALYSIS OF VARIANCE (ANOVA)

Consider a study in which a randomized trial is undertaken to compare a control group, an intervention group receiving a standard treatment, and an intervention group receiving a new treatment on a single continuous outcome measure, such as health status. How can it be determined whether there is a statistically significant difference in the mean outcome score among the three groups? The conventional method of analysis for these data is analysis of variance (ANOVA). ANOVA encompasses a broad collection of statistical procedures used to partition variation in a data set into components due to one or more categorical explanatory variables (i.e., factors). The topics covered in this entry are (a) a description of the applications of ANOVA in medical research, (b) a review of the computations for the ANOVA test statistic, and (c) criteria to assess the reporting of ANOVA results in medical literature.

Applications

Data arising from many different types of studies can be analyzed using ANOVA, including the following:

One-way independent groups design, in which two or more groups of study participants are to be compared on a single outcome measure. This is the simplest type of design in which ANOVA is applied.

One-sample repeated measures design, in which a single group of study participants is observed on

two or more measurement occasions. The measurements for each participant are typically correlated (i.e., related).

Factorial independent groups design, in which two or more factors are crossed so that each combination of categories, or cell of the design, comprises an independent group of study participants. Interaction and main effects will usually be tested in factorial designs. A statistically significant two-way interaction implies that the effect of one factor is not constant at each level of the second factor.

Mixed designs, which contain both independent groups and repeated measures factors. Within-subjects interaction and main effects, as well as the between-subjects main effect, may be tested in a mixed design. A significant within-subjects two-way interaction effect indicates that the repeated measures effect is not constant across groups of study participants.

Computing an ANOVA Test Statistic

The sidebar outlines the goal of ANOVA in a one-way independent groups design, the required computations, and the decision rule for the test statistic. The method is described for the simplest situation, in which all the group sizes are equal. A numeric example is also provided.

In an independent groups design, the assumptions that underlie validity of inference for the ANOVA F test are as follows:

1. The outcome variable follows a normal distribution in each population from which data are sampled.

2. Variances are equal (i.e., homogeneous) across the populations.

3. The observations that comprise each sample are independent (i.e., unrelated).

In one-sample repeated measures designs or mixed designs, measurements taken from the same study participant are correlated, but measurements from different study participants are assumed to be unrelated. In these designs, the data are assumed to follow a multivariate normal distribution and conform to the assumption of multisample sphericity. Multivariate normality means that the marginal

Computing the ANOVA F Test When Group Sizes Are Equal

Goal of ANOVA: To test the plausibility of the null hypothesis, H_0: $\mu_1 = \mu_2 = \ldots = \mu_J$, the hypothesis of equal population means for J groups, against the alternative hypothesis, H_A, at least one of the means is different from the others.

Computations: Compute the sample means, $\bar{y}_1, \bar{y}_2, \ldots, \bar{y}_J$; the grand (i.e., overall) mean, $\bar{y}$; and the sample variances $s_1^2, s_2^2, \ldots, s_J^2$. When the same number of study participants are in each group, n, the total number of study participants is $n \times J = N$. The numerator of the test statistic, the variability between groups, is

$$\text{MSBG} = \frac{n}{J-1}\left[(\bar{y}_1 - \bar{y})^2 + (\bar{y}_2 - \bar{y})^2 + \ldots + (\bar{y}_J - \bar{y})^2\right].$$

The farther apart the means of the groups, the larger this quantity will be.

The denominator of the test statistic, the variability within groups, is

$$\text{MSWG} = \frac{1}{J}\left[s_1^2 + s_2^2 + \ldots + s_J^2\right].$$

This quantity will be larger when there is more variability within groups.

Test statistic:

$$F = \frac{\text{MSBG}}{\text{MSWG}}.$$

Decision rule: Reject H_0 if F exceeds a critical value from an F distribution with numerator degrees of freedom $df_1 = J - 1$ and denominator degrees of freedom $df_2 = N - J$ for a prespecified level of significance (e.g., $\alpha = .05$). The F statistic will be large when H_0 is not true.

Example: Suppose that a researcher collects data for three groups of study participants, with 10 participants in each group. Let the group means be $\bar{y}_1 = 12.0$, $\bar{y}_2 = 8.0$, and $\bar{y}_3 = 11.5$. Then the grand mean, $\bar{y} = 10.5$. Let the group variances be $s_1^2 = 15.0$, $s_2^2 = 10.5$, and $s_3^2 = 18.0$. Then the numerator of the test statistic is MSBW = 47.5 and the denominator is MSWG = 14.5. The test statistic, $F = 3.28$, is compared with a critical value from the F distribution with $df_1 = 2$ and $df_2 = 27$, which is equal to $F_{crit} = 2.96$ when $\alpha = .05$. The p value is .0362. The null hypothesis, H_0: $\mu_1 = \mu_2 = \mu_3$, is rejected.

measurements have a common variance and also that this common variance is the same for all groups of study participants.

The F test is not robust to assumption violations; this means that it is sensitive to changes in those factors that are extraneous to the hypothesis being tested. In fact, the F test may become seriously biased when assumptions are not satisfied, resulting in spurious decisions about the null hypothesis.

The assumptions that underlie the ANOVA F test are unlikely to be satisfied in many studies. Outliers or extreme observations are often a significant concern and can result in a substantial loss of statistical power to detect study effects. Furthermore, study participants who are exposed to a particular healthcare treatment or intervention may exhibit greater (or lesser) variability on the outcome measure than study participants who are not exposed to it. Inequality of variances can have serious consequences for control of the Type I error rate, the probability of erroneously rejecting a true null hypothesis.

Researchers who rely on ANOVA to test hypotheses about equality of means may, therefore, unwittingly fill the literature with nonreplicable results or at other times may fail to detect effects when they are present. This is of concern because the results of statistical tests are routinely used to make decisions about the effectiveness of clinical interventions and to plan healthcare delivery. In this era of evidence-informed decision making, it is crucial that the statistical procedures applied to a set of data will produce valid results.

Researchers often regard nonparametric procedures based on rank scores, such as the Kruskal-Wallis test or Friedman's test, as appealing alternatives to the ANOVA F test when the assumption of normality is suspect. However, nonparametric

distribution for each measurement occasion, that is, the distribution of scores for each measurement occasion, ignoring all other occasions, is normal and the joint distribution of the measurement occasions (i.e., the distribution of all occasions together) is normal. Multisample sphericity means that the difference scores for all pairs of repeated procedures test hypotheses about equality of distributions rather than equality of means. They are therefore sensitive to heterogeneous variances; distributions with unequal variances will necessarily result in rejection of the null hypothesis. Rank-transform test procedures are also appealing because they can be implemented using existing statistical software packages. A rank-transform ANOVA F test is obtained by converting the original scores to ranks prior to computing the conventional F statistic. One limitation of rank-transform procedures is that they cannot be applied to tests of interaction effects in factorial designs. The ranks are not a linear function of the original observations; therefore, ranking the data may introduce additional effects into the statistical model. Furthermore, ranking may alter the pattern of the correlations among the measurement occasions in repeated measurement designs. Rank-transform tests, while insensitive to departures from normality, must therefore be used with caution.

Transformations of the data, to stabilize the variance or reduce the influence of extreme observations, are another popular choice. Logarithmic, square root, and reciprocal transformations are common. The primary problem with applying a transformation to one's data is that it may become difficult to interpret the null hypothesis when the data are no longer in the original scale of measurement. Also, a transformation may not accomplish the goal of getting rid of outliers.

When variance equality cannot be assumed, robust procedures such as the Welch test for the one-way independent groups design are recommended alternatives to the ANOVA F test. Welch's test does not pool the group variances in the computation of the test statistic denominator and modifies the degrees of freedom with a function of the sample sizes and the variances. Welch's test does, however, assume that the data are normally distributed. If normality is not tenable, then a modification of the Welch test should be considered. One alternative involves substituting robust means and variances for the usual means and variances in the computation of the test statistic. Robust means and variances are less affected by the presence of outlying scores or skewed distributions than the usual mean. There are a number of robust statistics that have been proposed in the literature; among these, the trimmed mean has received

substantial attention because of its good theoretical properties, ease of computation, and ease of interpretation. The trimmed mean is obtained by removing, or censoring, the most extreme scores in the distribution, which have the tendency to shift the mean in their direction. Current recommendations are to remove between 10% and 20% of the observations in *each* tail of the distribution. A consistent robust estimator of variability for the trimmed mean is the Winsorized variance, which is computed by replacing the most extreme scores in the distribution with the next most extreme observations. While robust measures are insensitive to nonnormality, they test a null hypothesis different from traditional estimators. The null hypothesis is about equality of trimmed population means. In other words, one is testing a hypothesis that focuses on the majority (i.e., central part) of the population rather than the entire population.

Finally, computationally intensive methods, such as the bootstrap method, have also been used to develop alternatives to the ANOVA F test. The bootstrap method can be described as follows: The usual ANOVA F test is computed on the original observations, but statistical significance is assessed using a critical value from the empirical distribution of the test statistic rather than a critical value from the F distribution. The empirical distribution is obtained by generating a large number (e.g., 1,000) of data sets; each data set is a random sample (sampling with replacement) from the original observations. Sampling with replacement means that any observation can potentially be sampled multiple times. The F test is computed for each bootstrap data set. The bootstrapped test statistics are ranked in ascending order; the critical value for assessing statistical significance corresponds to a preselected percentile of the empirical distribution, such as the 95th percentile. Bootstrap test procedures have good properties in the presence of assumption violations. For example, the bootstrapped ANOVA F test for repeated measures designs will control the rate of Type I errors to α, the nominal level of significance, under departures from both normality and sphericity.

Assessing ANOVA Results

For decision makers to have confidence in ANOVA results reported in the medical literature, it is important that the choice of test procedures is justified and the analytic strategy is accurately and completely described. The reader should be provided with a clear picture of the characteristics of the data under investigation. This can be accomplished by reporting exploratory descriptive analysis results, including standard deviations or variances, sample sizes, skewness (a measure of symmetry of the distribution) and kurtosis (a measure of peakedness of the distribution), and normal probability plots. As a general rule of thumb, skewness and kurtosis measures should be within the range from +1 to −1 to assume that the data follow a normal distribution. The normal probability plot is a graphic technique in which the observations are plotted against a theoretical normal distribution; if all the points fall on an approximate diagonal line, then normality is likely to be a tenable assumption.

While preliminary tests of variance equality, such as Levene's test, or tests of sphericity, such as Mauchly's test, are available in statistical software packages, their use is not recommended in practice. Many tests about variances are sensitive to departures from a normal distribution, and those that are insensitive to nonnormality may lack statistical power to detect departures from the null hypothesis of equal variances, which can result in erroneous decisions about the choice of follow-up tests.

For factorial designs, unless there is theoretical evidence that clearly supports the testing of main effects only, the analysis should begin with tests of interactions among the study factors. Graphic presentations of the cell means are often useful to characterize the nature of the interaction.

Each test of a main or interaction effect should be completely described. This includes reporting the numeric value of the test statistic, degrees of freedom, and p value or critical value.

A statistically significant ANOVA F test is routinely followed by multiple comparisons to identify the localized source of an effect. The choice of a multiple comparison test statistic and procedure for controlling the familywise error rate, the probability of making at least one Type I error for the entire set of comparisons, should be explicitly identified in the reporting of results. A simple Bonferroni approach may suffice, in which each of m comparisons is tested at the α/m level of significance.

However, this multiple comparison procedure is often less powerful than modified Bonferroni procedures, such as Hochberg's procedure.

Conclusion

ANOVA is one of the most popular test procedures for analyzing medical data because it can be used in a wide variety of research applications. Researchers may be reluctant to bypass the conventional ANOVA F test in favor of an alternative approach. This reluctance may stem, in part, from the belief that the F test is robust to departures from derivational assumptions. While Type I error rates may be relatively robust to the presence of nonnormal distributions, power rates can be substantially affected. This is a critical issue, particularly for small-sample designs, which are common in clinical trials. Departures from variance homogeneity and sphericity can result in seriously biased tests of between-subjects and within-subjects effects, respectively. Statistical procedures that are robust to assumption violations have been developed for both simple and complex factorial designs and are now routinely available in many statistical software packages.

Lisa M. Lix and H. J. Keselman

See also Analysis of Covariance (ANCOVA); Measures of Central Tendency; Multivariate Analysis of Variance (MANOVA); Variance and Covariance

Further Readings

Conover, W. J., & Iman, R. L. (1981). Rank transformation as a bridge between parametric and nonparametric statistics. *The American Statistician, 35*, 124–129.

Hill, M. A., & Dixon, W. J. (1982). Robustness in real life: A study of clinical laboratory data. *Biometrics, 38*, 377–396.

Hochberg, Y. (1988). A sharper Bonferroni procedure for multiple tests of significance. *Biometrika, 75*, 800–802.

Keselman, H. J. (2005). Multivariate normality tests. In B. S. Everitt & D. C. Howell (Eds.), *Encyclopedia of statistics in behavioural science* (Vol. 3, pp. 1373–1379). Chichester, UK: Wiley.

Keselman, H. J., Wilcox, R. R., & Lix, L. M. (2003). A generally robust approach to hypothesis testing in independent and correlated groups designs. *Psychophysiology, 40,* 586–596.

Lix, L. M., Keselman, J. C., & Keselman, H. J. (1996). Consequences of assumption violations revisited: A quantitative review of alternatives to the one-way analysis of variance *F* test. *Review of Educational Research, 66,* 579–619.

Scariano, S. M., & Davenport, J. M. (1987). The effects of violations of independence assumptions in the one-way ANOVA. *The American Statistician, 41,* 123–129.

Toothaker, L. E. (1991). *Multiple comparisons for researchers.* Newbury Park, CA: Sage.

Vickers, A. J. (2005). Parametric versus non-parametric statistics in the analysis of randomized trials with non-normally distributed data. *BMC Medical Research Methodology, 5,* 35.

Wasserman, S., & Bockenholt, U. (1989). Bootstrapping: Applications to psychophysiology. *Psychophysiology, 26,* 208–221.

Wilcox, R. R. (1995). ANOVA: A paradigm for low power and misleading measures of effect size? *Review of Educational Research, 65,* 51–77.

Wilcox, R. R., & Keselman, H. J. (2003). Modern robust data analysis methods: Measures of central tendency. *Psychological Methods, 8,* 254–274.

Zimmerman, D. W. (2004). A note on preliminary tests of equality of variances. *British Journal of Mathematical and Statistical Psychology, 57,* 173–181.

APPLIED DECISION ANALYSIS

Decision analysis (DA) is a methodology by which the various aspects of a decision are represented in an explicit and quantitative model to support or improve the procedure and/or outcome of decisions under uncertainty. The term *decision analysis* is used both for the domain and for the actual single exercise of construction and quantifying a model for a particular problem. DA can be used purely for the sake of knowledge itself (such as to increase one's own understanding or that of others in a teaching setting) and also with the purpose to apply that knowledge to real-life medical dilemma, where a choice has to be made. This is called *applied decision analysis,* although the more correct term might be *applicable decision analysis,* as, however one may be with the model, it remains to be seen whether it will convince doctors and patients sufficiently to be used in clinical practice.

In this entry, an overview is given of applied DA, its history, the why and how, and its present and future potential and limitations.

History

The history of applied DA starts with Stephen Pauker's famous "Clinical Decision Making Rounds at the New England Medical Center," which started in 1981 and filled the first 10 issues of the journal *Medical Decision Making.* Typically, these papers dealt with problems in individual patients and elaborated from that individual to more general issues. Since that pioneering time, the number of publications on clinically applied DA has increased strongly over time and keeps doing so. Papers on applied DA increase more than twice as fast as those on other clinical issues (with a doubling time of 4.2 years as compared with 9.9 years).

The "Why" of Applied Decision Analysis

Why one should perform a DA for a real-life clinical problem may not be clear to everyone in the first place. Normally, medical choices in healthcare are dealt with in a more or less implicit way, where doctors or other healthcare professionals rely on their knowledge or experience to estimate which choice alternative would (probably) provide the best outcome. Dissatisfaction with the subjectivity and the lack of transparency of this process and its outcomes has over several decennia led to the development of more explicit and quantitative methods of dealing with clinical issues that include not only DA but also evidence-based medicine (EBM). DA differs in its ambition from EBM.

EBM builds on the assumption that doctors only have an information problem that can be solved by providing them with the right data. EBM, and in particular the Cochrane collaboration, has therefore put an enormous effort in tracking that information and making the data available to doctors.

As has been argued by Arthur Elstein and others, DA goes one step further and assumes that in addition to the information problem, doctors also have a judgment problem. That judgment problem has to do with the complexity of integrating all the available information elements and their relations, and condensing it into the right choice, and with the fact that making choices entails taking into account not only probabilities but likewise valuing potential outcomes. That may be a reason why doctors may have a better feel about EBM (here is the info, so you can decide) than about DA (here is the info and the advice, because you cannot be trusted to make the right judgment). The added value that DA brings is in structuring and summarizing available knowledge and in supporting or steering actual decisions.

There are several advantages of using applied DA to tackle clinical problems. First, a global problem is dissected into parts, so that the intricacies and complexities of the decision problem are made clearer. Second, using data synthesis methods (an abundance of), available data will be combined and restructured into a limited number of variables that are essential to the (solution of the) problem, so that available knowledge is summarized in a clear and concise way. Third, far from being mechanistic or generalizing, the DA approach allows for individualization of choices if variables are used that characterize individuals and their (relevant) characteristics. Fourth, the root causes of clinical disagreement (if present) will become more clear by the process of dissecting the problem, building the model, and combining it with the available information. This will pinpoint why clinicians (if they do) differ in opinion and will allow for the testing of the arguments of each camp against available evidence. Finally, and perhaps most important for clinical purposes, the (ir)relevance of various elements of the problem may be tested by using sensitivity and threshold analysis. Thus, the understanding of the intricacies of the clinical issues may improve considerably, thanks to quantitative answers on "what if" questions (albeit about different patients, settings, and/or any key variables).

Self-evidently, there are also potential disadvantages to using DA to solve clinical problems. Real-life problems are inevitably simplified when they are translated into DA models, thus providing solutions that fit the model but do not necessarily solve the real-life problem. This means that other issues (such as feasibility, experience and expertise, safety, and acceptability), that go beyond the purely medical information represented in the model, but may be highly relevant, may not be taken into account in the model's advice. Then, the information necessary to quantify all the variables in the model may be

deficient, and the pragmatic use of low-quality data entails the risk of "garbage in, garbage out." One should not forget that building a decision model, and in particular collecting and summarizing available evidence into the necessary variables, requires decision analytic expertise and experience, and it may take a considerable amount of time. Finally, however careful a decision model is constructed, there is always the risk that errors within the model may go unobserved, which will jeopardize the validity of the answers supplied (example).

Thus, before one embarks on doing a DA, one should take heed. Building a decision tree and "playing with it" to better understand the various issues may be relatively easy. But upscaling it to something that is sufficiently convincing for incorporation into guidelines, or for publication in a peer-reviewed journal, is an endeavor of a different scale.

The "How" of Applied Decision Analysis

The technical execution of an applied DA can be subdivided into several stages or aspects:

1. Identifying the precise nature of the real-life medical problem, including
   a. the type of question (diagnosis, therapy, diagnostic-therapeutic management), the patient category, the setting (primary care, center of excellence);
   b. the relevant outcomes such as mortality, (quality-adjusted) life expectancy, disease-free survival, cost, and so on;
   c. the available policy alternatives, both the realistic ones, and the extremes of doing nothing and treating everyone always; and
   d. the various arguments in favor of, or against, each policy alternative.

2. Structuring the problem first in a flowchart or an algorithm (using "if-then-else" sequences only, and no variables yet), and only then in a full-fledged decision tree.

3. Obtaining the necessary data on underlying diseases and their natural histories on prior probabilities and relations with determinants in subgroups, on characteristics of available diagnostic tests and of relevant therapies, and on (the value of) relevant outcomes.

4. Performing calculations on expected outcomes and costs, and including sensitivity analysis (what matters?), threshold analysis (when should one choose differently?), and resulting in overall conclusions.

For the first stage, close cooperation with experts in the (clinical) field is of the utmost importance to make sure that the decision analyst understands why there is a problem and what the real-life options and outcomes may be. It is particularly important to identify the relevant stakeholders and to know their optimization criteria (what do they consider important, either as something to achieve or as something to avoid). To convince the stakeholders, and in particular the decision makers, one should know which issues and aspects of the problem and its potential solutions they hold important. Stage 2 requires adequate logical understanding and sufficient technical expertise to create a model in whatever technical context, while Stage 3 requires considerable experience with literature searching and data synthesis. Before calculations are performed and any conclusions may be drawn from them, all aspects of the model should be checked and double checked, ideally by two or more experts in the field. Most experienced decision analysts have had personal experience with the impact that mistakes in structure and formulas may have on model outcomes. In general, errors are weeded out before publication by rigid testing of the model through sensitivity analyses and other testing procedures and by having others check and double check the model. However, discussions about the correctness of model assumptions and details, in relation to the intricacies of the clinical problem, may be heated, and may continue even after publication.

Suitability for Real-Life Problems

The choice to perform an applied DA should not be taken lightly. One should have a clear idea of what a DA may add to the usual clinical (more implicit and less quantitative) way of dealing with a problem, used by experienced clinicians, and whether DA is suitable for the problem at hand. Not all clinical problems are ideally suitable for this approach, and the overall balance of advantages and disadvantages may strongly differ for

different clinical problems. In general, DA can be used more advantageously for clinical problems

- that concern risk or uncertainty,
- that are structurally complex,
- about which sufficient quantitative data are available,
- in which solutions differ for different patients or patient categories,
- in which different and conflicting interests have to be considered and weighed, and
- of which the frequency of occurrence or the magnitude of the problem justifies the effort of performing a DA.

Impact on Clinical Performance

The impact of applied DA, in particular to what extent papers on applied DA are actually changing medical practice, is not easy to assess. Likewise, it has long been unclear which factors contribute to success or failure in real-life clinical practice. In medication prescription, A. Holbrook found that factors such as system speed, convenience of use, quality, relevance to the task at hand, and integration with workflow are important determinants of success. Recent reviews on the effectiveness of clinical decision support systems in improving clinical performance have increased our insight in these matters. However, many of these decision support systems that are assessed in these systematic reviews differ from "classical decision analyses" with their decision trees and tables of variables. Four factors have been found to independently predict success: (1) automatic provision of decision support as part of clinician workflow, (2) provision of recommendations rather than just assessments, (3) provision of decision support at the time and location of decision making, and (4) computer-based decision support. These findings confirm what decision analysts have experienced over many years—that the results of formal decision tree calculations should be transformed into clinically more acceptable formats. In addition, automatic prompting to use the system is a success factor as it reduces the burden and threshold of use. Not surprisingly, most studies where the authors were the creators of the system are more positive about a system's ability to improve clinical performance.

Other Issues

Real-life clinical problems are not solved by the completion of a DA alone. In practice, actions have to be taken by the decision maker. In this process, several other issues may come into play, which have been described by decision psychologist Frank Yates. For any decision, he identifies 10 cardinal checks. They range (apart from the first question on whether there is the need to decide at all) from the "who and how" of the clinical decision, to more practical issues such as acceptability and implementation. All these checks emphasize the fact that there is a real-life world out there, beyond the model, and that for decisions to be successful, one should look beyond the model to real-life situations and to both their potential and their limitations.

Health Technology Assessment

Health technology assessment and cost-effectiveness analysis are next-generation family members of DA. By the fact that they take not only medical outcomes into account, but likewise costs and equity issues, they are becoming more and more relevant to healthcare systems that suffer from the strain that expanding medical technologies and increasing public demands put on the limited available healthcare resources in many countries. One of the most striking examples of the use of such methods at the macrolevel is the use of health technology assessment to steer policy making in the U.K. National Health Service by National Institute for Clinical Excellence (NICE). Whether new medications or other interventions are allowed and are paid for by the National Health Service is based on a rigid analysis of both the available evidence on their effectiveness and of the cost burden they would put on the National Health Service (and thereby on the British taxpayer). NICE's approach has set quite an example of methodological rigor and is a success story of practical potential of applied DA and health technology assessment methods. It is therefore all the more striking that NICE is quite regularly depicted as bureaucratically denying patients the access to "wonderful new drugs" on the basis of cost containment only. This contrast is an illustration of the fact that however right one may be from an intellectual point of view, the value of being able to explain clearly and simply through the right channels to all stakeholders (and maybe of using the right communication/PR methods while doing so) cannot be overestimated, and it confirms the relevance of Yates's warnings.

Success and Effectiveness

Applied DA and its descendants such as health technology assessment and clinical decision support systems have come a long way since their start in the early 1980s. Research as well as experience suggests that the success of applying DA methodologies to real-life problems depends on many factors, not least of all an intense exchange of ideas between analysts and potential users right from the start and the continuing realization that there is a reality beyond the model and its calculations and that feasibility, acceptability, and other implementation issues will codetermine the effectiveness of applied DA.

J. Kievit

See also Cost-Effectiveness Analysis; Evidence-Based Medicine

Further Readings

Beck, J. R., Plante, D. A., & Pauker, S. G. (1981). A 65-year-old Chinese woman with lymphadenopathy and progressive pulmonary infiltrates. One million Chinese women can't all have tuberculosis. *Medical Decision Making, 1,* 391–414.

Claxton, K., Ginnelly, L., Sculpher, M., Philips, Z., & Palmer, S. (2004). A pilot study on the use of decision theory and value of information analysis as part of the NHS Health Technology Assessment programme. *Health Technology Assessment, 8,* 1–103, iii.

Computerization of medical practice for the enhancement of therapeutic effectiveness. COMPETE Publications. Retrieved January 16, 2009, from http://www.compete-study.com/publications.htm

Elstein, A. S. (2004). On the origins and development of evidence-based medicine and medical decision making. *Inflammation Research, 53*(Suppl. 2), S184–S189.

Garg, A. X., Adhikari, N. K., McDonald, H., Rosas-Arellano, M. P., Devereaux, P. J., Beyene, J., et al. (2005). Effects of computerized clinical decision support systems on practitioner performance and patient outcomes: A systematic review. *Journal of the American Medical Association, 293,* 1223–1238.

Hanney, S., Buxton, M., Green, C., Coulson, D., & Raftery, J. (2007). An assessment of the impact of the NHS Health Technology Assessment Programme. *Health Technology Assessment, 11,* iii–xi, 1.

Kawamoto, K., Houlihan, C. A., Balas, E. A., & Lobach, D. F. (2005). Improving clinical practice using clinical decision support systems: A systematic review of trials to identify features critical to success. *British Medical Journal, 330,* 765.

National Institute for Clinical Excellence (NICE). http://www.nice.org.uk

Yates, J. F. (2003). *Decision management.* San Francisco: Jossey-Bass.

Artificial Neural Networks

Research on artificial neural network modeling started in the early 1940s when the first scientific paper by Warren McCulloch and Walter Pitts was published. The motivation came from the fields of artificial intelligence and neuroscience when initial investigators attempted to model the workings of neurons in the human brain. One of the hypothesized reasons for the brain's superiority compared with common computers lies in the fact that neurons function in parallel. There are approximately 10^{12} neurons in the human brain, all interconnected and receiving input from many other neurons, as well as stimulating many others in a conglomeration of complex interconnections. Thus, neural networks are able to perform highly complex computing tasks in an efficient and powerful manner. In addition, they are able to integrate newly acquired data, or experiences, into existing ones, thus allowing for efficient learning and inference. Figure 1 illustrates a basic representation of the neuron and how it gets activated to fire (stimulate) other connected neurons.

As shown in Figure 1, the neuron collects and processes input from structures referred to as dendrites. It then sends out electrical activity through a long strand called an axon. This axon splits into multiple branches, and at the end of a branch, a synapse converts the electrical activity from the axon and sends stimuli to the neighboring neuron. This activity is either excitatory or inhibitory. Prior information affects signal transfer functions and influences how neurons respond to any future stimuli; synaptic processing mimics learning in this sense. Information transmission and processing across multiple neurons influence the development of artificial neural network models.

The simplest representation of a single-layer artificial neural network is shown in Figure 2. Similar to neuronal processing, information is passed between nodes (neurons) interconnected by links (synapses) with modifiable weights. In the case of a single-layer neural network, input into the node is often represented as a vector of features $X = (x_1, x_2, \ldots, x_n)$. (A single-layer network is also referred to as a two-layer network corresponding to the number of layers of input and output units. Often, it is referred to as a single-layer because there is only one layer of modifiable weights.) Each of these feature values, x_i, is multiplied by a corresponding weight, w_i. Thus, the effective input at the output unit would be the sum of all the products $\sum w_i x_i$. Adding a constant bias term ($x_0 = 1$) with a corresponding weight w_0 produces the formula for a single-unit perceptron.

$$f(x, w) = w0 + \sum_{i=1}^{n} xiwi. \qquad (1)$$

This could then be represented as

$$f(x, w) = \sum_{i=0}^{n} xiwi. \qquad (2)$$

A clinical scenario where an artificial neural network would be useful would be in predicting mortality after a procedure (e.g., angioplasty) in patients with chronic renal failure. The input might comprise several clinical features, such as age, gender, hypertension, diabetes, heart failure, and coronary artery involvement. The output would be mortality after 6 months, which is binary in this example although not necessarily so for artificial neural networks. The artificial neural network is useful for achieving increased accuracy of prediction when the features might have nonlinear interactions.

The input into the node is then processed to generate an optimal output. This is determined by a function $y = g(f(x, w))$. Typically, $f(x, w)$ is linear as in Equation 1. The function g, on the other

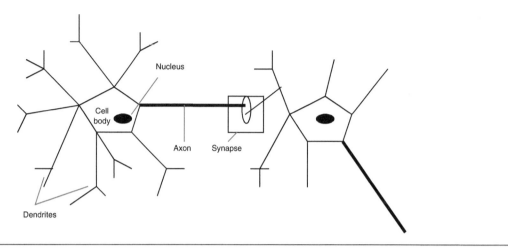

Figure 1   Structure of a typical neuron and a synaptic junction

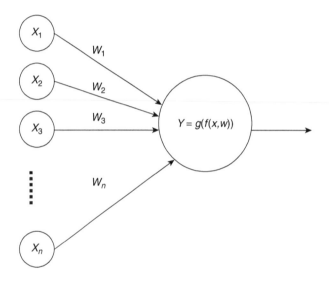

Figure 2   Single-layer artificial neural network

hand, is commonly referred to as the activation function. It is chosen from a selection of functions, including the following:

$$g(x) = x, \text{ a linear function.} \tag{3}$$

$$g(x) = x_+, \text{ producing a nonnegative value.} \tag{4}$$

$$g(x) = \tanh(x), \text{ producing}$$
$$\text{output between } -1 \text{ and } 1. \tag{5}$$

$$g(x) = \sin(x), \text{ where the}$$
$$\text{output is } 1 \text{ if } x \geq 0 \text{ and } -1 \text{ if } x < 0. \tag{6}$$

$$g(x) = [\sin(x) + 1]/2, \text{ where}$$
$$\text{the output is } 0 \text{ or } 1. \tag{7}$$

$$g(x) = [1 + e^{-x}]^{-1}, \text{ with a sigmoidal}$$
$$\text{output between } 0 \text{ and } 1. \tag{8}$$

The specifications for an artificial neural network are determined by two mechanisms, the architecture of the network and optimization of the network parameters generally based on performance in a given data set.

Architecture

Single Layer

A typical single-layer network is shown in Figure 2. As shown in this simplified example, artificial neural networks consist of layers with input nodes and corresponding modifiable weights. In a single-layer network, all nodes connect to the output node(s) where the activation function generates an output.

The learning process or network optimization involves recursive modification of weights as more training data get processed. The recursive algorithm is described as follows.

Taking the angioplasty example in the previous section, the network learns by adding examples from the training data set. Suppose a new observation datum is to be added into the model (x_m, z_m), where x_m corresponds to the feature vector for one patient (e.g., 60 years of age, male gender, nonhypertensive, diabetic, with heart failure and left main coronary artery involvement), and z_m corresponds to the actual output (e.g., death after 6 months). The weights for each of the current nodes would be modified as follows:

1. Calculate the error derived from the predicted output for each output unit, compared with the desired (actual) output, z_m. This could be represented as the mean squared error:

$$E(w) = \frac{1}{2} \sum_{r=1}^{N} (z_r - p_r)^2. \qquad (9)$$

Following matrix transposition of Equation 2, the predicted output for the training data, p_r, is obtained.

$$p_r = \sum_{i=0}^{n} x_i w_i = x_r^T w_r. \qquad (10)$$

2. Given the weights for the nodes in the single layer, $w_i = w_1, w_2, \ldots, w_n$, the weights change according to the following rule: $w_i = w_i + \Delta w_i$, where

$$\delta w_i = \eta E(w) x_i. \qquad (11)$$

η (greater than 0) is the learning rate. To minimize the error, E, using the gradient descent method for optimization, the steps include

$$\delta w_i = -\eta \frac{\partial E(w)}{\partial w_i}. \qquad (12)$$

To substitute E, where p_{mr} is the predicted output for the training data,

$$D = \{(x_r, z_r), r = 1, \ldots, N\}$$

$$E = \frac{1}{2} \sum_{r=1}^{N} (z_m r - p_m r)^2. \qquad (13)$$

Further substituting p_{mr} with Equation 10,

$$E = \frac{1}{2} \sum_{r=1}^{N} (z_m r - x_m r^T w_m r)^2. \qquad (14)$$

For some learning rate η (greater than 0), a recursive version of the steepest descent is obtained. Further substituting Equation 14 into Equation 12 results in $\Delta w_i = \eta(z_{mr} - x_{mr}^T w_{mr}) x_{mi}$, which is similar to Equation 11.

The single-unit perceptron convergence theorem states that if two classes in a training set can be separated by a hyperplane in $\mathbf{R}$, then the delta rule (Equation 11) converges to result in a single hyperplane in a finite number of steps. This has been further developed by investigators who worked on cases where the classes are not linearly separable and where there are greater than two classes. In 1969, M. Minsky and S. Papert released a research publication that basically stated that single-layer perceptrons were not able to solve simple problems, most notably the exclusive-OR (XOR) problem. This was addressed subsequently using multiple-layer perceptrons.

Multiple Layers

Neural networks typically have more than a single layer. The most common form has two layers, the second corresponding to a hidden layer. The architecture is arbitrarily designed, with the main components including the number of layers and the number of units in each layer. Figure 3 illustrates a two-layer neural network.

Feedforward Operation

A neural network that has more than a single layer typically proceeds forward to process input from one layer to the next. The only limitation is that each layer only sends signals to the next layer after it. In Figure 3, there is an input layer that processes the external stimuli. There is a second layer, also referred to as a hidden layer. The third column of nodes corresponds to the two output nodes. Weights are specified and modified for each

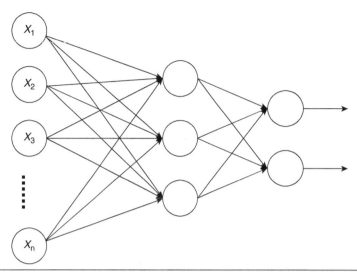

Figure 3   Two-layer artificial neural network with two output nodes

interconnection between nodes. In addition, the hidden layer(s) and output node(s) have activation functions and biases assigned, as described for single-layer artificial neural network. In the multiple-layer artificial neural network, each hidden node computes the weighted sum of all its input from the preceding layers. An activation function, in turn, computes the signal that it then sends to the next group of node(s), which would be another hidden layer or the output node(s). A single hidden layer is able to solve the XOR problem. In fact, A. N. Kolmogorov proved that any continuous function from input to output can be implemented in a two-layer network. However, practical considerations limit the applicability of this theorem. The activation functions would have to be very complex, and there is no principled way that has been suggested to find nonlinear functions based on training data. In addition, some functions are not smooth, which is important for gradient descent learning.

Backpropagation

Backpropagation is one of the most commonly used and simplest methods for training multilayer networks. The simplest way to describe the training method is to follow what happens when a new training datum is added into the network. Suppose the entire training data are represented as follows: $D = \{(x_r, z_r), r = 1, \ldots, N\}$, where x is the feature vector and z is the actual expected output. When a

new datum is added, (x_m, z_m), training of the network ensues. Similar to the method described in the single-layer network, the backpropagation proceeds in the following manner:

1. The output of the network is computed using the feedforward operation for each of the output nodes.

2. The training error between the predicted and actual output is calculated. Typically, it is based on the sum over the output units of the squared difference between the predicted and actual output (Equation 9), which will be referred to as *net*.

3. The weights are initialized with random values and are modified in a direction that will reduce the error, similar to that of Equation 12. The weight update or learning rule is calculated based on the first derivative of *f(net)*, the unit's nonlinear activation function.

4. As was previously done for the hidden-to-output weights, the input-to-hidden weights also get updated.

5. The steps are repeated until the error reaches a specified low threshold.

The description for the two-layer network can readily be generalized into more layers. The activation functions in each node can also vary apart from the bias units and the learning rates.

Special Considerations

Some techniques have been identified to optimize backpropagation and to guide the users in building neural networks. These techniques are briefly described below.

Activation Function

As noted previously, backpropagation should work with any activation function, given that there is continuity of the function and its derivative. However, in selecting an activation function, some guidelines include selecting functions that are nonlinear, that saturate (functions with a minimum and maximum output value), and that have continuity and smoothness. A sigmoid is one such activation function.

Criterion Function

The use of the squared error is described in Equation 10. There are, however, other alternatives that may be used, including cross-entropy error for comparing the separation between probability distributions and Minkowski error for distributions that have long tails.

Number of Hidden Layers

Any number of hidden layers is possible as long as the activation function in each unit is differentiable. However, since the two-layer network can implement any arbitrary function, the addition of an extra layer adds complexity and makes the network more prone to getting caught in local minima. A special condition for using an extra layer includes data transformations, such as rotation or lateral shifts in data.

Number of Hidden Units

The number of hidden units primarily influences the expressivity of the network and how complex the decision boundaries are. Thus, well-separated data will require fewer hidden units. The number of hidden units dictates the number of weights in the network (in addition to the dimensionality of the input vector). Thus, it should not be more than the total number of the training data, n. A rule of thumb is to use $n/10$ hidden units. This can then be adjusted up or down during training.

Initializing Weights

Weights have to be nonzero. The recommended range for the hidden-to-output weights is $-1\sqrt{h}$ to $+1\sqrt{h}$, where h is the number of hidden nodes connected to the output. Similarly, the range for the input-to-hidden weights is $-1\sqrt{d}$ to $+1\sqrt{d}$, where d is the number of input variables connected to the hidden unit.

Learning Rate

The learning rate influences the quality of the network in most instances where training does not reach the training error minimum. In practice, the learning rate is set at .1. It is lowered if the criterion function diverges during learning and is increased if learning is very slow.

Stop Training

Excessive training can lead to poor generalization, also called *overfitting* or *overtraining*. In practice, the goal is to stop training when the error in a separate validation set reaches a minimum.

Applications

Artificial neural network has been used in multiple domains and applications, including image processing, speech recognition, and prediction of financial indices. The use of artificial neural networks in medical decision making ranges from recognition of chromosomal abnormalities, detection of ventricular fibrillation, protein structure prediction, pharmacovigilance applications, and identifying clinical outcomes. Multiple publications review various networks that have been trained and validated in various clinical domains. In addition, many more studies publish the predictive performance of artificial neural network in comparison with other predictive modeling techniques. Artificial neural network has shown comparable performance to several predictive modeling techniques, including logistic regression, decision tree, and support vector machine.

In all, the use of artificial neural network should be tempered with the known constraints of the method. These include the ability to correctly specify the architecture and parameters of the network and, more important, the ability to measure the contribution of each of the components of the input vector in determining the output of the network. In many clinical domains, the "black box" is not ideally suited for understanding what factors influence specific clinical outcomes. This, in turn, is a deterrent to deciding what interventions to modify clinical factors might need to be recommended for clinical care. On the other hand, artificial neural network has been successfully used for clinical domains when nonlinear interactions need to be modeled in a complex manner. This was illustrated in the successful use of artificial neural network for computerized image analysis of Papanicolaou smears, used for rescreening for cervical abnormalities not previously identified by manual screening. In such clinical settings, more accurately predicting an outcome is of paramount importance in clinical decision making.

Ronilda Lacson and Lucila Ohno-Machado

See also Ordinary Least Squares Regression; Prediction Rules and Modeling

Further Readings

Cheng, B., & Titterington, D. (1994). Neural networks: A review from a statistical perspective. *Statistical Science, 9*(1), 2–54.

Duda, R., Hart, P., & Stork, D. (2001). *Pattern classification* (2nd ed.). New York: Wiley.

Kurkova, V. (1992). Kolmogorov's theorem and multilayer neural networks. *Neural Computation, 5*(3), 501–506.

Lacson, R. C., & Ohno-Machado, L. (2000). Major complications after angioplasty in patients with chronic renal failure: A comparison of predictive models. *Proceedings of the AMIA Symposium,* 457–461.

McCulloch, W. P. W. (1943). A logical calculus of ideas imminent in nervous activity. *Bulletin of Mathematical Biophysics, 5,* 115–133.

Minsky, M., & Papert, S. (1969). *Perceptrons.* Cambridge: MIT Press.

Penny, W., & Frost, D. (1996). Neural networks in clinical medicine. *Medical Decision Making, 16*(4), 386–398.

Ripley, B. D. (1996). *Pattern recognition and neural networks.* Cambridge, UK: Cambridge University Press.

Rosenblatt, F. (1962). *Principles of neurodynamics: Perceptrons and the theory of brain mechanisms.* Washington, DC: Spartan Books.

Ruján, P. (1993). A fast method for calculating the perceptron with maximal stability. *Journal de Physique, 3,* 277–290.

Rumelhart, D., Hinton, G., & Williams, R. (1986). Learning internal representation by back-propagating errors. *Nature, 323,* 533–536.

Williams, R. W., & Herrup, K. (1988). The control of neuron number. *Annual Review of Neuroscience, 11,* 423–453.

ASSOCIATIVE THINKING

Associative thinking is used to describe memory-based judgment processes that require the decision maker to infer a diagnosis or other category on the basis of the presence or absence of related features through the activation of associations—memories in which features and categories co-occur. Broadly speaking, the mind automatically associates in memory those experiences or concepts that co-occur. The decision maker later retrieves these associations (again, automatically, and typically unconsciously) in the performance of judgment and decision tasks. For example, when a pediatrician repeatedly sees children who present with persistent sore throat and fever and observes that they are often positive for strep throat, she or he may come to associate the symptoms and the diagnosis, and on the next presentation of a child with sore throat and fever, strep throat is likely to be high on her differential diagnosis. In essence, judgments are evoked by considering the similarity or representativeness of new stimuli to associations previously learned. More frequent and salient co-occurrences result in more memorable associations.

The study of association in thinking has a long history, dating back at least as far as the work of English empiricists in the 17th century. In modern dual-process theories of cognition, associative thinking is often considered to be characteristic of System 1 (intuitive) thinking. It is contrasted with the more effortful and rule-oriented System 2 (deliberative) thinking.

Determinants

According to dual-process theories, associative thinking is automatically performed, but associations may be suppressed or modified by later deliberation. Associative judgments are more likely to be expressed when deliberation is limited or infeasible. For example, time pressure or cognitive load may increase the likelihood of relying on associative thinking. In other cases, lack of appropriate information or information format may prevent deliberation. For example, Windschitl and Wells showed that eliciting judgments using verbal measures of uncertainty (e.g., "unlikely") evoked associative thinking more frequently than when numerical measures were used.

Associations vary in their strength. Hogarth notes that associations can be reinforced positively or negatively and offers three factors that lead to reinforcement. First, human beings may be genetically predisposed to create particular associations very quickly through operations similar to classical conditioning. Experiences of pain and fear, for example, often rapidly produce or reinforce strong associations with co-occurring events. Second, people can be motivated to increase the strength of an association. Motivation can take the form of either internal motivation to better understand the environment or external motivation (e.g., operant conditioning) from rewards or punishments provided by the environment. For example, associations that lead to decisions that result in approbation are likely to be reinforced. Third, associations are strengthened as the frequency of the association being observed increases. For example, a physician examining a patient within his or her specialty is likely to have developed strong associations between symptoms and diagnoses as a result of the frequency with which the physician examines such patients; a physician examining a patient with a novel diagnosis outside his or her specialty may have fewer and weaker relevant associations.

Advantages and Disadvantages

Because associative thinking allows for rapid categorization and judgment, it can be ecologically adaptive. This is particularly the case when the decision maker has considerable opportunity to develop valid associations and must make decisions in limited time or without other resources necessary to support a more deliberative process. For example, medical decision making in emergent conditions is often greatly facilitated by the ability of the physician to make correct associations rapidly.

On the other hand, when associative knowledge is developed that does not accurately match the actual state of the world, associative thinking can lead to systematic biases in judgment. In addition to such common heuristics for likelihood judgments as availability, representativeness, and value-induced bias, it is also possible to simply make incorrect associations. For example, medical students exposed to dermatological diagnoses and later tested on diagnostic skill have been shown to establish (irrelevant, and therefore incorrect) associations between diagnoses and the body part on which they first learned the diagnosis.

Improving Associative Thinking

Although faulty associative thinking can sometimes be overridden by analytic thinking, associative thinking itself can be improved by developing more veridical and useful associations. This requires either selecting or creating learning environments that provide sufficient exposure to an appropriate set of co-occurring events, information on whether correct associations have been learned (feedback), and suitable rewards for correct associations and adverse consequences for erroneous associations. Hogarth broadly divides learning environments into those that are kind and those that are wicked. Kind environments provide relevant feedback and have exacting consequences for errors; the former allows the learner to adjust associations through observation of their outcomes, and the latter ensures that the learner is well motivated to seek ongoing improvement in, and refinement of, the associations learned. Wicked environments, in contrast, provide either no feedback or distorted feedback, limiting the learner's ability to correct errors, and are lenient in their tolerance of error, reducing motivation to correct errors.

In medical education, learning environments can often be manipulated to provide better control over exposure to co-occurring events. For example, presentation of multiple teaching and practice cases for the differential diagnosis of heart failure in descending order of typicality has been shown to facilitate the development of better associations and improved diagnostic performance in medical students. Similarly, Ericsson has argued that the development and maintenance of expert-level performance in medicine relies on deliberate practice designed to ensure that the expert continues to seek, acquire, and assess appropriate associations on an ongoing basis.

Alan Schwartz

See also Biases in Human Prediction; Dual-Process Theory; Heuristics

Further Readings

Allen, S. W., Brooks, L. R., Norman, G. R., & Rosenthal, D. (1988). Effect of prior examples on rule-based diagnostic performance. *Proceedings of the Annual Conference on Research in Medical Education, 27,* 9–14.

Ericsson, K. A. (2004). Deliberate practice and the acquisition and maintenance of expert performance in medicine and related domains. *Academic Medicine Research in Medical Education Proceedings of the forty-third annual conference November 7–10, 79*(10), S70–S81.

Hastie, R., & Dawes, R. M. (2001). *Rational choice in an uncertain world: The psychology of judgment and decision making.* Thousand Oaks, CA: Sage.

Hogarth, R. M. (2001). *Educating intuition.* Chicago: University of Chicago Press.

Kahneman, D. (2003). Maps of bounded rationality: A perspective on intuitive judgment and choice. In T. Frangsmyr (Ed.), *Les Prix Nobel. The Nobel Prizes 2002.* Stockholm: Almqvist & Wiksell.

Papa, F. J., Stone, R. C., & Aldrich, D. G. (1996). Further evidence of the relationship between case typicality and diagnostic performance: Implications for medical education. *Academic Medicine, 71*(Suppl. 1), S10–S12.

Papa, F. J., Oglesby, M. W., Aldrich, D. G., Schaller, F., & Cipher, D. J. (2007). Improving diagnostic capabilities of medical students via application of cognitive sciences-derived learning principles. *Medical Education, 41,* 419–425.

Stanovich, K. E., & West, R. F. (2000). Individual differences in reasoning: Implications for the rationality debate? *Behavioral and Brain Sciences, 23,* 645–726.

Windschitl, P. D., & Wells, G. L. (1996). Measuring psychological uncertainty: Verbal versus numeric methods. *Journal of Experimental Psychology: Applied, 2*(4), 343–364.

ATTENTION LIMITS

Broadly defined, attention is the focus of cognitive resources on processing information. Research on attention addresses the following questions: (a) What initiates the focus of cognitive resources on objects of psychological concern? (b) What causes the focus of cognitive resources to shift from one object to another? (c) How many objects, or how much information, can be kept in cognitive focus at one moment in time?

The psychological study of attention has investigated the three questions of initiation, change, and capacity of cognitive focus at many levels of information processing. At the lowest level are studies of how cognitive resources are focused when processing sensory information in the visual, auditory, olfactory, gustatory, and tactile domains. At the highest level are studies of cognitive focus on the rich, meaningful content of human thought that underlies making complex, real-world decisions such as those involved in medical diagnosis and treatment.

Attention has relevance to medical decision making at many levels of information processing. At the lowest level of information processing, attention supports a physician's detection of the physical characteristics of a patient that lead to a medical diagnosis of the patient's condition. This might include visual information about the patient's coloration; auditory information from their heartbeat, breathing, and gastrointestinal processes; and tactile and olfactory information that are unique to the patient's condition.

The important factors that initiate attention and limit the capacity of a medical decision maker's attention to sensory input are different from those for simple sensory events in abstract laboratory studies. Whereas the physical characteristics of a stimulus (such as its intensity and duration) have been shown to influence attention in simple laboratory tasks, a medical decision maker's expertise (as defined by his or her background, beliefs, and understanding) creates a mental model (or a schema) that plays a central role in determining what information, and how much information, the decision maker attends to and how that information is interpreted.

A medical decision maker's expertise also plays a central role in determining what information he or she pays attention to when using executive, cognitive processes, in the absence of sensory input, to reason through a patient's medical conditions either to arrive at a diagnosis or to select a treatment program. The interplay between a decision maker's mental model of a medical problem and the effect of that mental model on directing the decision maker's attention is very important. The importance of the interplay is shaped by (a) a limit on how much information a decision maker can hold in mind at one moment (also known as span of apprehension) and (b) the need of the decision maker to incorporate the most relevant and important information within the span of his or her limited attention if he or she has to make a wise decision.

The practical importance of attention limits on medical decision making is great. Since 1956, psychologists have recognized that the capacity of human attention, or the span of human apprehension, is limited to between five and nine items. Thus, a decision maker presented with a complex medical problem is unlikely to be able to incorporate all the available information about that problem into his or her cognitive focus. Because of these limits, it is exceedingly important that the decision maker has sufficient expertise to prepare him or her to attend to the most important information. Otherwise, the quality of a medical decision is likely to be compromised by being based on a small set of less relevant information. The long medical education, internship, and residency that most doctors go through help develop and hone their mental models for making good medical decisions.

The practical importance of attention limits is especially great for patients involved in their own treatment decision making. Patients must acquire a reasonable understanding of the mental model that medical experts hold of their condition. In the absence of this mental model, patients are unlikely to discover what the most important issues are for understanding, diagnosing, and treating their own condition. Thus, patients interested in playing an active role in their medical treatment need to acquire a mental model that incorporates the set of variables medical experts agree are the most important for making a wise decision for their cases. Otherwise, patients are unlikely to appreciate the medical recommendations made to them

and may perhaps insist on following a course of treatment that is unwise.

David A. Walsh

See also Cognitive Psychology and Processes

Further Readings

Deutsch, J. A., & Deutsch, D. (1963). Attention: Some theoretical considerations. *Psychological Review, 70,* 80–90.

Hershey, D. A., & Walsh, D. A. (2000). Knowledge versus experience in financial problem solving performance. *Current Psychology, 19,* 261–291.

Kahneman, D. (1973). *Attention and effort.* Englewood Cliffs, NJ: Prentice Hall.

Miller, G. A. (1956). The magical number seven, plus or minus two: Some limits on our capacity for processing information. *Psychological Review, 63,* 81–97.

Treisman, A., & Gelade, G. (1980). A feature-integration theory of attention. *Cognitive Psychology, 12,* 97–136.

Wright, R. D., & Ward, L. M. (2008). *Orienting of attention.* Oxford, UK: Oxford University Press.

ATTRACTION EFFECT

The attraction effect (also known as the decoy effect or the asymmetric dominance effect) refers to a phenomenon in which adding an inferior alternative into an existing choice set increases the probability of choosing an alternative from the original set. The term *attraction effect* comes from the fact that an inferior alternative attracts attention or the choice share to one of the alternatives in the choice set. Because the attraction effect is caused by the addition of an inferior alternative, which is called a *decoy*, to a core choice set, it is also called the *decoy effect* (the decoy effect is a broader term than the attraction effect). Finally, the *asymmetric dominance effect* refers to a specific case of the attraction effect in which the decoy is asymmetrically dominated by one of the alternatives in the set.

The attraction effect has important theoretical implications because it violates some fundamental assumptions of many rational choice models. One such assumption is the *principle of regularity*, by which the probability of choosing one alternative from an initial choice set cannot be increased by adding a new alternative. The attraction effect also violates an assumption that choices are independent of irrelevant alternatives.

Experimental Paradigm

For the attraction effect to occur, several conditions must be met. In a typical experimental setting (decision environment) in which the attraction effect is demonstrated, alternatives are defined on a few (usually two) attributes (or dimensions) in a decision space (see Figure 1 for a two-attribute decision space). In this decision space, two alternatives (A and B) form a core choice set. These alternatives are selected so that they are nondominating or competitive to each other. In Figure 1, A is weaker on Dimension 1 (e.g., the quality dimension) and stronger on Dimension 2 (e.g., the price dimension), while the reverse is the case for B. Then an alternative that is inferior to only one alternative in the core set, which is called a decoy, is added to the set. The alternative that is directly superior to the decoy is called the *target* (B) and the other alternative that does not have a dominance relation with the decoy is called the *competitor* (A). The attraction effect is demonstrated when the proportion of people choosing the target significantly increases when the decoy is present compared with when the decoy is absent. The decoy is rarely chosen in most cases. The attraction effect has been demonstrated using both the between- and within-subjects designs.

Decoy Types

There are six types of decoys studied in the literature. These decoys can be broadly divided into two categories depending on whether there is an asymmetric dominance relation between the target and the decoy: asymmetrically dominated decoys and nonasymmetrically dominated decoys. There are three decoy types in each category. The asymmetrically dominated decoys have been studied more extensively in the literature because they produce a greater attraction effect.

Asymmetrically Dominated Decoys

The asymmetrically dominated decoys include the range (R), frequency (F), and range-frequency (RF) decoys (see Figure 1). The range (R) decoy extends the range of the target on the dimension on which the target is weaker than the competitor. The frequency (F) decoy increases the frequency of alternatives along the dimension on which the target is stronger than the competitor. The range-frequency (RF) decoy combines the effect of the range decoy with the effect of the frequency decoy. All these three types of decoys are directly dominated by the target but not by the competitor.

Nonasymmetrically Dominated Decoys

The nonasymmetrically dominated decoys include the compromise (C), inferior (I), and range with symmetric dominance (RS) decoys (see Figure 1). The range with symmetric dominance (RS) decoy increases the range downward on the dimension on which the target is weaker than the competitor but is symmetrically dominated by both the target and the competitor. The inferior (I) decoy is similar to the range decoy in that it increases the range on the dimension on which the target is weaker than the competitor. But its value on the dimension on which the target is stronger than the competitor is also raised so that there is no longer direct dominance relation between the target and the decoy. Although the inferior decoy is not directly dominated by the target, it is clearly inferior to the target.

The compromise (C) decoy is produced by raising the value of the inferior decoy further along the dimension on which the target is stronger than the competitor. The compromise decoy appears more attractive than the inferior decoy and helps increase the probability of choosing the target by making the target appear to be a good compromise between the two extreme alternatives (i.e., the decoy and the competitor). The effect produced by the compromise decoy is called the *compromise effect*. Although this effect is similar to the attraction effect in that the decoy increases the choice probability of the target (so categorized as the decoy effect), it is distinguished from the attraction effect because there is no dominance relation between the target and the decoy.

Phantom Decoy

A phantom alternative refers to a choice option that appears real but is unavailable at the time of

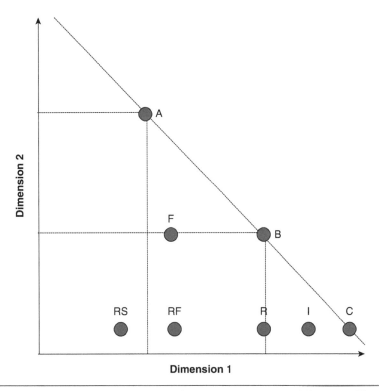

Figure I   Graphical representation of the attraction effect with competitor (A), target (B), and six decoy types: (1) range, R; (2) frequency, F; (3) range-frequency, RF; (4) compromise, C; (5) inferior, I; and (6) range with symmetric dominance, RS

decision making. Examples include consumer goods that are out of stock, show tickets that are sold out, a job candidate who accepted another job, and so on. The decoys described above (i.e., asymmetrically dominated and nonasymmetrically dominated decoys) are available decoys; they have a potential to increase the choice share of the target by being present along with the target and the competitor. However, it has been demonstrated that the phantom decoy, which is not available when making a choice, also has a similar influence as the physically available decoys. Although some phantom decoys can also increase the choice probability for dominated alternatives, the phantom decoy effect appears to be procedurally similar to the attraction effect.

Decision Domains and Populations

The attraction effect has been demonstrated in various domains with diverse groups of people.

The effect has been mostly studied in the consumer choice domain using product categories such as apartment, battery, beer, bicycle, boat, calculator, car, CD player, computer, film, gas barbecue grill, house, light bulb, lottery, microwave oven, mouthwash, orange juice, parking space, plane ticket, printer, restaurant, running shoes, video camera, sunscreen, toothpaste, TV sets, and wine. The effect has also been shown in the in-store and online purchases. In addition to numerous demonstrations of the effect in the consumer domain, it has also been shown in many other domains, such as the choices of partners, job candidates, political candidates in elections, investment options, and medicines. Furthermore, the effect has been shown with a wide range of people, including young adults ranging in age from the late teens to 30s and older adults in their 60s and 70s, undergraduate, graduate, and professional school students, grocery store customers, and internal medicine residents.

Factors Affecting the Attraction Effect

The size of the attraction effect is influenced by several factors, including perceived information relevance or meaningfulness of alternatives (mainly attribute values), product class knowledge, task involvement, perceived similarity between the decoy and the target, relative brand preference, choice share captured by the decoy, and perceived decoy popularity. More specifically, the attraction effect decreases with an increase in the perceived information relevance, product class knowledge (especially when attribute values are presented numerically), task involvement, and preference strength. Meanwhile, the effect increases with an increase in the perceived decoy-target similarity, choice share captured by the decoy, and perceived popularity of the decoy. Also, assuming that the two attributes on which alternatives are defined are quality and price, the attraction effect is stronger when the target is stronger on the quality dimension than the competitor compared with when the target is stronger on the price dimension than the competitor. Finally, the attraction effect (along with the compromise effect) is also influenced by motivational factors, such as prevention and promotion motivations. Specifically, prevention-focused people are more likely to show the compromise effect and less likely to show the attraction effect than promotion-focused people.

Theories and Explanations

Several theories and explanations have been proposed. They assume that the attraction effect occurs because people with limited knowledge do not have strong preformed preferences for attributes (because they do not know which attributes are important to them), and as a result, they are likely to focus on different attributes in different situations as the local decision context changes (as occurs when a decoy is present vs. not along with the core choice set).

Loss Aversion: Decoy as a Reference Point

Based on Tversky and Kahneman's reference-dependent theory of riskless choice that losses (or disadvantages) have greater impact on decision making than gains (or advantages), one explanation for the attraction effect is that a decoy may play a role of a reference point against which other alternatives are compared in terms of expected loss. According to the reference-dependent theory, an alternative with a moderate improvement on one attribute and no loss on the other is more attractive than another with a large improvement on one attribute and a small loss on the other. For example, if the range decoy is viewed as a reference point for both the target and the competitor, the target represents a small improvement on Dimension 2 and no loss on Dimension 1, whereas the competitor represents a large improvement on Dimension 2 and a small loss on Dimension 1 (see Figure 1 for the range decoy), and as a result, the target appears more attractive than the competitor in the presence of the decoy.

Weight Change: Context-Dependent Weighting

The weight-change model argues that adding a decoy changes the relative weights assigned to different attributes. That is, according to the weight-change model, the attraction effect occurs because the decoy causes decision makers to increase the relative weight they assign to the strong attribute of the target or decrease the relative weight they assign to the weak attribute of the target. For example, the relative weight given to a dimension decreases when the range of the value is extended because the attribute value differences become relatively smaller (see Figure 1 for the range decoy) or increases when the number of different attribute values on that dimension increases because the attribute value differences become relatively larger (see Figure 1 for the frequency decoy).

Value Shift: Perceptual Biases

The value-shift model argues that the subjective values assigned to each attribute value are shifted by the presence of the decoy, while weights on attributes remain constant. According to the value-shift model, a change in subjective evaluation of each attribute value leads to an increase in the overall value of the target relative to the competitor. This explanation is based on an idea that the decoy in the attraction effect operates in the same way as Parducci's range-frequency theory. For example, the addition of a decoy that has an extremely low value on the dimension on which the target is weaker than the competitor should reduce the difference between the target and the competitor in their subjective values on the dimension (see Figure 1 for the range decoy). In another example, the addition of a decoy that has an intermediate value on the dimension on which the target is stronger than the competitor should increase the difference between the target and the competitor in their subjective values on the dimension (see Figure 1 for the frequency decoy). As a result, in the above examples, these decoys increase the relative attractiveness of the target by making it appear less weak than the competitor on the previously weak dimension and stronger than the competitor on the previously strong dimension.

Value Addition: Dominance Heuristic

The value-added model argues that relations among alternatives, such as presence of dominance, add value to the target and, as a result, cause the attraction effect. More specifically, the addition of a decoy to the core choice set creates a dominance relation between the target and the decoy, and this dominance relation adds justifiability value to the target because choosing the target becomes easier to justify with the presence of dominance.

Sunghan Kim

See also Accountability; Choice Theories; Context Effects; Loss Aversion; Prospect Theory

Further Readings

Heath, T. B., & Chatterjee, S. (1995). Asymmetric decoy effects on lower-quality versus higher-quality brands: Meta-analytic and experimental evidence. *Journal of Consumer Research, 22,* 268–284.

Highhouse, S. (1996). Context-dependent selection: The effects of decoy and phantom job candidates. *Organizational Behavior and Human Decision Processes, 65,* 68–76.

Huber, J., Payne, J. W., & Puto, C. (1982). Adding asymmetrically dominated alternatives: Violations of regularity and the similarity hypothesis. *Journal of Consumer Research, 9,* 90–98.

Huber, J., & Puto, C. (1983). Market boundaries and product choice: Illustrating attraction and substitution effects. *Journal of Consumer Research, 10,* 31–44.

Mishra, S., Umesh, U. N., & Stem, D. E., Jr. (1993). Antecedents of the attraction effect: An information-processing approach. *Journal of Marketing Research, 30,* 331–349.

Parducci, A. (1974). Contextual effects: A range-frequency analysis. In E. C. Carterette & M. P. Friedman (Eds.), *Handbook of perception* (Vol. 2). New York: Academic Press.

Tversky, A., & Kahneman, D. (1991). Loss aversion in riskless choice: A reference-dependent model. *Quarterly Journal of Economics, 106,* 1039–1061.

Wedell, D. H., & Pettibone, J. C. (1996). Using judgments to understand decoy effects in choice. *Organizational Behavior and Human Decision Processes, 67,* 326–344.

ATTRIBUTABLE RISK

The concept of attributable risk (AR) is usually used in public health sciences to quantify the population impact of an exposure on overall disease burden. Such a population impact often has two determining factors: (1) strength of an association between the exposure and the disease and (2) the prevalence of exposure in the population of interest.

When exposure is simply binary, that is, exposed versus unexposed, a prototype measure of AR is defined by the so-called AR fraction:

$$AR = 1 - \Pr\{D\backslash\bar{E}\}/\Pr\{D\},$$

where $\Pr\{D\}$ is the probability of having a disease for anyone in the population, and $\Pr\{D\bar{E}\}$ is the probability of having a disease only for those unexposed in the population. From a disease prevention perspective, $\Pr\{D\}$ can also be considered as a measure of overall disease burden on the population, while $\Pr\{D\backslash\bar{E}\}$ is considered as the measure of disease burden on the same population but with all exposure eliminated ideally.

For example, information was obtained in Tasmania during 1988 to 1990 from the parents of 2,607 1-month-old infants regarding their baby's usual sleeping positions. Table 1 tabulates the cumulative incidence of crib death (a sudden infant death syndrome) through 1 year of age in these infants by their usual positions: sleep prone (on their

Table 1 Crib death by sleeping position among infants

		Crib Death		
		Yes (D)	No (D̄)	Total
Sleep Position	Prone (E)	9	837	846
	Other (Ē)	6	1,755	1,761
	Total	15	2,592	2,607

Source: Dwyer, Posonby, Newman, and Gibbons (1991).

stomach) and other position (side or back). In this example, the overall death rate is calculated as $\Pr\{D\backslash\bar{E}\} = 15/2,607 = 5.75/1,000$, while the death rate of other sleeping positions is calculated as $\Pr\{D\backslash\bar{E}\} = 6/1,761 = 3.41/1,000$. Therefore, the AR is calculated as $AR = (1 - 3,41/5.75) \times 100\% = 40.7\%$.

An alternative form of the AR defined above is obtained by an application of Bayes's theorem:

$$AR = \Pr\{E\}(RR - 1)/[1 + \Pr\{E\}(RR - 1),$$

where RR is the relative risk measured by the ratio of $\Pr\{D\backslash E\}/\Pr\{D\backslash\bar{E}\}$. From this form, it is clear that AR is determined by $\Pr\{E\}$ and RR jointly. The AR increases as either the prevalence of exposed or the strength of association becomes greater, while it decreases otherwise. A greater RR alone, however, may not necessarily lead to a greater AR, which in fact shall additionally depend on the prevalence of exposure in the population. As a result, AR usually does not have the similar "portability" to the RR in etiologic inferences of a disease association among different populations. AR may vary from population to population. Nevertheless, its ability to jointly assess the association and the prevalence of exposure may serve itself a good measure in policy making to prioritize prevention strategies.

Conceptual Use and Interpretation

In practice, AR is usually used to assess the potential impact of prevention programs aimed to modify the exposure distribution in a target population. It can be used as a guide to evaluate and compare different preventive strategies.

For a specific prevention program, AR can be considered as a measure of impact of modifying multiple risk factors at the same time, although it is seemingly calculated only for one risk factor. It may be interpreted in two ways: one interpretation is that AR measures the potential impact due to modifying the distribution of the exposure and its correlated risk factors in the population, and the other interpretation is that AR for all known risk factors measures what knowledge has been gained about the disease etiology. Specifically in the latter interpretation, AR measures the remaining portion of overall disease burden that is not explained by the known risk $1 - AR$ factors. For example, most of the researchers consider that an AR less than 50% for known exposure and risk factors means that there is a strong need for further research in a disease area.

However, AR itself does not entail a comparable meaning to any conventional terms for risk. A variety of alternative terms have been used for AR, such as *population attributable fraction, etiologic fraction,* and *attributable fraction.* Many of these terms can be misleading to infer causality. AR itself merely reflects the overall impact of an association and the prevalence of exposure in a population. To avoid such confusion in causal inferences of an association, researchers have used AR to quantify the proportion of disease that can be related or linked, rather than attributed, to an exposure.

Properties

When an exposure is hazardous, that is, with an RR greater than 1, AR as a percentage lies between 0 and 1. When either RR is 1 or no one is exposed,

AR is 0. When an exposure is protective, that is, with RR less than 1, AR is less meaningful with a range of $(-\infty, 0)$. In practice, researchers can recode the exposure by having RR to be always greater than 1 to avoid negative AR.

As a joint measure of prevalence of exposure and RR, AR increases as the prevalence of exposure increases. This means that the value of AR depends on how reference exposure is determined. When an exposure is measured on a continuous scale, more stringent choice of threshold for hazardous exposure usually leads to higher AR. For example, some authors found that the AR was estimated at 38% of esophageal cancer attributed to an alcohol consumption of more than 80 g/day with reference level of 0 to 79 g/day. When the reference level changed to 0 to 39 g/day, the value of AR jumped to 70%. Therefore, when applying AR in prevention of a continuous exposure, it is critical to clearly specify the reference exposure for any meaningful estimation and comparison.

When a reference exposure is determined and the rest of exposure is categorized into several mutually exclusive categories, the sum of ARs for these categories equals the AR for these categories combined. This is called the distributive property of AR. For example, some authors found that the AR estimates are 13%, 6%, and 64% for malignant mesothelioma attributed to moderately low, medium, and high likelihoods of exposure, respectively, and summed up to a total of 83% of nontrivial (moderately low, medium, and high combined) likelihood of exposure. Given this property, some researchers argue that there is no need to break the exposure into finer categories, if the overall AR is of main concern, even when risk appears to increase with higher exposure levels.

Estimation

The estimation of AR usually depends on the study design that dictates how data are collected. In three major types of study design that are often used in public health research, that is, cross-sectional, cohort, and case-control, AR is almost always estimable with proper assumptions.

In cross-sectional studies, all the quantities that define AR are estimable, and the estimation of AR is usually straightforward.

In cohort studies, $\Pr\{D\backslash E\}$, $\Pr\{D\backslash\bar{E}\}$, and $\Pr\{E\}$ are usually estimable from the observed data. When the sampled cohort is a random sample of the population of interest, the estimated $\Pr\{E\}$ is likely comparable with that in the population, and hence the estimated AR is meaningful to the population. When the cohort is sampled with a predetermined proportion of exposure, the value of AR may be less meaningful for the cohort studies.

For case-control studies, researchers often use an alternative form to estimate AR:

$$Ar = \Pr\{E \mid D\}(1 - 1/RR).$$

In this alternative form, $\Pr\{E/D\}$ can be estimated among the cases, that is, individuals with disease, and RR can be estimated by an approximation of the odds ratio (OR), assuming a rare disease.

When only one exposure is of sole concern without taking into account other factors, consider a prototype 2×2 table for observed data in Table 2, regardless of the underlying study design. Then a crude AR can simply be estimated by

$$AR = (bc - ad)/(nb).$$

Variance of this AR estimator can be estimated by the Delta method for various distributions that are assumed in individual study designs. As a result, $100(1 - \alpha)\%$ -level confidence intervals can be constructed with properly transformed AR, for example, $\log(1 - AR)$, or $\log\{AR/(1 - AR)\}$. Researchers have discussed extensively in statistical literature the merits of these transformations in confidence interval construction.

Crude AR tends to be biased when it ignores potential confounding factors for the association between exposure and disease. Adjusted AR has been advocated by researchers and methodologists to account for potential confounding factors. Similar to the usual adjustment techniques for RR estimation, adjusted AR can be calculated by a variety of nonparametric and model-based approaches.

One approach is by stratification. It is similar to the Mantel-Haensel approach in estimating OR from several strata. A crucial assumption is that a common RR or OR exists for all the strata. Based on the study designs, either $\Pr\{E\}$ or $\Pr\{D\backslash E\}$ can be

Table 2 A prototype 2 × 2 table in epidemiologic studies

	Disease (D)	No Disease ($\bar{D}$)	
Exposed (E)	a	b	E
Not Exposed ($\bar{E}$)	c	d	$n - e$
	f	$n - f$	N

calculated for each stratum. Then applying an estimate of RR or OR would lead to consistent adjusted AR estimates. Variance of the estimators obtained by this approach tends to be complex but can be computed by the Delta method or the maximum likelihood methods for their large sample asymptotic properties. Empirical simulation has shown that their bias and coverage probability tend to be satisfactory in large samples as well.

A second approach is by calculating the weighted sum of ARs over strata, for example, as in

$$AR = \sum_{s=1}^{S} w_s AR_s,$$

where $s = 1,2,\ldots, S$, are stratum indicators, and w_s are the assigned weights for stratum-specific AR_s. This weighted approach usually does not require common RR or OR and yields a variety of types of adjusted AR by choosing different sets of weights. For example, an adjusted AR can be called "caseload" adjusted if w_s is the proportion of cases in stratum s, and "precision-weighted" if w_s is inversely proportional to the variance of stratum-specific AR estimators. Variance of the weighted adjusted AR can be similarly computed by the Delta method in large sample.

Model-based adjusted approaches have been extensively studied as well in statistical literature. For example, one such is in the form of

$$AR = 1 - \sum_{s=1}^{S} \sum_{e=1}^{E} d_{se}/RR_{e|s},$$

where $e = 1,2,\ldots, E$ are the levels of exposure, d_{se} are the cases, and $RR_{e|s}$ are the adjusted RR. Note that this form is not exactly a maximum likelihood estimator. Alternative model-based estimators have also been proposed for case-control designs

under unconditional logistic regression model and for cohort designs under unconditional logistic regression model and the Poisson model. In practice, these approaches would yield similar results in both small and large samples.

Extensions

The prototype AR is mostly used when both disease and exposure are dichotomous. Extensions of the prototype AR have been studied in various scenarios.

When exposure is not limited to be dichotomous, that is, exposed versus unexposed, those who are exposed can be further categorized into multiple levels of exposure. Then the prototype AR can be extended to the so-called partial or level-specific AR that represents the level-specific AR, which may have practical implication for screening high-risk groups. In literature, extended AR has been developed for continuous exposure.

When there are several types of exposure, researchers have estimated exposure-specific AR and the overall AR for all the exposure types jointly. Usually the sum of exposure-specific AR does not equal the overall AR. When different types of exposures are mutually independent and their effect on disease is multiplicative, then the product of exposure-specific complement AR, that is, 1 − AR, equals the complement overall AR.

When disease outcome is time-to-event outcome, T, say, extensions of time-varying AR have been proposed, such as $AR(t) = 1 - F(t \mid \bar{E}) / F(t)$ at time t, where $F(t \mid \bar{E}) = \Pr\{T \le t \mid \bar{E}\}$ is the cumulative distribution function of unexposed, and $F(t)$ is the cumulative distribution function of overall. When T is subject to censoring, statistical methods have been developed for a similar quantity

$AR(t) - 1 - \lambda(t \mid \bar{E})/ \lambda(t)$, where $\lambda(t)$ is the hazard function of unexposed and $\lambda(t)$ is the hazard function of overall, under the widely used Cox proportional hazards model assuming that the relative hazards of $\lambda(t \mid E)/ \lambda(t \mid \bar{E})$ is constant. Additional prognostic factors can be included in this model to calculate adjusted $AR(t)$.

AR has also been extended to accommodate ordinal data and recurrent disease events. Other AR-related quantities include the so-called AR in exposed, that is, $AR_e = 1 - \Pr\{D \mid \bar{E} / \Pr\{D \mid E\}$, which essentially plays the same role as RR, and the so-called preventable fraction, that is, $PF = 1 - \Pr\{D\} / \Pr\{D \mid \bar{E}\}$, for a protective exposure or intervention, which measures the impact of an association between disease and the protective exposure at the population level.

More generally from a disease prevention perspective, a very important concept that generalizes AR is the so-called generalized impact fraction (IF), which is defined as $IF = 1 - \Pr\{D\} / \Pr\{D \backslash \wp\}$, where $\Pr\{D \backslash \wp\}$ is the target disease burden due to modifying the exposure distribution in the population. The generalized IF can be used to assess various interventions targeting all subjects, or subjects at specified levels, while aiming at modifying the exposure distribution but not necessarily eliminate exposure. This IF can also be extended to censored time-to-event outcomes.

Ying Qing Chen

See also Bayes's Theorem; Cox Proportional Hazards Regression; Logistic Regression; Maximum Likelihood Estimation Methods; Screening Programs

Further Readings

Basu, S., & Landis, J. R. (1993). Model-based estimation of population attributable risk under cross-sectional sampling. *American Journal of Epidemiology, 142,* 1338–1343.

Benichou, J. (2001). A review of adjusted estimates of attributable risk. *Statistical Methods in Medical Research, 10,* 195–216.

Chen, Y. Q., Hu, C., & Wang, Y. (2006). Attributable risk function in the proportional hazards model for censored time-to-event. *Biostatistics, 7,* 515–529.

Drescher, K., & Schill, W. (1991). Attributable risk estimation from case-control data via logistic regression. *Biometrics, 47,* 1247–1256.

Dwyer, T., Posonby, A. L., Newman, N. M., & Gibbons, L. E. (1991). Prospective cohort study of prone sleeping position and sudden infant death syndrome. *Lancet, 337,* 1244–1247.

Greenland, S., & Robins, J. M. (1988). Conceptual problems in the definition and interpretation of attributable fractions. *American Journal of Epidemiology, 128,* 1185–1197.

Levin, M. L. (1953). The occurrence of lung cancer in man. *ACTA Unio Internationalis Contra Cancrum, 9,* 531–541.

Miettinen, O. S. (1974). Proportion of disease caused or prevented by a given exposure, trait or intervention. *American Journal of Epidemiology, 99,* 325–332.

Walter, S. D. (1976). The estimation and interpretation of attributable risk in health research. *Biometrics, 32,* 829–849.

Whittemore, A. S. (1982). Statistical methods for estimating attributable risk from retrospective data. *Statistics in Medicine, 1,* 229–243.

AUTOMATIC THINKING

It is commonly said that components of medical diagnosis and decision making, as well as of procedural skills, are executed automatically. This is not always good news. Patients may not appreciate a physician diagnosing their illness without awareness. Physicians, likewise, may not like to view themselves as unconscious automatons. Nonetheless, performing some task components automatically has advantages of speed and efficiency. Indeed, expert performance may depend on this automaticity: Allocating some necessary tasks to unconscious subroutines frees up attention for the more difficult customization of plans accommodating for the particulars of the situation. Automatic thinking may have some disadvantages, however. As it is difficult to reflect on automated thought processes, physicians cannot explain what they are thinking or teach students how to think that way. They may not notice if an automatic process is not going well and hence lose the opportunity to correct an error or improve execution. Insofar as it requires conscious reflection to change the way one executes a skill, the automated aspects of a physician's cognition may not improve with experience. Finally, it is difficult for others, and even for the physicians themselves, to assess if their automated perception or decision making is biased by self-interest or is influenced by medical advertising or by their relations with manufacturer representatives.

Four varieties of automatic, unconscious thinking that have been described by cognitive psychologists can provide insight for understanding automated processes that occur in medical decision making. These characterizations conceive of automatic thinking (1) as a part of everyday skilled cognition, (2) as a problematic component of expertise, (3) as a characteristic of some motivational components of reasoning, and (4) as a feature of evolutionarily primitive cognition.

A common framework for all these views is the generic cognitive psychology model of knowledge and skill. For medicine, this holds that knowledge structures pertinent to diagnosis and treatment of patients, available in long-term memory, are activated into the physician's working memory when their pattern matches the pattern of the current situation, already attended in working memory. When the degree of fit seems adequate, that is, when the physician is confident that he or she understands the patient's illness, then the physician does the action available in the knowledge structure. When the knowledge does not seem to adequately fit the case, the physician does further work—gathering more case information, seeking more knowledge from other physicians or the literature, or problem solving by consciously reworking the available case information and knowledge. New knowledge structures built in this way are available for later use—whether or not they prove accurate for the present case. A knowledge structure that is useful because it helps explain a patient's disease or guide successful treatment may be more likely to be activated and relied on next time there is a similar patient. With experience, a larger set of specific knowledge structures is built up, so the physician can have a rapid, automatic yet appropriate response to a larger proportion of patients.

Automatic Thinking in the Execution of Everyday Skill

The first of cognitive psychology's explanations of automatic thinking in physicians is the account of ordinary learned knowledge or skill. Just as an experienced driver may arrive at a familiar destination

and realize that he or she can't remember making any particular turns today, a physician may realize at the end of a routine day that he or she does not remember examining any of the patients. A surgeon may not remember the details of each layer of stitching. Yet every decision was made adequately and each step of the operation executed competently. Factors that would seem to prevent a physician's work life from being completely automatic in this way include the necessity to explain treatments to patients and helpers, to dictate or type for the medical record, or to explain to students. Yet with enough practice, such acts of communication too can be handled automatically.

Physicians are said to use heuristic strategies to make medical judgments or decisions, although they may not be aware that they do so unless it is called to their attention. This is a distinct concept from automatic thinking. The task of the physician is difficult because of its unavoidable uncertainty. Even when the physician is fully attending to a decision—not thinking "automatically" at all— there remains the problem of how to determine what is best to do. We can articulate very high standards for rational decision making that require extensive computation. Shortcut strategies are unavoidable, and one hopes that physicians use shortcuts that are usually accurate. A physician might consciously apply a heuristic strategy, or that strategy might be well learned and incorporated into a script or knowledge structure that comes to mind as a unit and thus is applied automatically. Thus, the concept of a heuristic strategy is different from automated thinking, even though it might be empirically demonstrable that physicians' behavior is consistent with the use of heuristic strategies more often when they are responding automatically to routine patients than when deliberating about an unusual case.

Automatic Thinking in Expertise

The second account of automatic thinking, while recognizing it may be essential for efficient performance, views it as a barrier to the improvement of performance that is necessary in the attainment of expertise. To put it in perspective, while it may take 50 hours of coached training and self-reflective practice to learn to drive competently enough that one can tune out that familiar route, to attain a high level of driving skill (as required by a racer or a stunt driver) may require thousands of hours of supervised practice. If we assume that a skill that is executed automatically cannot be changed, then a physician diagnosing or managing a patient without attention cannot improve his or her skill. On the other hand, reaching high levels of skill may require that most of the constituent components of the skill have been overlearned so that they may be executed automatically, freeing up the physician's attention to focus on one particular element that needs to be adjusted and improved. Thus, automatic thinking is both a barrier to and a necessary precondition of the attainment of expertise.

Automatic Thinking in the Motivational Components of Reasoning

The third characterization of automatic thinking focuses on the human motivations and perceptions that imbue the setting in which the physician works. Factors in the external social context, mediated by internal motivations, may influence the thinking process without the physician's intending they do so and without the physician's awareness; these can be characterized as automatic processes. Unlike the automated rationality characteristic of everyday skill or expert cognition, where it is assumed that the physician previously performed these mental operations consciously and intentionally, this motivated automatic thinking may express all-too-human, irrational motives that the physician would not necessarily endorse if they were drawn to his or her attention.

The effect of irrelevant aspects of names is an example of nonrational automatic thinking. If a name carries a value-laden connotation, physicians may unwittingly react with respect to those values. Consider two physicians, Dr. Goode and Dr. Crapp. We might guess that other physicians may be more likely to refer patients to Dr. Goode. At a deeper level, Dr. Goode himself may have been subtly influenced his entire life to live up to his name, acquiring a fundamentally more sound mastery of medicine and a more conventionally upright value system than his colleague, unless the colleague became a gastroenterologist.

A more serious effect of the automatic response to names may be seen in the effect of the labels assigned to ventilation-perfusion scans used when pulmonary embolism is suspected. A patient with a "low probability" scan has a higher probability than normal of having a pulmonary embolism, but the automatic connotations of the "low probability" label—relief, relaxation, having nothing to worry about—may cause a physician to reduce vigilance below what would be appropriate.

Merely being reminded of money can change the way people think and act. Physicians in the United States are daily reminded of its importance, in their regular business meetings, phone calls they must make to protest insurance company denials and justify procedures that patients need, or conversations in which staff threaten to work elsewhere for higher pay. Studies have shown that when people are reminded of money, they tend to help other people less, to hold themselves more separate from others, and to work harder to solve intellectual problems. These automatic changes in their way of thinking can affect physicians' ways of gathering information and using it to make decisions for their patients, in ways that may either promote or impede their Hippocratic values.

The feelings and norms of friendship, social exchange, and mutual obligation can influence physicians' thinking without their awareness. Pharmaceutical detailers cordially and generously provide physicians food and small gifts in exchange for the privilege of delivering brief messages about the advantages of the medications they sell. Physicians, who feel uncomfortable being paid simply for listening, engage the sales representatives in friendly conversations to express their gratitude, and of course the friendliness is reciprocated. As an automatic effect of these friendly exchanges, shown in multiple studies, the physicians increase their use of the products after such visits. This increase occurs even when the physicians declare that they feel no obligation and that they listen to the marketing message with objective skepticism.

Automatic thinking underlies the observation that a physician who does not like a patient cannot be a good doctor for that patient due to the automatic effects of that dislike on each of the parties. The patient perceives some form of disinterest and, without intending, talks less, thus providing less information about the illness. The physician, responding both to sensed patient attitude and to own level of interest, is less likely to dig for more information or to spontaneously ruminate about the patient's case. These automatic social responses work together to reduce the quality of the cognition the physician applies to a disliked patient.

A similar confluence of automatic responses may underlie the effects of prejudice and stereotyped expectations in the structured apprenticeships of physicians' clinical education. A generation or less ago, for example, some older male surgeons had low expectations of female residents' performance, as well as conflicting social role expectations. This led to offering them less help and coaching and impeded the establishment of warm collegial relations. In this environment, the female residents' automatic thinking led them to make fewer requests for supervision. The result of these enmeshed automatic responses was less educational progress and lower evaluations for the residents. Similar tales have been told regarding African American medical students, residents who graduated from foreign medical schools, and even family medicine residents on specialty rotations.

An important class of automatic influence of the sociomotivational context on thinking is the influence of fear and anxiety. This is manifest in the widespread habit of excessive testing to protect against the remotest possibilities, picked up as a standard operating procedure, often without the physicians recognizing that this part of their script serves more to allay physician anxiety than to protect the patient.

A more vivid manifestation may be seen in physicians' thinking under the real threat of death, in the traditional approach to end-of-life care. When stunned patients and family members deal with the high probability of death, physicians naturally strive to do all they can do, to muster all their power in line with the traditional injunction to preserve life at all costs, despite its futility. Recently, new institutions have been developed to redirect the automatically activated motivations to exercise control in the face of anxiety and to adhere to authority's precepts in the face of the possibility of death. The alternative approach is embodied in the standards of palliative care, which provides a new set of skills to exercise to give the physician something useful to do when the patient is dying. It incorporates a new authoritative framework, including the laws authorizing Do Not Resuscitate orders and living wills, the legitimacy of the Advance Directive, and the proxy decision maker.

It is a good example of the design of institutions to cope with the automatic thinking elicited by the most challenging situations physicians face, demonstrating that this form of automatic thinking need not be opposed to rationality.

Automatic Thinking as a Feature of Evolutionarily Primitive Cognition

The fourth account of physicians' automatic thinking attributes the availability of particular types of knowledge structures or reasoning strategies to instincts inherited from our mammalian or reptilian ancestors. Consider, for example, that for eons we have had the capability to hold an object in each hand and sense which is heavier. From this, we speculate, arises our habit of making comparisons between just two treatment options at a time, rather than three or more. This unexamined tendency, traceable to how our minds are embodied, might lead physicians to pay insufficient attention to third or fourth options, the error of premature closure.

The generic cognitive model tells us that physicians may have several cognitive processes going on in parallel, some of them attended and others proceeding automatically. Among the automatic background processes may be evolutionarily primitive processes that scan the environment for danger or for items of appetitive interest. The physician may experience this when an ongoing diagnostic process is interrupted by an involuntary perception of the patient. A holistic assessment of the patient, such as "this patient looks sick," may trump the usual 20 Questions diagnosis game and lead directly to action. This kind of interruption has been characterized as a competition between two systems of thinking, although likely there are more than just two systems. It has been suggested, furthermore, that ideas from the simpler, more primitive system are more likely to control thinking when the physician is tired, distracted, under time pressure, or venturing into unfamiliar territory.

For physicians to make decisions at the optimal standard of rationality could require cognitively intense calculation using all available information, but instead physicians use shortcut strategies that refer to subsets of the information. Such strategies may be traced, it has been suggested, to our evolution in environments with multiple, partially redundant cues, which has endowed us with a special capability to learn particular types of decision strategy appropriate for such environments. (This is analogous to the claim that humans have an inborn capability to learn the grammar of language.) Thus, while experts might identify 50 signs or symptoms associated with the various causes of chest pain, those symptoms tend to be correlated with each other. One physician could attend to one subset of symptoms, another physician to a different subset, and each could diagnose chest pain accurately. Simple strategies, such as to choose a diagnosis by counting the arguments (features) for each, may be sufficient to support rapid yet accurate decisions that have important consequences.

There is disagreement about whether it is necessary to invoke evolutionary selection to account for the availability of such simple yet effective strategies. In computer simulations, such strategies produce adequate accuracy while using fewer resources and taking less time. With these advantages, even if evolution had not provided the strategies, we would have had to invent them. If physicians adopt such strategies because they are easy and effective, then we may not need to invoke an inbuilt grammar of decision making to explain their use. Nonetheless, the analysis of the fit between the physicians' simplified decision strategies and the structure of the disease environment provides a useful perspective on automatic cognition.

Implications

Physicians' automatic thinking is important because it potentially affects decisions whose outcomes matter, allowing gains in efficiency and providing helpful insights, or perhaps causing the physician to ignore some of the information available about a patient. With the four competing accounts of automatic thinking, there are many opportunities for researchers to describe, explain, and assess its role in physicians' decision making, and to resolve the unknowns concerning the source, role, and malleability of the automatic parts of cognition. Such research will be challenging, however; because automatic cognition is difficult to self-report, experts are reluctant to submit selves to intensive observation, and observing such behavior is likely to change it.

Robert M. Hamm

See also Associative Thinking; Cognitive Psychology and Processes; Context Effects; Decision Making and Affect; Dual-Process Theory; Heuristics; Intuition Versus Analysis; Irrational Persistence in Belief; Pattern Recognition

Further Readings

Abernathy, C. M., & Hamm, R. M. (1995). *Surgical intuition*. Philadelphia: Hanley & Belfus.

Bargh, J. A., & Ferguson, M. J. (2000). Beyond behaviorism: On the automaticity of higher mental processes. *Psychological Bulletin, 126*(6), 925–945.

Betsch, T., & Haberstroh, S. (Eds.). (2005). *The routines of decision making*. Mahwah, NJ: Lawrence Erlbaum.

Bilalić, M., McLeod, P., & Gobet, F. (2008). Inflexibility of experts: Reality or myth? Quantifying the Einstellung effect in chess masters. *Cognitive Psychology, 56,* 73–102.

Bursztajn, H., Feinbloom, R. I., Hamm, R. M., & Brodsky, A. (1981). *Medical choices, medical chances*. New York: Delacorte.

Cain, D. M., & Detsky, A. S. (2008). Everyone's a little bit biased (even physicians). *Journal of the American Medical Association, 299*(24), 2893–2895.

Ericsson, K. A. (2004). Deliberate practice and the acquisition and maintenance of expert performance in medicine and related domains. *Academic Medicine, 79*(Suppl. 10), S70–S81.

Gigerenzer, G. (1996). The psychology of good judgment: Frequency formats and simple algorithms. *Medical Decision Making, 16*(3), 273–280.

Stanovich, K. E., & West, R. F. (2000). Individual differences in reasoning: Implications for the rationality debate? *Behavioral and Brain Sciences, 23*(5), 645–726.

Vohs, K. D., Mead, N. L., & Goode, M. R. (2008). Merely activating the concept of money changes personal and interpersonal behavior. *Current Directions in Psychological Science, 17*(3), 208–212.

Wood, W., & Neal, D. T. (2007). A new look at habits and the habit-goal interface. *Psychological Review, 114*(4), 843–863.

AXIOMS

Axioms in the days of Euclid (Euclidian Geometry) were self-evident truths within logic and mathematics. Axioms today (as considered within a system or theory) are sets of rules that are internally consistent. For example, axioms in expected value decision making are a set of internally consistent rules for rational choice. Axioms are often described in terms of how plausible they are, in what sense(s) they may or may not be compelling, and how the axioms are stated. In the latter case, the phrase *elegantly simple* can be directed at the expression of a set of axioms that are viewed positively regarding their statement.

Axioms and Theories

One can start with a set of axioms and then move toward the development of a theory, or one can state a theory and look for or attempt to develop the set of axioms needed to support that theory. In the latter approach, an axiomatic method is proposed that contains a set of postulates (first principles). Within such a set of postulates, the postulates that are stated are "all and only" the necessary definitions and assumptions from which the theory can be derived.

The verb *to axiomatize* suggests that one can take a theory and attempt to derive first principles for or in support of that scientific or social scientific theory. For example, one can have a theory, such as a form of expected utility theory, and take that theory's claims and attempt to axiomatize that form of expected utility theory. Another claim is that an axiomatic method can be used to express all significant theories of any scientific or social scientific discipline and one can further argue that any scientific or social scientific discipline should be capable of such axiomatic expression.

The Axiomatic Versus the Empirical

Some might argue that "the axiomatic" is contrasted with "the empirical," where, for example, the axiomatic refers to logical deduction and the empirical refers to data derived from the real world (by observation alone, observation with measurement, or experimentation) to objectively study and test hypotheses. Here, experimentation includes baseline observation and measurement, introduction of an intervention, and then postintervention reobservation and remeasurement, analysis of data, interpretation of analyzed data, and the drawing of conclusions. Once tested in one

environment or setting, a central objective in the development of an empirical science is coherence in the application of theory obtained from this one source to a different source. This coherence then confirms the extensibility of the application of that theory.

The above proposed distinction between what is axiomatically driven and what is empirically driven seems to suggest that the axiomatic is based on consideration of first principles, while the empirical is based on consideration of observations and measurements at a time and over time with or without experimentation. However, this assumption can be challenged as an oversimplification on two grounds. First, a science or a scientific theory itself can be axiomatized. Second, an axiomatic theory can be tested as a framework for understanding a particular science or social science in its application to the real world. For example, as a social science, a theory of human decision-making behavior can be developed and tested in terms of the truth or falsity of its set of axioms as explaining real-world behavior.

Let us take an example of an attempt to explain human behavior on the basis of first principles. A theoretician can be approached about the behavior of humans in the real world and asked the question: Why do humans when placed in this particular setting behave in the fashion that they do? This was a question posed to Daniel Bernoulli: Why do gamblers behave as they do in the St. Petersburg paradox—a coin-flipping game in which most gamblers do not behave like rational bettors? This is a game that has a theoretical return on investment of an infinite sum of money, but it is counterintuitive to realize that. So a typical person won't appreciate the return on investment and will not be willing to pay much in order to play this game. Bernoulli's explanation was that gamblers behave in the St. Petersburg paradox as if they were maximizing the expectation of some utility function of the possible outcomes in the problem facing them. The classical resolution of the paradox involved the introduction of (a) a utility function, (b) the statement of an expected utility hypothesis, and (c) the presumption of diminishing marginal utility of money. Here, the gambling behavior existed (the St. Petersburg paradox was recognized as a problem needing a solution), and Bernoulli was asked to consider an explanation for the behavior (a solution of the paradox). Bernoulli then developed the set of first principles to explain the behavior (to attempt to solve the paradox). The main contributors to the axiomatic derivation of expected utility theory are John Von Neumann and Oskar Morgenstern, Frank Ramsey, Bruno de Finetti, and Leonard Savage.

Once one has an explanatory hypothesis involving human decision behavior (as in Bernoulli's solution to the St. Petersburg paradox), one can ask whether this hypothesis can be further broken down into a set of axioms that can be tested (one at a time) in the real world as verifiable or falsifiable. It also needs to be recognized that certain axioms, hypotheses, and theories can be true to a specifiable extent under one set of circumstances and false to a specifiable extent under another set of circumstances in terms of the real world.

Axioms of Expected Utility Theory

Axioms and what can be done to these first principles can perhaps be best represented by an "equality" and what can be done to both sides of the equality while still preserving the equality: What can be done to one side of an equal sign in an equality and to the other side of the equal sign of the equality and still maintain the equality? Or in the statement of an equation, it can be asked, "What can be done to both sides of the equation while still preserving the truth value of the equation?"

Two axioms of expected utility theory are (1) comparability (If A and B are in the alternative set S, then either $A > B$ or $B > A$, or both $A = B$); and (2) transitivity (If $A > B$, and $B > C$, then $A > C$).

Testing an Axiom in a System

Real-world settings can be used to test the viability of an axiom of a system or theory to ensure through the testing of the complete set of axioms used to express a system or theory that it is consistent with what is found in the real world. In such a testing setting, one needs to demonstrate that real-world decision makers behave according to the axioms (verification) or do not behave according to the axioms (falsification) of the system or theory. And one can proceed to test each axiom of the set of axioms in the system or theory under consideration.

Testing the Axioms of Expected Utility Theory

In testing the axioms of expected utility theory in the real world, one can start with the axioms and ask in a real-world setting whether humans behave according to the axioms. But how does one go about testing the axioms of expected utility theory in the real world?

Here, one needs to introduce a methodology (technique) for elicitation of preferences, for example, the standard gamble. Once one has the axioms and the methodology, one can test the axioms in terms of verification or falsification.

How would one identify the presence of a falsification of an axiom? If the fundamental value that humans place on any particular health outcome varies according to the position of the outcome in the procedure (i.e., the standard gamble) used to elicit that individual's preferences, then there would be a failure of an axiom in the system and, thus, an internal inconsistency in the system or theory. An internal inconsistency exists when one or more of the main axioms fail to be sustained on real-world testing.

Inconsistencies

What do internal inconsistencies look like in the case of the axioms of expected utility theory? If in a real-world economic setting, there is a divergence between what a human is willing to pay for a good that he or she does not possess and his or her willingness to receive compensation for giving up that same good when he or she does possess it, then there may be an inconsistency in one of the axioms in the system or theory used to explain human decision-making behavior in this economic decision-making setting.

If, in a real-world medical setting, a patient places a greater value on an outcome with a given probability when that outcome is described (framed, presented) in terms of the chance of "survival," then when it is redescribed (reframed, re-presented) in an equivalent way in terms of the chance of "dying," there may be an inconsistency in one of the axioms in the system or theory used to explain human decision-making behavior in this medical decision-making setting. For example, if a patient is willing to accept surgery when the risk of surgery is described as having a 90% chance of surviving the initial surgery and still being alive 6 months after the surgery but not when that same surgery is described as having a 10% chance of dying at the time of the surgery and not being alive 6 months after the surgery, then there may be an inconsistency in one of the axioms used to explain medical decision-making behavior.

Focusing on the question of the internal consistency of the standard gamble, one can ask, "What is to be done about the internal inconsistencies that are found with the use of the standard gamble?" One research goal is to achieve internal consistency within the standard gamble. Another research goal is an intermediate goal to limit the level of internal inconsistency found within the standard gamble. Here, research studies focus on the attempt to incorporate additional elements (e.g., weighting and probability transformation parameters) to the standard gamble valuation procedure in the attempt to limit internal inconsistency.

Future Directions

It is not the case that a theory is captured by one and only one set of axioms. In the attempt to axiomatize any scientific or social scientific theory, there is always a search under way for the most plausible, the most compelling, and the most elegantly simple set of axioms used to capture a theory in any domain. The search for such axioms is ongoing in every logical, mathematical, scientific, and social scientific field today. In the case of the sciences and social sciences, the search continues for the most plausible, most compelling, and the most elegantly simple set of axioms that can be applied to the real world attempting to successfully explain human behavior in decision making. Such a search should have as its ultimate goal not only describing human behavior but also optimizing that decision making to help

people achieve their goals as viewed from their perspectives.

Dennis J. Mazur

See also Expected Utility Theory; Gain/Loss Framing Effects; Risk Aversion

Further Readings

Allais, M. (1979). The foundations of a positive theory of choice involving risk and criticism of the postulates and axioms of the American School. In M. Allais & O. Hagen (Eds.), *Expected utility hypotheses and the Allais paradox*. Dordrecht, the Netherlands: Reidel.

Arrow, K. J. (1971). The theory of risk nearing. In *Essays in the theory of risk bearing*. Chicago: Markham.

Battalio, R. C., Kagel, J., & MacDonald, D. N. (1985). Animals' choices over uncertain outcomes. *American Economic Review, 75,* 597–613.

Camerer, C. (1989). An experimental test of several generalized utility theories. *Journal of Risk and Uncertainty, 2,* 61–104.

Chateauneuf, A., & Wakker, P. (1999). An axiomatization of cumulative prospect theory for decision under risk. *Journal of Risk and Uncertainty, 18,* 137–145.

Chew, S., & Waller, W. (1986). Empirical tests of weighted expected utility theory. *Journal of Mathematical Psychology, 30,* 55–62.

Edwards, W. (1955). The prediction of decisions among bets. *Journal of Experimental Psychology, 50,* 201–214.

Edwards, W. (1962). Subjective probabilities inferred from decisions. *Psychology Review, 69,* 109–135.

Ellsberg, D. (1961). Risk, ambiguity and the savage axioms. *Quarterly Journal of Economics, 75,* 643–669.

Machina, M. (1982). "Expected utility" analysis without the independence axiom. *Econometrica, 50,* 277–323.

Oliver, A. J. (2004). Testing the internal consistency of the standard gamble in "success" and "failure" frames. *Social Science & Medicine, 58,* 2219–2229.

von Neumann, J., & Morgenstern, O. (1944). *Theory of games and economic behavior*. Princeton, NJ: Princeton University Press.

B

Basic Common Statistical Tests: Chi-Square Test, *t* Test, Nonparametric Test

A statistical test provides a mechanism for making quantitative decisions about a process or processes. The intent is to determine whether there is enough evidence to "reject" a conjecture or hypothesis about the process. The conjecture is called the null hypothesis. In medical research, appropriate use of a test, correctly interpreting *p* values, and drawing valid conclusions may help to clarify the confusion between statistical and clinical significance and make judicious decisions. The rest of this entry is organized as follows: Beginning with the chi-square test, the most applicable test for categorical data, this entry introduces *t* test and analysis of variance (ANOVA) for quantitative outcomes, ending with the introduction of nonparametric tests.

Chi-Square Test

Chi-square test is a statistical test commonly used to compare observed data with data a researcher would expect to obtain according to a specific hypothesis. Chi-square tests can be used in tests of goodness of fit, testing if a sample of data came from a population with a specific distribution; or in tests of independence when a researcher wants to see if there is a relationship between categorical variables. In this case, the outcome is categorical—for example, whether people from different regions differ in the frequency with which they report that they support a political candidate.

Pearson Chi-Square

Pearson chi-square is used to assess the above two types of comparison. It is the most common test for significance of the relationship between categorical variables. The chi-square test becomes increasingly significant as the numbers deviate further from this expected pattern. The value of the chi-square and its significance level depend on the overall number of observations and the number of cells in the table. Relatively small deviations of the relative frequencies across cells from the expected pattern will prove significant if the number of observations is large.

The Pearson chi-square inherently tests the underlying probabilities in each cell; and when the expected cell frequencies fall, for example, below 5, those probabilities cannot be estimated with sufficient precision. Therefore, the assumption underlying the use of the Pearson chi-square is that the expected frequencies are not very small.

Maximum Likelihood Chi-Square

Based on maximum likelihood theory, the maximum likelihood chi-square tests the same hypothesis as the Pearson chi-square statistic, and in practice, it is usually very close in magnitude to the Pearson chi-square statistic.

Fisher Exact Test

When conducting a chi-square test in which one or more of the cells have an expected frequency of 5 or less, the Fisher's exact test is used. This test is only available for 2 × 2 tables and is based on the following rationale: Given the margins of the table, and assuming that in the population the two factors in the table are not related (null hypothesis), the probability of obtaining cell frequencies as uneven or worse than the ones that were observed can be computed exactly by counting all possible tables that can be constructed based on the marginal frequencies.

McNemar Chi-Square

This test is primarily used in a before-after design study; that is, it assesses the significance of the difference between two dependent samples. For example, researchers may count the number of students who fail a test of minimal math skills at the beginning of the semester and at the end of the semester. In a 2 × 2 table, the McNemar chi-square tests whether the counts in cells above the diagonal differ from counts below the diagonal. If the two counts differ significantly, this reflects change between the samples, such as change due to an experimental effect between the before and after samples.

t Test

A parametric test is a statistical test that assumes an underlying distribution of observed data. *t* test is one of the most common parametric tests and can be categorized as follows.

One-Sample t Test

One-sample *t* test is used to test whether the population mean of the variable of interest has a specific value (hypothetical mean), against the alternative that it does not have this value, or is greater or less than this value. A *p* value is computed from the *t* ratio (which equals the difference of the sample mean and the hypothetical mean divided by the standard error of mean) and the numbers of degrees of freedom (which equals sample size minus 1). If the *p* value is small, the data give more possibility to conclude that the overall mean differs from the hypothetical value.

Two-Sample t Test

The two-sample *t* test is used to determine if the means of the variable of interest from two populations are equal. A common application of this is to test if the outcome of a new process or treatment is superior to a current process or treatment.

t Test for Independent Samples

An independent samples *t* test is used when a researcher wants to compare the means of a variable of interest (normally distributed) for two independent groups, such as the heights of gender groups. The *t* ratio is the difference of sample means between two groups divided by the standard error of the difference, calculated by pooling the standard error of the means of the two groups.

t Test for Dependent Samples

If two groups of observations of the variable of interest (that are to be compared) are based on the same sample of subjects who were tested twice (e.g., before and after a treatment); or if the subjects are recruited as pairs, matched for variables such as age and ethnic group, and one of them gets one treatment, the other an alternative treatment; or if twins or child–parent pairs are being measured, researchers can look only at the differences between the two measures of the observations in each subject. Subtracting the first score from the second for each subject and then analyzing only those "pure (paired) differences" is precisely what is being done in the *t* test for dependent samples; and, as compared with the *t* test for independent samples, this always produces "better" results (i.e., it is always more sensitive). The *t* ratio for a paired *t* test is the mean of these differences divided by the standard error of the differences.

Assumptions

Theoretically, the *t* test can be used even if the sample sizes are very small (e.g., as small as 10) so long as the variables of interest are normally distributed within each group, and the variation of scores in the two groups is not reliably different.

The normality assumption can be evaluated by looking at the distribution of the data (via histograms) or by performing a normality test. The equality of variances assumption can be verified with the *F* test, or the researcher can use the more robust Levene's test.

Analysis of Variance

Analysis of variance (ANOVA) is a statistical test that makes a single, overall decision as to whether a significant difference is present among three or more sample means of the variable of interest (outcome). An ANOVA is similar to a *t* test; however, it can also test multiple groups to see if they differ on one or more explanatory variables. The ANOVA can be used to test between-groups and within-groups differences. There are two types of ANOVAs: one-way ANOVA and multiple ANOVA.

One-Way ANOVA

A one-way ANOVA is used when there are a normally distributed interval outcome and a categorical explanatory variable (with two or more categories), and the researcher wishes to test for differences in the means of the outcome broken down by the levels of the explanatory variable. For instance, a one-way ANOVA could determine whether class levels (explanatory variable), for example, freshmen, sophomores, juniors, and seniors, differed in their reading ability (outcome).

Multiple ANOVA (Two-Way ANOVA, N-Way ANOVA)

This test is used to determine if there are differences in two or more explanatory variables. For instance, a two-way ANOVA could determine whether the class levels differed in reading ability and whether those differences were reflected by gender. In this case, a researcher could determine (a) whether reading ability differed across class levels, (b) whether reading ability differed across gender, and (c) whether there was an interaction between class level and gender.

Nonparametric Test

Nonparametric methods were developed to be used in cases when the researcher knows nothing about the parameters of the variable of interest in the population. Nonparametric methods do not rely on the estimation of parameters (such as the mean or the standard deviation) describing the distribution of the variable of interest in the population.

Nonparametric methods are most appropriate when the sample sizes are small. In a nutshell, when the samples become very large, then the sample means will follow the normal distribution even if the respective variable is not normally distributed in the population or is not measured very well.

Basically, there is at least one nonparametric equivalent for each parametric general type of test. In general, these tests fall into the following categories.

One-Sample Test

A Wilcoxon rank sum test compares the median of a single column of numbers against a hypothetical median that the researcher enters. If the data really were sampled from a population with the hypothetical mean, one would expect the sum of signed ranks to be near zero.

Differences Between Independent Groups

Nonparametric alternatives for the *t* test for independent samples are the Mann-Whitney *U* test, the Wald-Wolfowitz runs test, and the Kolmogorov-Smirnov two-sample test. The Mann-Whitney *U* test, also called the rank sum test, is a nonparametric test assessing whether two samples of observations come from the same distribution. This is virtually identical to performing an ordinary parametric two-sample *t* test on the data after ranking over the combined samples. The Wald-Wolfowitz runs test is a nonparametric test of the identity of the distribution functions of two continuous populations against general alternative hypotheses. The Kolmogorov-Smirnov two-sample test is one of the most useful and general nonparametric methods for comparing two samples, as it is sensitive to differences in both location and shape of the empirical cumulative distribution functions of the two samples.

An appropriate nonparametric alternative to the one-way independent-samples ANOVA can be found in the Kruskal-Wallis test, which is applicable when the researcher has the outcome with two or more levels and an ordinal explanatory variable. It is a generalized form of the Mann-Whitney test method, since it permits two or more groups.

Differences Between Dependent Groups

For the *t* test for dependent samples, the non-parametric alternatives are the Sign test and Wilcoxon's matched pairs test. The sign test can be used to test that there is "no difference" between the continuous distributions of two random samples. The Wilcoxon test is a nonparametric test that compares two paired groups, through calculating the difference between each set of pairs and analyzing that list of differences. If the variables of interest are dichotomous in nature (i.e., "pass" vs. "no pass"), then McNemar's chi-square test is appropriate. If there are more than two variables that were measured in the same sample, then the researcher would customarily use repeated measures ANOVA. Nonparametric alternatives to this method are Friedman's two-way ANOVA and Cochran Q test. Cochran Q is an extension to the McNemar test and particularly useful for measuring changes in frequencies (proportions) across time, which leads to a chi-square test.

Relationships Between Variables

Spearman *R*, Kendall tau, and coefficient gamma are the nonparametric equivalents of the standard correlation coefficient to evaluate a relationship between two variables. The appropriate nonparametric statistics for testing the relationship between the two categorical variables are the chi-square test, the phi coefficient, and the Fisher exact test. In addition, Kendall coefficient of concordance is a simultaneous test for relationships between multiple cases, which is often applicable for expressing interrater agreement among independent judges who are rating (ranking) the same stimuli.

Li Zhang

See also Analysis of Covariance (ANCOVA); Analysis of Variance (ANOVA); Sample Size and Power

Further Readings

Agresti, A. (2007). *An introduction to categorical data analysis* (2nd ed.). New York: Wiley.

Agresti, A., & Franklin, C. (2007). *The art and science of learning from data*. Upper Saddle River, NJ: Prentice Hall.

Bishop, Y. M. M., Fienberg, S. E., & Holland, P. W. (1975). *Discrete multivariate analysis: Theory and practice*. Cambridge: MIT Press.

Fienberg, S. E. (1977). *The analysis of cross-classified categorical data*. Cambridge: MIT Press.

Kachigan, S. K. (1986). *Statistical analysis: An interdisciplinary introduction to univariate & multivariate methods*. New York: Radius Press.

Kendall, M., & Stuart, A. (1979). *The advanced theory of statistics* (Vol. 2, 4th ed.). London: Griffin.

Mendenhall, W. (1975). *Introduction to probability and statistics* (4th ed.). North Scituate, MA: Duxbury Press.

Runyon, R. P., & Haber, A. (1976). *Fundamentals of behavioral statistics* (3rd ed.). Reading, MA: Addison-Wesley.

Snedecor, G. W., & Cochran, W. G. (1989). *Statistical methods* (8th ed.). Ames: Iowa State University Press.

BAYESIAN ANALYSIS

Bayes's theorem is often used in decision analysis, so it would be natural to think that *Bayesian analysis* is a generic term to describe decision analyses using the Bayes's theorem. On the contrary, Bayesian analysis refers to a school of thought in statistical analysis. It differs both operationally and conceptually from the two other traditional ways of carrying out statistical analysis: frequentist and likelihood based. Statisticians who adhere to the principles of Bayesian analysis sometimes call themselves Bayesians.

The goal of most statistical analysis is to make inferences about population parameters. These parameters are not observable directly but can be estimated using data. For example, incidence of a particular disease in a given country is a parameter. It is practically impossible to find the true incidence, but it is quite possible to estimate it based on an appropriately chosen sample. In traditional statistical analysis only the information in the sample will be used for the purpose of estimation. In Bayesian analysis, information external to the sample, such as prior related findings, expert information, or even subjective beliefs can be incorporated into the analysis. Results of a Bayesian analysis will reflect a weighted combination of the information in the sample and the prior information. These weights are intrinsically chosen by the analyst based on the study design (especially sample size) and the precision of prior information.

Example

A simple example might help clarify the concepts and the process. Suppose we want to estimate the mean age of patients seen at a pediatric emergency care facility. Based on our knowledge about the patient profile of this particular institution, we expect the mean to be around 7. We think it could be as low as 5 or as high as 9. We can represent our prior information about the mean age in the form of a normal distribution with mean 7 and standard deviation 1. This means that, a priori, the probability that the mean age is below 5 or above 9 is approximately 5%. The data we collect on a particular day based on 10 consecutive admissions are 7, 6, 8, 12, 15, 10, 4, 8, 11, 9 (sample mean of 9). How can we reconcile our prior information with the observed data?

If we let μ denote the mean age (not the sample mean, but the population mean), and the prior information on μ with $\pi(\mu)$, then $\pi(\mu)$ is a normal distribution with mean 7 and variance 1, to be denoted by $N(7, 1)$. We are assuming that X (the observations) also follows a normal distribution $N(\mu, \sigma^2)$, where σ^2 is the (population) variance of age. Call this distribution $L(X|\mu, \sigma^2)$. For the time being, let us assume that we know that $\sigma^2 = 10$; we will comment later on how to handle the more realistic case of unknown variance. We can now use Bayes's theorem to find the distribution of μ, given X:

$$P(\mu|X) = \frac{\pi(\mu)L(X|\mu, \sigma^2 = 10)}{\int \pi(\mu)L(X|\mu, \sigma^2 = 10)\, d\mu}.$$

This is called the *posterior distribution* of μ (contrast with prior distribution). The fundamental premise of Bayesian analysis is that the posterior distribution contains all the available information about μ and hence should form the basis of all statistical inference.

The analytical evaluation of the integral in the denominator is tedious but possible. It turns out that $P(\mu|X)$ also follows a normal distribution with mean

$$m_p = \frac{(m_\pi/\sigma_\pi^2) + (n\bar{x}/\sigma^2)}{(1/\sigma_\pi^2) + (n/\sigma^2)},$$

and variance

$$\sigma_p^2 = \frac{1}{(1/\sigma_\pi^2) + (n/\sigma^2)}.$$

Here, n is the sample size, m_π and σ_π^2 are the prior mean and variance, and m_p and σ_p^2 are the posterior mean and variance, Substituting the values from the example, we have

$$m_p = \frac{(7/1) + (10 * 9/10)}{(1/1) + (10/10)} = \frac{16}{2} = 8;$$

$$\sigma_p^2 = \frac{1}{(1/\sigma_\pi^2) + (n/\sigma^2)} = \frac{1}{(1/1) + (10/10)} = .5.$$

By going through the calculations we see that the posterior distribution is $N(8, .5)$. A sensible estimate of the mean patient age in this facility, then, is 8. Notice how the sample mean of 9 is shrunk toward the prior mean 7. In fact, the equation for the posterior mean above can be seen to be a weighted average of prior and sample means, where the weights are inversely proportional to the variances. Since the variance of the sample mean (σ^2/n) decreases with the sample size, increasing the sample size will make the posterior mean closer to the sample mean. For example, if the sample size was 100 with the same mean (9) and variance (10), the posterior mean would be 8.8.

Figure 1 displays the three distributions at work for this example. The prior is shifted right to become the posterior because the bulk of the data lies to the right of the prior. But the variance of the posterior is largely determined by the prior. This suggests a weakness in this analysis, namely, that we were too confident in our prior information to begin with. We were absolutely sure that the mean age would be between 4 and 10, since the prior we chose places negligible mass of probability outside this range. Yet four of our data points were greater than 10. This could of course be due to pure chance, but there could be other reasons. Perhaps the sample was not representative. Since it reflects the experience on a single afternoon, it might have been biased by outside factors that we are not aware of (such as a soccer tournament of 10-plus-year-olds held nearby). Or we might have judged our confidence in the prior incorrectly. It behooves a good analyst to investigate this further.

We can also form a confidence interval based on this distribution. For example, μ will be within the interval $(\mu_p \pm 2\sigma_p)$ approximately 95% of the time, and hence this defines a 95% confidence interval for μ. Confidence intervals are usually called *posterior intervals* if they are calculated from a Bayesian perspective. In this case, the 95% posterior interval for μ is (6.61, 9.39). It is quite wide because it is based on 10 samples only. For purposes of comparison, the standard 95% confidence interval can be calculated as (2.8, 15.3). The Bayesian interval is narrower due to the contributions from the prior information as well as the data. Remember the discussion from the above paragraph suggesting that the prior was perhaps too precise (it had a small variance). If the prior had the same mean but a larger variance, for example, 10, then the posterior distribution would be N(8.8, 0.9) and the 95% posterior interval would be (6.9, 10.7). Notice how the posterior mean shifted closer to the sample mean. This is because the weight that the prior mean received is much smaller now because the prior variance is higher.

Finally, we can compute the posterior probabilities of a hypotheses. If we wanted to test, for example, the hypothesis that H_0: $\mu > 10$, we could simply compute $P(\mu > 10|X)$, that is, the posterior probability that μ is greater than 10. Based on the N(8, 0.5) posterior, this turns out to be .002. Since this probability is very small, we can safely conclude that μ is less than 10. Note that the small prior variance is influencing this inference in the same way in which it influenced the posterior intervals. If the prior variance had been 10, then the posterior probability of this hypothesis would have increased to .103, and it would have been likely for the analyst to conclude that there was not sufficient information to reject the hypothesis that $\mu > 10$ (although it is still less likely than the alternative $\mu \leq 10$). The practice of varying the prior parameters and observing the effects on the posterior is known as sensitivity analysis and is further discussed below in more general terms.

The interpretation of Bayesian findings is very different from the interpretation of traditional statistical results. For example, with a posterior interval, we can conclude that μ lies within the posterior interval with 95% probability. With a confidence interval, we have to resort to the frequentist interpretation that 95% of the intervals constructed in this manner will contain the true μ. Similarly, with hypothesis testing, we can directly conclude that the probability of the hypothesis is low or high. With a *p* value, however, the interpretation is more cumbersome: If the null hypothesis is true, then the probability of observing a result at least as extreme as what is observed is the *p* value. Most people find the Bayesian interpretations more palatable.

Generalization to Multiple Parameters

The ideas in this simple example can be generalized to any statistical model with an arbitrary number of parameters. If we let θ represent the set of parameters (θ will be a vector) we are interested in, and X denotes the observations in our sample, the same version of Bayes's theorem holds:

$$P(\theta|X) = \frac{\pi(\theta)L(X|\theta)}{\int \pi(\theta)L(X|\theta)\,d\theta}.$$

This time, both π and L will be multivariate distributions. In the example above, if we relax the assumption of known σ^2, despite the fact that we

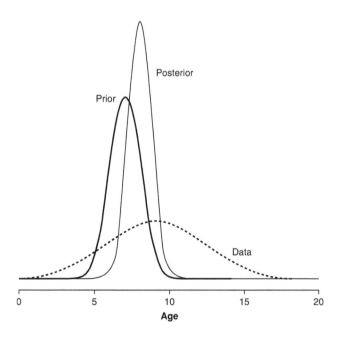

Figure 1   Prior, data, and posterior distributions

Note: Prior (--), data (..), and posterior (__) distributions for the pediatric emergency room example.

will have two parameters, we can apply the same principles to arrive at the posterior distribution.

If both π (the prior) and P (the posterior) are from the same family, then we have a *conjugate* family for L. For example, normal distribution is the conjugate for itself (i.e., if π and L are normal, then P will also be normal). A conjugate family makes calculations easier, and its use deserves serious consideration, if it exists. The problem is that for most problems of practical importance, such as regression and analysis of variance, there are no conjugate families. Since the integral in the denominator is often intractable, application of Bayesian methods in practice used to be very limited. The emergence of particular numerical methods that collectively came to be known as Markov chain Monte Carlo (MCMC) enabled statisticians to generate a sample from P without explicitly deriving an equation for it. Since this sample has distribution P, it can be used to mimic the properties of P. For example, one can form a 95% posterior interval from this sample by truncating it at the 2.5th and 97.5th percentiles. In other words, MCMC methods enable an analyst to bypass the integration in the denominator of the Bayes's theorem above. This has fueled an explosion of Bayesian applications, including the ones with very large numbers of parameters that cannot be solved within the regular statistical paradigm.

Objections to Bayesian analysis often include the difficulty of choosing a prior distribution. While most people will agree that some prior information exists in most real-world problems, they rarely agree on how to formulate it in the form of a probability distribution. It is ostensibly true that one can replace the prior of the analyst with another one and repeat the analysis to arrive at his or her own conclusions. This is rarely done, however, leaving Bayesian analysts with the responsibility of choosing a π that will be acceptable to most analysts (in addition to choosing such an L, which is the responsibility of most other statisticians as well) or performing an extensive sensitivity analysis with the hope that wide variations in π will not result in wide variations in conclusions. In the example above, we performed an informal (and highly incomplete) sensitivity analysis by changing the variance of the prior from 1 to 10 and recomputing the posterior distribution. In most cases, sensitivity analysis will define a range within which the inferences are robust to prior specifications, but this range can be unacceptably narrow.

Defenders of Bayesian analysis point to the flexibility it brings as well as the formal incorporation of external information. It is often argued that most scientists are implicit Bayesians, evaluating others' findings in light of their subjective outlook—something that can be explicitly done in the Bayesian framework. Another advantage is that, since θ is random, one can make probability statements about θ and the interpretation of Bayesian intervals and tests is very straightforward. In contrast, most nonstatisticians struggle with the appropriate definition of frequentist statistical results such as p values.

Mithat Gönen

See also Bayes's Theorem; Confidence Intervals; Likelihood Ratio

Further Readings

A Bayesian goes shopping [Editorial]. (1992). *Medical Decision Making, 12,* 1.

Berry, D. (1996). *Statistics: A Bayesian perspective.* Belmont, CA: Duxbury Press.

Berry, D. A. (2006, September). Bayesian statistics. *Medical Decision Making, 26,* 429–430.

Carlin, B., & Louis, T. (2000). *Bayes and empirical Bayes methods for data analysis* (2nd ed.). Boca Raton, FL: Chapman & Hall.

Efron, B. (1986). Why isn't everyone a Bayesian? *American Statistician, 40*(1), 1–5.

Gelman, A., Carlin, J., Stern, H., & Rubin, D. (2004). *Bayesian data analysis* (2nd ed.). Boca Raton, FL: Chapman & Hall.

Gilks, W. R., Richardson, S., & Spiegelhalter, D. J. (Eds.). (1996). *Markov chain Monte Carlo in practice.* London: Chapman & Hall.

Lee, P. (2004). *Bayesian statistics: An introduction.* London: Arnold.

Parmigiani, G. (2002). *Modeling in medical decision making: A Bayesian approach.* Chichester, UK: Wiley.

BAYESIAN EVIDENCE SYNTHESIS

Evidence synthesis has come to replace *meta-analysis* as a term referring to the statistical combination of multiple sources of evidence. In its simplest form, each evidence source is represented by a sufficient statistic, which may be, for example, a numerator and a denominator, a mean with its standard error, or a summary estimate such as an estimate of the log odds ratio and its standard error. The evidence synthesis is then the process of finding a suitable weighted average of these quantities. However, meta-analysis need not be restricted to summary statistics and has, for example, been extended to analyses of data from individual patients in multiple studies. Furthermore, evidence synthesis may be used to imply much more general forms of statistical synthesis, involving data sources of multiple types, each perhaps providing information on one or more parameters.

Bayesian evidence synthesis is then the use of Bayesian statistical methods in evidence synthesis. This can be formulated as follows: There are K unknown *basic* parameters, θ, and N data points Y_i, $i = 1, \ldots, N$, each representing, let us assume, a sufficient statistic from study i, in this case consisting of numerators r_i and denominators n_i. We may also define additional *functional* parameters $\theta_{K+1}, \ldots, \theta_M$. To rule out recursive definitions, it must be possible to define these as functions $G_{K+1}, \ldots, G_M$ of the basic parameters. Finally, each data point provides an estimate of a $G_i(\theta)$ that is some function of parameters.

One approach to computation, the maximum likelihood solution, assuming that the N data points are independent, would be to find values of θ that maximize

$$L = \Pi_{i = 1, \ldots, N} \, L_i \, (Y_i | \theta_1, \theta_2, \ldots, \theta_K), \qquad (1)$$

bearing in mind that the likelihood contribution from each study might take a different distributional form (normal, binomial, Poisson, etc.).

Bayesian evidence synthesis specifies a prior distribution for the basic parameters only $P(\theta)$. There is no requirement that the parameters be independent, so we may consider this to be a joint prior distribution, if necessary. We then find the joint posterior distribution by application of Bayes's theorem:

$$P(\theta_1, \ldots, \theta_K | Y_1, \ldots, Y_N) \propto P(\theta) \, L \qquad (2)$$

The data to be synthesized form a connected network that can be described in terms of a directed acyclic graph (DAG). However, the synthesis problems are capable of being reparameterized in many different ways, so that items of data that inform, for example, a basic parameter in one parameterization may inform a functional parameter in another. Hence, several DAGs may describe the same network. Some evidence networks may also be described in terms of graphs. One important feature that remains invariant under reparameterization is the inconsistency degrees of freedom, $N - K$. This can be thought of as representing the number of independent ways in which the evidence can be inconsistent under a given model. For example, in the DAG presented in Figure 1 and discussed in more detail below, there are three basic parameters and four independent data items to inform them. The inconsistency degrees of freedom is therefore $4 - 3 = 1$. The Bayesian formulation, which forces the investigator to be explicit about which parameters are basic, and therefore have a prior distribution, and which are functional, yields valuable insights into the structure and dynamics of the data and model.

The Bayesian framework is, of course, essentially the same in evidence synthesis as it is in other areas of statistics, but it takes a slightly different flavor in this context. Instead of combining a "prior" based, formally or informally, on the accumulated evidence so far, together with the likelihood in the latest study, the whole exercise is concerned with combining all the available evidence. For this reason, the priors put on most parameters are typically vague. Nevertheless, the focus on putting together all available evidence, to obtain the best possible estimates with the most realistic assessment of uncertainty, is very much in tune with the Bayesian spirit.

History

The origins and development of Bayesian evidence synthesis lie more in decision making than in traditional statistical inference. On the other hand, Bayesian methods have brought to decision modeling the advantages of formal posterior inference, and of statistical methods for model diagnosis, that have otherwise tended to be lacking. The decision-making context is inevitably associated with multiple parameters and multiple sources of uncertainty. Probabilistic methods were introduced in the 1980s at the time when the development of computers made it possible to evaluate complex models by Monte Carlo simulation. Each parameter is represented by a statistical distribution, one Monte Carlo cycle value is drawn from each distribution, and the costs and benefits are computed. The expected costs and benefits are then taken as an average over the simulated sequence. This scheme has been regarded as essentially Bayesian in that it focuses on the probability distributions of parameters. Essentially, it samples from a (informative) prior $P(\theta)$ but unlike Equation 2 does not update this with further data.

Forward simulation from a prior is, however, severely limited. Typically, each parameter represented by a separate distribution, as well as each distribution, is informed by a separate item from the data, either from a single study or from a meta-analysis. This means that the number of data sources must equal the number of parameters, no more and no less. A scheme with Bayesian updating, in contrast, can incorporate multiple functions of parameters so that, if the data are available, there can be more sources of data than there are parameters. Furthermore, Bayesian hierarchical models can be deployed to share information over the parameter space and thus to manage situations where there are fewer data items than there are parameters.

A related advantage of full Bayesian updating is that the ability to incorporate data on more functions of parameters than there are parameters represents an opportunity to validate the model. This can also be regarded as a form of probabilistic model calibration. Model diagnostics are available to check the consistency of the different sources of evidence with respect to any parameter.

The above formulation of the Bayesian evidence synthesis model is due to David M. Eddy and his colleagues, whose 1992 book, *Meta-Analysis by the Confidence Profile Method,* appears to have been the first systematic exposition of Bayesian evidence synthesis in the context of medical decision making. Although the book introduced extremely powerful statistical methods and ideas to a wider audience, it failed to have the impact it deserved. This was due, perhaps, to the somewhat stylized examples and the specialized software required.

In fact, Bayesian forms of statistical synthesis seem to have emerged independently in related fields, in each case based on different computational approaches. The Confidence Profile Method was based on a fully Bayesian computation using Monte Carlo simulation and on two further approximate methods that are not always accurate for small sample sizes. Another set of computational methods that have been used for synthesis, named Bayesian Monte Carlo, is based on weighted Monte Carlo sampling, where the weights were given by the likelihood of the data at each set of parameters. This approach became popular in the Environmental Health Risk Assessment field, beginning with simple accept-reject algorithms and then evolving to a fully Bayesian approach. Typical applications included updating prior distributions for contaminant release, environmental transport, and biological effects, with field data on pollution levels.

A further series of methods, called variously Bayesian Synthesis, Bayesian Melding, and Bayesian Pooling, were developed for deterministic models of animal and plant populations. These algorithms are also based on various types of noniterative reweighting schemes.

Bayesian Markov chain Monte Carlo (MCMC) has become the standard software for Bayesian evidence synthesis, certainly in the medical decision-making context. The development of freely available user-friendly MCMC software, such as WinBUGS, has opened the possibilities of Bayesian evidence synthesis to a wide range of researchers. Users of the package need only specify priors and likelihoods and define functional parameters. As a result, a wide and increasing range of applications is appearing in health technology assessment literature. The expression *multiparameter evidence synthesis,* coined by Victor Hasselblad, another founder of the Confidence Profile Method, is often used for applications of this sort.

Many of these are examples of *comprehensive decision analysis,* a term used when a Bayesian statistical synthesis is embedded within a decision analysis, an approach first seen in publications from Duke University in the 1990s. More recently, the increasing adoption of net benefit analysis has made this conceptually appealing, and the simulation format for MCMC, of course, fits in readily with the simulation approach that has become familiar from probabilistic modeling based on simple Monte Carlo methods.

Examples

This section outlines some examples of Bayesian evidence synthesis. Figure 1 shows a fragment of a model of HIV epidemiology in the form of an influence diagram, in which four sources of data inform three basic probability parameters. The basic parameters would most naturally be given Beta prior distributions. The three surveys that directly inform the basic parameters provide prevalence data and would, therefore, each contribute a binomial likelihood. The fourth source of evidence would provide the observed number of diagnosed cases, which would be represented as a

Poisson distribution. This type of evidence structure is quite common in epidemiology applications. Note that the model in effect "calibrates" the basic parameters so that their product is consistent with the routine surveillance data.

As noted earlier, the inconsistency degrees of freedom is 1. Therefore, the investigator can assess whether or not the four sources of data are consistent with each other, under this model. If they are not, this would suggest that one or more of the studies is not estimating the presumed target parameter but is biased. *Which* study is biased, of course, cannot be determined without further data or expert judgment, and very possibly more than one is biased.

Another very common structure for Bayesian evidence synthesis is illustrated in Figure 2. Mixed

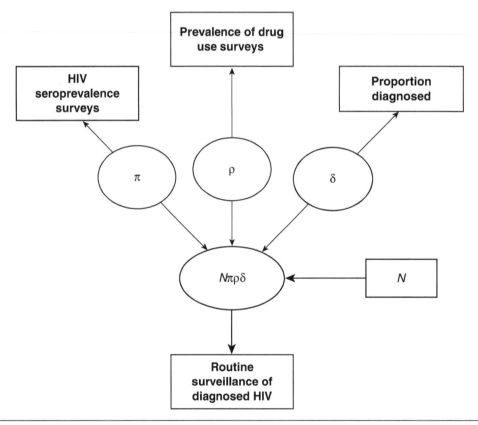

Figure 1   Schematic influence diagram (directed acyclic graph)

Note: Ellipses indicate stochastic nodes, rectangles constants or data, and edges the direction of influence. There are three *basic* parameters: HIV prevalence in injecting drug users (IDUs), π; proportion of the population who are IDUs, ρ; proportion of infected IDUs who are diagnosed, δ. With population size N, a constant, these define the product $N\pi\rho\delta$, a functional parameter, which is the number of diagnosed IDUs. There are four sources of data: Three directly inform the basic parameters; the fourth directly informs a functional parameter.

Treatment Comparison structures allow the synthesis of data from pairwise, or multiarm, randomized controlled trials of treatments. For example, the evidence base may consist of one or more trials making each of the following comparisons: A versus B, A versus C, B versus C, A versus B versus D, C versus D, and so on. If we arbitrarily choose A as the reference point, we may choose the relative treatment effects of B, C, D, and so on, relative to A as the basic parameters. All the other contrasts, d_{XY}, may then be expressed in terms of the basic parameters:

$$d_{XY} = d_{AY} - d_{AX} \qquad (3)$$

For example, if we take Streptokinase (SK) as reference treatment, then we can express the relative efficacy of percutaneous transluminal angioplasty (PCTA) relative to accelerated t-PA (At-PA) as follows:

$$d_{\text{PCTA, At-PA}} - d_{\text{SK, PCTA}} \quad d_{\text{SK, At-PA}} \qquad (4)$$

The key assumption being made of the data, of course, is that each of the randomized controlled trials included would, if all the treatments had been included, be providing estimates of the same relative effect parameters. If there are T treatments and information on N pairwise contrasts, then there are $(T - 1)$ basic parameters and the inconsistency degrees of freedom is $(N - T + 1)$. Equations 3 and 4 effectively reduce the parameter space from N unrelated comparisons to $(T - 1)$. In this case, we have $T = 7$ treatments and evidence on $N = 10$ contrasts, giving 4 degrees of freedom for inconsistency, though where multiarm trials are involved, this simple formula requires adjustment.

Bayesian methods have been used to synthesize many other evidence structures. These include, for example, collapsed frequency tables; regression models based on different subsets of variables; surrogate or intermediate endpoints in trials with clinical endpoints; multiple outcomes, or the same outcome reported at multiple time points in clinical trials; Markov rate models; and individual and aggregate data. Collapsed category methods are becoming increasingly common in genetic epidemiology.

Bayesian evidence synthesis in cost-effectiveness analysis is often associated with expected value of information analysis. Because multiple parameters are estimated from a common data set, their posterior distributions are invariably correlated. This can introduce additional complexity in expected value of information calculations.

A E Ades

See also Cost-Effectiveness Analysis; Expected Value of Perfect Information; Meta-Analysis and Literature Review; Net Benefit Regression

Further Readings

Ades, A. E., & Sutton, A. J. (2006). Multiple parameter evidence synthesis in epidemiology and medical decision making: Current approaches. *Journal of the Royal Statistical Society, Series A, 169,* 5–35.

Brand, K. P., & Small, M. J. (1995). Updating uncertainty in an integrated risk assessment: Conceptual framework and methods. *Risk Analysis, 15,* 719–731.

Dominici, F., Parmigiani, G., Wolpert, R. L., & Hasselblad, V. (1999). Meta-analysis of migraine headache treatments: Combining information from heterogenous designs. *Journal of the American Statistical Association, 94,* 16–28.

Eddy, D. M., Hasselblad, V., & Shachter, R. (1992). *Meta-analysis by the Confidence Profile Method: The statistical synthesis of evidence.* Boston: Academic Press.

Goubar, A., Ades, A. E., DeAngelis, D., McGarrigle, C. A., Mercer, C., Tookey, P., et al. (2008). Estimates of HIV prevalence and proportion diagnosed based on Bayesian multi-parameter synthesis of surveillance data (with discussion). *Journal of the Royal Statistical Society, Series A, 171,* 541–580.

Lu, G., & Ades, A. E. (2006). Assessing evidence consistency in mixed treatment comparisons. *Journal of the American Statistical Association, 101,* 447–459.

Raftery, A. E., Givens, G. H., & Zeh, J. E. (1995). Inference for a deterministic population dynamics model for Bowhead whales (with discussion). *Journal of the American Statistical Association, 90,* 402–430.

Spiegelhalter, D. J., Abrams, K. R., & Myles, J. P. (2004). *Bayesian approaches to clinical trials and health-care evaluation.* Chichester, UK: Wiley.

BAYESIAN NETWORKS

A Bayesian network is a graphical representation of a multivariate probability distribution on a set

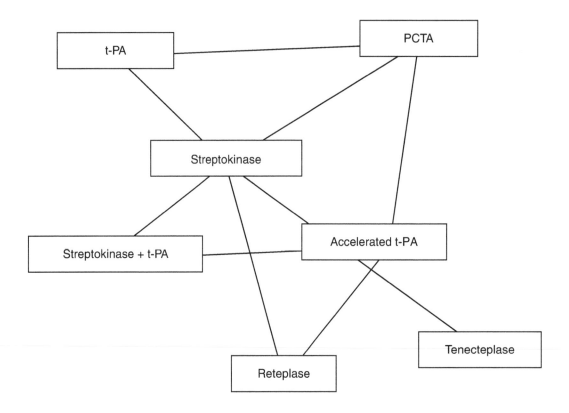

Figure 2   A Mixed Treatment Comparison network involving six thrombolytic treatments following acute myocardial infarction and one surgical treatment, percutaneous transluminal angioplasty (PCTA)

Note: Each edge indicates that the treatments have been compared in at least one randomized, controlled trial.

of discrete random variables. Representational efficiency is achieved by explicit separation of information about *conditional independence* relations between the variables (coded in the network structure) and information about the probabilities involved (coded as a set of numeric parameters or functions). The network structure is expressed as a directed acyclic graph (DAG) that makes the representation amenable to an intuitively appealing, causal interpretation. Algorithms exist for learning both network structure and parameters from data. Furthermore, Bayesian networks allow for computing any marginal or *conditional probability* regarding the variables involved, thus offering a powerful framework for

reasoning with uncertainty. Bayesian networks are also called *belief networks* and *causal probabilistic networks*.

Bayesian networks are suited to model the uncertainty that inheres in many biomedical domains and are, therefore, frequently used in applications of computer-assisted decision making in biomedicine. Furthermore, extensions of Bayesian networks (called *influence diagrams*) can be used to perform decision analyses.

This entry first sketches the historical background of Bayesian networks. Subsequently, it elaborates on model structure, approaches for network construction, inference methods, medical applications, and software.

Historical Background

Bayesian networks originated in the mid-1980s from the quest for mathematically sound and computationally tractable methods for reasoning with uncertainty in artificial intelligence. In the preceding decade, the first applications of computer-assisted decision making had found their way to the medical field, mostly focusing on the diagnostic process. This had required the development of methods for reasoning with uncertain and incomplete diagnostic information.

One popular method was the naive Bayesian approach that required specification of positive and negative predictive values for each of a set of predefined diagnostic tests and a prior (i.e., marginal) probability distribution over possible diagnostic hypotheses. The approach assumed that all test results were mutually independent markers of disease and used Bayes's theorem to compute posterior (i.e., conditional) probabilities on the hypotheses of interest. The approach is simple and fast and requires a relatively small number of marginal and conditional probabilities to be specified. However, the assumption of independence is mostly wrong and leads to overly extreme posterior probabilities.

Another approach arose in the field of expert systems, where algorithms had been devised to reason with so-called certainty factors, parameters expressing the strength of association in if-then rules. The underlying reasoning principles were mostly ad hoc and not rooted in probability theory, but large sets of if-then rules allowed for a domain representation that was structurally richer and more complex than naive Bayesian models. Bayesian networks bring together the best of both approaches by combining representational expressiveness with mathematical rigor.

Model Structure

Bayesian networks belong to the family of probabilistic graphical models (PGMs), graphs in which nodes represent random variables, and the (lack of) arcs represent conditional independence assumptions. Let $G = (V(G), A(G))$ be a directed acyclic graph, where the nodes $V(G) = \{V_1, \ldots, V_n\}$ represent discrete random variables with a finite value domain. For each node $V_i \in V(G)$, let π_i denote the set of parent nodes of V_i in graph G. A Bayesian network now is a pair $B = (G, \Theta)$, where $\Theta = \{\theta_i | V_i \in V(G)\}$ is a set of parametrization functions. The function θ_i describes a local model for node $V_i \in V(G)$ by specifying a conditional probability $\theta_i(v|s)$ for each possible value v of variable V_i and all possible value assignments s to its parents π_i. The Bayesian network B defines a unique multivariate probability distribution Pr on $V_1, \ldots, V_n$ using the factorization

$$\Pr(V_1, \ldots, V_n) = \prod_{i=1}^{n} \theta_i(V_i | \pi_i).$$

An example Bayesian network is shown in Figure 1. This network has eight variables and is a simplified representation of diagnosing a patient presenting to a chest clinic, having just come back from a trip to Asia and showing dyspnea. This symptom may be caused by tuberculosis, lung cancer, or bronchitis. In this example, the local model for the variable "dyspnea" specifies that there is a .80 probability that dyspnea is present when the patient has bronchitis but no tuberculosis or lung cancer and a .70 probability of dsypnea when the patient does have tuberculosis or cancer but no bronchitis.

It follows from the definition of Bayesian networks that each variable is conditionally independent of its nondescendants in the graph given its parents; this is called the *local Markov condition*. It induces a more general notion of conditional independence, the *global Markov condition*, which builds on the graphical criterion of *path blocking*. Let X, Y, and Z be nonintersecting sets of nodes in $V(G)$, and consider an arbitrary path from a node in X to a node in Y. The path is blocked by the set Z if it includes a node such that either (a) the arrows on the path meet head-to-tail or tail-to-tail at the node, and the node is in the set Z, or (b) the arrows meet head-to-head at the node, and neither the node, nor any of its descendants, is in the set Z. For example, the set {smoking, bronchitis} blocks the path lung cancer—smoking—bronchitis—dyspnea. Sets X and Y are conditionally independent given Z in probability distribution Pr if each path from a node in X to a node in Y in graph G is blocked by Z. In words, this means that once Z has been observed, knowing X will not influence our beliefs about Y and vice versa.

A Bayesian network represents the conditional independence relations between a set of variables,

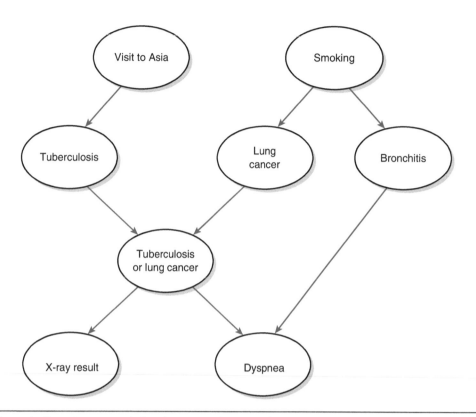

Figure 1   Example Bayesian network for diagnosing dyspnea after a visit to Asia

Source: From Table 2 (p. 164) of Lauritzen, S. L., & Spiegelhalter, D. J. (1988). Local computations with probabilities on graphical structures and their application to expert systems (with discussion). *Journal of the Royal Statistical Society, Series B, 50*(2), 157–224. Reprinted with permission of Wiley-Blackwell.

not their causal dependencies. Under certain conditions, however, one can assume that the arcs in a Bayesian network permit a causal interpretation. The crucial observation is that the occurrence of an uncertain event is independent of its noneffects, given its direct causes. Therefore, if a directed graph accurately depicts causality, it will also obey the local Markov condition, and one can use it as the graphical part of a Bayesian network. In such cases, one can basically think of conditional independence relations as byproducts of causality. This applies to the example network from Figure 1.

In the most basic representation, the parametrization function θ_i of each node $V_i \in V(G)$ is simply stored as a contingency table. The size of such a table, however, grows exponentially in the number of parents of V_i in the graph. There exist various ways of reducing the size of the representation. Popular examples are the noisy OR gate, which

assumes that the influence of each parent on V_i is independent of other parents, and local tree structures for representing the table.

Construction

Two different approaches to developing Bayesian networks can be distinguished. The first one is manual construction in collaboration with domain experts and was frequently applied in early medical applications of Bayesian networks. The second approach learns the network from data; this approach has become more feasible in the medical field with the large amounts of patient data that are currently recorded in information systems and is, consequently, being applied in more recent medical applications.

Manual construction of Bayesian networks involves the use of knowledge engineering techniques and, thus, resembles the manual construction of knowledge bases and decision models such as decision trees. In the development process, a number of stages can be distinguished that are iterated, inducing further refinement of the network under construction. The first stage is the selection of relevant variables that form the nodes in the network. Variable selection is generally based on expert opinion (interviews) and descriptions of the domain. Subsequently, dependency relationships among the variables are identified and added as arcs in the network. For this purpose, the notion of causality is generally employed in interviews with domain experts by asking for the causes and consequences of manifestations. In the third stage, qualitative probabilistic constraints (e.g., the probability of an adverse outcome with severe comorbodities is at least as high as with moderate comorbidities) and logical constraints (e.g., the occurrence of pregnancy is limited to females) among the variables are identified. These constraints are also helpful in the next stage of assessing the local (conditional) probability distributions for each variable and in their verification. Elicitation methods that originate from the field of medical decision making (e.g., for translation of verbal expressions of probabilities to numbers) can be used for deriving subjective probabilities from domain experts.

In the second approach of constructing Bayesian networks, both the graphical structure and the conditional probability distributions are learned from data. As an exhaustive search through the space of all possible network structures (DAGs) is computationally prohibitive, most algorithms apply a heuristic search strategy, starting with a single structure (either an empty or a randomly chosen graph) and incrementally modifying this structure until a termination condition is reached. There are two main types of algorithms. The first type of algorithm evaluates the current network structure and its closest resemblers using a goodness-of-fit scoring function and continues with the structure having the highest score. The second type of algorithm employs statistical independency tests on the data to determine, for each pair of variables, whether an arc should be added between them in the graph. After the network structure has been established, the parametrization functions are estimated from the data using maximum likelihood estimation; the expectation maximization (EM) algorithm can be used in case of incomplete data. In addition to network learning in a frequentist approach, Bayesian statistical methods can be used in which prior probabilities are assigned to the network structure and the probability distributions.

In practice, often mixtures of the above approaches are used for construction of Bayesian networks, for example, by employing data to estimate or update conditional probability estimates in an otherwise manual construction process or by placing constraints on the network structure based on domain knowledge before inducing a network from data. In each approach, construction of Bayesian networks is completed with the evaluation of the performance of the network constructed, preferably on independent data.

Inference

Given a Bayesian network $B = (G, \Theta)$, we can identify a number of probabilistic inference tasks. Let Pr denote the multivariate probability distribution that is defined by B, let e denote evidence (i.e., observed states) on a subset $V' \subset V(G)$ of network variables, and let $V'' \subset V(G) \backslash V'$ be a subset of variables of interest. Inference tasks fall into two categories.

Evidence Propagation: Given evidence e, what is conditional probability distribution on the set V''? Special cases are computation of the conditional probability $\Pr(h|e)$ of a particular state h of the set V'' and of the marginal (i.e., unconditional) probability $\Pr(e)$.

Maximum a Posteriori (MAP) Assignment: Given evidence e, what is the most likely state h of V''; that is, $h = \text{argmax}_s \{\Pr(s, e)\}$, where s ranges over all possible states of V''? The special case of MAP assignment, where V'' consists of all network variables except those in V', that is, $V'' = V(G) \backslash V'$, is called *most probable explanation*.

Generally speaking, both inference categories become more complicated when V'' gets larger because the associated set of possible states grows exponentially in size. The main difference between the categories is that evidence propagation infers probabilities for given states, while MAP assignment infers a state. In both cases, it does not matter whether the evidence variables V' are located above or below the variables of interest V'', because information can travel both in the direction of network arcs and against it. The former situation corresponds to causal (or predictive) reasoning, the latter situation to diagnostic reasoning.

Both inference categories constitute challenging computational problems. Much research effort has therefore been devoted to designing efficient inference methods. It is common to distinguish between *exact* and *approximate* inference. The most popular method for exact inference, the join tree algorithm, converts the Bayesian network into a tree structure in which each junction represents a cluster of network variables. Evidence propagation proceeds by applying a message-passing scheme to the join tree. The join tree representation may take a long time to construct and become very large when the network is densely connected. It need only be constructed once, though, and the message-passing phase is fast. Other exact inference methods are variable elimination and recursive conditioning.

Approximate inference methods can be used when exact inference methods lead to unacceptable computation times because the network is very large or densely connected. Popular approaches are simulation methods and variational methods. Simulation methods use the network to generate samples from the conditional probability distribution $\Pr(V''|e)$ and estimate conditional probabilities of interest when the number of samples is sufficiently large. Variational methods express the inference task as a numerical optimization problem and then find upper and lower bounds of the probabilities of interest by solving a simplified version of this optimization problem.

Medical Applications and Examples

In a medical context, Bayesian networks are mainly developed to support three types of problem solving: (1) diagnostic reasoning, (2) prognostic reasoning, and (3) therapy selection. Bayesian networks form a suitable formalism for modeling the uncertainties in diagnostic tests due to false-positive and false-negative findings and enable the computation of the conditional probability $\Pr(h|e)$ of a diagnostic hypothesis h given the evidence of diagnostic test results e by evidence propagation.

Early examples of diagnostic applications of Bayesian networks are the MUNIN system for diagnosis of peripheral muscle and nerve diseases, the Pathfinder system for diagnosis of lymph node diseases, and a network for diagnosis in internal medicine and neurology, a reformulation of the rule-based expert system, INTERNIST-1/QMR. Diagnostic Bayesian networks are often equipped with methods for determining the optimal order of diagnostic tests for reducing the uncertainty in a patient's differential diagnosis.

Prognostic Bayesian networks have a pronounced temporal structure with the outcome variable as final node in the network and pretreatment variables and treatment variable as its ancestor nodes. With MAP assignment, most probable prognostic scenarios can be determined using the network. In the literature, a relatively small number of prognostic applications of Bayesian network have been described, including applications for non-Hodgkin lymphoma, for malignant skin melanoma, and for cardiac surgery.

The medical task of therapy selection involves both diagnostic and prognostic reasoning. Bayesian networks for therapy selection are, therefore, usually extended to decision-theoretic models that include utility functions to guide the choice among different decisions. A suitable extension of Bayesian networks for representing probabilistic knowledge, decisions, and utility information are influence diagrams. Examples of this type of medical application include Bayesian networks for therapy selection for esophageal cancer and for treating infectious diseases in intensive care medicine.

Software

A large number of software packages are available for inference with Bayesian networks, manual construction, and network induction from data. A widely used package is Hugin, which includes algorithms for both inference and network induction (structure and parameter learning). Similar functionality is provided by the BayesiaLab software and the Bayes Net Toolbox that can be used within the Matlab mathematical software package. The Netica software supports parameter learning only. A Web directory of Bayesian network software is available at http://directory

.google.com/Top/Computers/Artificial_Intelligence/
Belief_Networks/Software.

Niels Peek and Marion Verduijn

See also Bayes's Theorem; Causal Inference and
Diagrams; Computer-Assisted Decision Making;
Conditional Independence; Conditional Probability;
Diagnostic Process, Making a Diagnosis; Diagnostic
Tests; Expert Opinion; Expert Systems; Frequentist
Approach; Influence Diagrams; Markov Models;
Probability; Probability, Verbal Expressions of;
Problem Solving; Subjective Probability

Further Readings

Cowell, R. G., Dawid, A. P., Lauritzen, S. L., &
Spiegelhalter, D. J. (1999). *Probabilistic networks and
expert systems*. New York: Springer.

Darwiche, A. (2008). Bayesian networks. In F. van
Harmelen, V. Lifschitz, & B. Porter (Eds.), *Handbook
of knowledge representation* (pp. 467–509).
Amsterdam: Elsevier.

Jensen, F. V., & Nielsen, T. D. (2007). *Bayesian networks
and decision graphs*. New York: Springer.

Lauritzen, S. L., & Spiegelhalter, D. J. (1988). Local
computations with probabilities on graphical
structures and their application to expert systems.
Journal of the Royal Statistical Society, Series B, 50,
157–224.

Lucas, P. J. F., Van der Gaag, L. C., & Abu-Hanna, A.
(2004). Bayesian networks in biomedicine and health
care. *Artificial Intelligence in Medicine, 30*, 201–214.

Murphy, K. (2005). Software packages for graphical
models/Bayesian networks. Retrieved January 23, 2009,
from www.cs.ubc.ca/~murphyk/Bayes/bnsoft.html

Pearl, J. (1988). *Probabilistic reasoning in intelligent
systems: Networks of plausible inference*. San
Francisco: Morgan Kaufmann.

BAYES'S THEOREM

A Bayesian approach to inference implies combining prior judgment with new information to
obtain revised judgment. Prior judgment is
expressed in a prior probability that a hypothesis
is true. The prior probability is subsequently
updated with new data that become available
to yield the revised posterior probability of the
hypothesis. Bayesian updating can be applied to
the results of diagnostic tests (which is explained
here), to a research hypothesis under investigation,
or to a parameter being estimated in a study.

Bayesian Updating of the Probability of Disease

Estimates of probabilities of disease conditional on
diagnostic test results are usually not readily available. One is more likely to have an assessment of
the probability of a test result among patients with
or without the disease. Converting conditional
probabilities of the latter type (test results given
disease) to probabilities of the type needed for
decision making (disease given test results) should
take into account the pretest (or prior) probability
of disease, $p(D+)$, the test characteristics (sensitivity and specificity), and the test result (positive or
negative) to obtain a posttest (revised or posterior)
probability of disease, $p(D+|T+)$ or $p(D+|T-)$. This
process is called Bayesian probability revision and
can be done using one of several methods.

As an example, consider a 47-year-old female
patient who presents with atypical angina in whom
you would like to exclude coronary artery disease
(CAD). Based on the literature, her pretest (prior)
probability of having CAD is 13%. You refer her
for a CT to determine her coronary calcium score
(CTCS), which is 0 (i.e., a normal/negative test
result). Now you wonder whether she still could
have CAD in spite of the negative CTCS result.
CTCS has a sensitivity of 96% and specificity of
60% for the diagnosis CAD.

Bayesian Probability Revision With a 2 × 2 Table

Given the prior probability of disease $p(D+)$, sen-
sitivity $p(T+|D+)$, and specificity $p(T-|D-)$, we can
construct a 2 × 2 table of a hypothetical population and, with the numbers of TP, FN, FP, and
TNs, calculate the posttest (revised) probabilities.
The steps are as follows:

1. Pick an arbitrary number n for the total
   hypothetical population (e.g., $n = 10,000$).

2. Using the prior probability $p(D+)$, partition the
   total number of patients across those with and

without the disease, that is, $n(D+) = n \cdot p(D+)$ and $n(D-) = n \cdot (1 - p(D+))$.

3. Using sensitivity $p(T+|D+)$, determine the number of patients with disease who have a true-positive versus a false-negative test result, that is, $TP = n(D+) \cdot p(T+|D+)$ and $FN = n(D+) \cdot (1 - p(T+|D+))$.

4. Using specificity $p(T-|D-)$, determine the number of patients without disease who have a true-negative versus a false-positive test result, that is, $TN = n(D-) \cdot p(T-|D-)$ and $FP = n(D-) \cdot (1 - p(T-|D-))$.

5. Calculate the posttest (revised or posterior) probabilities as follows:
   o Postpositive test probability of disease = $p(D+|T+) = TP/(TP + FP)$.
   o Postpositive test probability of absence of disease = $p(D-|T+) = FP/(TP + FP)$.
   o Postnegative test probability of disease = $p(D+|T-) = FN/(TN + FN)$.
   o Postnegative test probability of absence of disease = $p(D-|T-) = TN/(TN + FN)$.

Note:

Postpositive test probability of disease = positive predictive value.

Postnegative test probability of absence of disease = negative predictive value.

For our example patient, the 2 × 2 table is as follows:

	CAD+	CAD–	
CTCS+	1,248	3,480	4,728
CTCS–	52	5,220	5,272
	1,300	8,700	10,000

The postnegative CTCS probability of CAD = 52/5272 = 1%. In other words, with a 0 calcium score on CT, the likelihood of CAD in this patient is really very low.

Probability Revision Using Bayes's Formula

Consider a test result R, which may be any finding, for example, a positive or negative test result for dichotomous tests or a particular result on a categorical, ordinal, or continuous scale for tests with multiple results. Consider the true disease status D_j, which indicates a particular disease status j, one of a set of disease statuses $j = 1, ..., J$. From the definition of a *conditional probability* we know that

$$p(D_j|R) = p(R, D_j)/p(R);$$

that is, the probability of D_j (the disease status j) among patients with a test result R equals the proportion of those with R that also have D_j. Test result R can occur among patients with any disease status $j = 1, ..., J$; that is,

$$p(R) = p(R, D_1) + p(R, D_2) + p(R, D_j) + ... + p(R, D_J)$$

$$= p(R|D_1) \cdot p(D_1) + p(R|D_2) p(D_2) + p(R|D_j) \cdot p(D_j) + ... + p(R|D_J) p(D_J).$$

Substituting the expression for $p(R)$ in the first equation, we get the generalized version of Bayes's formula:

$$p(D_j|R) = \frac{p(R|D_j)p(D_j)}{\sum_j p(R|D_j)p(D_j)}.$$

For a dichotomous (+ or −) test, R becomes either $T+$ or $T-$, and for disease present versus disease absent, D_j becomes $D+$ or $D-$, in which case Bayes's formula becomes

$$p(D+|T+) = \frac{p(T+|D+)p(D+)}{p(T+|D+)p(D+) + p(T+|D-)p(D-)},$$

which is the same as

Postpositive test probability

$$= \frac{\text{Sensitivity} \times \text{Pretest probability}}{\text{Sensitivity} \times \text{Pretest probability} + [1 - \text{Specificity}] \times [1 - \text{Pretest probability}]}.$$

For our example, we are interested in the postnegative test probability of CAD, so the appropriate equation is

$$p(D+|T-) = \frac{p(T-|D+)p(D+)}{p(T-|D+)p(D+) + p(T-|D-)p(D-)}$$

$$= \frac{(1-.96) \cdot .13}{(1-.96) \cdot .13 + .60 \cdot (1-.13)}$$

$$= .01.$$

Probability Revision With the Odds-Likelihood-Ratio Form of Bayes's Formula

Consider a test result R and true disease status $D+$ and $D-$. From the definition of a *conditional probability*, we know that

$$p(D+|R) = p(R, D+)/p(R)$$
$$= p(R|D+) \cdot p(D+)/p(R),$$

and

$$p(D-|R) = p(R, D-)/p(R)$$
$$= p(R|D-) \cdot p(D-)/p(R).$$

Dividing the first by the second equation, we get

$$\frac{p(D+|R)}{p(D-|R)} = \frac{p(D+)}{p(D-)} \times \frac{p(R|D+)}{p(R|D-)},$$

which is Bayes's in odds-likelihood-ratio form and can also be rewritten as

Posttest (posterior) odds = Pretest (prior) odds × Likelihood ratio for R.

In plain English this means the following:

Our judgment that the patient has the disease after doing the test (posterior odds) equals our judgment that the patient has the disease before doing the test (prior odds), updated with the information we get from the test result R (likelihood ratio for R).

The *likelihood ratio* (LR) for test result R summarizes all the information we need to know about the test result R for purposes of revising the probability of disease. LR for test result R is the ratio of the conditional probability of R given the disease under consideration and the probability of R given absence of the disease under consideration.

The posttest (posterior) *odds* can be converted back to a probability using

$$\text{Probability} = \frac{\text{Odds}}{1 + \text{Odds}}.$$

In our example, we have a 0 calcium score, so we need to use the LR for a negative test result:

$$\text{Probability} = \frac{\text{Odds}}{1 + \text{Odds}}.$$

$$= (1 - .96)/.60 = .067.$$

Prior probability = .13

Prior odds = .13/(1 − .13) = .15

Posterior odds = Prior odds × LR(CTCS−) = .15 × .067 = .0100

Posterior probability = .01/(1 + .01) = .0099

Note that the posterior odds and posterior probability are practically equal because the probability is very low.

M. G. Myriam Hunink

See also Conditional Probability; Diagnostic Tests; Likelihood Ratio; Odds and Odds Ratio

Further Readings

Hunink, M. G. M., Glasziou, P. P., Siegel, J. E., Weeks, J. C., Pliskin, J. S., Elstein, A. S., et al. (2001). *Decision making in health and medicine: Integrating evidence and values*. Cambridge, UK: Cambridge University Press.

BENEFICENCE

In biomedical research, generally, the success of new therapeutic approaches relies on three conditions: specificity, efficacy, and lack of toxicity. These conditions are often tested in cell cultures, mouse models, and clinical trials before a drug is offered to patients. Hence, if biomedical approaches are to be used therapeutically, one should balance the possible harms and the possible benefits of these methods (perform a *risk-benefit analysis*). The terms *harms* and *benefits* are ethically relevant concepts, since ethical obligations or principles about not inflicting harm (*nonmaleficence*) and promoting good (*beneficence*) are generally accepted. The ethical principles of nonmaleficence and beneficence form part of several different ethical theories. For instance, they are the foundation of the utilitarian theory, which says that ethically right actions are those that favor the greatest good for the greatest number. Another example is the Hippocratic Oath, which expresses an obligation of beneficence and an obligation of nonmaleficence: I will use treatment to help the sick according to my ability and judgment, but I will never use it to injure or wrong them.

This entry analyzes the ethical principles of beneficence and nonmaleficence in biomedicine by drawing on the bioethical theory of principles of the American bioethicists Tom L. Beauchamp and James F. Childress. These ethicists have published their theory in several editions of the book, *Principles of Biomedical Ethics*.

Risk-Benefit Analysis

According to Beauchamp and Childress, the evaluation of risk in relation to possible benefit in biomedicine is often labeled *risk-benefit analysis*. They say that the term *risk* refers to a possible future harm, where *harm* is defined as a setback to interests, particularly in life, health, and welfare. Statements of risk are both descriptive and evaluative. They are descriptive because they state the probability that harmful events will occur, and they are evaluative because they attach a value to the occurrence or prevention of the events. Commonly in the field of biomedicine, the term *benefit* refers to something of positive value, such as life or health. Beauchamp and Childress state that the risk-benefit relationship may be conceived in terms of the ratio between the probability and magnitude of an anticipated benefit and the probability and magnitude of an anticipated harm. Use of the terms *risk* and *benefit* necessarily involves an evaluation. Values determine both what will count as harms and benefits and how much weight particular harms and benefits will have in the risk-benefit calculation.

Risk and benefit identifications, estimations, and evaluations are all stages in risk-benefit analysis; the next step is *risk management*, which Beauchamp and Childress define as the set of individual or institutional responses to the analysis and assessment of risk, including decisions to reduce or control risks. These ethicists believe that while risk-benefit analysis may seem like a technical issue, in which risks and benefits are defined, quantified, and compared, the definition of risk

and benefits and the evaluation of how much risk is acceptable (risk management) are clearly ethical issues. Beauchamp and Childress offer an example: Risk management in hospitals includes establishing policies aimed at reducing the risk of medical malpractice suits.

Required Actions

According to Beauchamp and Childress, the balancing of the general ethical principles of nonmaleficence and beneficence is not symmetrical, since our obligation not to inflict evil or harm (nonmaleficence) is more stringent than our obligation to prevent and remove evil and harm or to do and promote good (beneficence). These authors state that our obligation of beneficence requires taking action (positive steps) to help prevent harm, remove harm, and promote good, whereas our obligation of nonmaleficence only requires intentionally refraining from actions that cause harm; hence, nonmaleficence usually involves omissions. Thus, according to Beauchamp and Childress, possible harms associated with potential therapeutics are given more weight in a risk-benefit analysis than the possible benefits. For clarity, Table 1 presents a brief formulation of the principles of beneficence and nonmaleficence of Beauchamp and Childress.

Different Kinds of Beneficence

The question remains, however, whether we are obligated to sacrifice ourselves to benefit others. Beauchamp and Childress believe that there are limits to the demands of beneficence. They distinguish between *obligatory beneficence* (in the forms of general beneficence and specific beneficence) and *optional beneficence* (in the form of ideals of beneficence).

General Beneficence

According to Beauchamp and Childress, a person X has a determinate obligation of beneficence toward Person Y if and only if each of the conditions listed in Table 2 is satisfied (assuming X is aware of the relevant facts).

Specific Beneficence

Beauchamp and Childress state that obligations of specific beneficence usually rest on special moral

Table 1 Two of the four principles of biomedical ethics: beneficence and nonmaleficence (a brief formulation of the bioethical principles of beneficence and nonmaleficence of Beauchamp and Childress)

The principle of beneficence

- ☐ One ought to prevent and remove evil or harm.
- ☐ One ought to do and promote good.
- ☐ One ought to weigh and balance the possible goods against the possible harms of an action.

The principle of nonmaleficence

- ☐ One ought not to inflict evil or harm. Or, more specifically, one ought not to hurt other people mentally or physically.

Table 2 Conditions determining the obligation of general beneficence of Beauchamp and Childress

1. Y is at risk of significant loss of or damage to life or health or some other major interest.
2. X's action is needed (singly or in concert with others) to prevent this loss or damage.
3. X's action (single or in concert with others) has a high probability of preventing it.
4. X's action would not present significant risks, costs, or burdens to X.
5. The benefit that Y can be expected to gain outweighs any harms, costs, or burdens that X is likely to incur.

relations (e.g., in families and friendships) or on special commitments, such as explicit promises and roles with attendant responsibilities (such as healthcare professional and patient).

Ideal Beneficence

Beauchamp and Childress make a distinction between ideal beneficence and obligatory beneficence in terms of the costs and the risks to the agents of beneficence. Ideals of beneficence involve severe sacrifice and extreme altruism in the moral life (e.g., giving both of one's kidneys for transplantation). According to Beauchamp and Childress, persons do not have an obligation of ideal beneficence; other persons can admire those who fulfill the ideal, but they cannot blame or criticize those who do not practice it.

Strength of Principles

According to Beauchamp and Childress, ethical issues of biomedicine not only include the balance of the possible harms and the possible benefits (risk-benefit analysis), it also includes considerations about respecting the autonomy of the patient or the human subject and justice considerations

regarding healthcare allocation. They argue that the four ethical principles of (1) beneficence, (2) nonmaleficence, (3) respect for autonomy, and (4) justice are central to and play a vital role in biomedicine. Table 3 presents a brief formulation of the bioethical principles of respect for autonomy and justice of Beauchamp and Childress.

According to Beauchamp and Childress, no one principle ranks higher than the others. Which principles should be given most weight depends on the context of the given situation. Beauchamp and Childress consider the four principles as *prima facie binding*; that is, they must be fulfilled, unless they conflict on a particular occasion with an equal or stronger principle. These ethicists believe that some acts are at the same time prima facie wrong and prima facie right, since two or more principles may conflict in some circumstances. Agents must then determine what they ought to do by finding an actual or overriding principle. This means that the agents must find the best balance of right and wrong by determining their actual obligations in such situations by examining the respective weights of the competing prima facie principles. For instance, in modern medicine, patients' right to make judgments about treatment is valued. It is discussed in biomedical ethics whether respect for

Table 3   Two of the four principles of biomedical ethics: respect for autonomy and justice (a brief formulation of the bioethical principles of respect for autonomy and justice of Beauchamp and Childress)

The principle of respect for autonomy

- As a negative obligation: Autonomous actions should not be subjected to controlling constraints by others.
- As a positive obligation: This principle requires respectful treatment in disclosing information, probing for and ensuring understanding and voluntariness, and fostering autonomous decision making.

This principle does not count for persons who are not able to act autonomously: Infants and drug-dependent patients are examples. However, these persons are protected by the principles of beneficence and nonmaleficence.

The principle of justice

Beauchamp and Childress examine several philosophical theories of justice, including egalitarian theories that emphasize equal access to the goods in life that every rational person values. Beauchamp & Childress propose that society should recognize an enforceable right to a decent minimum of healthcare within a framework for allocation that incorporates both utilitarian and egalitarian principles.

the autonomy of patients should have priority over professional beneficence directed at those patients; hence, there are conflicts between beneficence and respect for autonomy (the problem of paternalism).

Beauchamp and Childress believe that the principles find support across different cultures. They claim that the principles are part of a cross-cultural common morality and that in all cultures people who are serious about moral conduct accept the norms of this common morality. However, even though these principles are generally acknowledged, this does not mean that there is consensus about what is good and bad; the principles are to be specified, balanced, and interpreted in different cultural settings.

Although Beauchamp and Childress's theory is widely used and outstanding in bioethics, it is also subject to much philosophical discussion. For example, in an attempt to criticize philosophical bioethics in general, the ethicist Adam M. Hedgecoe points to Beauchamp and Childress's theory in his 2004 article, *Critical Bioethics: Beyond the Social Science Critique of Applied Ethics*, because principlism is the dominant way of doing bioethics. Hedgecoe claims that philosophical bioethics gives a dominant role to idealized rational thought and tends to exclude social and cultural factors. He believes that principlism defends abstract universal

principles without empirical evidence and that principlism develops and justifies theories without paying attention to the practical application of those theories. As an alternative to principlism, Hedgecoe defends the position of what he calls *critical bioethics,* where the results of empirical research feed back to challenge and even undermine the theoretical framework of bioethics.

Some ethicists do not think that Hedgecoe's critique of Beauchamp and Childress's theory is justified. First of all, according to Beauchamp and Childress, there is no straightforward movement from principles to particular judgments. Principles are only the starting points and, as such, general guidelines for the development of norms of appropriate conduct. The principles need to be supplemented by paradigm cases of right action, empirical data, organizational experience, and so on. Beauchamp and Childress state that rights, virtues, and emotional responses are as important as principles for ethical judgment. Secondly, in his 2003 article, *A Defense of the Common Morality*, Beauchamp stresses the importance of empirical research for ethical principles. He claims that the usefulness of the four principles can be tested empirically and that the question of whether they are part of a cross-cultural common morality can be explored. Beauchamp does not present any empirical data generated systematically by qualitative research to support this position. But he does invite the design of an empirical research study to investigate the issue. For example, a Danish empirical study by Mette Ebbesen and B. D. Pedersen shows that the four bioethical principles of Beauchamp and Childress are reflected in the daily work of Danish oncologist physicians and Danish molecular biologists. Empirical research can likely improve the bioethical theory of principles by bringing it into concord with practice.

Mette Ebbesen

See also Bioethics; Risk-Benefit Trade-Off

Further Readings

Beauchamp, T. L., & Childress, J. F. (1989). *Principles of biomedical ethics* (3rd ed.). Oxford, UK: Oxford University Press.

Beauchamp, T. L., & Childress. J. F. (2001). *Principles of biomedical ethics* (5th ed.). Oxford, UK: Oxford University Press.

DeGrazia, D. (1992). Moving forward in bioethical theory: Theories, cases, and specified principlism. *Journal of Medicine and Philosophy, 17,* 511–539.

Ebbesen, M., & Pedersen, B. D. (2007). Using empirical research to formulate normative ethical principles in biomedicine. *Medicine, Health Care, and Philosophy, 10*(1), 33–48.

Ebbesen, M., & Pedersen, B. D. (2008). The principle of respect for autonomy: Concordant with the experience of oncology physicians and molecular biologists in their daily work? *BMC Medical Ethics, 9,* 5.

Engelhardt, H. T., Jr. (1998). Critical care: Why there is no global bioethics. *Journal of Medicine and Philosophy, 23*(6), 643–651.

Frankena, W. (1973). *Ethics* (2nd ed.). Englewood Cliffs, NJ: Prentice Hall.

Hedgecoe, A. M. (2004). Critical bioethics: Beyond the social science critique of applied ethics. *Bioethics, 18*(2), 120–143.

Holm, S. (1995). Not just autonomy: The principles of American biomedical ethics. *Journal of Medical Ethics, 21*(6), 332–338.

Lustig, B. A. (1998). Concepts and methods in recent bioethics: Critical responses. *Journal of Medicine and Bioethics, 23*(5), 445–455.

O'Neill, O. (2001). Practical principles & practical judgment. *Hastings Center Report, 31*(4), 15–23.

Pellegrino, E. (2008). *The philosophy of medicine reborn: A Pellegrino reader.* Notre Dame, IN: University of Notre Dame Press.

Strong, C. (2000). Specified principlism: What is it, and does it really resolve cases better than casuistry? *Journal of Medicine and Philosophy, 25*(3), 323–341.

BIAS

In statistics, *bias* generally refers to a systematic distortion of a statistical result. Bias can occur in both the process of data collection and the statistical procedures of data analysis. Very few studies can avoid bias at some point in sample selection, study conduct, and results interpretation. Analysis of results without correcting the bias can be misleading and harmful in decision making. With careful and prolonged planning, researchers may reduce or eliminate many potential sources of bias. Collaboration between the statistician and the domain expert is very important, since many biases are specific to a given application area. This entry discusses two different aspects that the term *bias* is commonly used to describe.

Bias in Sampling

Bias in sampling is the tendency that the samples differ from the target population from which the samples are drawn in some systematic ways. A few important concepts include the following.

Biased Sample

Most biases occur during data collection, often as a result of taking observations from an unrepresentative subset of the population rather than from the population as a whole. A sample is said to be a *biased sample* if the probability of a member in the population being sampled depends on the true value(s) of one or more variables of interest of that member. The sampling process that leads to a biased sample is called *biased sampling*. For example, if women with a family history of breast cancer are more eager to join a mammography program, the sample of women in the mammography program is a biased sample of all women. If the variable(s) is important to a study, conclusions based on biased samples may not be valid for the population of interest.

Sample weights can sometimes be used for correcting the bias if some groups are underrepresented in the population. For instance, a hypothetical population might include 50 million men and 50 million women. Suppose that a biased sample of 100 patients included 70 men and 30 women. A researcher can correct for this imbalance by attaching a weight of 5/7 for each male and 5/3 for each female. This would adjust estimates to achieve the same expected value as a sample that included exactly 50 men and 50 women.

Response Bias

Response bias is a type of cognitive bias that occurs when the sampled members from a population tend to produce values that systematically differ from the true values. It happens frequently in survey studies and affects the results of a statistical survey, especially when the questions on a survey are not properly worded or if the question relates to some variables that are sensitive to the members being surveyed, such as household income or drug history. In such situations, respondents answer questions in the way they think the questioner wants them to answer rather than according to their true beliefs.

Nonresponse Bias

Nonresponse bias is an extreme form of biased sampling. Nonresponse bias occurs when responses are not obtainable from all members selected for inclusion in the sample. Nonresponse bias can severely affect the results if those who respond differ from those who do not respond in important ways. Online and phone-in pools may be subject to nonresponse biases because many members in the target population may not have a phone or access to the Internet.

Measurement Bias

The term *measurement error bias* usually refers to systematic deviation from the true value as a result of a faulty measurement instrument, for instance, an improperly calibrated scale. Several measurements of the same quantity on the same experiment unit will not in general be the same. This may be because of natural variation in the measurement process. In statistical analysis, measurement error in covariates has three main effects: (1) It causes bias in parameter estimation for statistical models; (2) it leads to a loss of power, sometimes profound, for detecting interesting relationship among variables; and (3) it masks the features of the data, making graphical model analysis difficult.

Censoring Bias

Censoring bias occurs when a value occurs outside the range of a measuring instrument. Limitations in censoring at either end of the scale can result in biased estimates. For example, a bathroom scale might only measure up to 250 pounds. If a 320-pound individual is weighed using the scale, the observer would only know that the individual's weight is at least 250 pounds. Censoring bias is also common in survival analysis. Special techniques may be used to handle censored data.

Bias in Estimation

Another kind of bias in statistics does not involve biased samples but does involve the use of a statistic whose average value differs from the value of the quantity being estimated. In parameter estimation, bias refers to the difference between the expected value of an estimator and the true value of the parameter being estimated. An estimator with zero bias is called an *unbiased estimator*, and an estimator having nonzero bias is said to be a *biased estimator*.

Suppose a researcher is trying to estimate the parameter μ using an estimator $\hat{\mu}$ (i.e., a certain function of the observed data). The bias of the estimator μ is defined as the expected value of the difference between the estimator and the true value. This can be written mathematically as

$$\text{Bias}(\hat{\mu}) = E(\hat{\mu} - \mu) = E(\hat{\mu}) - \mu.$$

A famous example of a biased estimator is the sample variance. Suppose $X_1, X_1, \ldots, X_n$ are independent and identically distributed (i.i.d.) random variables with expectation μ and variance σ^2. The sample mean is defined as

$$\bar{X} = \frac{X_1 + X_2 + \cdots + X_n}{n},$$

and the sample variance is defined as

$$S^2 = \frac{1}{n}\sum_{i=1}^{n}(X_i - \bar{X})^2.$$

It can be shown that the sample mean is an unbiased estimator, while the sample variance is a biased estimator, where

$$E(\bar{X}) = \mu, \; E(S^2) = \frac{n-1}{n}\sigma^2 \neq \sigma^2.$$

Although biased estimators sound pejorative, they may have desirable statistical properties. For example, they sometimes have a smaller mean squared error than any unbiased estimator. Biased estimators are used in some special cases of statistical analysis.

Xiao-Feng Wang and Bin Wang

See also Bias in Scientific Studies; Probability Errors

Further Readings

Indrayan, A., & Sarmukaddam, S. B. (2001). *Medical biostatistics*. New York: Marcel Dekker.

Stewart, A., & McPherson, K. (2007). *Basic statistics and epidemiology: A practical guide* (2nd ed.). New York: Radcliffe.

BIASES IN HUMAN PREDICTION

In the language of cognitive psychology, the ability to predict is the ability to infer, estimate, and judge the character of unknown events. By this definition, a large part of clinical medicine requires that physicians make medical predictions. Despite its importance, it remains subject to many biases. There are a number of important biases affecting medical prediction in diagnosis, prognosis, and treatment choices. This is particularly true in emotionally intense medical circumstances at the end of life. Physicians, patients, and policy makers should be aware of these biases when confronted with decisions in all these circumstances to help avoid their consequences. This entry outlines ways in which cognitive biases often prevent accurate medical predictions across a number of decision-making situations.

Medical Prediction

One major type of medical prediction is the diagnosis of patients' disease. Diagnosis involves gathering and integrating evidence, testing hypotheses, and assessing probabilities. This requires that a clinician be able to generate accurate predictions from incomplete data about the underlying cause(s) of the patient's symptoms. For example, the symptom "pelvic pain" might be caused by a urinary tract infection, a sexually transmitted infection, or by cancer, among other possible diagnoses. A physician who sees a patient with this symptom must accurately predict the likelihood of multiple possible underlying causes to effectively gather evidence (i.e., ask about other possible symptoms and order appropriate tests), cognitively integrate that evidence, and determine the most probable diagnosis.

Once the physician has made a diagnosis, he or she must, along with the patient, make another medical prediction when they decide together on a treatment decision. Selecting the optimal treatment from multiple options requires that a clinician be able to predict which treatment will provide the patient with the best possible health outcome, accounting for both positive and negative effects. For example, a patient with localized prostate cancer has multiple treatment options available, including surgery, radiation therapy (of two types), hormone deprivation therapy, and surveillance. To make a treatment recommendation, a physician must predict the patient's response to various treatments, both in terms of disease control and potential burden from treatment side effects. The physician must also consider the patient's overall health, comorbidities, resources, social support, and preferences for possible health states.

Physicians also make medical predictions when necessary to provide prognoses, which are predictions of the likely duration, course, and outcome of a disease based on the treatment chosen. This is particularly important in diseases, such as terminal cancer, where patients and their families wish to form appropriate timelines for goals of care and to have access to certain types of care, such as hospice, when they would most benefit from them. Unfortunately, as Nicholas Christakis has shown, prognosis is particularly difficult in emotionally intense situations such as this.

Given the centrality of accurate predictions to medical decision making and the common assumption that medical training improves physician's decisions, it is disheartening that research has repeatedly shown that physicians' medical predictions are as susceptible to cognitive biases as others are in nonmedical domains. The mistakes are systematic, not random, errors that are likely due to the difficulty of the prediction task combined with human psychology. Thus, these biases are not significantly reduced by current medical training. As Reid Hastie and Robyn Dawes argue, one of the most persistent of these biases is overconfidence concerning one's predictions. The danger of overconfidence is that one cannot begin to correct other biases affecting the quality of one's predictions; simply recognizing their existence is something that overconfidence prevents. For example, an overconfident surgeon might regularly predict better surgical outcomes for his or her patients and perform surgeries on patients who are poor candidates for surgery. This overconfidence bias will go uncorrected because it is unrecognized as a systematic error.

Biases Affecting Diagnosis

The way in which possible diseases are represented has been shown to give rise to systematically different probability predictions in diagnosis. In one study, house officers were given a case description of a 22-year-old woman with right lower quadrant abdominal pain of 12 hours' duration. Half were asked to estimate the probabilities of the competing diagnostic possibilities gastroenteritis, ectopic pregnancy, or neither. The other half were asked to estimate the probabilities of five diagnoses: (1) gastroenteritis, (2) ectopic pregnancy, (3) appendicitis, (4) pyelonephritis, (5) pelvic inflammatory disease, or "none of the above." Although physicians in both groups were told that their probabilities must sum to 100%, the judged probability of "none of the above" was significantly smaller in the shorter list (50%) of diagnoses than in the longer list (69%). Logically, the opposite should be true, since the additional choices decrease the chances of none of the available diagnoses being correct.

This suggests that physicians do not think enough about diagnoses that are either not listed or that are not what they are currently thinking that the underlying problem might be, and that they don't pay close enough attention to probabilistic

information such as the "base rate" of the disease in the population. In medicine, this can lead to inappropriate confirmatory testing, where physicians increase costs without increasing the likelihood of a correct diagnosis. That is, they order tests that will confirm what they already know, making them overly confident of their diagnoses without actually providing any new information. In the long term, overconfidence and failure to correct for cognitive biases cause more experienced physicians to be more confident, but not more accurate, than less experienced physicians. It is easy to see how this can perpetuate a pattern of misdiagnosed and inappropriately treated patients because, as findings from social psychology have demonstrated, less confident and experienced people are more likely to defer to more experienced experts than to try to find alternative explanations.

The first step in correcting such biases is to demonstrate their existence and to alert physicians to their presence. However, another common cognitive bias, the hindsight bias, makes it difficult to learn from cases that show the errors of others. This bias has been demonstrated experimentally in physicians. In the relevant experiment, five different groups of physicians were presented with a challenging diagnostic case describing a patient with a mix of symptoms along with four potential diagnoses. Physicians in the control group were asked to predict the likelihood of each of the four diagnoses given the symptoms. Those in the other four groups were told which of the potential diagnoses was the "actual" one (each group was given a different one) and asked for the probabilities that they would have assigned to each of the four diagnoses. Physicians in each of the four "hindsight" groups inflated the probability that they would have assigned to the diagnosis they were told was correct. This has an important clinical implication because of the similarity of the experimental conditions to teaching rounds presentations. Challenging diagnostic cases presented authoritatively at teaching rounds may seem far more obvious than they really are because of hindsight bias, leading medical team members to fail to learn the difficulty of prediction illustrated by the case because they "knew it all along."

Biases Affecting Prognosis

Physicians also often commit the value-induced bias in medical prediction in which they unknowingly distort relevant probabilities regarding patient prognosis so as to justify poorly justified treatment choices. This bias helps explain why such a high percentage of the U.S. healthcare budget is spent on patients in the last 6 weeks of life. No physician wants to give up on a desperately ill patient (who may be cured) by stopping treatment, so physicians exaggerate the likelihood of success from treatment. This often leads to prolonging invasive (and often painful) treatments in the face of overwhelming odds against success in the belief that the patient might benefit, even though statistics are clearly against such an outcome.

Accurate prognosis is most valuable to patients and their families, and most difficult for physicians, in life-limiting illnesses such as terminal cancer. Physicians are remarkably poor at predicting the life expectancies of patients with terminal illnesses. In his book on medical prognosis at the end of life, Christakis points out that while prognosis can be a technically difficult task for physicians in many circumstances, the emotional difficulties associated with prognosis at the end of life make their prognoses in such cases even worse.

One of the biases that Christakis emphasizes is the superstitious belief in self-fulfilling prophecies of prognoses. In these situations, physicians seem to feel that by acknowledging a limited prognosis and treating appropriately with palliation, physicians will hasten a patient's demise. Evidence demonstrates that this is not the case; patients undergoing palliative care live just as long (or longer) as similarly diagnosed patients who have been given overly optimistic prognostic information. He demonstrates that physicians are far more likely to ameliorate patient pessimism or provide encouragement, even when unwarranted, than they are to correct unrealistic optimism. Although the motivation to provide hope to one's patients that motivates this response is largely a positive and compassionate one, the responsibility to provide accurate prognostic information and appropriate treatment planning is equally important, something this bias prevents.

Biases Affecting Treatment

To select the best treatment for a patient, a physician must predict the patient's adherence to the therapy. This is more challenging than it might at first appear, because even though patients generally do want to adhere to their treatment regimes, it is much easier to talk about changing a future behavior (e.g., taking a medicine regularly) than it is to actually do it. This "empathy gap" between one's current situation and one's future situation makes it very hard for physicians to appreciate the power of various visceral factors causing patients to make choices that they know are not good for their health.

For example, studies show that adherence to a medication schedule drops with the number of pills a patient is to take. So a physician might prescribe a blood pressure medication to a hypertensive patient (who is already taking several other medications), only to find out at a follow-up visit that the patient's hypertension has not improved. The problem may be that the patient needs a higher dose of the medication. However, there is also a substantial probability that the patient has not managed to adhere to the medication schedule. Nevertheless, studies comparing physician-prescribing behavior with patient prescription-filling behavior indicate that physicians almost always respond by prescribing the higher dosage, even when the prescription for the lower dosage is not being refilled. Physicians fail to predict that patients are not taking the currently prescribed dose.

Most people, including physicians, tend to underweight statistical evidence relative to other forms of evidence such as personal experience. Even though physicians are now trained in evidence-based medicine (EBM), which emphasizes following statistical guidelines based on the medical literature, they often fail to apply relevant statistical data. For example, statistical data tell us that there is no survival advantage to using pulmonary artery catheterization in the intensive care unit to guide fluid management for patients, making this an unnecessary procedure for guiding treatment choices. However, it is still commonly practiced because it is experientially convincing to closely monitor a patient's pulmonary artery pressures, even knowing that doing so does not improve patient outcomes. Before EBM, monitoring pulmonary arterial pressures via catheterization seemed like a logical thing to do based on pathophysiology; however, data do not support this practice. Thus, the practice continued beyond its statistical justification.

William Dale, Liz Moliski,
and Joshua Hemmerich

See also Diagnostic Process, Making a Diagnosis;
    Physician Estimates of Prognosis; Prediction Rules and
    Modeling

Further Readings

Chapman, G. B., & Sonnenberg, F. A. (Eds.). (2000).
    *Decision making in health care: Theory, psychology,
    and applications.* Cambridge, UK: Cambridge
    University Press.
Christakis, N. (1999). *Death foretold: Prophecy and
    prognosis in medical care.* Chicago: University of
    Chicago Press.
Glare, P., Virik, K., Jones, M., Hudson, M., Eychmuller,
    S., Simes, J., et al. (2003). A systematic review of
    physicians' survival predictions in terminally ill cancer
    patients. *British Medical Journal, 327,* 195–198.
Hastie, R., & Dawes, R. M. (2001). *Rational choice in
    an uncertain world: The psychology of judgment and
    decision making.* Thousand Oaks, CA: Sage.
Loewenstein, G., Read, D., & Baumeister, R. F. (Eds.).
    (2003). *Time and decision: Economic and
    psychological perspectives on intertemporal choice.*
    Thousand Oaks, CA: Sage.
The National Heart, Lung, and Blood Institute Acute
    Respiratory Distress Syndrome (ARDS) Clinical Trials
    Network. (2006). Pulmonary-artery versus central
    venous catheter to guide treatment of acute lung injury.
    New England Journal of Medicine, 354, 2213–2224.
Stone, P. C., & Lund, S. (2007). Predicting prognosis in
    patients with advanced cancer. *Annals of Oncology,
    18,* 971–976.

Bias in Scientific Studies

In empirical science, bias is any factor that may
systematically distort quantitative or qualitative
conclusions and recommendations. Psychological
sources of biases have separate encyclopedia
entries.

Delimitation

Bias must be distinguished from fraud, oversights,
misunderstandings, and nonsense arithmetic. It must
further be distinguished from the field of statistical
pitfalls, illusions, and paradoxes, though each of
these, when unrecognized, may bias perceptions and
recommendations.

The classical borderline between random error
and bias is sometimes fuzzy. The label "bias" is
often used about poor data recording, regardless
of whether it will affect conclusions and, if so,
how. Moreover, blunt procedures (imprecise measurements) may delay the recognition of a health
hazard, or benefit, and in that sense pure randomness is itself "biased" against public interests.

Recognition of Bias

Just as, while there is no checklist for the quality of
poems, one can develop one's flair for good poetry,
the field of bias is open ended. Notwithstanding
attempts, it is impossible to devise an exhaustive
list of mutually exclusive bias types. Even broad
categories such as selection bias and information
bias meet at hazy frontiers. But everybody can
train his or her flair for detecting bias.

Overly critical readers sometimes find bias
where it isn't (*bias bias*), or reject investigations on
grounds of bias even when the bias is obviously
negligible or purely hypothetical.

Texts often explain a bias by means of hypothetical examples from which all unnecessary
adornment has been peeled off. This is the strength,
not the weakness, of such examples. "Real patients
do not look like that!" is an often-heard but invalid
objection. Precisely, the complexity of clinical data
often lies behind an investigator's failure to realize
that his or her research procedure is biased.

The Estimand

One cannot discuss hits and misses without a
bull's-eye. So any discussion of bias presupposes a
defined target, the estimand. Not until agreement
about the estimand has been reached can the statistician and client proceed to discuss bias and,
subsequently, random uncertainty. Key questions
are as follows: What do we want to measure? What
is a rational measure thereof? For example, What is
a rational measure of successful rehabilitation after
multitrauma? What precisely is meant by "the
waiting time for liver transplantation in 2006"?

There are four rules of thumb for establishing
the estimand. (1) It should be conceptually well-
defined (often by imagining an ideal method being
applied to 10,000 truly representative cases). (2) Its
definition should be detached from study design

(i.e., it should parameterize the object process, not the inspection process, with its potential sources of bias). (3) In predictive settings, prospectivity should be built into the definition. This calls for a notion of "a population of naturally occurring identical-looking instances" (*case stream*), to which predictions are meant to apply. Anything that requires hindsight should be weeded out. Care must be taken to define the right units of prediction (women vs. pregnancies; bladder tumors vs. control cystoscopies). (4) Biased and data-driven agendas should be avoided. These remarks apply, *mutatis mutandis*, to qualitative research questions as well.

In studies whose key purpose is comparative, *internal validity* refers to the comparison being fair and *external validity* to the comparison's matching an envisaged target population. *Generalizability* (a broader term) refers to the applicability of study results outside the population sampled.

Formal Definitions of Bias

In theoretical statistics, the bias of a data-summarizing estimator is defined as the amount by which its expected value departs from the population (object-process) parameter, the estimand:

$$\text{Bias} = E(\text{Estimator}) - (\text{Estimand}).$$

An estimator is unbiased when the departure is zero for all values of the parameters in the statistical model of the object process. As an example, for the purpose of estimating a population mean, any average of independent observations is—provably—unbiased, no matter what their common distribution looks like. Their median, on the other hand, is rarely unbiased, except when the distribution is symmetric.

The logarithm of an unbiased estimator is not an unbiased estimator of the log estimand; the same holds true for other nonlinear transformations. In practical biostatistics, many ratio statistics, such as epidemiological odds ratios (OR), are unbiased on log scale, at least approximately. Neither the estimated OR nor its inverse is then unbiased for its estimand. However, unlike the biases engendered by methodological flaws, these "mathematical" biases are often small and tend to zero as sample sizes increase (*asymptotic unbiasedness*) typically faster than the associated standard error (*SE*).

Bias-variance trade-off: In moderately complicated statistical models, the analyst may face a choice between two or more estimator statistics, one of which has little bias, another a low variance. If the loss associated with misestimation is proportional to squared error, [(Estimator) − (Estimand)]², one would choose the estimator that minimizes the mean square error (*MSE*). The way this quantity depends on estimator bias and variance is simple:

$$MSE = E\{[(\text{Estimator}) - (\text{Estimand})]^2\} = \text{Bias}^2 + \text{Variance}.$$

Typical applications are those with an inherent risk of overfitting the data: probability density estimation, multivariate discrimination (statistical diagnosis), recursive partitioning trees, and so on.

Conditional bias and unbiasedness, given a (hidden or observable) event E, refer to the conditional distribution of the estimator given that E is present.

A *median-unbiased* estimator overrates and underrates the estimand equally often.

A *significance test* is said to be *biased* if the probability of rejecting the null hypothesis is sometimes smaller when it is false than when it is true: With a test at the 5% level, certain alternatives enjoy a power <5% (Type II error risk > 95%). Everyday statistical tests are designed to maximize power and have little or no bias.

Confidence limits: Confidence intervals around a biased estimator typically inherit the bias, but there is no standard notion of bias in connection with confidence limits. Relevant concerns include the following. Incorrect coverage is when a nominal 95% interval will straddle the true value of the estimand either more or less than 95 times out of 100. More appropriately, an upper 97.5% limit can be said to be biased if the probability that it exceeds the estimand is not .975: The limit is either misleadingly large or does not offer the claimed protection. Analogous remarks apply to the lower limit. Confidence intervals offer protection against random variation only; protection against bias must rest on plausible assumptions concerning systematic errors, preferably built into sensitivity analyses. If a data summary is beset with a bias of unknown magnitude, the protection offered by a confidence interval is spurious, unless the bias is obviously small relative to the width of the interval.

Biases in the Scientific Process

Biased Agendas

Sticking to easy, noncontroversial, and fundable aspects of a health problem could count as biased question asking. Health outcomes, for example, are easier to handle than questions of patient-physician rapport.

Data-Driven Agendas

The decision of what questions to answer and what parameters to estimate should be made beforehand (frequentist statistical theory presupposes that estimates and tests are reported no matter how the observations turn out). When clinical trialists selectively report those outcomes that have produced statistically significant differences, we have an instance of data-driven question asking, and their report should be received with skepticism due to the perils of *multiplicity* (multiple tests bombarding the same null hypothesis) and data dredging. Selective reporting also presents a severe obstacle to meta-analyses that try to amalgamate several studies.

Data Dredging

Data dredging is when researchers keep ransacking their data set until something "significant" turns up. One can have equally little trust in diagnostic indices, or indices of therapeutic success, constructed by combining the variables on file in myriad ways and choosing the "best" fit (almost certainly an overfit). *Repeated peeking* at the data as they accrue is similar: When trends in the data themselves codetermine when to stop and produce a report, we have an *"informative"* (bias-prone) *stopping rule.* Stopping as soon as, but only when, the data look sufficiently promising will bias results in an optimistic direction.

Conceptual Bias

The interpretation of a given data set is restricted—one may say biased—by narrowness of theoretical outlook (or Kuhnian paradigm). One straight-jacket is the idea of the natural course of a disease

process. Cholecystectomy was once suspected of causing gastrointestinal cancer. This reflected a failure to realize that premonitory cancerous dyspepsia plus silent gallstones sometimes triggered a cholecystectomy: The association was the diagnosticians' own fault! In sum, disease processes—and the hypotheses formed about them—are shaped, in part, by healthcare culture, its imperfections, and its self-image.

Publication Bias

Investigations having something new or significant to tell are more promptly and widely published. Hence the published literature on any particular date remains biased relative to the body of data analyses actually completed. *Double publication* adds a further slant, as does *citation bias*: Not only are investigators likely to cite preferentially the studies they agree with, but there also appear to be much-cited papers that become cited just because everybody else cites them. The net effect is a self-perpetuating body of knowledge, or prejudice, with insufficient built-in bias correction.

Additional Biases

Unlike the preceding "sociological" topics, the flaws that follow are primarily the responsibility of the individual research team. Again, dishonest action and simple oversights will be bypassed, as will breaches of good research practice.

Bias-prone handling of numerical data includes rounding problems (e.g., age on last birthday vs. exact age). *Misleading design of graphs and tables* should be caught by senior authors or at peer review. Narrow-minded interpretation, or an attempt to save words, may lie behind *misleading conclusions.* A statistical association may easily become "Young taxi drivers were more accident prone," suggesting causality. "Analgesic A proved superior to B" deprives readers of a chance to question the choice of doses.

Blunt analyses are biased toward the "nothing new" conclusion:

1. Unnecessary dichotomization is wasteful of information.

2. Chopping up the data set, with the laudable aim of comparing like with like (*stratification*), may

produce several nonsignificant tests and leave a cross-stratum effect undocumented.

3. Investigators taught to observe certain rules, such as reserving *t* tests for normally distributed data, give up halfway due to "violated assumptions" instead of exploiting the robustness of most statistical procedures. Again, results will be valid but vague. Replace the virtuous stance with a valiant one, and the data will speak.

Biased Data Collection

Overall distortions of answers or measurements may or may not bias results, as in the case of observer-interviewer effects, including interactions (elderly people may balk at the jargon and manners of young interviewers); Hawthorne effects (disciplined behavior when under observation); framing effects (wording of questions); or effects of embarrassing questions and forced choices.

Changes in data collection over time lead to treacherous biases. Examples include training and fatigue effects when interviewers have to conduct interviews over several months and unnoticed slippage or change of reagents in the lab.

Selection bias is a common term for bias due to the sampling of study units being misaligned with the intended population (despite a random or exhaustive sampling scheme). The little fish slip through the net; the big fish tear it apart. Death notices in newspapers are a biased source of longevity data.

Ascertainment bias refers to the data source: Telephone interviewing was notorious for reaching mostly middle-class people. Clinical materials that comprise a woolly mix of prevalent and incident cases are not representative of any recognizable population and, therefore, are biased regardless of study purpose. People who volunteer are self-selected and probably special.

In clinical studies, consecutive enrollment is the primary safeguard against selective forces. Randomized allocation serves to prevent skewed recruitment of comparison groups, and, by facilitating blinding, it helps prevent other types of bias. Concealment of allocation extends the veil of blinding backward to cover enrollment deliberations.

Chronic-disease trials preferentially recruit those who are dissatisfied with their current treatment; the result is a potential bias in favor of any new drug and a selection skew relative to an unselected stream of "my next patient" (first-time as well as chronic cases).

Healthy-worker, or healthy-survivor, *effects* refers to the notion that those who do not give in or succumb to occupational and other stresses are the strong and healthy; even after years of toil and exposure, they may still be healthier, or appear sturdier, than others.

Once selected, cases may be subjected to flawed intervention or flawed data recording. Flawed interventions lead to *performance bias* (think of unequal surgical skills) and *collateral treatment bias* due to secret use of supplementary medication.

As to data recording, *information bias* arises when the study objects "influence" the amount, kind, or quality of their data records. When chemical exposure is documented through labor union records, comparisons may end up being misleading because some trades are associated with less organized lifestyles (even in the absence of solvent-induced brain damage). *Recall bias* in a narrower sense would exist if those with neuropsychological impairment were, or were helped to become, more aware of past exposure. *Missing data* will cause bias if reluctance to provide data is somehow related to the study question (if an eligible subject's very existence also remains unrecorded, a selection problem is added).

Unequal contact with healthcare providers may skew the records (*surveillance, detection, verification, workup, access bias*). The risk of endometrial neoplasia in women on menopausal hormone replacement therapy once seemed high, but the excess was explained by occasional curettage prompted by bleeding.

Attrition bias: Dropouts from clinical trials pose a major problem, whether unbalanced or not, as the strict intention to treat (ITT) paradigm requires all outcomes to be recorded and utility assessed, preferably with equal precision.

Investigator-induced information bias: In the context of diagnostic test evaluation, *discrepant analysis* consists in trying to resolve discrepancies between the study test and the reference test by appealing to one or more arbiter tests in the hope of proving the reference test wrong; cases of agreement are not similarly challenged. An optimistic bias ensues.

Purity bias: Clinical investigators are sometimes obsessed with purity. They are reluctant to delve into the muddy waters of everyday case streams. Patients are thrown out arbitrarily when they look "atypical," even retrospectively. The resulting biases mostly involve violations of prospectivity. Downright short-circuits may occur, for example, when drugs intended to reduce infarct size suppress the infarct markers and lead to a final diagnosis of no infarction. Here, the prospective indication (clinical problem) was, and should remain, presumptive infarction.

In a quest for precision—a variant of purity—an oncologist in one study chose to disregard cancer recurrences not datable within ±2 months. As X-ray intervals rose to 6 months after 2 years without recurrence, many late recurrences were discarded, biasing not just the frequency and timing of recurrences but also the ratio between symptomatic and silent ones.

Uncertain Predictors and Covariates

Borrowing a term from radio engineering, statisticians use the word *noise* as a shorthand for unwanted random variation, regardless of source and cause. Noise affecting predictors or covariates gives rise to bias problems quite different from those connected with noisy response variables. One distinguishes between nondifferential and differential misclassification/distortion; that is, given the true predictor, is the noise independent of the response, or not?

Nondifferential Distortion

In a linear regression context, proportional misrepresentation of the predictor causes a proportional change in the apparent regression coefficient (in the opposite direction), whereas a fixed additive term is innocuous; tests are unaffected. Independent measurement variation (additive noise) attenuates the regression coefficient by a factor $S^2/(S^2 + s^2)$, where S is the SD of the true predictor and s the noise SD; tests also lose power. Other regression models are affected in roughly the same way. Multivariate-covariate adjustments also bias regression coefficients, but there is no general rule about the direction. In two-group comparisons, group differences are also attenuated or destroyed by misclassification.

However, additive noise in predictors may interact with data selection to produce insidious biases, especially when the protocol requires a predictor, such as fasting blood glucose, to stay within the normal range.

Differential Misclassification

Differential misclassification is serious and always subtle. A dietary habit that has been falsely accused of being harmful is given up by those who want to lead, and do lead, a healthy life. The incidence of a disease now proves higher among those who confess to the habit: False suspicion = Conviction (due to population [self-]manipulation). Related is the *treatment paradox*: When known danger signals during pregnancy prompt referral and special care, neonatal outcomes are equalized, falsely suggesting that referrals are unnecessary.

Dependent Observations

Dependent observations may bias comparisons, in addition to invalidating the SE formulae. For example, in an individually randomized trial of intensive versus standard poststroke support, patients in the gym share their experiences, producing correlated follow-up interviews; cross-talk between the randomization arms weakens the apparent intervention effect. So neither the observed effect nor its nominal SE can be trusted.

Special Bias Mechanisms

Time-related phenomena cause bias if ignored, *censoring* being a familiar example. Similar information biases arise when what happens outside a time window is unobservable or when enrollment is conditional on some event occurring within the window (a *truncation*). For example, conditionally on giving birth within a study window, women are interrogated concerning time to conception; subfertile women are thereby preferentially excluded.

Length bias, *size bias*: The larger the stone on the beach, the more seagull droppings, but not because the gulls take aim. The longer the duration of a condition, the less likely it is that the case will escape admission or notification. Chronic cases dominate cross-sectional snapshots (*prevalence*).

Conversely, rapidly growing cancers arc unlikcly to be caught at screening.

Cross-sectional surveys of outpatient clienteles conducted on January 1 will be dominated by chronic and late-autumn cases, whereas an analysis of treatments begun and ended within a calendar year are dominated by quick recoveries or by winter cases (in the northern hemisphere). A September case-control study comparing miscarriages with childbirths would show that hay fever at the time of conception is a cause of fetal loss. Even in all-year studies, seasonal variation is warped by weekends and holidays, both on the patient and on the healthcare side.

Lack of *observational synchronization*: Screen-detected cancer patients live longer after diagnosis than other patients even if death dates are unaffected by therapy (*lead bias*). Responders to cancer therapy live longer than nonresponders, if only because the predicate "responder" takes some time to acquire.

Berkson's fallacy concerns a bias in hospital studies. To statisticians, the distinguishing feature is this: An attempt to compare the frequencies of some property A given presence and absence of disorder B is made in a clinic that receives patients with B or C (note the *disjunction*!), thereby effectively comparing $P\{A|B\}$ with $P\{A|(C \text{ but not } B)\}$ instead of $P\{A|\text{not } B\}$.

Regression toward the mean: An outlying lab value probably holds a random swing, so when the test is repeated, a less extreme value is normally obtained. The pitfall is that of thinking that the change requires a biological explanation. Patients with fluctuating diseases are seen during exacerbations: Improvement follows, even without treatment; causal speculations are misplaced.

Noisy stratification inherits the regression problem: A drug made the heart beat faster in some subjects and slower in others, due to random fluctuation. Convinced that it was a real difference between two classes of people, the pharmacologist documented his result with a t test. Not biology, however, but his sorting of subjects into high and low had made the no-difference hypothesis false. Had he repeated the experiment, the two groups would have slipped back toward a joint mean. (Had another inactive drug been added in the second round, he would have discovered an antidote!) Groupings based on noisy criteria are dangerous.

Biased matching: In designs with individual matching, a tiny person will often get a somewhat taller control, and so on. A "sister closest in age" control scheme preferentially picks the middle sister of three, so mid-sib characteristics will be prevalent among controls. With "best friend" schemes, friends-making personalities will be over-represented among controls.

Jørgen Hilden

See also Bias; Biases in Human Prediction; Confidence Intervals; Confounding and Effect Modulation; Hypothesis Testing; Numeracy; Worldviews

Further Readings

Andersen, B. (1990). *Methodological errors in medical research*. Oxford, UK: Blackwell.

Armitage, P., & Colton, T. (2005). *Encyclopedia of biostatistics* (2nd ed.). Chichester, UK: Wiley Interscience.

Gluud, L. L. (2006). Bias in clinical intervention research. *American Journal of Epidemiology, 163*, 493–501.

Gøtzsche, P. C. (1990). *Bias in double-blind trials*. Copenhagen, Denmark: Lægeforeningens Forlag.

Gøtzsche, P. C. (1990). Bias in double-blind trials. *Danish Medical Bulletin, 37*, 329–336.

Hill, A. B. (1961). *Principles of medical statistics*. London: Lancet.

Mainland, D. (1963). *Elementary medical statistics*. Philadelphia: Saunders.

Porta, M. S. (2008). *A dictionary of epidemiology* (5th ed.). New York: Oxford University Press.

Sackett, D. L. (1979). Bias in analytic research. *Journal of Chronic Diseases, 32*, 51–63.

BIOETHICS

Ethics or moral philosophy is the branch of philosophy that concerns itself with the analysis of moral propositions and judgments. Bioethics, a neologism first used in the late 1960s, is currently used to describe two slightly different fields of applied ethics: (1) as a broad term covering the ethics of the life sciences and all their applications, including environmental and animal ethics—this is the common usage in Europe—and (2) as a narrower term covering the ethics of new biotechnological developments and medical/health-care ethics—this is the common usage in North America. It is the second, narrower, use of the term that is adopted in this entry.

Bioethics differs from traditional medical professional ethics, or medical deontology, in its emphasis on the role of the patient in decision making and the need to respect the patient's self-determination. Ethical considerations play a role in many medical decisions and form part of the background to many kinds of healthcare regulation. Areas where bioethics play a major role in decision making include reproductive medicine, end-of-life decision making, decision making for incompetent patients, and research ethics.

The involvement of bioethics and bioethicists in the development of healthcare regulation may sometimes lead to confusion, especially if the eventual regulation or regulatory body has "ethics" as part of its title. This does not necessarily mean that all the regulations are justified by good ethical reasoning. Research ethics as a regulatory system does, for instance, contain many elements that are not easily derivable from ethical analysis of research practices.

In the present entry, the focus is on bioethics as a branch of applied moral philosophy of use to individual healthcare professionals in their clinical decision making.

One specific feature that sets bioethics somewhat apart from other fields of applied ethics is the development of a number of bioethical frameworks specifically designed to be of direct use in clinical decision making. The most prominent of these is the "four principles" approach.

The Four Principles Approach

The four principles approach was initially developed in the United States. The impetus for the development of this approach was the observation that people can often agree on what should be done, that is, agree on a specific course of action, without being able to agree on why this course of action is the right one.

The basic idea in the four principles approach, or *principlism,* as it is often called by its critics, is that a healthcare professional should consider four ethical principles when making a clinical decision:

1. Respect for autonomy

2. Nonmaleficence (do not cause harm)

3. Beneficence (do good)

4. Justice

The principles are not ranked and none of them is absolute. They are all prima facie in the sense that they can be overridden if there are stronger reasons for following one of the other principles.

When making a decision with ethical implications, a healthcare professional should consider the following: (a) which of these principles are engaged in the decision, (b) how the principles are engaged, and (c) if two or more principles are engaged, whether they point to the same decision or whether they are in conflict and have to be balanced against each other.

In a conflict situation, three questions need to be answered: (1) Does the situation really fall within the scope of the principles? (there may, for instance, be no autonomy to respect if the patient is a fetus or is in a coma), (2) What is the exact entailment of each principle? (What does it tell us to do?), and (3) What is the right decision when the principles are weighed against each other? These three steps are referred to as determining *scope, specification,* and *balancing.*

Within moral theory, the four principles occupy a space in between overarching moral theories and specific moral judgment, and they are, in this sense, midlevel principles (see Figure 1). They can be derived top-down from moral theory. Any serious moral theory must support some version of these principles. No moral theory could, for instance, claim that harming others was not bad. The principles can also be derived bottom-up from the concrete judgments of everyday, common morality. If we reflect on these judgments and try to systematize them, we will also reach the four principles. After the derivation of the principles, we can then dispense with both in-depth consideration of moral theory and the messiness of common morality and use the principles instead.

The claim for the four principles is thus that they can resolve or mediate two kinds of moral disagreement, disagreement at the theoretical level and disagreement at the level of concrete judgments. They are furthermore useful for structuring

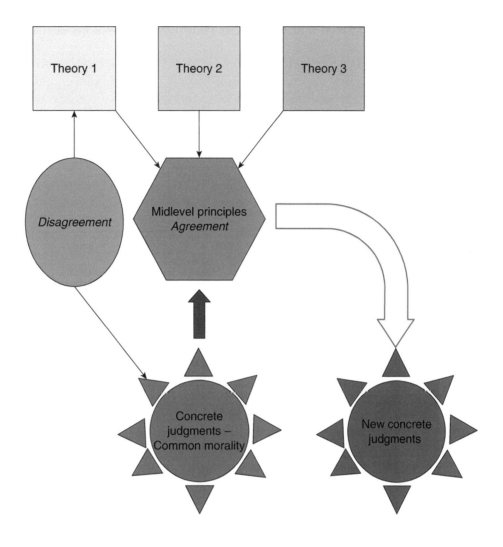

Figure I   The justification of the four principles

moral reflection and discussion concerning specific decisions.

Critiques of Principlism

The four principles approach has been the subject of considerable criticism focusing on two issues: (1) The principles may hide various forms of moral disagreement and (2) the decision process when two or more principles cannot be satisfied at the same time is unclear.

The first set of criticisms point out that the level at which we can agree on the principles is the level of contentless labels but that if we dig deeper disagreement reappears. Whereas we can all agree that we should be beneficent, that is, that there is some obligation to help others in need, we disagree concerning how strong this obligation is. How much of my wealth should I give to disaster relief, or how strong is my obligation to be a good healthcare Samaritan outside working hours? Many critics link this point to an ambiguity in the bottom-up derivation of the principles from common morality. Is common morality the same everywhere, and will we get similar content in the principles if derived from the common morality of the United States as we get when derived from the common morality of one of the Scandinavian welfare states? Or, put more strongly: Are the four principles really the principles of *American* bioethics?

The second set of criticisms focuses on the decision procedure when principles are in conflict.

There are many situations in healthcare where, for instance, the principle of respect for autonomy will be in conflict with considerations of justice, and to be action-guiding, the four principles approach needs an unambiguous decision procedure to resolve such conflicts. It has been argued that the three steps of determining scope, specification, and balancing are neither individually nor in combination sufficiently clear to provide unambiguous and unbiased decisions. It has especially been pointed out that it is unclear how principles are to be balanced against each other and that intuitions about this may be culturally specific. This links to a further criticism that, although the proponents of the four principles claim that there is no intrinsic or explicit ranking of the principles, there is an implicit ranking, with respect for autonomy and nonmaleficence trumping beneficence and justice. This trumping effect comes about because respecting the autonomy of others and not harming others are what moral philosophers call perfect duties—duties where it is possible to fulfill them completely. But doing good and being just are imperfect duties; there is always something more that can be done, and it is difficult to say precisely when a person is doing too little in respect of one of these duties. In any given situation, it is therefore easier to identify and estimate the importance of a breach of one of the perfect duties than of one of the imperfect duties.

Proponents of the four principles approach respond to these criticisms by claiming that (a) there is actually substantial agreement concerning the content of the principles, despite the protestations of the critics and (b) healthcare professionals find the approach helpful in making decisions, so it must be sufficiently action-guiding despite any inherent vagueness.

Variants of Principlism and Other Frameworks

Several variations on the principlist theme have been developed. These include the Ethical Grid and a transposition of the four principles into an ethics of love.

One impetus behind the development of the Ethical Grid is the argument that it is not enough to respect autonomy. An important element of healthcare practice is to create, promote, and support autonomy in patients and clients. Another is

that nonmaleficence and beneficence are two sides of healthcare's central focus on needs and not wants. Based on these considerations and the perceived need to provide more guidance concerning how to think through an ethical problem, a graphical aid—the Ethical Grid—has been developed for analyzing ethical problems in clinical practice and healthcare policymaking. In the grid, core ethical values in healthcare are at the center, more specific rules in the next level, considerations of beneficence in the third level, and more general considerations at the outer level. In using the grid, the first step is to identify which boxes are engaged in the problem at hand. If a problem, for instance, has no resource implications and no other repercussions for anyone else than the patient and the healthcare team, a number of boxes are irrelevant and can be left out of further consideration. In the second step, the implications of the possible choices are then considered for each relevant box in light of the core values in the center. This will identify the reasons for and against each possible choice. Based on this, it should then be possible to reach a conclusion concerning which action is best supported in the present context.

The Ethical Grid has been developed into a more comprehensive Web-based tool for exploring values, The Values Exchange.

Because of the focus on creating and promoting autonomy, the Ethical Grid has become popular in nursing and other professions allied to medicine, where care is seen as equally important to treatment.

Another variation on the principles theme proceeds from the following arguments: (a) that the basis for any ethics must be love in both its emotional and cognitive sense and (b) that the four principles as originally proposed appeal exclusively to the cognitive elements of our relationship with ourselves and with others. It is suggested that we will gain a better understanding of the scope and importance of the principles by understanding them as four different aspects of love, according to the following transposition:

1. Respect for autonomy = Love of self

2. Nonmaleficence = Love of life

3. Beneficence = Love of good

4. Justice = Love of others

Other frameworks that have been proposed for clinical bioethics are the 10 so-called moral rules:

1. Do not kill.
2. Do not cause pain.
3. Do not disable.
4. Do not deprive of freedom.
5. Do not deprive of pleasure.
6. Do not deceive.
7. Keep your promises.
8. Do not cheat.
9. Obey the law.
10. Do your duty.

The primary difference between the 10 moral rules and the four principles is that the rules are more specific and that positive obligations to benefit others are less prominent. The implications of the moral rules for healthcare practice have been explicated in a number of publications.

Liberal Utilitarianism

Within academic bioethics, there is considerable skepticism toward the use of bioethics decision frameworks. Many professional academic bioethicists suggest that the search for midlevel principles or similar devices is misguided and that any proper bioethical decision making needs to be based on moral theory. There is, however, significant disagreement concerning which moral theory to choose.

In what can broadly be described as Anglo-American bioethics (including the north of Europe, Canada, Australia, and New Zealand), liberal utilitarianism has become the preferred approach. Utilitarianism, which is a type of consequentialism, states that the morally right action is the one that maximizes net good consequences. It is, however, well known that unmodified utilitarianism can lead to strongly counterintuitive and very illiberal results.

In contemporary bioethics, utilitarianism is therefore almost always combined with some form of liberal restriction on allowable state or societal action, most often in the form of John Stuart Mill's so-called harm principle:

That principle is, that the sole end for which mankind are warranted, individually or collectively in interfering with the liberty of action of any of their number, is self-protection. That the only purpose for which power can be rightfully exercised over any member of a civilized community, against his will, is to prevent harm to others. His own good, either physical or moral, is not a sufficient warrant.

If this principle is accepted as a restriction on allowable actions by the state or by individual actors, then individuals have liberty to pursue their own projects as long as they do not harm others, although they may still be morally obligated to sacrifice their own interests for the maximization of good consequences. This has the desirable consequence for the liberal that most decisions made by patients are protected from interference even if they do not maximize good consequences overall. In the healthcare setting, this means that a healthcare professional should respect a patient's choices even if they seem to be to the detriment of the patient.

Liberal utilitarianism does, however, face problems in the context of resource allocation or priority setting in healthcare. Standard utilitarianism is broadly consistent with welfare economics and with health economics approaches to resource allocation, for instance in the form of maximization of quality-adjusted life years (QALY maximization). But the consistency with welfare economics is lost in liberal utilitarianism because of its emphasis on the liberty rights of persons. This has led some liberal utilitarians to argue that any allocation that deprives a person of a treatment that has health benefits is problematic, unless the allocation is done through some kind of lottery that provides everyone a chance to get the treatment that will benefit them, irrespective of resource implications.

Bioethics, the Embryo, and the Fetus

Reproductive decision making has been considerably influenced by bioethical analysis of the status and moral importance of the human embryo and fetus. It is traditionally assumed that embryos and fetuses are morally important in themselves or intrinsically, but this is denied by many writers in bioethics, who hold that they are not morally important and that there is nothing morally problematic in terminating them.

The arguments for the view that embryos and fetuses have no intrinsic moral importance but are only important if others (e.g., their progenitors) value them vary in their details. The main line of argument is, however, fairly constant and based on the idea that what is wrong with killing an entity is that it frustrates a preference or conscious interest that that entity has. It is thus only wrong to kill people who do not want to be killed, and voluntary euthanasia is by implication acceptable. But embryos and fetuses have no preferences or conscious interests concerning their future existence, either because they are not conscious at all (embryos or early fetuses) or because they do not have the concept of a future existence (late fetuses).

On this view, the creation and destruction of embryos for good reasons, for instance, as part of assisted reproduction or for stem cell research, is morally neutral as is abortion on demand. Although no country has legislation on reproductive medicine that is as liberal as this view of embryos and fetuses requires, it has influenced the move toward liberalization in many countries. Critics of this line of argument point to the fact that it has very wide application. Not only does it entail that abortion on demand is acceptable at any time during a pregnancy but also that infanticide, or the killing of normal infants, on the request of their parents becomes a morally neutral action, since infants are unlikely to have the conscious concept of a future existence. It also entails that persons with severe cognitive deficits are without intrinsic moral value.

Søren Holm

See also Cultural Issues; Rationing; Religious Factors; Shared Decision Making

Further Readings

Beauchamp, T. L., & Childress, J. F. (2001). *Principles of biomedical ethics* (5th ed.). New York: Oxford University Press.

Gert, B. (1973). *The moral rules: A new rational foundation for morality*. New York: Harper & Row.

Gert, B., Culver, C. M., & Clouser, K. D. (1997). *Bioethics: A return to fundamentals* (2nd ed.). New York: Oxford University Press.

Häyry, M. (1994). *Liberal utilitarianism and applied ethics*. London: Routledge.

Holm, S. (1995). Not just autonomy: The principles of American biomedical ethics. *Journal of Medical Ethics, 21*, 332–338.

Macer, D. R. J. (1998). *Bioethics is love of life: An alternative textbook*. Retrieved from http://www .eubios.info/BLL.htm

Mill, J. S. (1879). *On liberty and the subjection of women*. New York: Henry Holt. Retrieved January, 23, 2009, from http://oll.libertyfund.org/title/347

Seedhouse, D. (1998). *Ethics: The heart of health care* (2nd ed.). Oxford, UK: Wiley/Blackwell.

Steinbock, B. (Ed.). (2007). *The Oxford handbook of bioethics*. New York: Oxford University Press.

The Values Exchange: http://www.values-exchange.com/ news

BIOINFORMATICS

We are on the cusp of an explosion of biological data generated by the human genome project and sequencing projects in multiple organisms, coupled with advances in both experimental and information technologies. All this is contributing to a new era of personalized medicine, using a deeper understanding of our bodies and their diseases at the molecular level. The huge demand to manage, analyze, and interpret these various data has led to the growing stature of the field of information science that is called bioinformatics.

Bioinformatics encompasses all aspects of biological information—acquisition, processing, storage, distribution, analysis, and interpretation—and combines the tools and techniques of mathematics, computer science, and biology with the aim of furthering the understanding of diseases. The National Institutes of Health defines bioinformatics as "research, development, or application of computational tools and approaches for expanding the use of biological, medical, behavioral or health data, including those to acquire, store, organize, archive, analyze, or visualize such data."

Bioinformatics can be viewed as a bottom-up approach, working with molecular data to determine physiological information. In contrast, medical informatics can be viewed as a top-down approach, working with patient clinical data to determine underlying physiological processes. Together, bioinformatics and medical informatics are key methods shaping the future of personalized medicine. This means that, due to bioinformatics analysis of genomic data, medical decision making is evolving to be based on a person's individual genomic information instead of on studies relying on statistics about the general population.

History

As a field of biological and information science, bioinformatics has been present since the discovery of DNA, when proteins and cell forms became known as the building blocks of life. The cardinal functions of bioinformatics have been (a) handling and presentation of nucleotide and protein sequences and their annotation; (b) development of databases to store, analyze, and interpret these data; and (c) development of algorithms for making predictions based on available information. To address these topics, the field drew from the foundations of statistics, mathematics, physics, computer science, and molecular biology. Bioinformatics still reflects this broad base.

The Human Genome

The genome's language is a DNA code containing an alphabet of just four letters, or bases: G, C, A, and T. Remarkably, the entire human genome contains 3 billion of these DNA bases. While sequencing the human genome to decode these billions of bases in multiple people from different ethnicities, bioinformatics technologies were used and improved to view, combine, compare, and find patterns across this enormous amount of data. By comparing sequences of known and unknown genes, bioinformatics programs were developed that used probabilities and modeling to predict the function and roles of previously unknown genes. This vast amount of completed genomic sequence data and individual gene information now also needed to be stored, bringing about the creation of various gene databases that are publicly available.

During this genomic era, bioinformatics tools played a pivotal role in allowing researchers to generate and compare the DNA sequences of many genes to identify their roles and to determine whether a particular gene sequence has different

DNA bases than seen normally. This information has provided insights into many biochemical, evolutionary, and genetic pathways. It has also provided an important building block for potential medical decision making by making it possible to identify whether a patient's specific gene is normal or mutated.

Bioinformatics in the Postgenomic Era

The map of the human genetic code provides information that allows researchers and physicians to pursue new options for diagnosing and eventually treating many diseases, symptoms, and syndromes. Bioinformatics has enabled these discoveries via analysis and comparison of the various data sets of the genomic era.

Advances in experimental technologies for detecting the multiple levels of biological organization (DNA, RNA, or protein) on a high-throughput scale have required the bioinformatics field to develop increasingly more sophisticated methods and systems for analyzing and storing data. The emerging era of medicine depends strongly on a broad array of these new technologies, such as DNA sequencing, gene expression profiling, protein profiling, and developing new algorithms for finding patterns across large, sometimes dissimilar data sets. Bioinformatics methodologies are useful due to their ability to sift through this vast array of information to converge on a few relevant facts. Together, these new high-throughput technologies and bioinformatics analyses are providing the ability to understand and predict the behavior of complex biological systems, giving rise to the field of systems biology. We have arrived at a point in biology where the underlying mechanisms behind diseases are becoming known.

Gene expression microarrays and single nucleotide polymorphism (SNP) genotyping are two major areas where bioinformatics plays a vital role in interpreting the data generated from these high-throughput technologies. Analysis of the gene-expression profiles from healthy and diseased persons can provide the identification of what genes may be responsible for that disease, which can be investigated further using several technologies. Genotyping identifies an individual's DNA sequence, and bioinformatics analysis across genotypes provides a measurement of the genetic variation between those genotypes, or between members of a species. SNPs are changes in a single base of the DNA sequence, and these are often found to be the etiology of many human diseases and are becoming particularly important in pharmacogenetics. SNPs can also provide a genetic fingerprint for use in identity testing.

Scientific advances coupled with novel bioinformatics algorithms have helped uncover other functional elements of the genome such as miRNAs (microRNAs), RNAi (RNA interference), and so on, depicting the complex nature of the genome and its regulation. As newer molecules are discovered, the need to manage, analyze, and interpret them is also being addressed, using bioinformatic tools.

In the postgenomic era, bioinformatics has helped create integrated resources of databases, pathways, functions, and visualization tools to assimilate and integrate multiple layers of a person's molecular data. These resources and capabilities are enabling researchers to understand how the molecular processes of cells are linked to higher physiological functions.

Applications of Bioinformatics in Medical and Health-Related Research

Bioinformatics has the potential to influence a wide range of medical and health-related research, with subsequent downstream effects translated into more individualized medical decision making.

The mining, or comparison, of similar sets of patient gene expression data from microarray chips can find which genes are differentially expressed in patients as compared with the normal population. To further understand how changes in certain genes are linked to the clinical outcome, bioinformatics can be leveraged to provide information on the genes of interest, such as their processes, functions, interactions with other genes or proteins, genetic pathways, and any known drug targets associated with them.

Genotyping and bioinformatics play a key role in the search for genes that increase the susceptibility to specific diseases; for their genetic variations (SNPs); for SNP patterns that can be used to predict patient response to medicines; for identifying tractable drug targets; and for defining the function of the genes and proteins they produce.

Understanding the relationship between genetic variation and biological function on a genomic scale is expected to provide fundamental insights into the biology, evolution, and pathophysiology of humans and other species. Analyzing and comparing the genetic material of different species is an important method for studying the functions of genes and the mechanisms of inherited diseases. For example, by comparing the sequences in newly identified genes with those of genes whose functions are already known, scientists can make educated interpretations about which genes might be related to specific biochemical pathways in the body and how they might affect the occurrence or treatment of the disease. This information can also be used to experimentally model those sequence changes to verify these gene functions and to test if there is a better or worse response to drug treatment. Based on the differences in the genetic variants among ethnic groups, one can predict the appropriate dosage for a drug to be effective or to avoid serious side effects. This growing body of information from bioinformatics analysis is the basic foundation of the field of pharmacogenomics.

Pharmacogenomic approaches, which involve the study of how an individual's genetic inheritance affects the body's response to drugs, are emerging across broad classes of therapeutics to assist practitioners in making more precise decisions about the correct drugs to give to the appropriate patients to optimize their benefit-to-risk ratio. Bioinformatic analysis of data helps eliminate false-positive leads in the early stages of the drug discovery process, thus substantively compressing the time, resources, and costs needed in the drug discovery efforts. These approaches are continuously evolving to address the complexity and multivariate nature of increasing amounts of data. There are many clinical drug trials, sponsored by the pharmaceutical industry, that leverage bioinformatics with medical informatics, which will undoubtedly continue to change and improve therapeutic decisions for patients.

Classification of clinical syndromes by bioinformatics molecular profiling can advance the use of *gene* testing in the broadest sense (as a molecular diagnostic tool) in the diagnosis, therapy, and counseling of individuals affected with genetic disorders. For these advances to have real use, there needs to be equally robust phenotypic data that are meticulously mapped to DNA, RNA, and protein genotype. Databases have been and are being made available for storing, indexing, and querying patient data, clinical phenotypes, and genotypic data; however, an understanding of the types of data to be objectively documented, and the standards to be adopted regarding terminologies and storing data in query-compatible forms, is still evolving. With the proliferation of all these biological databases, tools, and resources, there is a high likelihood of compromised data quality and reliability; thus, caution is the watchword while using these resources judiciously for decision making.

Personalized Medicine

Personalized medicine is the use of information and data from a patient's genotype, or level of gene expression, to stratify disease, select a medication, provide a therapy, or initiate a preventive measure that is particularly suited to that patient at the time of administration. In addition to genetic information, other sources of information, including imaging, laboratory tests, and clinical knowledge about the disease process and the patient play equally important roles.

Translational bioinformatics has emerged as a field that bridges bioinformatics and medical informatics, with the potential of immense benefit for the medical community in reaching the personalized medicine era. This field uses translational tools and techniques to analyze and integrate the data resulting from high-throughput technologies to facilitate smooth translation of important information. This brings the information from bench to bedside by enabling medical providers to incorporate information into their routine medical practice of diagnosis and treatment.

Together, these tools will enable a paradigm shift from genetic medicine—based on the study of individual inherited characteristics, most often single genes—to genomic medicine, which by its nature is comprehensive and focuses on the functions and interactions of multiple genes and gene products, among themselves and with their environment. The information gained from such analyses, in combination with clinical data, is now allowing us to assess individual risks and guide clinical management and decision making, all of which form the basis for genomic medicine.

As medical technology has advanced rapidly over the past century to cure major diseases and discover drugs and therapies, there also has been major variability in therapeutic responses and ensuing side effects. The new insights from studying human diseases from an information science perspective helps in understanding that humans are a system of interconnected and dynamically organized cells, proteins, and genes. The new molecular data have given evidence that the variability in drug response is genetically determined, with age, sex, nutrition, and environmental exposures also playing contributory roles. Thus, classifying patient data among these various parameters and studying genetic distinctions in different subclasses of relevant data, via bioinformatics, will facilitate a more direct route to a patient's wellness and disease prevention than has yet been possible.

Future Direction

Sequencing of the human genome has ushered in prospects for personalized care. There is growing evidence that the practice of medicine might soon have a new toolbox to predict and treat disease more effectively. The Human Genome Project has spawned several important "omic" technologies that allow "whole genome" interrogation of sequence variation ("genomic"), transcription ("transcriptomic"), proteins ("proteomic"), and metabolites ("metabolomic"), which all provide more exacting detail about the disease mechanisms being investigated. In the field of molecular imaging, researchers are developing chemical and biological probes that can sense molecular pathway mechanisms that will allow medical professionals to monitor health and disease on an individual basis.

As genetic and genomic data proliferate from various public and government efforts worldwide, notably in the United States, Europe, and Japan, the push to cull meaningful insights from these mountains of data has also gathered speed, necessitated by seeking cures for elusive diseases and by pharmaceutical companies' desire for breakthroughs in drug discovery. This gold hunt for the perfect molecule and perfect drug target is largely facilitated by bioinformatics tools and technologies employed in the early phases of the drug discovery and development process.

As innovators race toward getting a person's DNA sequenced for $1,000, down from $100 million a decade ago, the field of bioinformatics has paralleled this rapid technology advancement. Leveraging bioinformatics and medical informatics is crucial for giving medicine and medical care a preventive, predictive, and personalized form in the near future.

Banu Gopalan and Petra Platzer

See also Genetic Testing

Further Readings

Augen, J. (2005). *Bioinformatics in the post-genomic era: Genome, transcriptome, proteome, and information-based medicine.* Boston: Addison-Wesley.

Bioinformatics Definition Committee. (2000). *NIH working definition of bioinformatics and computational group.* Retrieved January 23, 2009, from http://www.bisti.nih.gov/docs/CompuBioDef.pdf

Kanehisa, M. (2000). *Post-genome informatics.* Oxford, UK: Oxford University Press.

Kuhn, K. A., Knoll, A., Mewes, H. W., Schwaiger, M., Bode, A., Broy, M., et al. (2008). Informatics and medicine: From molecules to populations. *Methods of Information in Medicine, 47*(4), 283–295.

Liebman, M. N. (2002). Biomedical informatics: The future for drug development. *Drug Discovery Today, 7*(20 Suppl.), S197–S203.

Maojo, V., & Kulikowski, C. A. (2003). Bioinformatics and medical informatics: Collaborations on the road to genomic medicine? *Journal of the American Medical Informatics Association, 10*(6), 515–522.

Martin-Sanchez, F., Iakovidis, I., Nørager, S., Maojo, V., de Groen, P., Van der Lei, J., et al. (2004). Synergy between medical informatics and bioinformatics: Facilitating genomic medicine for future health care. *Journal of Biomedical Informatics, 37*(1), 30–42.

National Center for Biotechnology Information: http://www.ncbi.nlm.nih.gov

Teufel, A., Krupp, M., Weinmann, A., & Galle, P. R. (2006). Current bioinformatics tools in genomic biomedical research (Review). *International Journal of Molecular Medicine, 17*(6), 967–973.

Valafar, F. (2003). Techniques in bioinformatics and medical informatics. *Annals of the New York Academy of Sciences, 980,* 41–64.

Yan, Q. (2008). The integration of personalized and systems medicine: Bioinformatics support for pharmacogenomics and drug discovery. *Methods in Molecular Biology, 448,* 1–19.

BOOLEAN ALGEBRA AND NODES

A Boolean, or logical, variable is one that can take the values **T** (true) or **F** (false); and the Boolean, or logical, algebra pioneered by George Boole (1815–1864) holds the formal machinery that allows such *truth values* to be logically combined. Boolean principles offer a framework for handling questionnaire and symptom data of the common *binary* kind (yes vs. no, normal ["negative"] vs. abnormal ["positive"], etc.), for clinical decisions, even measurements, probabilities, and so on, often have to be *dichotomized (binarized)*. Library searches exploit Boolean AND, OR, and NOT, and the digital computer is essentially a huge number of electronic switches (on vs. off) connected in a Boolean manner, marching to the beat of a clock. Boolean principles also underlie logical checking of rule-based decision support systems for inconsistencies, incompleteness, and redundancy.

The Algebra

Let $A, B, C, \ldots$ be diagnostic tests or, more precisely, the Boolean variables that hold the answers to "Did test A come out positive?" and so on. Boolean *negation*, alias NOT, swaps **T** and **F**, indicating, in our example, whether a test came out negative:

$$\neg A = (\text{not } A) = (\text{false if } A \text{ is true; true if } A \text{ is false}) = (\text{F if } A, \text{ otherwise } \text{T}).$$

Note that $\neg(\neg A) = A$. Other basic operations are AND and OR:

AND ("Did both A and B come out positive?"):

$$A \wedge B = (A \text{ and } B) = (\text{T if both } A \text{ and } B, \text{ otherwise } \text{F});$$

OR ("Did A, B, or both, come out positive?"):

$$A \vee B = (A \text{ or } B) = (\text{F if neither } A \text{ nor } B, \text{ otherwise } \text{T}) = \neg(\neg A \wedge \neg B).$$

The mirror image of the rightmost identity also works:

$$A \wedge B = \neg(\neg A \vee \neg B) = (\text{F if one or both of } A \text{ and } B \text{ are false, otherwise } \text{T}).$$

Set theory involves set intersection ($\cap$), union ($\cup$), and complementing, which are the precise analogs of $\wedge$, $\vee$, and $\neg$, respectively.

OR and AND are *associative* operations: More than two terms can be ORed (or ANDed), in arbitrary order, to reflect "at least one true" ("all true"). *Distributive* properties include

$$(A \wedge B) \vee (A \wedge C) = A \wedge (B \vee C),$$
$$(A \vee B) \wedge (A \vee C) = A \vee (B \wedge C).$$

The former may be read: To be a "female diabetic or female with hypertension" means to be a "female with diabetes or hypertension." Self-combination:

$$(A \wedge A) = (A \vee A) = A.$$

Finally, test A must be either positive or negative, but cannot be both:

$$(A \vee \neg A) = \mathbf{T}, \quad (A \wedge \neg A) = \mathbf{F}.$$

The former expression is a *tautology*, that is, a necessarily true proposition.

The OR described so far is the inclusive OR, as in the "or both" above. Informatics (checksums, cryptography) makes frequent use of the *exclusive* OR, abbreviated EXOR. *Equivalence* ($\equiv$), in the sense of having the same truth value, and EXOR are each other's negations:

$$(A \equiv B) = (A \text{ and } B \text{ are both true or both false});$$

$$(A \text{ EXOR } B) = \neg(A \equiv B) = (\text{one of } A \text{ and } B \text{ is true, not both}).$$

Now, ((A EXOR B) EXOR C) is true if just one or all three terms are true. Extending this rule to repeated EXORs of multiple Boolean terms, one finds that the result is true if the number of true terms is odd and false if it is even.

The Implication Symbol

The implication symbol ($\rightarrow$) is a treacherous abbreviation:

$$(A \rightarrow U) = (A \text{ "implies" } U) = (U \vee A) = (\text{if } A, \text{ then } U; \text{ otherwise } \mathbf{T}).$$

That is, if A, then the expression reproduces the truth value of U; if not A, then the result is $\mathbf{T}$—*regardless* of U!

This is different from "A causes U," however construed. It is also different from the language of decision recommendations and deductions in rule-based decision support systems. When you come across a statement such as "If symptom A is present, diagnosis U is applicable," you take it to be telling you nothing about patients without symptom A. If told that the statement is untrue, you take that to mean that A alone should not trigger label U. This is exactly how a rule-based system would react to cancellation of "If A, then U." The Boolean negation $\neg(A \rightarrow U) = (\neg U \wedge A)$, on the other hand, would claim that, despite symptom A, diagnosis U was not made (in a particular case), or every patient has symptom A and diagnosis U is never made (when read as a general rule).

Physical Analogs

A and B may be gates. When they must be passed one after the other, entry is possible if and only if both gates are open. Symbolically, $E = A \wedge B$. If, on the other hand, A and B are alternative routes of entry, $E = A \vee B$ (Is at least one gate open?). Electrical switches connected "in series" or "in parallel" are analogous.

Boolean Data in Programming: Boolean Nodes

Most programming languages make available a Boolean, or logical, data type. It may look thus:

```
Boolean L; #declares L to be a Boolean
variable#
  L: = (n < 20); #L becomes true or false
depending on the value of n#
  if(L)print("n  small"); #to  be  printed
only if n is below 20#
```

Programming languages have different ways of writing AND and OR. Often, however, it is convenient to let $\mathbf{T}$ and $\mathbf{F}$ be represented by 1 and 0, leading to

$$\neg A = (1 - A),$$

$$A \wedge B \wedge C \wedge \Lambda = ABC \quad \text{[an ordinary product of 0s and 1s]}$$

$$= \min(A, B, C, \ldots),$$

$$A \vee B \vee C \vee \Lambda = \max(A, B, C, K).$$

Conversely, mathematicians often write $\wedge$ and $\vee$ for min and max; so $x \wedge y = \min(x, y)$, the smaller of x and y. Checksum calculations, involving EXORing of multiple 0 or 1 digits, produce the result 1 precisely when the number of component 1s is odd, as stated above; that is, when their ordinary sum is odd:

$$\text{EXOR}(A, B, C, K) = (1 \text{ if } A + B + C + \wedge \text{ is odd};$$
$$\text{otherwise, 0}).$$

Boolean Nodes

A standard decision tree has a stem (clinical problem) and two types of splits: chance nodes and decision nodes. Between the stem and the leaves, each of which represents a possible clinical diary, the tree gets increasingly bushy because there is no way branches can rejoin. In practice, many subtrees are nearly identical and can be drawn, and programmed, just once. They can then be entered from various points as subroutines, with arguments that let them inherit patient features from the calling point.

Numerical arguments allow probabilities and utilities to be context dependent (e.g., age dependent); Boolean arguments allow the subtree to be structurally modified. They govern special *Boolean nodes*, which act as switches. The Boolean argument "Has the patient already had a hemicolectomy?" may govern a switch that blocks a decision branch involving hemicolectomy. Likewise, in modeling an annual screening program, the same annual subtree may have to be entered recursively: A Boolean switch may serve to prevent endless recursion.

Boolean nodes allow compact, minimally redundant trees to be drawn—sometimes at the expense of intelligibility. (Some authors have used the term for other kinds of two-way nodes.)

Boolean Matrices

Consider a graph of N interconnected nodes (*vertices*). An $N \times N$ matrix $C = \{C_{ij}\}$ of Boolean elements may represent the interconnections (*arcs, edges*),

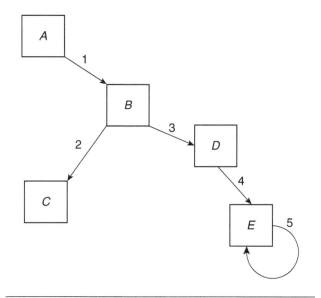

Figure 1   Boolean graph

C_{ij} being **T** if and only if node i is directly connected to node j. Both directed and nondirected graphs may be represented in this way; in the latter case, the matrix is symmetric ($C_{ij} = C_{ji}$). The diagonal elements, C_{ii}, are set to **F** unless self-referring nodes make sense, as they do in state-progression models, including Markov chains. Matrix C is called the *adjacency matrix* of the graph.

The matrix product $D = CC$, with addition and multiplication replaced with OR and AND, now answers the question of whether one can pass in precisely two steps from node i to node k. Readers familiar with matrices will see that

$$D_{ik} = \bigvee_{j = 1, K, N} \{C_{ij} \wedge C_{jk}\} = (C_{i1} \wedge C_{1k}) \vee$$
$$(C_{i2} \wedge C_{2k}) \vee \Lambda.$$

$$= (\text{Is there at least one node } j \text{ that can be used as a stepping stone?}).$$

This idea can be elaborated to answer many types of connectedness questions. For example, in the directed graph in Figure 1, the arcs are numbered for convenience, and in Figure 2, the elements in matrix C that go into the calculation of $D_{A,D}$ are shaded.

The Boolean Approach to Diagnostic Tests

The 2^k possible outcomes of k binary tests and the $k!$ possible sequences of execution may render

Adjacency matrix C (edge absent marked with a dot; edge numbers shown for clarity)

To From	A	B	C	D	E
A	.	T (1)	.	.	.
B	.	.	T (2)	T (3)	.
C	.	.	.	.	.
D	.	.	.	.	T (4)
E	.	.	.	.	T (5)

Matrix D = CC (by aligning the "From A" row with the "To D" column in matrix C, both shaded, one sees that the only match is in the second position, implying that node B is the only stepping stone from A to D, i.e., route 1–3)

To From	A	B	C	D	E
A	.	.	T (12)	T (13)	.
B	.	.	.	.	T (34)
C	.	.	.	.	.
D	.	.	.	.	T (45)
E	.	.	.	.	T (55)

Figure 2   Boolean tables

ordinary decision trees unmanageable: One ends up with $2^k k!$ leaves, or 48 when $k = 3$ (80 when tests may be executed simultaneously). A shortcut is offered by the following, much simpler, Boolean procedure, supplemented, if necessary, by an ad hoc analysis to find the least costly or risky execution scheme (*flowchart*).

After tabulating the 2^k outcomes and the associated clinical actions found by utility maximization, suppose it turns out that intervention U is recommended when, and only when, Tests A, B, and C have the result patterns: $(+ + +)$, $(+ + -)$, $(- + +)$, or $(- - +)$. The Boolean representation $U = (A \wedge B \wedge C) \vee (A \wedge B \wedge C) \vee (A \wedge B \wedge C) \vee (A \wedge B \wedge C)$ reduces to $U = (A \wedge B) \vee (A \wedge C)$, suggesting that test A should be performed first and, depending on the result, B or C will decide. However, it also reduces to $U = (B \wedge C) \vee ((B \text{ EXOR } C) \wedge (A \equiv B))$,

suggesting that one should begin with B and C and, if they disagree, check whether A sides with B.

The former execution scheme is attractive when A is inexpensive and risk-free, the latter when A is costly or risky. Unless the choice is obvious, one must go through all contingencies and calculate expected money and utility costs. These concerns, as well as the constraints that arise when tests are technically intertwined, can be handled in a decision tree, but the answer found by the Boolean procedure is otherwise exactly the one a decision tree would give.

In other words, the two procedures lead to the same *test interpretation scheme*, but the Boolean procedure may require ad hoc supplementary calculations to find the optimal *test execution scheme*. *Warning:* Speaking of Tests A and B being applied in parallel (in series) may refer to the tests being *executed* simultaneously (vs. one after the other). Some authors, thinking of the gate analogy above, therefore use the parallel versus series terminology to characterize two *interpretation* schemes, namely, $U = (A \vee B)$ versus $U = (A \wedge B)$.

As a by-product, the Boolean procedure reveals whether any tests are mandatory (needed in all cases) or redundant (dispensable). In the small artificial example, this did not happen.

The 1986 paper that popularized these techniques also illustrated some geometric features that the ROC diagram will possess when the *lattice* of all Boolean combinations of several binary tests is plotted.

Jørgen Hilden

See also Causal Inference and Diagrams; Diagnostic Tests; Markov Models; Receiver Operating Characteristic (ROC) Curve; Subtrees, Use in Constructing Decision Trees

Further Readings

Boole, G. (1854). *An investigation of the laws of thought.* London: Macmillan.

Garcia-Remesal, M., Maojo, V., Laita, L., Roanes-Lozano, E., & Crespo, J. (2007, August). An algebraic approach to detect logical inconsistencies in medical appropriateness criteria. *Proceedings of the 29th Annual International Conference of the IEEE Engineering in Medicine and Biology Society, 1,* 5148–5151.

Glasziou, P., & Hilden, J. (1986). Decision tables and logic in decision analysis. *Medical Decision Making, 6,* 154–160.

Lau, J., Kassirer, J. P., & Pauker, S. G. (1983). Decision Maker 3.0: Improved decision analysis by personal computer. *Medical Decision Making, 3,* 39–43.

BOUNDED RATIONALITY AND EMOTIONS

The rational decision maker with limitless capacities to process information does not exist. People's cognitive and emotional resources are bounded (limited), thereby motivating them to engage in strategies to maximize effective use of these resources. It has been increasingly recognized that deliberation and intuition are two resources essential for adequate decision making. This entry discusses not only rationality and emotions but also the role they play in decision making and the strategies people use to approach decision problems.

Bounded Rationality

In 1957, Herbert Simon proposed the notion of *bounded rationality* to account for the fact that perfectly rational decisions are often not feasible in practice due to the finite information-processing capacities of humans. Simon points out that most people are only partly rational and are in fact emotional or irrational in the remaining part of their actions. Human beings are limited in their capacity for storing and processing information. As a consequence, people process information sequentially and use heuristics, or rules of thumb, to keep the information-processing demands of complex tasks within the bounds of their cognitive capacities. These heuristics are procedures for systematically simplifying the search through the available information. The use of heuristic strategies improves the performance of the individual as a limited information processor and is, as Simon argues, "at the heart of human intelligence." In this vein, Gerd Gigerenzer and colleagues argue that simple alternatives (i.e., heuristics) to a full rational analysis as a mechanism for decision making frequently lead to better decisions than the theoretically optimal procedure. These heuristics are generally successful,

but in certain situations they lead to systematic cognitive biases.

Heuristics

People use heuristics for multi-attribute decision problems such as choosing a car or choosing a hospital for treatment as well as for risky decision making such as the choice between an operation and a wait-and-see policy with different mortality risks. Two approaches to the use of heuristics in decision making can be distinguished: the *accuracy/effort approach* and the *heuristics-and-biases approach.* According to the accuracy/effort approach, people process and evaluate only a part of the information and use noncompensatory decision rules to limit the information-processing demands of multi-attribute decision problems. For instance, people eliminate options because of an unsatisfactory score on one attribute, as, for example, when choosing among cars, a decision maker eliminates all options above a certain price, irrespective of the evaluation of the other attributes. John Payne and colleagues see humans as adaptive decision makers who weight the benefits of a decision strategy (i.e., the probability that a strategy will select the best alternative) against the costs (i.e., the mental effort, time, and money needed).

Another approach is the heuristics-and-biases approach. This approach is most prominently represented by the research of Amos Tversky and Daniel Kahneman and emphasizes the biases and errors in human judgment that are due to the use of heuristics. Contrary to the earlier approach, it does not consider the use of heuristics as a rational trade-off between accuracy and effort but as a failure to recognize the "correct" solution. Tversky and Kahneman consider these heuristics as highly economical and usually effective but add that in some cases they may lead to systematic and predictable errors. An example of such a heuristic is the availability heuristic: Objects or events are judged as frequent and probable or causally efficacious to the extent that they are readily available in memory. This heuristic is likely to erroneously affect the evaluation of information whenever some aspect in the environment is made disproportionally salient or available to the perceiver.

These two approaches are both related to the limited information-processing capacities or the bounded rationality of people. The heuristics-and-biases approach focuses on the first stage of the decision process, that is, the editing phase, which occurs in a more or less automatic way. The accuracy/effort approach is concerned with the stages after the initial coding process, which seem more controlled. According to this approach, people resort to the use of heuristics if an analytical approach to decision making becomes too demanding. A more complete understanding of decision making should include the accuracy/effort as well as the heuristics-and-biases approach, as decision behavior is likely to consist of multiple systems that interact in various ways.

Dual-Processing Theories

It is an old idea in psychology that human processing of information takes place on many levels that can operate simultaneously and relatively independently. These dual-process models of human reasoning and decision making have become more popular in the past decade or so. In a recent article, Kahneman relates the heuristics-and-biases research to the dual-processing theories about reasoning and decision making. This ancient idea that cognitive processes can be distinguished into two main categories, roughly corresponding to the everyday concepts of intuition and reason, is now widely embraced under the general label of dual-process theories. These two categories of cognitive processes can be distinguished by their speed, their controllability, and the contents on which they operate. The dual-process models distinguish cognitive operations that are quick and associative from others that are slow and governed by rules. Intuitive or System 1 thinking is closely related to perception and quickly proposes intuitive answers to judgment problems as they arise. Operations are fast, automatic, associative, and effortless, and they are often emotionally charged. They are also governed by habit and are therefore difficult to control or modify. Deliberative or System 2 reasoning monitors the quality of these proposals, which it may endorse, correct, or override. The processes of System 2 are slower, serial, effortful, and deliberatively controlled. They are also relatively flexible and potentially rule governed. A characteristic of System 2 is that it is limited or bounded by working memory capacity and is assumed to be linked to general intelligence, while System 1 functions independently of working memory. These characteristics that have been attributed to the two modes are related to consciousness (unconscious and holistic vs. conscious and analytic) and functionality (e.g., associative, automatic, and parallel vs. rule-based, logical, and sequential). In a recent article, Jonathan Evans gives an overview of the several dual-processing theories of reasoning, judgment, and social cognition.

Emotions: Immediate Emotions

Emotional processing, although not included in all dual-processing theories, is placed in System 1 rather than in System 2. In several theories, a fast emotional basis for decision making is contrasted with a slower and more deliberative cognitive basis. The emotional side of judgment and decision making has recently received more attention in judgment and decision research. Research shows that every stimulus evokes affective evaluation that is not always conscious. *Affective valence* is a natural assessment and can, according to Paul Slovic and colleagues, be used as a heuristic attribute for making complex decisions. They propose that representations of objects and events in people's minds are tagged, to varying degrees, with affect. When making a judgment or a decision, people consult or refer to an "affect pool" containing all the positive and negative tags consciously or unconsciously associated with the representations. Affect may serve as a cue to judgments in the same way as availability.

Slovic and colleagues argue that the affect heuristic guides the perception of risk and benefits in the sense that a positive affect generalizes to other aspects of the activity or technology. Thus, when benefits of a technology are seen as high, this positive affective evaluation generalizes to a positive evaluation of the risk associated with this technology, that is, to a lower perceived risk. Conversely, technologies with low perceived individual benefits are associated with higher perceived risks. The affect heuristic may also work with other heuristics. Slovic and colleagues suggest that the availability heuristic may work not only through ease of recall or imaginability but also because remembered images are associated with affect. As is the case with other heuristics, the affect heuristics, presented by Slovic and colleagues as the centerpiece of experiential or System 1 thinking, may also have drawbacks leading to erroneous judgments. When emotional responses to risky situations (e.g., worry, fear) diverge from cognitive evaluations, these may have a greater impact on risk-taking behavior than do cognitive evaluations. Risks of positive-valued activities, such as fast driving (for some people), may be underestimated, while negative-valued activities, such as flying in airplanes, may lead to an overestimation of risks. When emotions are more intensive, they can even overwhelm deliberative decision making altogether. Some people experience intense fear when they think about flying in airplanes, even though they recognize that the risks are low.

Immediate emotions can have a direct effect, as is the case in the affect heuristic in which affect is used as information for judgment, or an indirect effect. The indirect influence of immediate emotions occurs by influencing people's judgments of expected consequences and their emotional reactions to these outcomes. For instance, when people are not hungry or not in pain, they underappreciate what it will feel like to be hungry or in pain. Furthermore, immediate emotions can bias the interpretation of information in such a way that decision makers selectively attend to and retrieve emotionally relevant information. Studies have found that negative emotions narrow attentional focus, while positive emotions broaden attentional focus. Negative emotions are also found to trigger more systematic processing than positive emotions. One explanation given by George Loewenstein and Jennifer Lerner for this is that negative emotions alert the individual to the possibility that something is wrong and action has to be taken. Happiness or positive mood may have the meaning that everything is all right and, therefore, may lead to more heuristic processing. It has been found, for instance, that happiness increased reliance on stereotypes, which indicates a categorical, holistic way of processing information rather than an analytical way.

Emotions: Anticipatory Emotions

The effect of immediate emotions on decision making should be distinguished from anticipatory emotions. People often compare the consequences of their decisions with what could have happened under different circumstances, which results in counterfactual emotions. One of these emotions is anticipatory regret that results from the comparison between the outcome one will experience as a consequence of a decision and the outcome one would experience if one were to choose differently. For instance, women may choose to attend public health screening for breast cancer in spite of very low chances of having breast cancer because not going may result in strong negative feelings in case they might have a cancer that would then be detected much later. Anticipatory emotions may also explain the finding that patients having to make decisions that are emotionally charged, such as whether to go for prenatal testing or have an operation, usually do not take into account the probabilities. An explanation of people's lack of responsiveness to probabilities is that anticipatory emotions arise as reactions to mental images of the outcome of a decision. Such images are discrete and not very much affected by probabilities. The impact of the image of having a probability of 1 out of 50 of carrying a child with Down syndrome may be the same as the impact of the image of having a probability of 1 out of 500. The decision of women to opt for or against prenatal testing may therefore be more influenced by how they feel about having a child with Down syndrome than by the probabilities. These anticipatory emotions are partly cognitive, in the sense that people may think of them consciously and take them into account when weighing the pros and cons of several options. On the other hand, as they are affect laden, they are part of System 1 thinking and largely intuitive.

Danielle R. M. Timmermans

See also Bias; Dual-Process Theory; Emotion and Choice; Heuristics; Intuition Versus Analysis

Further Readings

Evans, J. St. B. T. (2008). Dual-processing accounts of reasoning, judgment and social cognition. *Annual Review of Psychology, 59,* 255–278.

Gigerenzer, G., & Todd, P. M. (1999). *Simple heuristics that make us smart.* Oxford, UK: Oxford University Press.

Kahneman, D. (2003). A perspective on judgment and choice. Mapping bounded rationality. *American Psychologists, 58*, 697–720.

Loewenstein, G., & Lerner, J. S. (2003). The role of affect in decision making. In R. J. Davidson, K. R. Scherer, & H. H. Goldsmith (Eds.), *Handbook of affective sciences* (pp. 619–642). Oxford, UK: Oxford University Press.

Payne, J. W., Bettman, J. R., & Johnson, E. J. (1992). Behavioral decision research: A constructive processing perspective. *Annual Review of Psychology, 43*, 87–131.

Slovic, P., Finucane, M. L., Peters, E., & MacGregor, D. G. (2002). The affect heuristic. In T. Gilovic, D. Griffin, & D. Kahneman (Eds.), *Heuristics and biases: The psychology of intuitive judgment* (pp. 397–420). Cambridge, UK: Cambridge University Press.

Brier Scores

Brier scores are used to assess the precision of probability predictions. For an event that can only occur in a set of mutually exclusive categories, the Brier score is the sum of the squared differences between the predicted probabilities that the event will occur in a specific category (numbers in the interval from 0 to 1) and the observed outcomes (1 if the event occurs in a specific category, 0 otherwise). Brier scores were originally proposed as a means to describe the precision of probabilistic weather forecasts (e.g., categories "rain," "no rain"). Here, they were appreciated because they allow for a finer assessment of a forecaster's ability to generate accurate predictions than mere counts of numbers of correct predictions. For the same reason, Brier scores have been proposed in the medical context as an alternative to receiver operating characteristic (ROC) methods in diagnostic testing for the calibration of the quality of medical decision makers, for tuning statistical prediction rules, and for the assessment of predictions in survival analysis.

General

Consider an event that can only occur in one of r distinct categories. For example, a medical decision maker might assign probabilities to each category, where the probabilities should sum up to

1. Let $\pi_j \in [0,1]$ denote the prediction for the probability that the event occurs in category j, for $j = 1,\ldots, r$, and let Y_j denote the random outcome, where $Y_j = 1$ if the event occurs in category j and $Y_j = 0$ if it does not. The Brier score is a loss function that has been proposed as a measure to quantify the loss incurred if π is predicted, and Y is the outcome. It is the squared difference $(\pi - Y)^2$. In a sample of size n where π_{ij} and y_{ij} are the ith prediction and the ith actually observed outcome for category j, respectively, the *empirical Brier score* is given by $(1/n)\sum_i \sum_j (\pi_{ij} - y_{ij})^2$. For example, when the events "relapse" versus "no relapse" are of interest, and there are two patients, the first with a relapse and the second without, a naive predicted probability of .5 for both patients results in a Brier score of $1/2 \times (((.5 - 0)^2 + (.5 - 1)^2) + ((.5 - 1)^2 + (.5 - 0)^2)) = .5$. If, however, for the patient with relapse, the predicted probability of relapse is .6, and for the patient without relapse the predicted probability of relapse is .3, then the Brier score reduces to $1/2 \times (((.4 - 0)^2 + (.6 - 1)^2) + ((.7 - 1)^2 + (.3 - 0)^2)) = .25$.

Brier Scores With Dichotomous Data

In a setting with dichotomous data, that is, with only $r = 2$ categories (e.g., when one predicts whether a patient will survive for a certain period of time), it is common to consider only one of the categories for calculation (dropping the subscript j). While in the original formulation, the Brier score takes values in the range from 0 to 2 when there are only 2 categories, the modified version ranges from 0 to 1; that is, the resulting value is only half of the original Brier score.

Brier scores can generally be applied to predictions π_i with $0 \leq \pi_i \leq 1$. These predictions may have been derived from a careful statistical model-building process. They can, however, stem from diverse sources and might also, for example, constitute a summary of expert guesses. For calculating the Brier score, predicted probabilities are needed. When only classifications are available and these are taken as predicted probabilities, so that all π_i are 0 or 1, the squared differences take only the values 0 and 1, and the Brier score is the proportion of observations where classification and outcome are identical. Therefore, in these cases, the empirical Brier score coincides with the misclassification rate.

Properties

The Brier score is a *strictly proper scoring rule*. This means that, when prediction error is quantified by the Brier score, the best predictor is the true probability of the event: Let $p = P(Y = 1)$; then $E(\pi - Y)^2$ attains its unique minimum for $\pi = p$. This can be seen by the following decomposition of the expected Brier score, $E(\pi - Y)^2 = E(p - \pi)^2 + E(p - Y)^2$, which means that inaccuracy (measured by the Brier score) can be split into imprecision and inseparability. Using the Brier score to judge prediction error, thus, forces forecasters to give their best probabilistic predictions, not just classifications. However, imprecision and inseparability primarily are theoretical quantities that cannot be measured directly.

Comparison With ROCs

Another popular technique for judging the performance of medical decision makers is ROC curves. These are obtained from the predicted probabilities π_i by using a cutoff for arriving at actual predictions and then varying this cutoff. For each value of the cutoff, the proportion of correctly classified observations with outcome $y_i = 1$ is recorded and plotted against the proportion of wrongly classified observations with $y_i = 0$ for that cutoff. The area under the resulting ROC curve is an indicator for the performance of the decision maker, with larger values indicating better performance. However, since ROC curves are a rank-based method, two decision makers who rank the observations in the same order will have identical ROC curves, even if their actual predicted probabilities differed. Since it has been argued that the predicted probabilities might be even more important than the actual classification in medical settings, a technique for evaluating performance should be more focused on the former, and therefore, the Brier score should be preferred over ROC curves.

Calibration of Medical Decision Makers

Given predicted probabilities from decision makers, feedback should not only be given on accuracy, that is, on how effective objects could be assigned to the correct category (using a cutoff on the probabilities), but also on precision, that is, on how close the predicted probabilities are to the true probabilities. While the misclassification rate only gives information on accuracy, the Brier score also considers precision. For the dichotomous setting, it is a sum of a measure of imprecision (a property of the decision maker) and a measure of inseparability (a property of the situation at hand). The difference of the Brier scores for two decision makers in the same situation therefore gives their difference in precision.

There are several decompositions of the Brier score that result in explicit values for precision, which in this context is also called reliability or calibration. These decompositions, therefore, also provide for estimates of the theoretical quantities of imprecision and inseparability. Similar to the procedure used for constructing calibration plots, the predictions are grouped by the value of the predicted probabilities; that is, predictions with the same or similar predicted probability are combined into groups j, where $j = 1, \ldots, J$, for which the predicted probability is d_j and the proportion of events is p_j. With n_j being the number of observations in group j, the Brier score can be decomposed into a reliability component $(1/n)\sum_j n_j (d_j - p_j)^2$ and a resolution component $(1/n)\sum_j n_j p_j (1 - p_j)$. The former indicates how close the predicted probabilities are to the true probabilities (with smaller values indicating better calibration of the decision maker), while the latter indicates the ability of the decision maker to sort the observations into categories such that the proportions of outcomes p_j are maximally diverse. From this decomposition, it can again be seen that the Brier score takes its minimum value when the true probabilities are used as predictions.

Assume that there are 20 patients, where a predicted probability of relapse is wanted and that 8 of these patients actually suffer a relapse. If the predicted probability is .5 for all patients, there is only one group ($J = 1$) with predicted probability $d_1 = .5$ and proportion of events $p_1 = .5$. The reliability component therefore is $1/20 \times 20 \times (.5 - .4)^2 = .01$, which seems to be very good. However, the resolution, which is $1/20 \times 20 \times .4 \times .6 = .24$, is rather poor, resulting in a Brier score of .25. If, in contrast, a decision maker provides two predicted probabilities, .6 for a group of 10 patients, where 5 have an event, and .2 for the remaining 10 patients, where 3 suffer relapse, the value of the reliability component will also be equal to .01, that is, very good. However, the resolution now is $1/20 \times ((10 \times .5 \times .5) + (10 \times .3 \times .7)) = .23$, resulting in a Brier score of 0.24, indicating better overall prediction performance.

Reliability, either by explicitly reporting its value or by means of calibration plots, which graph p_j against d_j, has often been used for giving feedback to decision makers, that is, for improving calibration, while resolution seems to have been neglected. In addition, there exist several other decompositions that allow for detailed analysis of decision-maker performance.

Evaluation of Statistical Prediction Rules

Besides analyzing the performance of decision makers, the Brier score can also be used for evaluating statistical prediction rules. The basis for the latter is formed by statistical models, which are typically built from some training data, where, in addition to the outcome for each observation, a set of informative variables is given (e.g., "age" and the concentration of some biomarker for patients, for which survival up to some time is the event of interest). Many statistical models can not only provide classification for new observations (given the information from the variables), thus comprising prediction rules, but also predicted probabilities. Using a cutoff for classification on the latter, performance could be judged by misclassification rate on new data. However, many statistical models require choice of some tuning parameters, which should be selected to maximize performance. Optimizing by means of misclassification rate may easily result in overfitting; that is, use of tuning parameters results in more complexity than is supported by the data, as this criterion is most sensitive to the fit of a statistical model for observations with large ambiguity (i.e., which have true probabilities close to the classification cutoff). When it is expected, for example, that the cutoff for classification might be changed later, the Brier score is a more reasonable criterion for selecting tuning parameters, as it is sensitive to the model fit for all observations, regardless of their true probability. Therefore, it is also more appropriate if interpretation of the prediction rule is wanted, as the structure of the fitted model will be equally valid for all observations.

Brier Scores With Survival Data

In survival analysis, the outcome of interest Y is the time until a specific event (e.g., death) occurs. Here, probability predictions often refer to the survival status $Y(t^*)$ at a specific time t^*, $Y(t^*) = 0$ meaning dead/event occurred, $Y(t^*) = 1$, alive/event not yet occurred at t^*. Let $\pi(t^*)$ denote the prediction for the survival status at t^*.

Brier Score at a Specific Time and Integrated Over Time

The *Brier score at t^** is $[\pi(t^*) - Y(t^*)]^2$, if survival status $\pi(t^*)$ is predicted and $Y(t^*)$ is the outcome. When predictions are to be assessed over a period from time 0 to time t^* rather than for one specific time t^*, the prediction error at t can be averaged over this interval, yielding the *integrated Brier score*, $\int_0^{t^*} [\pi(t) - Y(t)]^2 dW(t)$, where $W(t)$ is a suitable weight function, for example, t/t^*. For a sample of size n, the empirical versions are given by $(1/n)\sum_i [\pi_i(t^*) - y_i(t^*)]^2$ and $(1/n)\sum_i \int_0^{t^*} [\pi_i(t) - y_i(t)]^2 dW(t)$, respectively.

Censoring

In studies of survival time data or time-to-event data, a common problem called *censoring* occurs when some, but not all, individuals can be followed up until death (or until the event of interest occurs). This may happen for many reasons, for example, when a medical study on mortality is evaluated before all patients have died. In that case, the outcome data are (Y, δ), where Y denotes the observation time when the individual was observed to survive, and δ is the event indicator containing the censoring information: $\delta = 1$ indicates that death was observed after Y time units, whereas $\delta = 0$ means that the individual was observed to survive for Y time units before it was censored, so that the exact time of death is unknown.

Empirical Brier scores can be devised to estimate the true expected Brier score even in the presence of censoring, which, however, needs to be accounted for. To this end, the individual contributions to the empirical Brier score are weighted according to the censoring information. Thus, the empirical Brier score at t^* in the presence of censoring is $(1/n)\sum_i w_i(t^*) [\pi_i(t^*) - y_i(t^*)]^2$, where $w_i(t^*)$ is the weight for individual i. In the simplest case, where censoring can be assumed not to depend on the individual's survival chances, the weights incorporate the Kaplan-Meier estimator G of the censoring or potential follow-up distribution, which is obtained from $(Y, 1 - \delta)$ by exchanging the roles of censored and uncensored observations. Then $w_i(t^*) = \delta_i/G(Y_i)$ if $y_i \leq t^*$, and $w_i(t^*) = 1/G(t^*)$ if $y_i > t^*$. With this approach, individuals whose survival status at t^* is unknown due to censoring receive weight 0 (these individuals contribute indirectly to the empirical Brier score, because they are used in the calculation of G). Individuals whose survival status at t^* is known receive weights >1, so that they represent the contributions of individuals whose Brier score is unobservable in addition to their own contribution. Again, to average prediction error at t over an interval from 0 to t^*, an integrated version of the empirical Brier score can be used: $(1/n)\sum_i\int_0^{t^*}w_i(t)[\pi_i(t) - y_i(t)]^2dW(t)$.

Dynamic Predictions

Similar techniques can be used to devise empirical Brier scores when the predictions for a survival status are updated as time progresses. Such updated predictions can arise, for example, when physicians' probability estimates of survival are updated during daily morning rounds or from joint statistical models of longitudinal biomarkers and survival data. Here, the survival status at time t^* is predicted at time s with $0 \leq s < t^*$ by the probabilistic predictor $\pi_i(s;t^*)$.

Evaluation of Statistical Prediction Rules

Similar to the selection of tuning parameters for statistical prediction rules with a categorical outcome, the Brier score can also be used for model complexity selection for survival models. When the empirical version of the Brier score (with proper weights) is obtained for a range of times and plotted against time, this results in prediction error curves. The tuning parameter of a statistical prediction rule should then be chosen such that the area under this curve, that is, the integrated Brier score, is minimal. However, as with a categorical outcome, the empirical version of the Brier score should not be calculated from the data that the prediction rule was fitted to. One can, for example,

set aside a test set, but this has the disadvantage of losing observations for the fitting of the prediction rule. An attractive alternative is provided by the bootstrap procedure, where the drawing of new data sets is imitated by randomly drawing observations from the original data set. The statistical prediction rule is then fitted to each of these bootstrap data sets, and the empirical version of the Brier score is calculated separately for each one based on the observations that are not in the respective bootstrap data set. The final prediction error curve estimate is then obtained from the averaged Brier score over all bootstrap samples. This can then be used not only for selecting tuning parameters for one statistical prediction rule but also to compare the prediction performance of several prediction rules.

Harald Binder and Erika Graf

See also Calibration; Diagnostic Tests; Kaplan-Meier Analysis; Prediction Rules and Modeling; **Receiver Operating Characteristic (ROC) Curve; Survival Analysis**

Further Readings

Brier, G. W. (1950). Verification of forecasts expressed in terms of probability. *Monthly Weather Review, 78,* 1–3.

Gerds, T. A., & Schumacher, M. (2007). Efron-type measures of prediction error for survival analysis. *Biometrics, 63,* 1283–1287.

Graf, E., Schmoor, C., Sauerbrei, W., & Schumacher, M. (1999). Assessment and comparison of prognostic classification schemes for survival data. *Statistics in Medicine, 18,* 2529–2545.

Hilden, J., Habbema, J. D. F., & Bjerregard, D. (1978). The measurement of performance in probabilistic diagnosis III: Methods based on continuous functions of diagnostic probabilities. *Methods of Information in Medicine, 17,* 238–246.

Schoop, R., Graf, E., & Schumacher, M. (2007). Quantifying the predictive performance of prognostic models for censored survival data with time-dependent covariates. *Biometrics, 64*(2), 603–610.

Yates, J. F. (1982). External correspondence: Decompositions of the mean probability score. *Organizational Behavior and Human Performance, 30,* 132–156.

C

CALIBRATION

Calibration refers to the degree of correspondence between probabilities and observed relative frequencies. Suppose that when a patient is admitted to an intensive care unit (ICU), a physician assesses the probability that the patient will survive until hospital discharge. If data on these probabilities and the resulting outcomes (survival or death) are collected for a large number of patients, the data can be organized by the numerical probabilities. For example, the relative frequency of survival among all the patients for whom a probability of 70% was assessed can be determined. If this relative frequency is 70%, and the relative frequencies for other probability values also match those probabilities, the probabilities are said to be perfectly calibrated. If the probabilities and their associated relative frequencies differ, the probabilities are miscalibrated, with the degree of miscalibration increasing as the differences increase.

The relevance of calibration relates to the use of probabilities in decision making. Medical decisions are typically made under uncertainty, such as the uncertainty about whether a surgical procedure will be successful if performed on a particular patient. The likelihood of success quantifies this uncertainty and should be a key factor in the decision about whether to perform the surgery. Thus, the calibration of the numerical probability assessed for success is relevant. If the relative frequency of success is only 40% among patients for whom a probability of success of 70% had been assessed, a decision based on a probability of 70% could be suboptimal.

Measuring Calibration

Measures of calibration are based on pairs of probability values p_i and the corresponding relative frequencies $r_i = 100(f_i/n_i)$, where n_i is the number of times the probability value p_i is used and f_i is the number of times the event occurs when the probability is p_i. For example, if the probability of survival is assessed to be 70% for 100 of the patients who are admitted to an ICU, and 68 of those patients survive, $r_i = 100(68/100)$, or 68%. If there are m probability values $p_1, \ldots, p_m$, there will be m pairs (p_i, r_i).

Calibration is often studied graphically, through a plot of r_i as a function of p_i. This plot is called a *calibration diagram*, and an example of such a plot is shown in Figure 1. Here the values of p_i (expressed in percentages) are 0, 10, 20, ..., 100, and each square represents a pair (p_i, r_i). If the probabilities were perfectly calibrated, the squares would all be on the line from (0, 0) to (100, 100). Of course, a statistical variation in r_i given p_i is likely to cause some deviation from this perfect-calibration line, and such deviations will tend to be larger for small values of n_i (small samples with probability value p_i).

The calibration diagram shown in Figure 1 demonstrates good calibration, although it does reflect a bit of a tendency for r_i to be greater than p_i for lower probability values and to be less than p_i for higher probability values. This tendency is

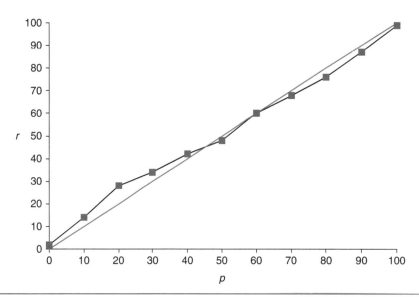

Figure 1   A calibration diagram

often called *overconfidence* because the probabilities are more extreme (lower than the relative frequencies for low probabilities and higher for high probabilities) than justified by the data. Many empirical studies of calibration display overconfidence to varying degrees, whereas other studies demonstrate better calibration.

Calibration diagrams are quite informative, providing at a glance an indication of how far the data points are from the perfect-calibration line, which points are more distant from the line, and whether they are above or below the line. Summary measures of overall calibration are also used, just as summary statistics such as a mean are used in addition to histograms in statistics. The most common summary measure is the weighted average of the squared differences between the probabilities and relative frequencies, with the weights proportional to the sample sizes for the different data points:

$$C = \sum_{i=1}^{m} w_i (p_i - r_i)^2, \text{ with } w_i = n_i / \sum_{j=1}^{m} n_j.$$

Here $(p_i - r_i)^2$ is a measure of the calibration of the probability value p_i, and the *calibration score* C is a weighted average of these calibration measures for the m probability values. A lower value of C indicates better calibration, with perfect calibration corresponding to $C = 0$.

A measure such as C is especially useful in comparing the calibration of probabilities from different sources. Probabilities in medical decision making are often subjective in nature, being assessed by experts such as physicians. It can be informative to compare the calibration of probabilities from different physicians or from different groups of physicians. Probabilities can also be generated through models or from past data, in which case comparisons between physicians' subjective probabilities and model-based or data-based probabilities are possible. The methods used to measure calibration can be used regardless of the source of the probabilities.

Calibration and Sharpness: The Evaluation of Probabilities

What characteristics are of interest in the evaluation of probabilities? Calibration is a characteristic that often receives much attention. But it is not the whole story.

It is possible for probabilities to be very well-calibrated but not very informative. For example, suppose that the overall success rate of a surgical procedure at a given hospital is 80% and that the rate has remained quite steady over the past several years. To aid in decisions about whether to perform this procedure on particular patients, a physician assesses the probability of success for each patient. Information from a patient's records and an examination of the patient should be helpful in assessing the probability for that patient. But if good calibration is the only measure of how good the probabilities are, the physician could just assess a probability of 80% for each patient and be confident of good calibration. Here 80% is the *base rate*, and the expertise of the physician should make it possible to distinguish between patients for whom the surgery is more likely to be successful and patients for whom the surgery is less likely to be successful. A base rate forecast ignores this expertise and is uninformative in the sense of not distinguishing among different patients.

In this example, what would be "perfect" probabilities? A physician would be perfect in predicting the outcomes if the assessed probability was 100% for all patients who then had successful surgery and 0% for all patients with unsuccessful surgery. Of course, this is an ideal that is not likely to be achieved in practice. Nonetheless, it provides a benchmark indicating the most informative probabilities, just as base rate probabilities provide a benchmark indicating relatively uninformative probabilities. To the extent that a set of probabilities can move away from the base rate toward the ideal of perfect forecasts, the probabilities are considered more accurate.

A class of measures called *scoring rules* has been developed to measure the accuracy of probabilities. The most frequently used scoring rule is a quadratic scoring rule, sometimes called the Brier score. For the surgery example, let p be expressed in percentage terms and let the outcome, e, of the surgery for a particular patient be coded as 100 if it is successful and 0 if it is not successful. Then the quadratic score for that patient is a squared-error function: $Q = (p - e)^2$. A lower score is better, with the best possible score being 0 for a perfect probability.

Letting e_{ij} denote the outcome (0 or 100) for the jth patient among the n_i patients for whom the probability, p_i, was assessed, the average quadratic score across all patients is

$$\bar{Q} = \sum_{i=1}^{m} \sum_{j=1}^{n_i} (p_i - e_{ij})^2.$$

This average score can be decomposed into two terms and written as

$$\bar{Q} = \sum_{i=1}^{m} w_i r_i (100 - r_i) + \sum_{i=1}^{m} w_i (p_i - r_i)^2 = S + C.$$

Here C is the calibration score defined earlier, and $S = \sum_{i=1}^{m} w_i r_i (100 - r_i)$ is a measure of the *sharpness* of the relative frequencies, with a lower S indicating greater sharpness. The term $r_i(100 - r_i)$ relates to the sharpness of the relative frequency corresponding to the probability value p_i, and the *sharpness score, S,* is a weighted average of these sharpness measures for the m probability values. The best possible $\bar{Q}$ is 0, and less-than-perfect sharpness ($S > 0$) or calibration ($C > 0$) lead to a worse score.

To understand the sharpness and calibration terms better, think about the assessment of a probability of successful surgery for a patient as if it were separated into two steps. First, the patient is classified into a "bin" with other patients perceived to have roughly the same likelihood of successful surgery. Then a label is assigned to each bin in the form of a probability number. Suppose that some patients are put into a bin with probability value 80%, which means that each of them is judged to have an 80% probability of successful surgery. If they all undergo the surgery, with success for 74% of them, the calibration measure for the bin is $(80 - 74)^2 = 36$, and the sharpness measure is $74(100 - 74) = 1924$. If we calculated these measures for all m bins and then took weighted averages, we would get S and C, from which we could find $\bar{Q} = S + C$. The sharpness, S, is related to how discriminatory the bins are and not to the probability values; note that S does not depend on the p_i values. The calibration, C, on the other hand, has to do with how consistent the probability values are with the relative frequencies. In other words, the sharpness has to do with the effectiveness of the separation of patients into bins, and the calibration has to do with the fidelity of the bin labels (the probability numbers) to the data.

A scoring rule such as the quadratic score, then, measures overall accuracy, taking into account both the sharpness and calibration. If just a single bin is used, with a base rate probability assigned to all cases, the calibration should be excellent but the sharpness weak. If the separation into bins is very effective but the labeling of the bins is poor, the sharpness can be excellent while the calibration is poor. An extreme example of the latter occurs when all patients are given probabilities of 0 or 100 but those with a probability of 0 have successful surgery and those with a probability of 100 have unsuccessful surgery. Sharpness measures the true discriminatory power of the division into bins, but poor calibration can render that power ineffective by causing poor decisions if the probability labels are taken at face value. For the extreme example just given, those assigned probability labels of 100 would most likely go ahead with the surgery, only to see it fail, whereas those assigned probability labels of 0 would avoid the surgery, not knowing that it would be successful if performed.

If probabilities are quite sharp but poorly calibrated, perhaps their calibration can be improved. Training through relevant experience and feedback might help an individual improve calibration. Alternatively, a decision maker can recalibrate probabilities as deemed appropriate. Essentially, this amounts to relabeling the bins. If past data on the probabilities from a particular physician indicate a tendency toward overconfidence, future probabilities might be adjusted, making low probabilities a bit higher and high probabilities a bit lower, in an attempt to calibrate the physician's probabilities. The difficulty is that the decision maker may not be aware of the degree of miscalibration.

A goal to strive for in probability assessment is to make the probabilities as sharp as possible while still maintaining good calibration. The sharpness indicates the true discriminatory power of the probabilities, and the calibration guarantees that this power can be used appropriately by decision makers. In a sense, sharpness is more important than calibration because it is possible to try to improve calibration, as noted above. Improvements in sharpness are more difficult, requiring additional information (e.g., more tests) or greater effort in understanding the implications of the existing information; they cannot be gained by mere relabeling. Nonetheless, miscalibrated probabilities can send misleading messages to decision makers, so striving for good calibration as well as sharpness is desirable.

Robert L. Winkler

See also Brier Scores; Expert Opinion; Judgment; Subjective Probability; Uncertainty in Medical Decisions

Further Readings

Budescu, D. V., & Du, N. (2007). Coherence and consistency of investors' probability judgments. *Management Science, 53,* 1731–1744.

Lichtenstein, S., Fischhoff, B., & Phillips, L. D. (1982). Calibration of probabilities: The state of the art to 1980. In D. Kahneman, P. Slovic, & A. Tversky (Eds.), *Judgment under uncertainty: Heuristics and biases* (pp. 306–334). Cambridge, UK: Cambridge University Press.

McClelland, A. G. R., & Bolger, F. (1994). The calibration of subjective probabilities: Theories and models 1980–94. In G. Wright & P. Ayton (Eds.), *Subjective probability.* Chichester, UK: Wiley.

Murphy, A. H., & Winkler, R. L. (1977). Reliability of subjective forecasts of precipitation and temperature. *Applied Statistics, 26,* 41–47.

O'Hagan, A., Buck, C. E., Daneshkhah, A., Eiser, J. R., Garthwaite, P. H., Jenkinson, D. J., et al. (2006). *Uncertain judgements: Eliciting experts' probabilities.* Chichester, UK: Wiley.

Sox, H., Blatt, M. A., Higgins, M. C., & Marton, K. I. (2006). *Medical decision making.* Philadelphia: American College of Physicians.

von Winterfeldt, D., & Edwards, W. (1986). *Decision analysis and behavioral research.* Cambridge, UK: Cambridge University Press.

Winkler, R. L. (1996). Scoring rules and the evaluation of probabilities. *Test, 5,* 1–60.

Winkler, R. L., & Poses, R. M. (1993). Evaluating and combining physicians' probabilities of survival in an intensive care unit. *Management Science, 39,* 1526–1543.

Yates, J. F. (1990). *Judgment and decision making.* Englewood Cliffs, NJ: Prentice Hall.

CASE CONTROL

Case-control studies are a nonexperimental form of medical research that informs cause-effect relationships. Their main purpose is the identification of risk factors for events of interest. Most famously, case-control studies provided the first evidence of a strong association between cigarette smoking and lung cancer. However, findings from a number of recent case-control studies have been subsequently contradicted or found to overestimate the strength of relationships compared with more robust epidemiological study designs. An example is the case-control finding that hormone replacement therapy (HRT) had a protective effect against coronary heart disease, following which randomized trial evidence identified a small increased risk associated with HRT.

Case-control studies identify cases as patients who already have a disease or condition of interest, and then attempt to identify characteristics of these patients that differ from those who do not have the condition of interest (the controls). For a defined exposure (e.g., walking alongside golf courses) and a defined outcome (e.g., experience of head injury), Table 1, a 2×2 table, represents hypothetical findings and informs analysis of an odds ratio.

The odds are expressed as the ratio of the probability that the event of interest occurs to the probability that it does not. In the example, the probability that a golf course walker experiences a head injury is 10/100 or .1, and the probability that he or she does not suffer such an injury is 90/100 or .9. The odds are therefore 10/90, or .11 (the number of events divided by the number of nonevents). The corresponding odds for non–golf course walkers are 5/150, or .03.

The odds ratio is estimated as the odds in the case group divided by the odds in the control group, that is, .11/.03 or 3.67 in the hypothetical golf course example. This is interpreted as golf course walkers being at more than 5 times the odds of suffering a head injury compared with non–golf course walkers.

Traditional case-control studies only inform estimates of the odds ratio between exposure states; they do not enable the estimation of absolute or relative risk because the full size of the population from which the cases (with and without the exposure(s) of interest) are drawn cannot be estimated in a straight case-control study.

Table 1   Hypothetical 2×2 table

	Cases (Head Injury)	Controls (No Head Injury)
Exposed (walk by golf course)	10	90
Nonexposed (do not walk by golf course)	5	150

Accounting for Bias

The strength and interpretation of identified relationships is first dependent on a study's ability to match the cases and controls, such that both groups can be defined as random samples from the same underlying population. A second significant issue in the application of case-control studies is the accurate identification of the existence or absence of all potentially relevant factors. The exclusion of factors that are associated with both included exposures and the outcome of interest may introduce a bias in the association estimates due to confounding. A third form of bias is labeled *recall bias* and may occur when the outcome acts as a stimulus to aid the recall of the experience or timing of exposures in cases, which tends to inflate risk estimates in case-control studies.

To illustrate these issues, the study of the safety effects of bicycle helmets is used. The representation of the issues is necessarily brief, and the interested reader is referred to a lively discussion in the journal *Accident Analysis and Prevention*. Case-control studies in this area have generally defined cases as persons experiencing head injuries following a bicycle accident. Control groups have included random samples from a population of bicyclists, as well as patients presenting at an emergency department with nonhead injuries sustained following a bicycle accident. Selecting controls from the full population of bicyclists reflects a random sample from the same underlying population from which the cases were drawn and so avoids selection bias. However, such a control group may be subject to both confounding and recall bias. Confounding may occur if cyclists who wore helmets were generally more careful riders than nonwearers (and therefore less likely to experience a bicycle accident), and so more careful riders would be overrepresented in the control group. If this was the case, then one would want to control for riding care in the analysis. A potential solution could involve the elicitation of risk-taking characteristics from the cases and controls, so as to control for differences in the data analysis. Recall bias may not be perceived as a significant problem but would occur if the controls were less likely to accurately recall their use of a helmet.

The nonrandom selection of controls as individuals presenting with nonhead injuries was the more common approach. As the research question specifies the effect of helmets on reducing head injuries following bicycle accidents, the population of interest is cyclists who crashed, and this is a reasonable approach if hospital presentation by controls is not related to helmet wearing. The use of hospital-based controls may also reduce the effects of recall bias as all respondents have a similar stimulus (hospital visit) to aid recollection. It also may reduce the impact of differential risk-taking characteristics between controls and cases as a confounding factor as both groups were hurt sufficiently to seek medical care. However, risk differences may remain: For example, cases and controls may have differing distributions of cycle speed at the point of accident.

There are various methods available to control for possible confounding factors (assuming they can be identified and measured). In the bicycle example, analysis can be restricted to accidents occurring at high speed (or low speed) only. Alternatively, cases and controls could be matched with respect to accident speed. Both these approaches require the specification of sufficiently narrow speed categories that represent important differences. A more flexible approach is to use regression analyses to statistically adjust the risk ratio of interest to capture the effect of potential confounders.

Nested Case-Control Studies

An adaptation to the traditional case-control study design is the nested case-control study, which involves applying a case-control study within the confines of an established cohort. Cohort studies follow individuals over time to observe outcome(s) of interest as they occur, with exposure status being defined at the beginning of the study (i.e., prospectively). Advantages of cohort studies (over case-control studies) include the fact that all individuals in the study analysis are automatically derived from the same population (the cohort) and that there is no uncertainty around the time sequence of the exposure preceding the outcome in the establishment of a cause-effect relationship.

A nested case-control study selects cases on the basis of events occurring (either prospectively or retrospectively). A risk set is defined for each case that includes individuals at risk of the event at the time of the observed case (on the cohort time axis)

and may include some matching criteria. One or more controls are then randomly selected from the defined risk set for each case.

The advantages of this study design include the natural satisfaction of the requirement that controls are randomly sampled from the same population within which the cases occurred (selection bias) and the fact that data on all individuals in the cohort are more easily obtained (recall bias). The nested approach also enables the estimation of relative risks, as well as odds ratios.

Establishing Causal Relationships

Evidence on the existence of a causal relationship between an exposure and an outcome is required to directly inform public health decisions and the design of clinical interventions. The likelihood of confounding can never be completely eliminated (even in a randomized trial), particularly so in case-control studies, and so the presentation and interpretation of study results should always be accompanied by an open and explicit assessment of the probability that results may be confounded and of the direction and size of any confounding bias.

If an association is adequately demonstrated by a case-control study, the next step is to assess whether the observed association is likely to be causal. A range of criteria have been proposed for testing the existence of a causal relationship:

Detailed Review of Potential Confounders

A detailed and explicit consideration, involving literature reviews, of factors that could be related to the exposure and outcome will increase the credibility of proposed causal relationships.

Temporal Relationship

The exposure will always occur before the outcome in a case-control study, but if the outcome develops too soon after the exposure, then the likelihood of causality is reduced.

Size of Odds Ratio

A higher odds ratio (greater than 1) or a lower odds ratio (less than 1) is, ceteris paribus, indicative of a greater probability of causation. However, levels of uncertainty should also be considered when interpreting the size of the mean odds ratio.

Etiological Plausibility

Further evidence is provided if the observed odds ratio and hypothesized causal relationship is supported by existing knowledge around the pathway to the outcome.

Repeated Findings

Similar findings of significant differences between cases and controls in alternative populations increase the chances that an association is causal.

Dose-Response Relationship

Further evidence of causality is provided if a consistent trend showing the odds ratio increases or decreases with increasing or decreasing levels of exposure.

Application to Technology Assessment

In the context of intervention evaluation studies, case-control studies have a limited role in the evaluation of therapeutic interventions as such studies generally evaluate homogeneous populations within which interventions have the same expected effect. There may be some scope for case-control studies to inform downstream effects in decision model-based evaluations; for example, post–disease recurrence pathways may be related to factors observed between treatment initiation and point of recurrence. In breast cancer, the likelihood of progression to metastases following locoregional recurrence is influenced by the duration of the prior disease-free interval.

Case-control studies have much greater potential in secondary evaluations of preventive and screening interventions. Such evaluations describe the pathway of full populations with respect to a disease, and often an important component is the description of separate pathways for different risk groups within an aggregate population. For example, a screening program for anal cancer in homosexual men might differentiate between HIV-negative and HIV-positive men.

Advantages and Disadvantages

The main advantage of case-control studies is that they can be undertaken at relatively low cost and within a shorter time frame than other prospective study designs, particularly around outcomes that are rare. However, case-control studies are generally less reliable than either randomized controlled trials or cohort studies, and causal relationships are often difficult to establish. The results of case-control studies are most often used to generate hypotheses that can be tested using more robust study designs.

Jonathan Karnon

See also Attributable Risk; Bias in Scientific Studies; Causal Inference and Diagrams; Causal Inference in Medical Decision Making; Confounding and Effect Modulation; Odds and Odds Ratio, Risk Ratio

Further Readings

Cummings, P., Rivara, F. P., Thompson, D. C., & Thompson, R. S. (2006). Misconceptions regarding case-control studies of bicycle helmets and head injury. *Accident Analysis and Prevention, 38,* 636–643.

Curnow, W. J. (2006). The Cochrane Collaboration and bicycle helmets. *Accident Analysis and Prevention, 37,* 569–573.

Essebag, V., Genest, J., Suissa, S., & Pilote, L. (2003). The nested case-control study in cardiology. *American Heart Journal, 146*(4), 581–590.

Koepsell, T. D., & Weiss, N. S. (2003). *Epidemiologic methods: Studying the occurrence of illness* (pp. 105–108, 247–280, 374–402). New York: Oxford University Press.

Lawlor, D. A., Smith, G. D., & Ebrahim, S. (2004). The hormone replacement-coronary heart disease conundrum: Is this the death of observational epidemiology? *International Journal of Epidemiology, 33,* 464–467.

Rothman, K. J., & Greenland, S. (1998). *Modern epidemiology* (2nd ed., pp. 62, 93–161, 255–259). Philadelphia: Lippincott-Raven.

Thompson, D. C., Rivara, F. P., & Thompson, R. (2004). Helmets for preventing head and facial injuries in bicyclists (Cochrane Review). In *The Cochrane Library* (Issue 2). Chichester, UK: Wiley.

CAUSAL INFERENCE AND DIAGRAMS

Causal inference is the science of attributing a particular outcome (or effect) to one or more particular causes. In addition to concluding that there is an association between two variables, causal inference implies that the effect is the direct result of a measurable cause. In medical research, the cause is often an intervention or treatment, and the outcome is often a disease or complication. Outcomes from those receiving the intervention, perhaps a particular drug, are often compared with those of a control group. When the difference in outcomes between the experimental and control groups is attributed to the intervention, causal inference is being made.

Causal inference is made most cleanly in a randomized, blinded study. However, even in a nonrandomized setting, some degree of qualified causal inference may be possible. This depends on the extent of thorough understanding of the relationships involved, careful design, and data collection and analysis. Causal inference relationships can be visualized and clarified using causal diagrams—modern tools that use arrows to visualize the purported relationships between causal variables, outcome variables, and confounding variables in both randomized and nonrandomized studies.

Randomized Studies

In a randomized research study, each subject is randomly assigned to receive one of the interventions to be compared. At randomization, but before receiving intervention, randomized groups are very similar to each other with respect to baseline predictors of outcome, the only systematic difference being the assigned intervention. Unless the process of randomization has been systematically altered, other baseline differences would be due to chance.

Thus, in a properly conducted randomized study, there is no selection bias or treatment assignment bias; neither patients nor doctors choose which intervention an individual will receive. Because a *confounder* is a variable that is associated with both intervention and outcome, and because there is usually no association between treatment assignment and baseline predictors of outcome in a randomized study, confounding does not usually exist. Differences in outcome between randomized groups are correctly interpreted as cause-effect.

Fundamental Problem of Causal Inference

Causal inference is a missing-data problem. It has its basis in individuals, not group averages. Let Y^1 and Y^0 represent an individual's potential (or hypothetical) response on treatment and control, respectively. An individual causal effect is defined as the difference between these two potential outcomes at the same point in time, or $\delta = Y^1 - Y^0$. The average of the individual causal effects, or the average causal effect (ACE), can be written as $E[Y^1 - Y^0] = E[\delta]$, where E is the expectation sign, indicating the average of all subjects. Causal effects may well differ across individuals.

However, individual causal effects are never observable because more than one intervention cannot be independently given to the same individual at the same time. In a parallel-group randomized study, each patient receives only one intervention, either treatment or control, and so the outcome is observed for only one of the potential outcomes for that patient. Causal inference is thus a huge missing data problem, in which half of the data for each individual is unobserved. How, then, can causal inference be made? This is the Fundamental Problem of Causal Inference.

Average Causal Effect

While individual causal effects cannot be observed, the average of the individual causal effects, the ACE, is estimated in a randomized study. If the individual causal effects were observable, it is mathematically true that the average of the individual differences (i.e., causal effects) would equal the difference in average response for treatment and control, ignoring individuals, such that $E[\delta] = E[Y^1 - Y^0] = E[Y^1] - E[Y^0]$. Thus, although no patient receives both treatments, in a randomized study, researchers can estimate the ACE from the difference in mean outcome between the treatment and control groups. This is true because treatment assignment is independent of potential confounders, and as a result, patients in the two groups are very similar, on average, on factors that might affect outcome. When randomized groups are compared on the outcome, the estimated difference between groups estimates the ACE for *individuals*.

Nonrandomized Studies

Researchers sometimes strive to make causal inference from nonrandomized studies in which patients have received either one or another of two interventions. The major problem with achieving this goal is selection bias since the treatment assignment has not been random and the groups to be compared likely differ on variables (other than the treatment) that cause the outcome of interest. Selection bias results in confounding, or distortion, of the causal effect of interest. In some situations, it may not be possible to conduct a randomized study due to time, resources, or ethics, making the option of causal inference in a nonrandomized study appealing.

Because it is quite difficult to make causal inference in a nonrandomized study, the traditional practice in biomedical research has been to *not* try to make causal inference. Instead of a cause-effect relationship, researchers have typically made inferences about the *association* between an intervention and an outcome in nonrandomized studies. For example, researchers might conclude that patients taking Drug A during surgery are less likely to have a postoperative complication than are patients taking Drug B. They would be less likely to conclude that Drug A *causes* a reduction in outcome compared with Drug B, and rightly so. However, special methods are available to attempt some degree of valid causal inference in nonrandomized studies.

Correlation Does Not Imply Causation

It is critical to remember that *correlation* does not imply causation. Other than a true cause-effect relationship, there are four main reasons why a statistically significant result might be obtained in a nonrandomized study: chance (random error), bias (systematic error), effect-cause relationship, and confounding. To entertain causal inference, each of these four reasons must be considered and ruled out to the best of a researcher's ability.

Random error and bias can lead to spurious findings that do not represent true effects in the population. Random error may occur as a result of measurement error or from the variability inherent in sampling (i.e., Type I error). Significant results due to systematic bias may result from off-target measurements by the observer, the instrument, or the patient. These errors can also occur in randomized studies.

Effect-cause and confounding are based on true effects, but they are not cause-effect. A positive or negative association between an exposure and an outcome might represent a true *effect-cause* relationship, instead of *cause-effect*. For example, researchers might conclude that maintaining deep anesthesia (vs. light) causes poor intraoperative and postoperative outcome for patients, when in truth patients who are already developing complications intraoperatively are the ones who require (or "cause") deeper anesthesia to keep them stable during surgery.

Finally, confounding by one or more variables might explain the association between the exposure and outcome, where a confounder is a variable associated with both. In confounding, a third factor (e.g., smoking) is a cause of the outcome (e.g., cancer) and also of the exposure (e.g., coffee drinking), resulting in an association between coffee drinking and cancer that is real but not causal. Confounding is often due to the unavoidable selection bias or treatment assignment bias in nonrandomized studies. Patients are likely to differ on variables responsible for them being in one treatment group versus the other. Since some of these variables are also likely to be related to the outcome of interest, the treatment effect of interest is confounded, or distorted, by these baseline variables unless addressed in the design or analysis phase.

Adjusting for Confounding in Design Stage

In the design phase of a nonrandomized study, confounding can be tackled by narrowing the inclusion criteria to focus on certain level(s) of a confounder, or by matching. In matching, nonexposed patients may be chosen to be very similar to the exposed patients on important confounding variables (e.g., age, sex, body mass index). Alternatively, case-control designs might match diseased and nondiseased on important confounders. Matching can be done on individual patients (1:1 or 1:k) or by choosing patients so that distributions are similar (i.e., frequency matching). However, it is logistically difficult to match on a large number of confounders. To the extent that all confounders are accounted for, and explanations other than cause-effect have been ruled out, some degree of cause-effect relationship may be inferred when matched groups are compared on outcome.

Adjusting for Confounding in Analysis Stage

In the analysis phase, confounding can be addressed by stratification, multivariable regression models, and propensity score methods. More complex methods, including instrumental variable analysis and structural equation models, may sometimes be used when the above are not adequate or feasible. A common concern is whether all confounding variables are known and observed.

Stratification analysis consists of estimating the relationship of interest between a hypothesized cause and an outcome within levels of a variable believed to confound the relationship. For example, if patients are selected to receive one intervention versus another based on baseline severity, analysis comparing intervention and outcome could be done within each level of baseline severity, and results averaged across levels.

Multivariable regression statistically adjusts for confounding variables by including them in the statistical model used to assess the relationship between the intervention and outcome.

Propensity score analysis is becoming mainstreamed as one of the best ways to remove confounding via selection bias in nonrandomized studies. First, a logistic regression model predicting treatment assignment from available baseline potential confounders is used to assign each patient a score representing the probability that he or she would receive treatment (vs. control). Intervention and control patients are then compared on the outcome(s) of interest after adjusting for the propensity scores through stratification, matching, or weighting.

There is a growing body of literature and practice using special statistical methods where researchers are sometimes able to legitimately make some degree

of causal inference in nonrandomized studies. The extent to which causal inference is justified in a nonrandomized study depends on the nature and knowledge of the research question, design of the study, knowledge and availability of all true confounding variables, quality of the available data, and skill with which analytical methods are employed.

Causal Diagrams

A causal diagram is a concise way to explore and explain causal relationships among variables. It was popularized by Judea Pearl as a method of displaying adjustment for a third variable or set of variables (Z) to allow causal inference between a cause (X) and effect (Y). Confounding of a causal relationship of interest and the correct (or incorrect) adjustment for confounding can be visualized in a causal diagram. Causal diagrams depend on subject matter experts to guide the plausibility of the postulated relationships. The most common and basic causal diagram is called a directed acyclic graph, or DAG.

Directed Acyclic Graph

A DAG is a graphical description of causal relationships among variables. Many different statistical models would fit any particular DAG. A DAG consists of vertices or nodes representing variables, edges connecting some of the variables, and arrows indicating the direction of relationships among variables. An edge marked by a single arrow is "directed" and indicates the direction of the causal relationship. For example, $X \rightarrow Y \rightarrow Z$ implies that X causes Y, Y causes Z, and X causes Z only through its effect on Y. Variables that are not directly connected in the DAG are assumed to not be *causally* related. *Acyclic* indicates that the DAG does not allow representation of mutual causation or feedback processes such as $X \rightarrow Y$, $Y \rightarrow X$. Each causal relationship can only go in one direction in a DAG, and, typically, only causal relationships are of interest.

Conditioning on variables that block backdoor paths from causal variables to outcome is the first and most widely used strategy to adjust for confounding. A backdoor path is a connected set of variables going from the cause to the effect of interest through an indirect route. A backdoor path indirectly connects the exposure and outcome, and includes at least one variable pointing to (i.e., causing) the exposure and one to the outcome.

For example, researchers may want to compare two anesthetic regimens for a particular type of surgery on a postoperative complication outcome by analyzing a patient registry. Patients with higher baseline severity are more likely to receive regimen A than B, and severity is also a strong indicator of outcome apart from its effect on treatment assignment. The causal diagram in Figure 1 displays the relationships between severity, regimen, and outcome, with backdoor path $D \leftarrow C \rightarrow Y$.

Severity (C) confounds the relationship between treatment (D) and outcome (Y) because it is a cause of both D and Y. The confounding effect of C could be removed by conditioning on C in one of several ways. In stratification, the $D \rightarrow Y$ effect of interest would be estimated within levels of C and then averaged. Multivariable regression could account for the $C \rightarrow Y$ relationship when assessing $D \rightarrow Y$ and would simultaneously compare levels of D at the average value of C. Finally, propensity score analysis could be used to match patients who did and did not receive D on the predicted probability that they would receive D, based on severity. Each of these methods would enhance the validity of making a causal inference between D and Y by conditioning on C.

When conditioning strategies are not feasible, instrumental variable (IV) techniques can sometimes be used. An IV has a causal effect on outcome Y only through its effect on the treatment variable D, as in the DAG IV $\rightarrow D \rightarrow Y$. Such variables are rare since variables responsible for

treatment assignment are often related to outcome through additional causal paths. A true instrumental variable can be used to estimate the causal effect of D on Y by assessing IV $\rightarrow D$ and IV $\rightarrow Y$ and then using the ratio between these two effects to isolate the relationship between D and Y.

Finally, structural equation models can establish an isolated and exhaustive mechanism that relates the causal variable to the outcome and then calculate the causal effect as it propagates through the mechanism.

Using a DAG to Decide Which Variables to Condition On

Causal diagrams are useful in deciding which variables need to be adjusted for, to remove confounding in the cause-effect relationship of interest. First, all arrows emanating *away from* the exposure of interest are removed. Then, if there remains a backdoor path connecting the exposure and outcome, one adjusts for variables on the path. Variables not on a backdoor path do not need to be adjusted for.

A *D-separation* criterion, also called *blocking*, was introduced by Pearl as a method to determine if confounding has been removed from a causal pathway in a DAG. A set of variables (or nodes) Z is said to D-separate a set of confounders X from Y if and only if Z blocks every path from a node in X to a node in Y. D-separation requires either causal chains or causal forks or both. Z must not include so-called collider variables (see Figure 2), which can unblock a backdoor path by adjusting for them, thus introducing confounding.

Causal chains ($i \rightarrow m \rightarrow j$) and causal forks ($i \leftarrow m \rightarrow j$) show D-separation because the two extreme variables are marginally dependent but become independent of each other, or blocked, once the researchers condition on (i.e., adjust for) the middle variable, m. In a causal chain, after conditioning on m, the potential confounder, i, has no effect on the probability of outcome, j.

Figure 1 is an example of a causal fork. Adjusting for severity of disease, the middle variable in the fork, removes the confounding on the relationship between the treatment and outcome. The relationship between treatment and outcome can then be estimated free of confounding by m.

Inverted forks ($i \rightarrow m \leftarrow j$), which include colliders, act the opposite way (Figure 2). A collider is

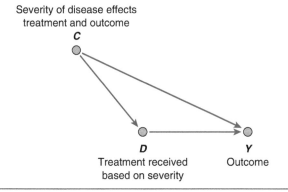

Figure 1   Directed acyclic graph showing confounding of *D-Y* causal effect by *C*

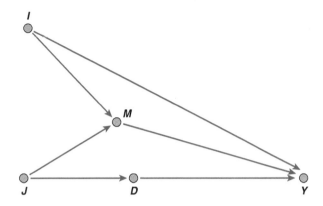

M is a collider. Conditioning on it will create confounding between *I* and/or *J* with the *D-Y* relationship by unblocking the backdoor path *D*←*J*→*M*←*I*→*Y*

Figure 2   Conditioning on a collider variable

variable *m* on a backdoor path that is caused by two or more known or unknown variables. If the extremes, *i* and *j*, are independent, they will *become* dependent once *m* or any of its descendents is conditioned on. This dependence will create confounding if, for example, *i* is also a cause of the outcome, *Y*, and *j* is also a cause of the exposure, *D*. So if a backdoor path between the cause and effect of interest includes a collider variable, confounding will be introduced if researchers adjust for *it alone*.

Consider the potential causal relationship between anesthetic technique *D* and postoperative complication *Y*. Suppose covariables severity of disease, *I*, and surgeon, *J*, are causes of an intraoperative variable *M* (blood loss), which is also a cause of outcome *Y*. Furthermore, suppose the variables are related as in Figure 2, with *J* also causing *D* and *I* also causing *Y*. There would be no confounding if we adjust for all three variables—*I*, *J*, and *M*—since that would completely block the backdoor path between *D* and *Y*. Also, there would be no confounding if we adjust for none of the three variables, since *I* and *J* are independent. However, confounding would be introduced if we *only* adjust for the intraoperative variable, *M*, since that would introduce dependence between surgeon (*J*), a cause of *D*, and severity of disease (*I*), a cause of *Y*. This underappreciated problem due to colliders often surfaces when the variable *M* is observable, such as at baseline measurement

of outcome, but there exist unobserved variables (*I* and *J*) causing *M* and also related to the exposure and the outcome.

In analyses attempting causal inference in the nonrandomized setting, a crucial limitation is that all confounding can usually not be accounted for because variables are either unknown or unavailable. In nonrandomized studies, causal inference can only be attempted with this important qualification.

Ed Mascha

See also Bias in Scientific Studies; Causal Inference in Medical Decision Making; Conditional Independence; Confounding and Effect Modulation; Counterfactual Thinking; Propensity Scores; Randomized Clinical Trials

Further Readings

Angrist, J. D., Imbens, G. W., & Rubin, D. B. (1996). Identification of causal effects using instrumental variables. *Journal of the American Statistical Association, 91,* 444–455.

Blackstone, E. (2002). Comparing apples and oranges. *Journal of Thoracic and Cardiovascular Surgery, 123,* 8–15.

Cox, D. R. (1992). Causality: Some statistical aspects. *Journal of the Royal Statistical Society A, 155,* 291–301.

Dawid, A. P. (2000). Causal inference without counterfactuals (with discussion). *Journal of the American Statistical Association, 95,* 407.

Hulley, S., Cummings, S., Browner, W., Grady, D., & Newman, T. (2007). *Designing clinical research.* Philadelphia: Lippincott Williams & Wilkins.

Morgan, S., & Winship, C. (2007). *Counterfactuals and causal inference: Methods and principles for social research.* Cambridge, UK: Cambridge University Press.

Pearl, J. (1995). Causal diagrams for empirical research. *Biometrika, 82,* 669–688.

Pearl, J. (2000). *Causality: Models, reasoning and inference.* Cambridge, UK: Cambridge University Press.

Rosenbaum, P., & Rubin, D. (1983). The central role of the propensity score in observational studies for causal effects. *Biometrika, 70,* 41–55.

Rubin, D. B. (1974). Estimating causal effects of treatments in randomized and nonrandomized studies. *Journal of Educational Psychology, 66,* 688–701.

CAUSAL INFERENCE IN MEDICAL DECISION MAKING

One of the most important tasks of decision analysts is to derive causal interpretations, on both the level of decision modeling and the level of statistical analyses of original data sets. Usually, an intervention, action, strategy, or risk factor profile is modeled to have a "causal effect" on one or more model parameters (e.g., probability, rate, or mean) of an outcome such as morbidity, mortality, quality of life, or any other outcome.

This entry introduces the key concepts of causal inference in medical decision making and explains the related concepts such as counterfactuals, causal graphs, and causal models and links them to well-known concepts of confounding. Finally, two examples are used to illustrate causal inference modeling for exposures and treatments.

Background

Decision analyses on risk factor interventions frequently include parameters derived from clinical or epidemiologic studies such as single relative risks or multivariate risk prediction functions (e.g., Framingham risk index for coronary heart disease, cancer risk scores, osteoporosis score). When applied in a decision model, changes in risk factors are then translated to causal effects on the risk of a disease or other outcome in the model. Thus, the causal interpretation of the modeling results strongly depends on the causal interpretation of each modeled risk factor. Therefore, this entry has a strong focus on epidemiologic modeling, which yields the parameters for the decision model.

Study Designs

The gold standard design to evaluate causal effects is the randomized controlled clinical trial. However, most decision models include (at least some) parameters or risk functions derived from epidemiologic (i.e., observational) studies, which have the potential for confounding. It is, therefore, crucial that all model parameters derived from epidemiologic studies be properly adjusted for confounding if one wants to use the results to derive causal interpretations.

Confounding

Definition of Confounding

Time-Independent Confounding

Standard textbook definitions of confounding and methods to control for confounding refer to independent risk factors for the outcome that are associated with the risk factor of interest but are not an intermediate step in the pathway from the risk factor to disease.

Time-Dependent Confounding

The more complicated (but probably not less common) case of time-dependent confounding refers to variables that may vary over time and simultaneously act as confounders (e.g., common cause of both exposure and disease) and intermediate steps (on the causal pathway from exposure to disease). In other words, confounder and exposure of interest mutually affect each other. For example, in a model evaluating the effect of weight loss on the risk of coronary heart disease, physical activity could be a time-dependent confounder because it is an independent risk factor for coronary heart disease, it influences weight, and it can also be influenced by weight.

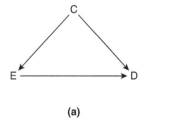

(a)

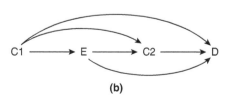

(b)

Figure I   (a) Time-independent confounding and (b) time-dependent confounding

Control for Confounding

Traditional textbook techniques to control for time-independent confounding include restriction, stratification, matching, and multivariate regression analysis. However, these methods have been criticized for being inadequate to control for time-dependent confounding. Other methods such as g-computation, marginal structural models, or structural nested models have been suggested as approaches to this problem.

Relevant Questions

To do a proper causal analysis, one must answer three questions:

1. Which a priori assumptions can be made about the causal relationships between the variables of an epidemiological study?
2. Under these assumptions, are the observed data sufficient to control for confounding?
3. What methods are appropriate to control for confounding?

Causal graphs can guide us in answering these questions.

Causal Graphs

Causal diagrams have a long history of informal application. More recently, formal concepts and rules have been developed for the use and interpretation of causal graphs, for example, in expert systems and operational research. Causal graphs can guide the process of identification of variables that must be measured and considered in the analysis to obtain unbiased (unconfounded) effect estimates. In their milestone paper "Causal Diagrams for Epidemiologic Research," published in 1999 in the journal *Epidemiology*, Sander Greenland, Judea Pearl, and James M. Robins provide an introduction to these developments and their use in epidemiologic research.

Use of Directed Acyclic Graphs in Epidemiology and Medical Decision Making

Directed acyclic graphs (DAGs) are a specific form of causal graph that can be used to understand and explicitly state causal a priori assumptions about the underlying biological mechanisms. DAGs consist of a set of nodes and directed links (arrows) that connect certain pairs of nodes. In medical decision-making research and epidemiology, nodes are used to represent variables, and arrows denote causal relationships. A set of formal and precise graphical rules and assumptions for DAGs has been developed, including a graphical method called d-separation, the causal Markov assumption, and a graphically oriented definition of confounding named the backdoor criterion. These methods allow researchers to determine

- whether they can estimate an unbiased effect from the observed data,
- which variables must be adjusted for in the analysis, and
- which statistical methods can be used to obtain unbiased causal effects.

Specific Applications of Directed Acyclic Graphs

Besides helping with the questions mentioned above, DAGs offer a readily accessible approach to understanding complex statistical issues, including the fallibility of estimating direct effects (i.e., controlling for intermediate steps), the rationale for instrumental variables, and controlling for compliance in randomized clinical trials (when both "intention to treat" and "per protocol" analyses can fail to yield the true causal intervention effect).

Key Lessons Learned From Causal Graphs

There are several lessons to be learned from causal graph theory. In particular, applying the formal rules of DAGs, one can derive four key messages.

Key message 1: Controlling for nonconfounders can induce severe bias in any direction.

The second lesson follows directly from message 1.

Key message 2: The selection of confounders must be based on a priori causal assumptions.

Further messages follow.

Key message 3: Estimating direct effects (i.e., controlling for a known intermediate step variable) can be problematic.

As traditional regression analysis can either control for a variable or not, it cannot appropriately adjust for confounders that are simultaneously affected by the intervention or risk factor of interest (i.e., time-dependent confounding). This leads to the last message.

Key message 4: Traditional adjustment methods (e.g., stratification or multivariate regression analysis) may fail to control for time-dependent confounding.

The following section provides some cases.

Quantitative Models of Causal Inference

Counterfactual Principle

Whereas causal graphs allow for deducting qualitative information about causal effects, medical decision making usually needs quantitative results to inform decisions. One type of quantitative model originating with Neyman and Fisher in the early 20th century is the counterfactual model. In such a model, an association is defined as causal when it is believed that, had the cause been altered, the effect would have changed as well. This definition relies on the so-called counterfactual principle, that is, what would have happened if, contrary to the fact, the risk factor or intervention had been something other than what it actually was.

Classes of Quantitative Causal Models

There are several classes of quantitative models for causal inference that are able to deal with both time-independent and time-dependent confounding. The following model classes are the most recent innovations and increasingly used in medical decision making and epidemiology:

- inverse probability of treatment weighting (marginal structured models),
- g-estimation, and
- parametric g-formula.

In the case of time-dependent confounding, all three of these methods require longitudinal data. This is not—as has been erroneously mentioned—a weakness of these modeling techniques. It is rather quite obvious that disentangling the causality of the feedback loop between the intervention of interest and the time-dependent confounder (which is a cause and effect of the intervention of interest) requires repeated measurements of the same variable. Hence, it is due to the inherent causal nature that observational data with time-dependent confounding can only be solved with longitudinal data.

All these techniques are quite complex and require special programming. The following paragraphs give an overview of how the key approaches differ between these models.

Inverse Probability of Treatment Weighting (Marginal Structured Models)

The imbalance regarding the confounder variable in each of the treatment (or exposure) categories is resolved in the following way: The technique of inverse probability of treatment weighting creates a pseudo population (i.e., counterfactual population); that is, for each subject receiving treatment, another (counterfactual) subject that does not receive the treatment but has the same properties regarding the past variable history is added to the data set. This weighting procedure yields a balanced (unconfounded) data set, and the crude effect estimates derived from this data set represent causal effects. In the presence of time-depending confounding, this step is repeated for each repeated measurement time.

g-Estimation

This approach is based on the assumption of no unmeasured confounding. Under this assumption, the outcome is independent of the exposure, given the past history of covariables. The g-estimation procedure is started with assuming a mathematical model. Then the model parameters are systematically varied in a grid search until the outcome is in fact independent of the exposure in the data set. The final values of the parameters are the ones with a causal interpretation.

Parametric g-Formula

The data set is divided into intervals. For each interval, traditional multivariate regression analysis can be performed (separately or pooled) controlling for the past history of variables but not including future measurements into the regression model. Subsequently, simulation techniques (e.g., Monte Carlo simulation) can be used to simulate the overall effect of one exposure or treatment versus another based on the parametrized regression equations.

Examples

Causal Analysis of Risk Factors: The Causal Effect of Public Health Interventions on the Risk of Coronary Heart Disease

Background

The World Health Organization (WHO) has established a project on comparative risk assessment for coronary heart disease (CHD) that evaluates the

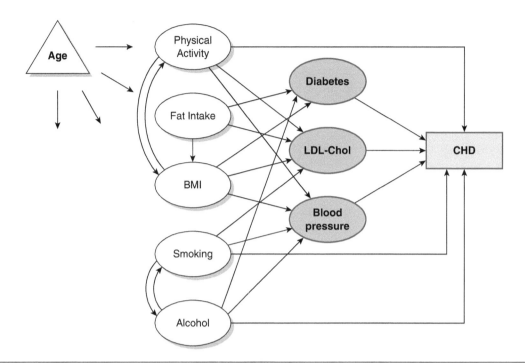

Figure 2 Causal diagram for CHD

overall impact of several public health interventions on the risk of CHD. The causal diagram for CHD was defined by a WHO panel of epidemiologists. This diagram represents the prior knowledge about the causal links among CHD risk factors, potential risk factors, confounders, intermediate variables, and the outcome, CHD.

Given that multiple direct and indirect risk factors are part of the causal web of CHD, such an evaluation not only must consider the direct effect of the risk factors under intervention but should also include their effects mediated through other risk factors. As various risk factors simultaneously act as confounders and as intermediate steps, traditional regression analysis is not an appropriate method to control for confounding, and a causal method must be used.

Methods

The analysis was based on the Framingham Offspring Study longitudinal data ($n = 5,124$) with a 20-year follow-up. The parametric g-formula was used to adjust for time-dependent confounding and to estimate the counterfactual CHD risk under each intervention. Pooled logistic regression models were used to predict risk factors and CHD distributions conditional on given risk factor history. The Monte Carlo technique and the bootstrap method

were used to estimate relative CHD risks with 95% confidence intervals. Evaluated strategies included interventions on smoking, alcohol consumption, body mass index (BMI), and low-density lipoprotein (LDL), and a combined strategy.

Results

The simulated 12-year risk of CHD under no intervention was about 8% for males and 3% for females. Smoking cessation at baseline in all smokers had a statistically significant relative risk of .8 in males and females ($p < .05$). The relative risk after shifting the LDL distribution to the distribution of the Chinese population was .7 for men and .5 for women (both $p < .05$). Shifting alcohol consumption to moderate alcohol intake or constantly lowering BMI to 22 kg/m² did not change CHD risk significantly. The combined intervention on smoking cessation, BMI, and LDL reduced the CHD risk by more than 50% in men and women ($p < .05$).

Conclusions

The parametric g-formula could be applied in a multiple risk factor analysis with time-dependent confounding, where traditional regression analysis fails. It showed that combined interventions have a joint potential of reducing CHD risk by more than 50%.

Causal Analysis of Treatment: The Adherence-Adjusted Effect of Hormone Therapy on Coronary Heart Disease

Background

The Women's Health Initiative (WHI) randomized trial found greater CHD risk in women assigned to estrogen/progestin therapy than in those assigned to a placebo. Observational studies had previously suggested reduced CHD risk in hormone users.

Methods

Miguel A. Hernán and colleagues used the data from the observational Nurses' Health Study. They emulated the design and intention-to-treat (ITT) analysis of the WHI randomized trial. Because the ITT approach causes severe treatment misclassification, the authors also controlled for time-dependent confounding and estimated adherence-adjusted effects by inverse probability weighting. Hazard ratios of CHD were calculated comparing initiators versus noninitiators of estrogen/progestin treatment.

Results

The results showed ITT hazard ratios of CHD similar to those from the WHI. The results from inverse-probability of treatment weighting analysis suggest that continuous hormone therapy causes a net reduction in CHD among women starting therapy within 10 years of menopause, and a net increase among those starting later. However, the authors mentioned that it cannot be excluded that either of these effects could be due to sampling variability.

Conclusions

These findings suggest that the discrepancies between the WHI and Nurses' Health Study ITT estimates could be largely explained by differences in the distribution of time since menopause and length of follow-up. The probability of treatment analysis allowed adjustment for adherence and determination of the CHD risks of hormone therapy versus no hormone therapy under full adherence.

Uwe Siebert

See also Applied Decision Analysis; Bias in Scientific Studies; Causal Inference and Diagrams; Confounding and Effect Modulation

Further Readings

Cole, S. R., & Hernán, M. A. (2002). Fallibility in estimating direct effects. *International Journal of Epidemiology, 31*(1), 163–165.

Cole, S. R., Hernán, M. A., Robins, J. M., Anastos, K., Chmiel, J., Detels, R., et al. (2003). Effect of highly active antiretroviral therapy on time to acquired immunodeficiency syndrome or death using marginal structural models. *American Journal of Epidemiology, 158*(7), 687–694.

Greenland, S., & Brumback, B. (2002). An overview of relations among causal modelling methods. *International Journal of Epidemiology, 31,* 1030–1037.

Greenland, S., Pearl, J., & Robins, J. M. (1999). Causal diagrams for epidemiologic research. *Epidemiology, 10*(1), 37–48.

Hernán, M. A., Hernandez-Diaz, S., Werler, M. M., & Mitchell, A. A. (2002). Causal knowledge as a prerequisite for confounding evaluation: An application to birth defects epidemiology. *American Journal of Epidemiology, 155*(2), 176–184.

Pearl, J. (2000). *Causality.* Cambridge, UK: Cambridge University Press.

Robins, J. M. (1998). Marginal structural models. In *1997 proceedings of the American Statistical Association.* Section on Bayesian Statistical Science (pp. 1–10). Washington, DC: American Statistical Association.

Robins, J. M., Hernán, M. A., & Siebert, U. (2004). Estimations of the effects of multiple interventions. In M. Ezzati, A. D. Lopes, A. Rodgers, & C. J. L. Murray (Eds.), *Comparative quantification of health risks: Global and regional burden of disease attributable to selected major risk factors* (pp. 2191–2230). Geneva: World Health Organization.

Tilling, K., Sterne, J. A. C., & Moyses, S. (2002). Estimating the effect of cardiovascular risk factors on all-cause mortality and incidence of coronary heart disease using g-estimation. *American Journal of Epidemiology, 155*(8), 710–718.

CERTAINTY EFFECT

Within decision making, the certainty effect is used to describe the impact of certainty on the decision maker. People are drawn to certainty, giving higher preference to options that have high levels of certainty. An option with high certainty (close to 0% or 100%) is more appealing to people than a complex or ambiguous probability. This causes many decision makers to choose options that go against the expected utility of the problem. A reduction in probability has a greater impact on the decision maker if the initial outcome is certain. For example, a reduction in survivability from 100% to 90% would have a greater impact than a reduction in survivability from 70% to 60%.

The underlying reason for the certainty effect falls on a person's preference for certain or absolute values. People will bear psychological effects from feelings both of certainty and of uncertainty. They prefer certainty, rather than complexity and ambiguity. Most decision makers cannot clearly define the difference between two probabilities, especially if they are ambiguous. Rather than consider exact probabilities, people often lump outcomes into categories such as "likely" and "unlikely." This makes comparison between two "likely" probabilities difficult. For example, if a healthcare provider explains two courses of treatment to a patient, he or she may present some probability of full recovery. If both options presented a midrange probability, it would be difficult for the patient to decipher the true difference between them. Consider the case where the first course of treatment presents a 70% chance of full recovery, whereas the second presents a 60% chance of full recovery. Most people would be unable to differentiate between these two probabilities but would rather refer to them as "good chances," "likely," or "better than average." If one course of treatment had extreme certainty (close to 100% in this example), the decision maker would put a higher weight on the certain treatment. This is due to the fact that decision makers tend to eliminate uncertainty altogether by overweighting the certain outcomes.

Consider the following case, originally presented by Amos Tversky and Daniel Kahneman. Treatment A leads to a 20% chance of imminent death and an 80% chance of normal life, with a longevity of 30 years. Treatment B leads to a 100% chance of normal life with a longevity of 18 years. According to expected utility theory, rational decision makers would choose Treatment A as it provides a higher utility in terms of lifespan (24 years compared with 18 years). However, the majority of decision makers choose Treatment B. This is a prime example of the certainty effect in

practice. Decision makers, be they physicians or patients, have a high preference for certain outcomes, regardless of the comparative utilities associated with them.

Decision makers are confident when handling extreme probabilities (near 0 or 1.0). When the probabilities are not as certain, however, the weighting of alternatives becomes disproportionate. Decreasing a risk from 5% to 0% should have the same utility as decreasing that risk from 20% to 15%. However, decision makers greatly prefer the first.

An experiment introduced by Richard Zeckhauser illustrates the certainty effect phenomenon. Respondents in the experiment were asked to imagine that they were compelled to play Russian roulette. They were given the opportunity to purchase the removal of one bullet from the loaded gun by choosing one option. Option 1 allowed them to reduce the number of bullets from four to three. Option 2 allowed them to reduce the number of bullets from one to zero. The respondents were asked to how much they would be willing to pay for each option. The result was that a majority of respondents would pay much more for the second option. This is the option that reduced their chances of being shot to 0.

On examination of both options, it is clear that the utility of each option is equal. Option 1 has a probability of being shot of 67%, which is reduced to 50% on removal of one bullet. Option 2 has a probability of being shot of 17%, which is reduced to 0% on removal of one bullet. Both options experienced a reduction of probability (or risk) of 17%. From the perspective of utility, both options are the same. However, people strongly preferred the option that led to certainty: Option 2.

The certainty effect is noticeable in situations that have positive prospects as well as those with negative prospects. In the positive domain, decision makers address scenarios in which there is a probability of a gain. Examples could include winning money in a lottery or increasing life expectancy. The key component of the certainty effect, one's overweighting of certainty, favors risk aversion in the positive domain. The decision maker would prefer a sure gain over a larger gain that is merely probable. In the negative domain, decision makers consider effects when presented with a loss scenario. This could include loss of life, increased illness, or side effects. The overweighting of certainty favors risk seeking in the domain of losses.

In the negative domain, the same effect leads to a risk-seeking preference for a loss that is merely probable over a smaller loss that is certain.

The certainty effect is a demonstration of how humans do not make rational decisions. This is not to say that they make incorrect decisions but rather that they have a stated preference toward things that are absolute. The certainty effect should be considered when evaluating how people make decisions.

Lesley Strawderman and Han Zhang

See also Allais Paradox; Certainty Equivalent; Expected Utility Theory; Prospect Theory

Further Readings

Cohen, M., & Jaffray, J.-Y. (1988). Certainty effect versus probability distortion: An experimental analysis of decision making under risk. *Journal of Experimental Psychology: Human Perception and Performance, 14,* 554–560.

Kahneman, D., & Tversky, A. (1979). Prospect theory: An analysis of decision under risk. *Econometrica, 47,* 263–292.

Tversky, A., & Kahneman, D. (1981). The framing of decisions and the psychology of choice. *Science, 211,* 453–458.

Tversky, A., & Kahneman, D. (1986). Rational choice and the framing of decisions. *Journal of Business, 59,* 251–278.

CERTAINTY EQUIVALENT

When examining the potential outcomes a given event may hold, a person is likely to approximate the probability of each possible result. Taken into consideration by the individual is the degree to which any of these outcomes may be certain. That is, although the benefit derived from an event with a lesser or unknown likelihood of occurring may be much greater, people often tend to opt for the less advantageous, although more certain, outcome. An influential variable, however, is to what degree the individual finds the certain outcome to be of value. Thus, certainty equivalents are the amount of utility, or usefulness, that a person will consider to forgo an offered gamble. When the person becomes indifferent between the choice of a certain event and a probabilistic one, the value of the certain event is called the *certainty equivalent.*

Certainty equivalents are used most frequently in an outward sense within the realm of economic ventures, though individuals may subconsciously use the framework for any scenario in which a gamble presents itself. The utility terms will therefore vary with the application as what is considered beneficial is highly circumstantial. Within medical decision making, however, certainty equivalents could include financial aspects relating to choices in care, various measures of quality of life for the self and for others, or potential recovery periods. The difference between the expected value of indefinite outcomes and the certainty equivalent is referred to as the risk premium.

Finding Certainty Equivalents

A number of mathematical methods exist for finding the certainty equivalent based on the utility function being presented. However, in practice, a person's certainty equivalent can be found more pragmatically by asking a series of questions. Each question should ask the person to choose one of two options. The first option presents a gamble, whereas the second option presents a certain outcome. If the person chooses the gamble, a second question is posed. This time, the first option remains the same, but the conditions of the gamble are altered. The question is presented to the individual so that the perceived benefit or the probability of such has been increased. This line of questioning continues until the person either chooses the second option (a given payout) or says he or she cannot decide. At this point, the value of the payout becomes the certainty equivalent.

Responses to Risk

Enhancements to actual gain or likelihood ratios will produce varying responses, many of which are dependent on the individual's bearing. While one person may be inclined to accept a gamble for a larger disbursement based on a lower probability, another may require a large probability for even the lowest of disbursements. While these variances are indeed environmentally produced, it has been suggested that inherent personality differences affect an individual's willingness to entertain the idea of a gamble over a more certain outcome.

Most people are considered risk-averse. That is, they avoid risk whenever necessary, rather opting for a certain outcome. For a risk-averse person, the certainty equivalent is generally lower than the expected value of the gamble. This condition is present in individuals who desire to behave in a way so as to reduce potential uncertainties. That is, people of this nature are likely to respond to expected outcomes, however smaller the advantage of a less assured event may be. The risk premium for a risk-averse person would be positive. He or she would require an extra incentive to take the gamble, usually found in the form of an increase in the probability of a given event occurring rather than an augmentation of the prospective payout.

A risk-seeking person, however, would have a certainty equivalent that is higher than the expected value of the gamble, indicating his or her preference for scenarios in which the outcome is less certain. The risk premium for a risk-seeking person would be negative. He or she would require an extra incentive to not take the gamble. It should be noted, however, that people who possess this characteristic are more likely to respond to rewards than to punishments. For example, given the same outcome for two given events, one certain and one probabilistic, an individual who is risk-seeking is unlikely to be deterred by the potential loss or detriment caused by an unsuccessful gamble. That is, the payout is of more importance than the probability; decreasing the likelihood of success in the gambling scenario is unlikely to dissuade that choice. Rather, a more efficient discouragement would come in the form of increasing the payout of the certain event or decreasing the payout of the gamble.

A risk-neutral person would have a certainty equivalent equal to the expected value of the gamble, leading to a risk premium of zero. Whereas people averse to risk require alterations in probabilities, and people attracted to risk require alterations in perceived benefits, those who are risk-neutral may respond to either of these variants. Individuals exhibiting indifference toward two more or less certain outcomes will be equally influenced by alterations to probability as well as to benefit. As opposed to other scenarios, within medical decision making it should also be considered that individuals are apt to take into account not only the expected benefit but the prospective harm that may result as well.

Application to Healthcare

As with other concepts within expected utility theory, frameworks of certainty equivalents can be applied to healthcare. Particularly when a patient is capable of receiving treatment through multiple options, the treating physician as well as the individual and his or her family are likely to consider certainty equivalents. The utility at hand becomes the treatment outcomes (recovery period, additional life expectancy), rather than the traditional financial outcomes. Therefore, within healthcare, although financial considerations are certainly taken into account when determining courses of treatment, the degrees of likelihood and their associated risks and benefits are more influential. Within more conventional gambling scenarios, the perceived benefit is often what drives the decision to participate or forgo the opportunity. When considering medical decision making, however, patients are likely to weigh equally the potential risks, such as the amount of pain expected or the risks associated with a given course of treatment.

For example, consider a patient who is presented with two treatment options. Treatment A is a lottery. Treatment A gives the patient a 50% chance of living an additional 10 years and a 50% chance of living an additional 5 years. Treatment B, however, is certain, giving the patient a 100% chance of living X years. According to expected utility theory, these two treatment options would have equal utility when $X = 7.5$ years. If the patient is risk-averse, their certainty equivalent would be lower, possibly $X = 6$ years. This means that he or she would choose Treatment B only if $X \geq 6$. A risk-seeking patient, however, would have a higher certainty equivalent, possibly $X = 8$ years. In this case, the patient would choose Treatment B only if $X \geq 8$ years. Otherwise, he or she would opt for Treatment A, preferring to take a gamble. The above example assumes, however, that the most important consideration when determining courses of medical treatment is the additional life expectancy gained. A more holistic approach realizes that multiple considerations are often influential within medical decision making, such as the expected quality of life associated with varying treatments.

Lesley Strawderman and Lacey Schaefer

See also Certainty Effect; Expected Utility Theory; Risk Aversion

Further Readings

Benferhat, S., & Smaoui, S. (2007). Hybrid possibilistic networks. *International Journal of Approximate Reasoning, 44*(3), 224–243.

Feeny, D. H., & Torrance, G. W. (1989). Incorporating utility-based quality-of-life assessment measures in clinical trials. *Medical Care, 27*(3), 190–204.

Hennessy, D. A., & Lapan, H. E. (2006). On the nature of certainty equivalent functionals. *Journal of Mathematical Economics, 43*(1), 1–10.

Hsee, C. K., & Weber, E. U. (1997). A fundamental prediction error: Self-others discrepancies in risk preference. *Journal of Experimental Psychology, 126*(1), 45–53.

Quiggin, J., & Chambers, R. G. (2006). Supermodularity and risk aversion. *Mathematical Social Sciences, 52*(1), 1–14.

CHAINED GAMBLE

Chaining (also called indirect linking) as used in the expression *chained gamble* or *chained lottery* is best conceived of as a strategy of adjusting preference measurement used within preference elicitation techniques such as the standard gamble and time trade-off methodologies. The approach of chaining gambles (or chaining lotteries) has been offered as a solution to the problem of within-technique inconsistency found with real-world use and testing of the standard gamble as a preference elicitation methodology in economic and medical decision making. The goal here is to understand why such chaining is proposed as an attempt to solve problems of lack of internal consistency (presence of internal inconsistency) in preference elicitation methodologies. This entry illustrates chained gambles for the standard gamble.

Detecting a Lack of Internal Consistency

Internal consistency can be examined in the following way. One technique is based on a more direct value preference elicitation. This more basic technique is used to generate values based on a "basic reference exercise," which is in fact the basic technique used to generate (elicit from patients) values across a set of outcomes. Such a basic reference exercise may invoke a simple elicitation exercise where the individual is asked to rank order outcomes on a scale from most desirable to least desirable. The second strategy, indirect

value elicitation through a chained exercise, generates values based on the use of the standard gamble technique. Adam Oliver, who has examined the internal consistency of a variety of techniques, including standard gambles, argues that if the first and the second strategies yield results that do not significantly or systematically differ from one another, then one might be able to say that the strategies are each internally consistent in that they yield the same ordering of preferences. If individuals distinguish between and among states on the basis of the basic simple direct rank ordering of preferences strategy but are unable to distinguish between their preferences for outcomes in the preference elicitation procedure, then there are potential problems.

Once an inconsistency is found in the use of a preference elicitation methodology, the search is on for what is causing this inconsistency. Initial considerations may fall on issues related to the patients as respondents whose preferences are being elicited and who may lack experience with the use of the technique. To eliminate the inexperienced respondent as the potential source of the problem, an attempt is then made to seek out and to study more experienced respondents, for example, more experienced professionals more familiar with the use of such techniques, to see if the experienced professionals also have problems with internal consistency of results using the techniques. If the same problems (or roughly the same problems) are found with both groups, then the next question that comes up is whether the problem is with the technique being used in preference elicitation itself.

If the same type of inconsistency is found in the elicitation of preferences from both inexperienced respondents and experienced professionals, then the technique itself may be causing the inconsistency. Chaining is a technique aimed at amending the inconsistencies found in the use of the standard gamble as a preference elicitation technique.

It should be noted, though, that any time one has to introduce a technique (a methodology or a procedure) into an arena of decision making of any sort, one needs to recognize that the arena being studied is of such a level of complexity that simply straightforward asking and answering of questions cannot always be employed to achieve the desired result, that is, the understanding of what the individual's (the patient's) preferences are across a set of outcomes.

Cross-Technique Inconsistencies

Inconsistencies between techniques and among techniques may exist, but the question that needs addressing is inconsistency within techniques. If an inconsistency between or among techniques is found, one still needs a counting procedure for determining answers to the following three questions: (1) What is to count as an inconsistency? (2) When does an inconsistency exist within a technique? (3) What is to be used as the gold standard for a consistent technique? Here, there must be an agreement on some basic preference ordering tool (instrument) that then serves as the basis for deciding which technique is "better" and on what grounds. In the example of chaining, *better* is defined in terms of more degrees of agreement with the results of the basic ordering tool.

Within-Technique Inconsistency and Standard Gamble

Using a basic ordering tool, within-technique inconsistency has been found with the standard gamble technique. Before elucidating the type of within-technique inconsistency that has been demonstrated with the standard gamble, it is important to understand the following definitions and concepts that exist within contemporary standard gamble discussions.

To understand chained gambles, one needs to understand the following basic assumptions about the division of healthcare states: extreme states, moderate states, and minor states. Extreme, moderate, and minor health states may be described in terms of severity of state, in terms of permanence (degree of irreversibility) of state, or in terms of severity and permanence of state.

Extreme States

Typically, in the decision sciences, there are two extremes of health states considered. At the negative extreme, there is death (considered in many frameworks as "immediate death"); at the other, positive extreme, there is "full or perfect health." Yet there are questions whether the state "immediate death" is itself the extreme end of the negative range of ill health states. More extreme states than death as considered by reasonable patients may include (a) end-staged neurodegenerative disease processes or severe cerebrovascular accidents (strokes) causing loss of memory, loss of thinking capacity, and progressive motor loss, and (b) end-stage cardiopulmonary disease (heart and lung failure) where there is a tremendous work of breathing and inability to carry out any exertion in one's daily life.

Moderate States

In neurology, any "less severe" state of loss of memory, loss of thinking capacity, loss of motor abilities, or less severe sensory loss may be considered a more moderate state of impaired health. In cardiology, states of increasingly severe chest discomfort or increasing limitations on one's abilities to exert oneself in walking can be described by some individuals as moderate states of ill health.

Minor States

Minor states are impaired states of a much lower intensity or severity or shortened temporal course than moderate states. In neurology, a minor degree loss of motor strength, 4.9 on a scale of 5.0, or in cardiovascular disease, 5 minutes of mild chest discomfort per week, may be considered as minor health states. However, as one walks patients down from extreme to moderate to minor health states and then on down to full or perfect health, some patients may find it hard to distinguish between minor states of impaired health and states of full or perfect health.

Interestingly, within-technique inconsistency has been found as a problem within standard gambles when minor states are being considered by the patient whose preferences are being elicited.

When individuals are asked their willingness to trade chance of survival for improvements in health status in a standard gamble, oftentimes they are unwilling to trade *chances of survival* for *improvements in health status*. In a basic simple direct rating exercise given prior to a preference elicitation of an individual, the individual reports that he or she is able to distinguish between states, but then when approached with a standard gamble, he or she reports that he or she is unwilling to trade. For example, an individual who is able to order full or perfect health as "better than" (more desirable than) a state of minor adverse or poor health in the basic reference exercise above is unwilling to trade chances of survival for improvements in health status in a standard gamble.

In the case of medical decision making, the approach of standard gambles has been found to be inconsistent in the following way: When minor or temporary states of health, most notably negative (adverse) states of ill health (poor health), are being evaluated, it is difficult for patients to evaluate the preferences for minor states of poor health as different from states of full or perfect health. Thus, there is an inability to truly assess minor states of poor health through the standard gamble elicitation methodology.

Chained Gambles

One way that has been proposed to improve on the standard gamble as a preference elicitation technique is to use chained gambles. Chaining links minor or temporary health states to death through intermediate states that then all become the links of a chain. Here, instead of valuing a minor or temporary health state against immediate death, one values the minor state with a moderate (intermediate) state and then the moderate (intermediate) state with immediate death.

For example, in neurology, if a slight hand tremor is the adverse outcome being valued, the treatment failure outcome in the chained comparison could be hand paralysis. The hand paralysis could then be "chained" in to form a further gamble where the paralysis of a hand is valued against a treatment that offers a chance of full or perfect health or immediate death. Another example can be found in the area of vascular surgery and peripheral vascular disease. If an individual is considering a state of intermittent claudication (cramplike discomfort felt in the lower legs and thighs often due to blockages in the supply of blood to the lower legs), intermittent claudication could be valued as the intermediate state in the chain against the loss of the ability to walk.

Here, minor and temporary adverse health states are valued relative to moderate and severe health states that are then valued against full or perfect health and immediate death. This use of chaining then assumes that through the use of such intermediate states, preferences will be preserved (more matching of preferences with the standard gamble when compared with preferences elicited by the basic reference exercise) and will be detected and picked up in a standard gamble that had previously been considered as "sufficiently insensitive" to pick up key nuances in patient preferences. Oliver

phrases the goal of chaining as the achievement of a consistent methodology where "direct value preference elicitation through a basic reference exercise" and "indirect value elicitation through a chained exercise" generate values that do not significantly or systematically differ from one another.

Future Use and Research

There is much need for preference elicitation strategies beyond disease states requiring surgery of terminal medical conditions. Possible uses of chaining are with patients with chronic illnesses, such as rheumatoid arthritis. Here, many patients are in chronic states of compromised health and need help with comparing management or treatment strategy states of consideration of "degree of increase in bodily versus mental functioning" on one therapy versus another therapy, without consideration of immediate death or full (or perfect) health because immediate death or full perfect health are not reasonable short- or medium-term outcomes in these patients with chronic diseases.

More research needs to be done in states of function through all their degrees of severity and states of permanence (degrees of irreversibility) as chronic diseases will continue to progress in these individuals over time throughout their lives. Challenges also exist in the area of developing new techniques for preference elicitation that aim to further reduce or eliminate internal inconsistency as a problem within preference elicitation methodologies.

Dennis J. Mazur

See also Expected Utility Theory; Utility Assessment Techniques

Further Readings

Baker, R., & Robinson, A. (2004). Responses to standard gambles: Are preferences "well constructed"? *Health Economics, 13,* 37–48.

Jones-Lee, M. W., Loomes, G., & Philips, P. R. (1995). Valuing the prevention of non-fatal road injuries: Contingent valuation vs. standard gambles. *Oxford Economic Papers, 47,* 676–695.

Llewellyn-Thomas, H., Sutherland, H. J., Tibshirani, R., Ciampi, A., Till, J. E., & Boyd, N. F. (1982). The measurement of patients' values in medicine. *Medical Decision Making, 2,* 449–462.

McNamee, P., Glendinning, S., Shenfine, J., Steen, N., Griffin, S. M., & Bond, J. (2004). Chained time trade-off and standard gamble methods: Applications in oesophageal cancer. *European Journal of Health Economics, 5,* 81–86.

Oliver, A. (2003). The internal consistency of the standard gamble: Tests after adjusting for prospect theory. *Journal of Health Economics, 22,* 659–674.

Oliver, A. (2004). Testing the internal consistency of the standard gamble in "success" and "failure" frames. *Social Science & Medicine, 58,* 2219–2229.

Oliver, A. (2005). Testing the internal consistency of the lottery equivalents method using health outcomes. *Health Economics, 14,* 149–159.

Rutten-van Mölken, M. P., Bakker, C. H., van Doorslaer, E. K., & van der Linden, S. (1995). Methodological issues of patient utility measurement: Experience from two clinical trials. *Medical Care, 33,* 922–937.

Torrance, G. W. (2006). Utility measurement in healthcare: The things I never got to. *Pharmaco-Economics, 24,* 1069–1078.

Witney, A. G., Treharne, G. J., Tavakoli, M., Lyons, A. C., Vincent, K., Scott, D. L., et al. (2006). The relationship of medical, demographic and psychosocial factors to direct and indirect health utility instruments in rheumatoid arthritis. *Rheumatology (Oxford), 45,* 975–981.

CHAOS THEORY

A major breakthrough of the 20th century, which has been facilitated by computer science, has been the recognition that simple rules do not always lead to stable order but in many circumstances instead lead to an apparent disorder characterized by marked instability and unpredictable variation for reasons intrinsic to the rules themselves. The phenomenon of rules causing emerging disorder, counterintuitive to many people, is the environment currently being explored as *self-organization, fractals* (a fragmented geometric shape that can be split into parts, each of which is a reduced-size copy of the whole, a property called self-similarity), *nonlinear dynamical systems,* and *chaos.*

Chaos theory, also called nonlinear systems theory, provides new insights into processes previously thought to be unpredictable and random. It also provides a new set of tools that can be used to analyze physiological and clinical data such as the electric signals coming from the heart or from the brain.

Chaos theory was born originally as a branch of mathematical physics in the 20th century thanks to the work of Edward Lorenz in meteorology. Chaos theory is concerned with finding rational explanations for such phenomena as unexpected changes in weather and deals with events and processes that cannot be modeled or predicted using conventional mathematical laws and theorems, such as those of probability theory. The theory basically assumes that small, localized perturbations in one part of a complex system can have profound consequences throughout the system. Thus, for nonlinear systems, proportionality simply does not hold. Small changes can have dramatic and unanticipated consequences. The fascinating example often used to describe this concept, which is known as the butterfly effect, is that the beating of a butterfly's wings in China can lead to a hurricane in Brazil, given a critical combination of air pressure changes.

The key word is *critical,* and many of the efforts of scientists working on chaos theory are concerned with attempts to model circumstances based on specific conditional conjunction. Unpredictable events in medicine, such as ventricular arrhythmias and sudden cardiac death in athletes, the course of certain cancers, and the fluctuations in frequency of some diseases, may be attributable to chaos theory.

Nonlinear Dynamics in Human Physiology

Chaos theory can be considered a paradigm of the so-called nonlinear dynamics. The issue of nonlinearity of medical data has very rarely been raised in the literature. Clearly, epidemiologists and statisticians devoted to the medical field are quite happy with linear techniques since they have been trained from the beginning with them; physicians and other health professionals, due to their proverbial poor mathematical competence, are also happy, provided that statisticians and regulatory agencies do not think differently.

What does a linear function signify? If one considers a Cartesian chart in which axis x represents the money a person gets and axis y measures the degree of happiness that person obtains as a result, then the more money a person has, the happier he or she is. In this scenario, one can easily predict the value of one variable by the value of the other, with a simple (linear) equation. However, this scenario, as with many others in real life, is actually more an exception than a rule. In real life, the relations are generally more complex. In fact, as many people can witness, an increase in earning can sometimes produce fears of losing money or uncertainties on how to invest this money, and this can reduce the feeling of happiness. This complex (nonlinear) relation does not permit one to understand, at first glance, from data gathered experimentally, the relationship between money and happiness.

Therefore, persisting in the linear approach is not without danger: If, for instance, for two given variables a correlation coefficient of .018 is calculated under the linear hypothesis and a p value of .80 is added, a relationship between the two is ruled out. Revisiting the relationship between these two variables through the nonlinear approach could change the situation dramatically since fuzzy and smooth interactions may determine significant effects through a complex multifactorial interplay.

Mathematical analyses of physiological rhythms, such as those of Jerry Gollub, show that nonlinear equations are necessary to describe physiological systems. The physiological variation of blood glucose, for example, has traditionally been considered to be linear. Recently, a chaotic component has been described both in diabetic patients and in normal subjects. This chaotic dynamic has been found to be common in other physiologic systems. Table 1 summarizes some of the best examples of nonlinear dynamics in human physiology. It has, for instance, been shown that the interbeat interval of the human heart is chaotic and that a regular heart beat is a sign of disease and a strong predictor of imminent cardiac arrest.

The work of Ary L. Goldberger has pointed out how traditional statistics can be misleading in

Table I   Examples of nonlinear dynamics in human physiology

Processes With Chaotic Behavior	Processes With Complex Fractal Fluctuations
Shape of EEG waves	Heart frequency
Insulin blood levels	Respiration
Cellular cycles	Systemic arterial pressure
Muscle action potential	Gait control
Esophagus motility	White blood cells number
Bowel motility	Liver regeneration patterns
	Uterine pressure

Source: Glass, L., & Mackey, M. C. (1988). *From clocks to chaos: The rhythms of life*. Princeton, NJ: Princeton University Press.

evaluating heart time series in health and disease. In fact, there are circumstances in which two data sets belonging to two subjects can have nearly identical mean values and variances and, therefore, escape statistical distinction based on conventional comparisons. However, the raw time series can reveal dramatic differences in the temporal structure of the original data, wherein one time series is from a healthy individual and the other from a patient during episodes of severe obstructive sleep apnea. The time series from the healthy subject reveals a complex pattern of nonstationary fluctuations. In contrast, the heart rate data set from the subjects with sleep apnea shows a much more predictable pattern with a characteristic timescale defined by prominent, low-frequency oscillations at about .03 Hz. Both the complex behavior in the healthy case and the sustained oscillations in the pathologic one suggest the presence of nonlinear mechanisms.

Other researchers such as Bruce McEwen and John Wingfield have introduced the concept of allostasis—maintaining stability through change—as a fundamental process through which organisms actively adjust to both predictable and unpredictable events. *Allostatic load* refers to the cumulative cost to the body of allostasis, with *allostatic overload* being a state in which serious pathophysiology can occur. In this regard, chaos theory seems to fit quite well with biological adaptation mechanisms.

The importance of chaotic dynamics and related nonlinear phenomena in medical sciences has been only recently appreciated. It is now quite clear, as noted by David Ruelle, that chaos is not mindless disorder—it is a subtle form of order—and that approximate results of treatment can be predicted.

Chaotic dynamics are characterized most of the time by what is called a strange attractor. This roughly means that during the chaotic evolution, the variables characterizing the state of the system remain in a restricted range of values. This leads to the possibility of characterizing the system evolution in terms of probabilities.

Applications to Medical Settings

One promising application of dynamic analysis involves strategies to restore complex biological variability, including fractal fluctuations (i.e., harmonic changes to self-similar heart rhythms), to cardiopulmonary systems. Initial results using artificial ventilation in experimental animals and clinical settings suggest the possibility of improving physiologic function with "noisy" versus "metronomic" parameter settings. The use of dynamic assays to uncover basic and clinical information encoded in time series also promises to provide new, readily implemented diagnostic tests for prevalent conditions such as sleep-disordered breathing. The extent to which dynamic measures and complexity-informed models and interventions will enhance diagnostic capabilities and therapeutic options in chronic obstructive lung disease is an intriguing area for future study.

Another paradigmatic area of interest and application is represented by electroencephalography (EEG). The 19 channels in the EEG represent a dynamic system characterized by typical asynchronous parallelism. The nonlinear implicit function that defines the ensemble of electric signals series as a whole represents a meta-pattern that translates into space (hypersurface) what the interactions among all the channels create in time.

The behavior of every channel can be considered as the synthesis of the influence of the other channels at previous but not identical times and in different quantities, and of its own activity at that moment. At the same time, the activity of every channel at a certain moment in time is going to influence the behavior of the others at different times and to different extents. Therefore, every multivariate sequence of signals coming from the same natural source is a complex asynchronous dynamic system, highly nonlinear, in which each channel's behavior is understandable only in relation to all the others.

The neurophysiologic community has had the perception that in the EEG signals there is embedded much more information on brain function than is currently extracted in a routine clinical context, moving from the obvious consideration that the sources of EEG signals (cortical postsynaptic currents at dendritic tree level) are the same ones attacked by the factors producing symptoms of chronic degenerative diseases such as dementia. The main problem, then, is the signal (relevant information)-to-noise (nonrelevant information) ratio, in which at the present moment the latter is largely overwhelming the former. As an example, when considering the EEG fluctuations at the 19 recording electrodes, it is like the fluctuation of 19 stock exchange securities in time (minutes, hours, days, etc.) due to the purchases/sales ratios as carried out by millions of invisible investors,

following a logic that is unknown to the analyzer but that is based on the intrinsic mechanism regulating the market. In this context, the "analyzer" ignores all the following variables:

1. why at each time the value of a given security (EEG signal) is going up or down;

2. how many investors (neurons, synapses, synchronous firing) are active on that security at a given time; and

3. when new investors, eventually organized, suddenly enter the market that is regulating that security and significantly alter the trend of the previous fluctuations (i.e., the subject's condition is altered because of an external or internal event).

The only two variables that the analyzers know for sure are the following:

1. The chaotic stock market entirely depends on the interplay of a large number of investors (brain, neurons, synapses).

2. Within the dynamics (variability) of the stock securities are embedded the investors' styles and abilities.

A 2007 article by Massimo Buscema and colleagues presents the results obtained with the innovative use of special types of artificial neural networks (ANNs) assembled in a novel methodology named IFAST (Implicit Function as Squashing Time) capable of compressing the temporal sequence of EEG data into spatial invariants (patterns of structures that remain stable across time). The principal aim of the study was testing the hypothesis that automatic classification of mild cognitive impairment (MCI) and Alzheimer's disease (AD) subjects can be reasonably corrected when the spatial content (the inherent structure) of the EEG voltage is properly extracted by ANNs.

Resting eyes-closed EEG data were recorded in 180 AD patients and in 115 MCI subjects. The spatial content of the EEG voltage was extracted by the IFAST stepwise procedure using ANNs. The data input for the classification operated by ANNs were not the EEG data but the connections weights of a nonlinear auto-associative ANN trained to reproduce the recorded EEG tracks. These weights represented a good model of the peculiar spatial features of the EEG patterns at the scalp surface. The classification based on these parameters was binary

(MCI vs. AD) and was performed by a supervised ANN. Half of the EEG database was used for the ANN training, and the remaining half was used for the automatic classification phase (testing).

The results confirmed the working hypothesis that a correct automatic classification of MCI and AD subjects can be obtained by extracting the spatial information content of the resting EEG voltage by ANNs and represents the basis for research aimed at integrating the spatial and temporal information content of the EEG. The best results in distinguishing between AD and MCI reached up to 92.33%. The comparative result obtained with the best method so far described in the literature, based on blind source separation and Wavelet preprocessing, was 80.43% ($p < .001$).

Future Outlook

The advancement of knowledge and progress in understanding the nature of bodily rhythms and processes have shown that complexity and nonlinearity are ubiquitous in living organisms. These rhythms arise from stochastic (involving or containing a random variable or variables), nonlinear biological mechanisms interacting with fluctuating environments.

There are many unanswered questions about the dynamics of these rhythmic processes: For example, how do the rhythms interact with each other and the external environment? Can researchers decode the fluctuations in physiological rhythms to better diagnose human disease? Mathematical and physical techniques combined with physiological and medical studies are addressing these questions and are transforming our understanding of the rhythms of life.

Enzo Grossi

See also Complexity

Further Readings

Buscema, M., Rossini, P., Babiloni, C., & Grossi, E. (2007). The IFAST model, a novel parallel nonlinear EEG analysis technique, distinguishes mild cognitive impairment and Alzheimer's disease patients with high degree of accuracy. *Artificial Intelligence in Medicine, 40*(2), 127–141.

Firth, W. J. (1991). Chaos, predicting the unpredictable. *British Medical Journal, 303,* 1565–1568.

Glass, L., & Mackey, M. C. (1988). *From clocks to chaos: The rhythms of life.* Princeton, NJ: Princeton University Press.

Goldberger, A. L., Amaral, L. A. N., Hausdorff, J. M., Ivanov, P. C., Peng, C. K., & Stanley, H. E. (2002). Fractal dynamics in physiology: Alterations with disease and aging. *Proceedings of the National Academy of Sciences of the United States of America, 99,* 2466–2472.

Goldberger, A. L., & Giles, F. (2006). Filley lecture: Complex systems. *Proceedings of the American Thoracic Society, 3*(6), 467–471.

Gollub, J. P., & Cross, M. C. (2000). Nonlinear dynamics: Chaos in space and time. *Nature, 404,* 710–711.

Kroll, M. H. (1999). Biological variation of glucose and insulin includes a deterministic chaotic component. *Biosystems, 50,* 189–201.

Lorenz, E. N. (1963). Deterministic non periodic flow. *Journal of the Atmospheric Sciences, 20,* 130–141.

McEwen, B. S., & Wingfield, J. C. (2003). The concept of allostasis in biology and biomedicine. *Hormonal Behavior, 43*(1), 2–15.

Ruelle, D. (1994). Where can one hope to profitably apply the ideas of chaos? *Physics Today, 47,* 24–30.

Singer, D. H., Martin, G. J., Magid, N., Weiss, J. S., Schaad, J. W., Kehoe, R., et al. (1988). Low heart rate variability and sudden cardiac death. *Journal of Electrocardiology, 21,* S46–S55.

CHOICE THEORIES

Choice theories can be classified in a number of ways. *Normative* theories seek to clarify how decisions should be made; *descriptive* theories try to understand how they are made in the real world. Theories may also concentrate on decisions made by individuals, groups, or societies. Normative theories tend to emphasize rational decision making and provide the underpinnings for economic evaluations, decision analysis, and technology assessment. Variations, including shared decision making, often focus on who should be making decisions but retain the assumptions of rationality. In contrast, descriptive models often emphasize psychological factors, including heuristics and biases. At the policy-making level, however, the recognition of the difficulties in constructing social welfare functions has led to intermediate models with both normative and descriptive elements, including bounded rationality, incrementalism, and mixed scanning.

Normative Theories

Rational Decision Making

Rational choice theory assumes that individuals act to maximize their own utility. A rational individual must therefore

1. determine the range of possible actions that might be taken,
2. determine the possible outcomes that might result from each of these actions,
3. affix a probability to each possible outcome (these must sum to 1.0),
4. affix values to the costs and consequences of each possible outcome, and
5. do the math.

The rational choice will be the one that produces the "best" outcome, as measured in terms of costs and consequences.

Rational decision making is highly data-intensive. It requires a decision maker to collect extensive information about all potential choices, outcomes, costs, and consequences. He or she must be able to order his or her preferences for different outcomes, and these preferences must satisfy the requirements of being complete (i.e., all potential outcomes are assigned preferences) and transitive (i.e., if someone prefers A to B, and B to C, he or she must prefer A to C). In the real world, these assumptions are often unrealistic.

Economists have adopted the theory of revealed preferences to omit some of these steps. Rather than attempt to measure preferences directly, this approach assumes that if someone has chosen a particular outcome, he or she must, by definition, prefer it to the alternatives. Associated with Paul Samuelson, this approach has been highly influential in the study of consumer behavior. It is also tautological and does not leave much room for improving choices (e.g., through providing additional information).

Rational Choice in Medical Decision Making

Decision Analysis

Medical decision making relies heavily on rational choice theory. One common way of analyzing treatment choices, decision analysis, employs the same structure. Constructing a decision tree requires specifying the possible actions ("choice nodes"), specifying the possible outcomes of each action ("chance nodes"), attaching probabilities to each outcome (which must sum to 1.0), and then affixing costs and consequences to each outcome. The tree is then "folded back" by computing the expected value at each node by multiplying the probability by the costs and by the consequences.

For example, in their five-part primer, *Medical Decision Analysis*, Allan Detsky and colleagues work through the example of how to model the choice of management strategies for patients presenting with clinical features that suggest giant cell arteritis (GCA). In this simplified model, the only treatment considered is treating with steroids, which can involve side effects. The rational model they employ thus involves a choice between three possible actions at the choice node—treating, not treating, and testing and treating only if the test result is positive. The possible outcomes can be simplified to four possibilities, depending on whether or not there was an adverse outcome as a result of the disease (in that case, blindness), and whether or not the person had side effects as a result of the treatment. Note that some of these outcomes cannot occur on some branches—for example, someone who did not receive treatment could not experience any outcomes involving side effects. The next step for the decision maker is to determine how likely each of these possible outcomes would be at each choice node (e.g., how likely would an untreated individual with those symptoms be to experience blindness if the person was not treated). Next, the decision maker would affix costs and utilities to each possible outcome. For example, these papers assigned a value of 1.0 to the state with no disease and no side effects, and a value of .5 to the state of having the disease without treatment (or side effects) but ending up with blindness. Sensitivity analysis can be used to modify these values (e.g., change the probability of adverse outcomes or the value attached to particular outcomes) and see how much they affect the resulting choices.

One way to simplify decision trees is to see whether any alternatives are "dominated" by others. Dominated choices are clearly inferior. In a condition of strong dominance, other alternatives are both less costly and of greater benefit. Rational decision makers can accordingly "prune" their decision trees to eliminate all dominated alternatives.

There is an extensive literature relating to how best to model these decisions (including the use of

Markov models) and how to compute costs and consequences. Sensitivity analysis can allow systematic variation in the values assigned to probabilities and outcomes. The underlying assumptions, however, are of rational decision makers maximizing their expected utilities.

Economic Analysis

Economic analysis refers to a family of related methods for weighing costs against consequences. All involve costing the potential outcomes; they vary only in how they assess consequences.

1. *Cost minimization* assumes that the outcomes are identical. In that case, it is not necessary to value them. The decision can be based solely on costs, and a rational decision maker will select the lowest-cost alternative.

2. *Cost benefit* assumes that consequences can also be valued in monetary terms. In that case, the rational decision maker will determine return on investment and select the alternative that produces the highest ratio of consequences to costs.

3. *Cost-effectiveness* assumes that consequences can be valued in a single, albeit nonmonetary, measurement of outcome. Again, the rational decision maker will select the alternative producing the highest ratio of consequences to costs.

4. *Cost utility analysis* is a variant of cost-effectiveness, which computes the "utility" attached to each outcome (on a scale of 0 to 1).

Again, there are many details about how to conduct these analyses, including how to value costs and consequences occurring in the future (e.g., discounting) and how to incorporate different ways of valuing risk. The underlying model, however, continues to assume that rational individuals will act to maximize their expected return, however defined and measured.

Technology Assessment

Technology assessment shares the underlying premise that rational individuals will seek to maximize outcomes for the given inputs. It can be considered a subset of economic models, and presents similar variation in which costs to include (and whose costs), and how to measure consequences.

Modern technology assessment is heavily influenced by such organizations as the Cochrane Collaboration and places considerable emphasis on ensuring that data are of high quality. Accordingly, there is often considerable dispute as to where to gather the data and what counts as evidence. Nonetheless, the underlying model remains rational choice.

Decision Makers

Multiple Decision Makers

An additional complexity occurs if there are multiple decision makers. In that case, the decision makers must be able to determine preference orderings that apply to the society. These are referred to as *social welfare functions;* Kenneth Arrow won a Nobel prize for demonstrating the General Possibility Theorem, which proves that, under many circumstances, it is not possible to construct a transitive preference ordering for a society, even given that all members of that society have individual preference orderings satisfying this requirement. For that reason, choice theories for multiple decision makers differ from those for individuals.

Shared Decision Making

If individuals are considered consumers, then the person paying for a particular service should be sovereign. Professionals may provide expert advice but would not determine the preference ordering. If there are externalities, however, such that one person's choice affects the outcomes for others, it is less simple to decide whose preferences should count. If costs are pooled (e.g., through insurance or public financing), then presumably those paying would have some say in the matter. If the consumer is misinformed (e.g., wants a clinical intervention where professionals do not believe that the benefits outweigh the risks), again, there may be disputes about whose preferences should matter. Note that these models do not necessarily require that there be a social welfare function but do require some methods for dispute resolution. Raisa Deber and colleagues have suggested distinguishing between *problem-solving* tasks (defined as preference-independent, where expertise is required) and *decision-making* tasks (which involve deciding based on personal preferences). A substantial literature has attempted to examine shared decision making in medicine; note that it assumes that patient preferences should be decisive. These models can be seen as subsets of rational models.

Descriptive Models

Heuristics and Biases

In contrast, another set of models seeks to understand how choices are actually made. These models draw heavily on psychology. One key literature examines the simplifying assumptions (often termed *heuristics and biases*) often made by individual decision makers. Even here, the strong dominance of rational decision making persists; the theory of cognitive dissonance stresses that people tend to be adept at justifying choices they have made, even when this requires distorting facts to convince themselves that they are being rational.

Other descriptive models examine how decisions are made within groups and how various pressures exist to influence the choices made.

Modification of the Model

Bounded Rationality

Another set of modifications recognize that it may not be rational to collect full information. Whereas a rational decision maker seeks to maximize, what Herbert Simon terms *administrative man* seeks to "satisfice" and select the first alternative that is "good enough." Some of this literature incorporates the information about cognitive limitations.

Incrementalism and Mixed Scanning

Policy analysts have suggested that most policies begin with what is. Charles Lindblom suggested that policy making is usually incremental, consisting of a series of small adjustments to existing policy resulting from a series of "successive limited comparisons." In this model, rather than beginning by setting goals and objectives, policy makers will perform limited analyses of immediate issues and implement a series of small decisions. This model has the advantage of being low-risk; smaller decisions have fewer short-term consequences and are less likely to elicit opposition. Continuous feedback allows the policies to be modified as required. The weakness is that the big picture is rarely examined. The incremental model is both normative and descriptive. It describes how policy usually occurs. However, some authors also consider it a desirable normative model, particularly under circumstances where bounded rationality is likely to be appropriate, where the risks of error are high, or where interest groups are highly invested.

Amitai Etzioni has suggested an intermediate stance he termed *mixed scanning*. In this model, incrementalism is the default mode, but policymakers are scanning for areas where more in-depth, rational decision making could be beneficial. His analogy is the job of a sentry, who scans the landscape to see where there is movement that calls for further investigation.

Social psychologists have noted the importance of the system within which decisions are made. The patient safety movement, for example, has noted that improving clinical performance is less a matter of removing bad apples than it is a matter of ensuring that systems are set up to encourage optimal performance. These models thus draw on the descriptive material and seek to set up models within which optimal choices are more likely to be made.

Raisa Deber

See also Applied Decision Analysis; Bounded Rationality and Emotions; Cognitive Psychology and Processes; Decision Psychology; Heuristics; Treatment Choices

Further Readings

Berwick, D. M. (1989). Continuous improvement as an ideal in health care. *New England Journal of Medicine, 320*(1), 53–56.

Deber, R., & Goel, V. (1990). Using explicit decision rules to manage issues of justice, risk, and ethics in decision analysis: When is it not rational to maximize expected utility? *Medical Decision Making, 10*(3), 181–194.

Deber, R., Kraetschmer, N., & Irvine, J. (1996). What role do patients wish to play in treatment decision making? *Archives of Internal Medicine, 156*(13), 1414–1420.

Detsky, A. S., Naglie, G., Krahn, M. D., Naimark, D., & Redelmeier, D. A. (1997). Primer on medical decision analysis: Part 1. Getting started. *Medical Decision Making, 17*(2), 123–125.

Detsky, A. S., Naglie, G., Krahn, M. D., Redelmeier, D. A., & Naimark, D. (1997). Primer on medical decision analysis: Part 2. Building a tree. *Medical Decision Making, 17*(2), 126–135.

Gold, M. R., Siegel, J. E., Russell, L. B., & Weinstein, M. C. (Eds.). (1996). *Cost-effectiveness in health and medicine.* New York: Oxford University Press.

Hastie, R., & Dawes, R. M. (2001). *Rational choice in an uncertain world.* Thousand Oaks, CA: Sage.

Krahn, M. D., Naglie, G., Naimark, D., Redelmeier, D. A., & Detsky, A. S. (1997). Primer on medical decision analysis: Part 4. Analyzing the model and interpreting the results. *Medical Decision Making, 17*(2), 142–151.

Naglie, G., Krahn, M. D., Naimark, D., Redelmeier, D. A., & Detsky, A. S. (1997). Primer on medical decision analysis: Part 3. Estimating probabilities and utilities. *Medical Decision Making, 17*(2), 136–141.

Naimark, D., Krahn, M. D., Naglie, G., Redelmeier, D. A., & Detsky, A. S. (1997). Primer on medical decision analysis: Part 5. Working with Markov processes. *Medical Decision Making, 17*(2), 152–159.

CLASSIFICATION AND REGRESSION TREE (CART) ANALYSIS

See Recursive Partitioning

CLINICAL ALGORITHMS AND PRACTICE GUIDELINES

Clinical algorithms and practice guidelines may be viewed as a targeted effort to provide the best clinical advice about specific management conditions. They are most useful if clinicians incorporate them as additional tools to specifically improve patient outcomes while offering holistic clinical care to patients.

Clinical Algorithms

Definition

Algorithms are branching-logic pathways that permit the application of carefully defined criteria to the task of identifying or classifying different types of the same entity. Clinical algorithms are often represented as schematic models or flow diagrams of the clinical decision pathway described in a guideline.

Clinical findings, diagnostic test characteristics, and treatment options are abbreviated into their basic components. Algorithmic flow diagrams are then constructed as branching logical pathways with decision points represented as yes/no nodes. Such a flowchart sequence is useful in identifying or classifying entities based on carefully devised criteria (Figure 1). Application of clinical algorithms is most defensible when the evidence supports choices in the decision tree. Although very useful for clinical decision making, algorithms cannot account for all patient-related variables. Therefore, algorithms are not intended as a substitute for the clinician's best judgment.

Proposed Standards

The Society for Medical Decision Making Committee on Standardization of Clinical Algorithms has proposed certain standards for construction of clinical algorithms. Their technical note has specific recommendations on the types and shapes of algorithm boxes (clinical state box—*rounded rectangle*; decision box—*hexagon*; action box—*rectangle*; and link box—*small oval*), titles, abbreviations, annotations and their format, and schemes for arrows, numbering, and paging.

Classification

Simple Classification Algorithms

Simple classification algorithms serve only as diagnostic aids and do not advocate any clinical intervention. They contain question nodes (algorithmic boxes) leading to yes or no exit arrows.

Management Algorithms

Management algorithms encompass both diagnostic and treatment modalities. They employ decision-relevant yes/no question nodes. Each question node in turn leads to an instruction node, denoted by a single exit arrow. Instruction nodes advocate for specific interventions. Thus, patients get classified into distinct clinical subgroups that would benefit from specifically targeted management strategies.

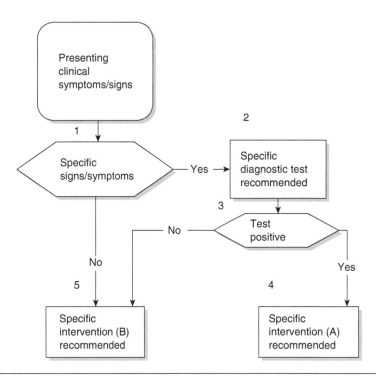

Figure 1   Schematic model of a management clinical algorithm

Note: Management algorithm for a patient with a hypothetical set of presenting symptoms/signs.

Outcome studies are essential to providing support for each management strategy.

Validity and Flexibility

It is often argued that algorithms are not always backed by empirical data, are infrequently linked to the literature, and are not adequately flexible when dealing with clinical uncertainties. To circumvent these inadequacies, two important modifications have evolved.

First, in an attempt to enhance the validity, *annotated management algorithms* have been devised. Here, each node concerned with specific findings, characteristics, or interventions is annotated with the intent of summarizing the guideline's detailed textual material. The textual material is in turn replete with citations. Thus, in this fact-based approach, the algorithm links the recommendations of the guideline to systematic literature reviews or, when appropriate, to expert consensus. The Agency for Health Care Policy and Research guideline development process exemplifies this approach.

Second, *counseling and decision nodes* are specifically implanted in the algorithm where therapeutic decisions are expected to be constrained due to a gap in current knowledge. This is particularly relevant when patient preferences vary with respect to two (or more) different therapeutic options (e.g., medical vs. surgical management). At each decision node, the expected outcome associated with each option is indicated to the extent possible. Thus, counseling and decision nodes facilitate therapeutic deliberations between physician(s) and patient.

Methodological Considerations

Four methodological issues are commonly cited as influencing the development of annotated management algorithms.

1. *Selection of a descriptor variable:* The best descriptor variables are easily observed and have great discriminatory power to categorize patients into different subtypes suited for separate management strategies. Discriminatory power of the variable

is gauged in terms of its sensitivity, specificity, and predictive value. So, ideally, these data should result from controlled studies. Often, evidence is sparse and expert panels develop a consensus about the best discriminatory variables to be used, based on certain stated rationales. Nevertheless, future research should aim to address such gaps in knowledge.

Variables can be optimally selected using sound statistical techniques. Regression analyses are the most common statistical methods used for estimating the discriminatory power of a variable. They quantify the impact of a given variable on outcome probabilities. Recursive partitioning, on the other hand, is an algorithmic strategy that identifies homogeneous, meaningful patient subtypes for guideline/algorithm development. Here, the patient population is reclassified into ever smaller subgroups based on Boolean combinations of variables. An example cited in the literature is as follows: age > 65 years and hematocrit < 30 and systolic blood pressure > 160 mmHg.

2. *Incomplete literature and consequent uncertainties:* Annotated algorithms depicting the lowest common denominator on which there is reasonable consensus may be used to clarify algorithms when uncertainty exists. In addition, the expert panel may identify and explicitly delegate possible management strategies into one of the four prototype categories defined in the literature: (1) necessary care (practice standard, recommendation), (2) appropriate, but not necessary care (option), (3) equivocal care (not recommended), and (4) inappropriate care (recommendation against use).

3. *A dilemma may be encountered when attempting to integrate qualitative descriptor variables* (e.g., increased postvoid residual urine) *with quantitative information* (e.g., specific cutoff volume for increased postvoid residual urine): Often, such an approach may not be backed by literature or panel consensus. Such dilemmas should be highlighted in the algorithm. Additionally, the annotation should include a tally of panelists' quantitative recommendations and any ensuing discussion of factors that permit the calculation of such variables.

4. *Optimal representation of health outcomes:* Health outcomes must be precisely defined and properly annotated, and they should be relevant to

the algorithm. Therapeutic side effects and their estimated occurrence risk should also be reported.

Technical Suggestion

Algorithms should be logically and succinctly laid out with carefully selected nodes representing the lowest common denominator. Nodes should apply to a significant proportion of patients. Otherwise they should be incorporated as annotations or combined with other nodes to reduce excessive and unnecessary detail.

Practice Guidelines

Definition

Clinical practice guidelines (CPGs) attempt to transform evidence into practice to improve patient outcomes. The approach of evidence-based CPGs is to define clinical questions, review current evidence, and determine grades of recommendation. Patient questions are also addressed. While CPGs reflect a broad statement of good practice with little operational detail, *protocols* are the result of their local adaptation.

Contents of High-Quality Clinical Practice Guidelines

This is best exemplified by the National Guideline Clearinghouse (NGC) Guideline Summary Sheet, available from the NGC's Web site. The Web site also provides links to NGC's Brief and Complete Guideline Summary, Guideline Comparison, Guideline Synthesis, and Classification Scheme.

The NGC Complete Guideline Summary describes the guideline's title, scope (includes disease/conditions, intended users, and target population), methodology, recommendations (major recommendations and clinical algorithms), evidence supporting the recommendation(s) and benefits and risks of its implementation, contraindications, qualifying statements, implementation strategy, and Institute of Medicine (IOM) national healthcare quality report categories. In addition, identifying information and availability of the guideline is provided, including details about bibliographic sources, adaptation from any previous guidelines, date of release, guideline developers, committees and endorsers involved, funding source(s), financial disclosure, guideline status and availability, and patient resources.

Characteristics of High-Quality Clinical Practice Guidelines

The IOM expert committee on guidelines has identified validity as the most important attribute. Validity is based on strength of scientific evidence underlying the recommendations and their impact on health and cost outcomes. Reproducibility, reliability, clinical applicability, clinical flexibility, cost-effectiveness, and clarity are other key aspects. CPGs should be a multidisciplinary process, with documentation of participants, assumptions, and methods, and be subjected to *scheduled reviews*.

Strength of Recommendation Taxonomy

Strength of recommendation is graded based on evidence into A (consistent and good-quality patient-oriented evidence), B (inconsistent or limited quality patient-oriented evidence), and C (consensus, usual practice, opinion, disease-oriented evidence, or case series for studies of diagnosis, treatment, prevention, or screening). The quality of a study measuring patient outcome(s) is similarly graded into levels 1 (*good quality evidence*), 2 (*limited quality evidence*), and 3 (*other evidence*).

Grades of Recommendation

It is controversial whether the level of evidence and grade of recommendation (GOR) should be standardized across CPGs in different areas. One such GOR proposed by the Joint Committee of Development of Clinical Practice Guidelines for the Treatment of Stroke is as follows: A (*strongly recommended*), B (*recommended*), C1 (*acceptable although evidence is insufficient*), C2 (*not recommended because evidence is insufficient*), and D (*not recommended*).

Role and Utility of Clinical Practice Guidelines

CPGs play an important role in enhancing clinicians' knowledge by keeping them abreast of the latest developments in medicine. This is intended to change their attitude about standard of care and shift their practice pattern, leading to improved patient outcomes. Healthcare policy makers can use CPGs to assign resources to the most needed areas. CPGs also guide plan administrators and insurers to arrive at reimbursement decisions for patients. In addition, public and patient education, research priorities, and medicolegal issues are influenced by CPGs.

Perspective of Clinicians and Patients

Most clinicians agree that CPGs are helpful educational tools intended to improve quality of care. Nevertheless, CPGs have been variously described as anti-intellectual, impractical, limiting clinical autonomy and discretion, cost-cutting, standardizing practice around the average, and causing increased litigation. Apart from negative attitudes and resistance to change, other barriers to CPGs include administrative and financial obstacles as well as limited time and resources for education and implementation. Sometimes, patients' choices may also be in conflict with the guidelines.

Successful Implementation

Successful implementation involves organizational commitment and raising awareness among intended users through dissemination of information (conferences, meetings, and publications), alongside education and preparation of staff. Other useful strategies include use of local clinical leadership; inclusion of CPGs within the contracting process; support of practitioners, including information giving and feedback; reminders and incentives; audit and feedback of results; and patient/client-mediated interventions.

Chenni Sriram and Geoffrey L. Rosenthal

See also Decision Making in Advanced Disease; Decision Modes; Decision Tree: Introduction; Diagnostic Process, Making a Diagnosis; Recursive Partitioning

Further Readings

American College of Physicians. (2009). *Algorithms* [Electronic version]. Retrieved October 7, 2008, from http://www.acponline.org/clinical_information/ guidelines/process/algorithms

Duff, L. A., Kitson, A. L., Seers, K., & Humphris, D. (1996). Clinical guidelines: An introduction to their development and implementation. *Journal of Advanced Nursing, 23,* 887–895.

Ebell, M. H., Siwek, J., Weiss, B. D., Woolf, S. H., Susman, J., Ewigman, B. D., et al. (2004). Strength of Recommendation Taxonomy (SORT): A patient-centered approach to grading evidence in the medical literature. *American Family Physician, 69,* 548–556.

Greer, A. L., Goodwin, J. S., Freeman, J. L., & Wu, Z. H. (2002). *International Journal of Technology Assessment in Health Care, 18,* 747–761.

Hadorn, D. C. (1995). Use of algorithms in clinical guideline development. In *Clinical practice guideline development: Methodology perspectives* (AHCPR Pub. No. 95-0009, 93-104). Rockville, MD: Agency for Health Care Policy and Research.

Lohr, K. N., Eleazer, K., & Mauskopf, J. (1998). Health policy issues and applications for evidence-based medicine and clinical practice guidelines. *Health Policy, 46,* 1–19.

Nakayama, T. (2007). What are "clinical practice guidelines"? *Journal of Neurology, 254*(Suppl. 5), 2–7.

Natsch, S., & van der Meer, J. W. M. (2003). The role of clinical guidelines, policies and stewardship. *Journal of Hospital Infection, 53,* 172–176.

Society for Medical Decision Making, Committee on Standardization of Clinical Algorithms. (1992). Proposal for clinical algorithm standards. *Medical Decision Making, 12,* 149–154.

Welsby, P. D. (2002). Evidence-based medicine, guidelines, personality types, relatives and absolutes. *Journal of Evaluation in Clinical Practice, 8,* 163–166.

COGNITIVE PSYCHOLOGY AND PROCESSES

Cognitive psychology is the study of the thinking mind. It emerged as a field of psychology in the 1980s and includes perception, attention, memory, decision making, problem solving, reasoning, and language among its areas of study. Using theory and empirical study, cognitive psychology aims to understand the cognitive processes used and what influences their use. In medical decision making, for decisions relevant to individuals, systems, and society, understanding the cognitive processes that people typically use, and why, would help (a) developers of decision support interventions target the interventions most effectively and (b) identify

outcomes appropriate for judging the effectiveness of particular decision-making strategies.

Decision making in cognitive psychology focuses on how people make choices. The field is distinct from problem solving, which is characterized by situations where a goal is clearly established and where reaching the goal is decomposed into sub-goals that, in turn, help clarify which actions need to be taken and when. In the medical world, making a diagnosis, for example, typically requires problem-solving processes. Decision making is also distinct from reasoning, which is characterized as the processes by which people move from what they already know to further knowledge. Although historically, decision making, problem solving, and reasoning were studied independently within cognitive psychology, it is recognized that in complex decisions both reasoning and problem-solving processes can be required to make a choice.

Decision making requires the integration of information with values. The information in a medical decision is often about a health state and the options for addressing it. Values are the qualities that underlie worth or desirability. A decision maker's values determine the particular subset of information that is most germane to his or her decision. Although both information and values are part of most medical decisions, the particular cognitive processing required can vary significantly from one decision to another.

Levels of Decisions

Four levels of decisions have been described—the higher the level, the greater the energy required and the more complex the decision processes.

Level 1—simple, familiar decisions: They are made quickly and largely automatically (unconsciously). An example occurs when people prone to headaches automatically reach for a particular painkiller in response to early headache signs.

Level 2—decisions that use static mappings when evaluating options: An example occurs when people choose particularly invasive treatments only because they believe that the more a treatment makes one suffer, the more likely it is to be successful.

Level 3—decisions that belong to a class of decision that is familiar to the decision maker, although the particular instance is not and can include options that have both pros and cons: An example occurs when people choose a family doctor after losing their doctor for the third time and therefore know what is important to them in the decision, but they need to learn about the new choices.

Level 4—decisions in unfamiliar situations when the choices are also not familiar: These decisions often require problem-solving (and possibly reasoning) processes to learn about the situation and the options. An example is a person, newly diagnosed with a relatively unfamiliar medical condition, needing to choose a treatment.

Cognitive Processes

Making decisions beyond lower-level decisions is typically protracted in time, requiring many types of cognitive processes. Ola Svenson is an early pioneer in describing decision processes, and he still provides one of the most comprehensive descriptions of those processes. He suggests that the process goal of decision making is to select one option that is superior enough over the other options that it can protect the decision maker from experiencing cognitive dissonance (discomfort from having values that conflict with the decision) and regret later. He describes three phases of processing: the initiation phase, differentiating the options, and after the decision.

Initiation Phase

Decision-making processes begin with the decision maker establishing the goal(s) of the decision and identifying options and attributes of the options that are important. Salient aspects of the situation tell the decision maker where to start. This phase structures the decision in the decision maker's mind. Therefore, the early-identified salient aspects can have important implications for the processing that follows. For example, a diagnosis of cancer generating fear of death can trigger the automatic elimination of a do-nothing-for-now option. Early screening of options is not unusual in situations where there are many options.

The initiation phase can include singling out one option. Sometimes it is a reference option, against which other options can later be compared.

When there are many options to consider, the singled-out option tends to be a preliminary preferred choice. Such a strategy limits energy demands that can become huge very quickly in situations where there are multiple options.

In addition to possible screening or selection of a preliminary preferred option, this early stage can involve information search. Exactly what information is searched for and retained can follow, to some extent, the salient attributes mentioned above.

Differentiating the Options

The major cognitive processing involved in decision making focuses on differentiating the options, one from the other. Svenson has identified three types of differentiating processes:

1. *Holistic differentiation* is quick, automatic (not within conscious control) processing.

2. *Structural differentiation* involves changes to the way the decision problem is represented in the mind of the decision maker. The structure can be altered by changing
   a. how attractive a particular aspect of an option is judged to be (e.g., shifting from a judgment that saving 10 of 100 people is not significant to considering that it is significant),
   b. the importance given to a specific attribute (e.g., shifting from being very concerned about possible incontinence to not being concerned about it),
   c. the facts about an option (e.g., shifting from believing that most men diagnosed with prostate cancer die of the disease to learning that most men do not die of their prostate cancer), and
   d. the particular set of attributes used to describe the options (e.g., shifting from interest in only treatments' effects on survival to their impact on quality of life).

3. *Process differentiation* involves using information about the options to arrive at a decision, following decision rules. Some rules involve combining all available information in a process of weighing pros against cons, while other rules involve using only some of the information, such as judging an attribute against a threshold.

For complex decisions, differentiation can be intermingled with information searches. In new situations, the decision maker may also need to discover which values are relevant to the decision, sometimes needing to figure out what their values are and, when values are in conflict with one another, their relative weightings. Because these processes are extended in time, research at different time points can suggest that values shift from one time to the next. Evidence suggests, however, that the processes eventually stabilize.

After the Decision

After the decision is made, the decision maker continues cognitive processing of the decision. Postdecision processes can include both the structural and process differentiation described above. Both implementation of the decision and outcomes of the decision can also be followed by yet further differentiation, though the specifics of what is processed may be altered. The postdecision processes manage the emotional consequences of having made the decision, potential cognitive dissonance, or regret.

Factors That Complicate Cognitive Decision Processes

Several factors about decision situations complicate both the actual processes used and our ability to learn about what is being done.

Uncertainty

Situations with information missing about a potential outcome are often distinguished from situations where an outcome is known but has a less-than-certain chance of occurring. People find it hard to act in the first type of situation; bad news is better than no news. In medical decision making, when making a decision for an individual, the two types of situations are not very different; knowing that, of a particular group of people, some will experience an outcome but others will not does not clarify what will happen to the individual. Discomfort with uncertainty can lead some patients, for example, to decide that they know what will happen to them.

Structure of the Environment

People are sensitive to the structure of the environment when judging a situation; thus, changing one aspect of the environment can change responses. Framing effects, where responses shift according to how a situation is described, is one example of such a change; an example of a framing effect in medical decisions is the response shift seen when an outcome is described as numbers of lives saved rather than numbers of lives lost. People's sensitivity to the environment means that asking questions in one way can produce different results compared with asking the apparently same question in a different way. It has been suggested, for example, that issues around compatibility between inputs (how the problem is described, an environmental structure) and outputs (the responses requested, another environmental structure) contribute to a broad range of what have been identified as nonnormative "biases" in human decision making.

Stress

Stress describes people's responses to what they judge to be threats. While mild stress can actually improve cognitive performance, high stress is generally seen as detrimental. It can increase distraction, making it harder to focus attention that can, for example, reduce the numbers of options or the numbers of attributes of each option being considered. It can also compromise the organization of the information in the decision maker's mind.

Intuition

Intuition has been defined as thinking processes that occur when the input is mostly knowledge acquired automatically (without conscious control) and the output is a feeling that can then be used as the basis for judgments and decisions. In some types of situations, intuitive decisions are more accurate than deliberate (with conscious control) decisions, but in other types of situations, deliberate decisions are more accurate. Intuition seems favored when people have prior experience with the relevant options and when the automatically acquired knowledge matches the demands of the decision. Intuitive attitudes are more likely to reflect the entire corpus of information acquired about the options, whereas attitudes related to deliberate learning are more likely to reflect only part of that information.

Heuristics

Heuristics are general rules of thumb that people use in cognitive processing to reduce mental energy demands. While the general thinking has been that using heuristics reduces the accuracy of processing, evidence now suggests that in some situations heuristics can actually improve the accuracy of decisions. Heuristics include simple rules about how to search for more information, when to stop the search, and estimating the likelihood of an event. For example, the representative heuristic can lead a teenager to ignore warnings about smoking because the typical image is that people with lung cancer are old.

Why Understand Cognitive Decision-Making Processes?

Understanding the cognitive processing used can naturally provide several types of guidance in the field of medical decision making. It can help identify the specific challenges that make a particular decision difficult, which, in turn, clarifies how to make decision support interventions most effective. Understanding the cognitive processing also reveals important complexities in human behavior that should be considered when creating interventions. For example, sensitivity to environmental structure implies that how information is presented (not just what is presented) can make a big difference in whether an intervention is helpful or not.

Understanding the particular processes people use and why they use them can also help guide selection of outcomes that indicate good quality decisions. For example, people naturally aiming their decision processes to protect them from experiencing cognitive dissonance and postdecisional regret suggests that measures of value concordance and of regret are important quality indicators.

Deb Feldman-Stewart

See also Decision Making and Affect; Decision Rules; Regret

Further Readings

Gigerenzer, G., Todd, P. M., & ABC Research Group. (1999). *Simple heuristics that make us smart.* New York: Oxford University Press.

Plessner, H., & Czenna, S. (2008). The benefits of intuition. In H. Plessner, C. Betsch, & T. Betsch (Eds.), *Intuition in judgment and decision making.* New York: Lawrence Erlbaum.

Selart, M. (1997). Aspects of compatibility and the construction of preference. In R. Raynard, W. R. Crozier, & O. Svenson (Eds.), *Decision making: Cognitive models and explanations.* London: Routledge.

Svenson, O. (2001). Values and affect in human decision making: A differentiation and consolidation theory perspective. In S. L. Schneider & J. Shanteau (Eds.), *Emerging perspectives on judgment and decision making research.* Cambridge, UK: Cambridge University Press.

COINCIDENCE

A coincidence is a random co-occurrence of two or more events that are perceived to be meaningfully associated with each other, even though there is no meaningful causal relationship linking them. A collision between an ambulance carrying an injured bullfighter and a cattle truck would constitute a coincidence, while internal bleeding following ingestion of broken glass would not. The need to distinguish true associations from coincidences is critical to good medical decision making, yet the human mind is ill equipped to make this distinction.

Co-occurrences of events can be perceived as meaningful when they happen along a number of dimensions, such as time (e.g., when a patient develops symptoms shortly after taking a drug), space (e.g., when multiple cases of a rare disease occur in the same town), or heredity (e.g., when several members of a family tree are found to have the same disorder).

While co-occurrences often indicate the existence of a direct causal relationship or a common underlying factor, many are simply the result of chance, and their constituent events should be considered independent of each other. However, determining whether a co-occurrence reflects meaningful or random covariance is often difficult. In fact, research shows that the human mind is limited in its ability to distinguish meaningful associations from coincidences. People (even those with medical degrees) tend to commit predictable errors when trying to distinguish random chance events from meaningful causal processes. As a result, we often overreact to coincidences and underreact to co-occurrences that deserve our attention.

Some events are, by their very nature, especially likely to capture our attention and generate an emotional response. Accordingly, they are more likely to be initially encoded in memory and are later more accessible for recall. As a result, we tend to notice their co-occurrences much more and infer more from these than from co-occurrences of other events. For example, we are overly influenced by the probability of each event occurring on its own. The more unlikely each of the events is thought to be, the more surprising we find their individual occurrences, and this makes their *co*-occurrence seem all the more surprising and meaningful. Taking vitamins and experiencing mild stomachaches are both relatively common events, so their co-occurrence is likely to go unnoticed. In contrast, taking a new experimental drug and experiencing acute abdominal pains are both relatively uncommon events, so their co-occurrence is likely to raise suspicion of a causal link. Another closely related factor is the number of events co-occurring: The greater the number of events that co-occur, the more we tend to find this co-occurrence meaningful. A physician is more likely to suspect the presence of a disease when his or her patient shows five unusual symptoms than when the patient shows two unusual symptoms.

While these two factors can provide rational bases for judging the meaningfulness of co-occurrences (though not always), others are much less justifiable. For example, co-occurrences are perceived to be more indicative of a causal relationship when they are experienced firsthand than when they are experienced by others. This helps explain why patients and their loved ones are more likely to see, in the co-occurrence of symptoms, the threat of a serious medical condition, where the physician sees harmless coincidence.

The need to distinguish meaningful co-occurrences from simple coincidences regularly arises across a variety of medical decision-making contexts. Physicians and other medical professionals are often confronted with the difficult task of recognizing when co-occurrences are meaningful or coincidental: Does the simultaneous occurrence of certain symptoms imply the presence of a disease, or did it happen by chance? Does the apparent relationship between administration of a new medical drug and improved health signal effectiveness, a placebo effect, or a meaningless coincidence? Should a physician be concerned when his or her patient reports experiencing unpleasant symptoms following a medical procedure, or is this mere happenstance? Are multiple outbreaks of a rare disease within a small geographic area the sign of a growing epidemic or just random clustering?

Separating coincidence from causality is a problem that also confronts patients and nonmedical professionals: Are feelings of nausea following a dining experience the first signs of serious food poisoning, which calls for a trip to the emergency room, or are they unrelated? Are the higher rates of surgical death associated with a particular hospital the result of malpractice or bad luck? Even when medical professionals are able to recognize coincidences, they must confront the objections of patients and loved ones who are quick to see meaningful associations in the co-occurrence of significant events (e.g., two family members dying from a rare disease) and resistant to the possibility that these could happen by chance alone.

A number of real-life examples illustrate the importance of distinguishing causation from coincidence. One striking case is the controversy that erupted in a number of Western countries, when many parents were convinced, by anecdotal evidence, that vaccination for measles, mumps, and rubella (MMR) caused autism. A number of studies were carried out in response to the resulting public outrage, with the majority of them finding no association between MMR vaccination and the occurrence of autism. As it turns out, children tend to be diagnosed with autism around the time they turn one, which also happens to be when they are administered the MMR vaccine. As result, a number of children who would have been diagnosed with autism, even without the vaccine, received this diagnosis shortly after receiving the MMR vaccine, leading many parents to perceive a direct link between the two.

Because of biases in human probabilistic reasoning, medical professionals and their patients are subject to misunderstanding coincidental occurrences as causally related. For this reason, teaching medical professionals to be aware of these biases is a prerequisite for good medical decision making and effective communication with patients.

Christopher Y. Olivola and
Daniel M. Oppenheimer

See also Biases in Human Prediction; Causal Inference in Medical Decision Making; Judgment; Probability Errors

Further Readings

Gilovich, T. (1993). *How we know what isn't so: The fallibility of reason in everyday life.* New York: The Free Press.

Griffiths, T. L., & Tenenbaum, J. B. (2007). From mere coincidences to meaningful discoveries. *Cognition, 103,* 180–226.

Hastie, R., & Dawes, R. M. (2001). *Rational choice in an uncertain world: The psychology of judgment and decision making.* Thousand Oaks, CA: Sage.

Nickerson, R. S. (2004). *Cognition and chance: The psychology of probabilistic reasoning.* Mahwah, NJ: Lawrence Erlbaum.

COMPLEXITY

Complexity science is the study of systems characterized by nonlinear dynamics and emergent properties. In contrast, simple mechanical systems are describable by sets of linear equations lending themselves to conventional scientific methods. But living systems and systems composed of living things display and adapt to changes in unpredictable ways. Complexity science studies systems as complete wholes instead of components or subsystems to effectuate better decisions that are more realistic for clinical and policy decisions.

Complexity is a term that describes how system components interact with one another. For instance, conventional medical science may be less able to predict which patients will experience unanticipated side effects from a new drug. Likewise, healthcare delivery and its many elements are not likely to respond predictably to policy or reimbursement changes.

As knowledge of health and illness progressed through the 20th century, Cartesian notions of a mechanical and predictable universe were inadequate to describe some natural phenomena. Researchers believed that multifaceted and complex findings associated with the health sciences might benefit from more advanced or comprehensive frameworks than the mechanical ones typically employed. To this end, a science of complexity was sought to improve predictability and quality of medical decision making with the use of specialized scientific methods.

Healthcare interventions draw on accumulated knowledge and wisdom concerning disease processes, formalized as science, to prevent, ameliorate, or cure conditions. Given that diseases, treatment options, and patients are often complex and unpredictable systems, perhaps clinical decision making could benefit through a deeper understanding of the system dynamics impinging on individual patients to a greater or lesser degree. For instance, complex patient ecologies include in addition to physiology, the cultural, local community, social, psychological, genetic, emotional, and relational domains, all of which can augment or impede treatment.

A science of complexity is attractive because of a potential to describe and predict systems phenomena more congruently with what is known about actual living system attributes and behaviors. For instance, the inputs, processes, and outputs associated with living systems are often described as *nonlinear* since system inputs yield unpredictable outputs. Furthermore, system behaviors may be *deterministic, stochastic,* or *random responses* to environmental challenges and changes; and all types of system responses may appear similar. Also, describing the "essence" of a given system through conventional repeated sampling methods of system outputs may never converge on fixed system *parameters.* Furthermore, living whole systems are *logically irreducible* to description and prediction by simple "reductionist" methods. Slicing a system conceptually or literally for study has limits. At some threshold, the emergent and nonlinear properties of a whole system cease to function normally, and the subject of inquiry is lost.

Important too is the tendency for conventional scientific tools that tend to favor group responses over individual or *idiographic* ones. Emergent or unexpected clinical or policy system behaviors are likely to be dismissed as measurement errors under conventional research methods.

Complex systems share some characteristics: (a) many nonlinearly interacting components; (b) system ordering initiated from the bottom up; (c) emergent structures to meet environmental demands; (d) self-organization; and (e) nonstationary characteristics. Paul Plsek challenges us when he says that "the real power [in understanding systems] lies in the way the parts come together and are interconnected to fulfill some purpose" (p. 309). Plsek further charts the domain of command and control, chaos, and complexity in Figure 1.

History

The scientific method and discourse since Descartes (1596–1650) progressed under two main assumptions: (1) System components could be analyzed as independent entities and then (2) added linearly together to describe and predict the behavior of the entire system. Thus was the Cartesian mechanistic worldview a radical and welcome departure from the previous *scholastic* forms of inquiry. Cartesian mechanics carried scientific inquiry for nearly three centuries and persists in various forms to this day.

Pierre Simon de Laplace formalized the continuity of a Cartesian "clockwork" universe over time by suggesting that the current system state is a consequence of its state in the moment immediately preceding the current one. Thus, by comprehending all nature's laws, a system's past may be described all the way back to its *initial state* and its future predicted. Over a century later, Henri Poincaré disagreed. He said that subtle factors in complex systems are amplified over time, leading to difficulty in perceiving earlier system state conditions and making long-range prediction of the future impossible. Importantly, both Laplace and Poincaré described deterministic models—but the Laplacian universe was defined as stable and predictable through time and a thorough understanding of individual system components. The universe described by Poincaré was more uncertain and best understood from its most recent states. But Poincaré did assert that complex-appearing system outputs might be produced by simple deterministic mechanisms but that some systems may be so sensitive to initial and slight perturbations that long-term prediction of a system is nearly impossible. While

Poincaré's ideas led the way for modern chaos theory, Werner Heisenberg was showing that at least subatomic systems were unpredictable and best describable in probabilistic—or *stochastic*—terms.

Cartesian mechanics (Descartes's *The World*, 1633) became inadequate to the task of explaining scientific observations as the 20th century began. In 1928, Ludwig von Bertalanffy proposed a *general systems theory* to correct Cartesian assumptions of reductionism and linear additivity. By 1951, he had extended general systems theory specifically to biology. In 1956, Kenneth Boulding classically defined general systems theory as "a level of theoretical model-building which lies somewhere between the highly generalized construction of pure mathematics and specific theories of specialized disciplines" (p. 197).

Meanwhile, two other forms of systems science were emerging. Economists adopted system dynamics, which studied information amplified through systems, circular causality, and the self-regulating and self-influencing of systems. System dynamics found that systems can be self-destructive or self-sustaining. Engineers found useful the system properties of information feedback and transmission between system components for describing, predicting, and modifying system behavior—the field of cybernetics.

Ultimately, complexity science emerged from systems theory with computer-based weather simulations by Edward Lorenz in 1961. Lorenz found that complex systems are highly sensitive to initial conditions, making nearly impossible accurate predictions for complex systems, depending on system stability. Thus, according to Kerry Emanuel, Lorenz had driven "the last nail into the casket of the Cartesian universe." Complexity science might offer a more realistic model of systems as stochastic and ever changing, rather than mechanical and stable from the beginning of time. Decision making about systems required a new set of parameters and tools to estimate them.

Complex Systems: Description and Measurement

Ruben McDaniel and others remind us that the terms *complexity* and *chaos* do not refer to the same phenomena. Three types of systems output illustrate the differences: (1) noncomplex deterministic (simple

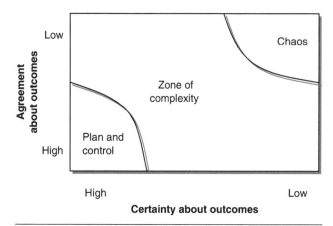

Figure 1   Depiction of the decision domains of plan and control, chaos, and complexity

Source: Stacey, Ralph D., *Strategic Management and Organizational Dynamics*, 2nd Edition, © 1996, p. 47. Adapted by permission of Pearson Education, Inc., Upper Saddle River, NJ.

mechanical), (2) complex deterministic (a chaos or chaotic system), and (3) complex random (from a complex system). Automobile engines are mechanical, noncomplex deterministic systems. All future behaviors of a specific automobile are predictable, given enough data.

Chaotic systems produce complex output that can be generated by a simple deterministic process. The formal definition and notion of a chaotic system is that a chaotic system is very sensitive to initial conditions. Chaotic processes describe electrical heart activity and nerve impulse transmission. The weather is a classic example of a chaotic system.

Chaotic systems, though deterministic, cannot be predicted over the long run. This is because of their sensitivity to initial conditions. Chaotic system behavior "drifts" over the course of time. The best predictor of tomorrow's weather is today's weather, and not the weather of 2 weeks ago. Equations that could predict system behavior yesterday become increasingly unstable or poor predictors into the future. Thus, each chaotic system's behavior is a consequence of, and best predicted by, its behavior in the preceding moment—a property called *dynamical* (see below).

Complex systems produce deceptively simple looking output from either complex or random processes. The problem is that chaotic (complex output/simple generator) and complex systems (simple or complex output/unknown processes)

are difficult to distinguish by simple observation. Biological and genetic evolution is an example of an ongoing random process in a complex system.

Not unexpectedly, measurement of complex systems may require some unconventional descriptors and tools. *Fractals* can describe dynamic processes or output outside familiar fixed Gaussian parameters that are assumed to converge to fixed or "true" values in conventional research. For instance, increasing the numbers of fractal samples causes fractal parameters to approach zero or positive infinity as their asymptotic limits, rather than an estimate of central tendency with dispersion of measurement errors. *Fractal dynamics* are used to describe bacterial growth in an inoculated petri dish, recapillarization after muscle trauma, or other biological space-filling potentials. The *fractal dimension* is a ratio of the number of branches produced by a living system compared with the resolution of measurement. For instance, how fast does respirable anthrax grow in lung tissue, and how much of the lung will be damaged irreparably in how much time? On a more constructive note, how much reperfusion of damaged heart muscle may occur if a heart attack victim is administered a certain drug within a certain time?

System bifurcation is graphic evidence that the behavior of a complex system is undergoing a major shift from extreme environmental pressures. *Dissipative structures* are distinctive physical changes observed in a system as it moves into a new equilibrium state after taking on too much information or energy for a system to maintain its current state. Boiling water is such an example, as liquid water becomes steam. Figure 2 is a graphical depiction of system bifurcation for the relation $x_{n+1} = rx_n(1 - x_n)$.

System state or type distinctions become crucial when attempting to predict system behavior. Clinicians may have to infer the kind of system they are dealing with based only on immediate observation. System behaviors determined only by previous states are *dynamical systems*. Dynamical systems output is not random, though it may appear to be. However, it is nearly impossible to identify all dynamical influences of chaotic system output. Five dynamical determinants constitute a natural upper limit for modeling chaotic systems. Some dynamical systems are more *stable* than others, that is, they generate self-similar outputs over

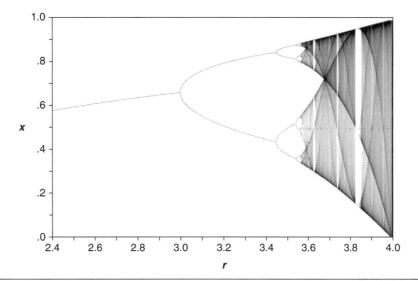

Figure 2   Graphic depiction of a system in bifurcation from environmental challenges

Note: The patterns of angled lines to the right represent dissipative structure as the system changes in outputs. A homogeneous pattern without lines would depict a system not undergoing bifurcation.

longer times. Dynamical stability is measured with low *Lyapunov* exponents, lambda (λ) in the dynamical function $f(x) = x^\lambda$. High Lyapunov exponents indicate less stable systems, and shorter time horizons for decision making. Variance in time horizons and individual patient outcomes are not captured in conventional reductionistic science.

Phase spaces and *attractors* are also complex system concepts. Phase space sets are plots of output variables as a function of either time of observation or its immediate prior state. Observing system output over a *phase space set* yields clues to the nature of the system processes. While random and chaotic data appear similar when plotted in a phase space set over time, a chaotic deterministic pattern may emerge when each output datum is plotted as a function of the previous one (Figure 3).

Random output homogeneously fills the phase space. Chaotic system output also may appear to fill phase space randomly. However, when each event is plotted as a function of the event immediately preceding it, the "noise" reveals a serial determinacy *if* the system is truly chaotic and not just random. Poincaré originally formalized the *strange attractor*, a type of dynamical system output. New information or vectors entering into an attractor system tend to settle into a small range of values, giving the appearance of attraction to a

"center of gravity" (see Figure 4). If the center is described as a fraction and not an integer, the attractor is called *strange*. If the attractor parameter (called a *fractal dimension*) is not an integer, the attractor is called *strange*. Normally one, two, three, or more dimensions are conceivable for locating an observation in space and time; it is indeed *strange* to conceive of 1.2619, or some other noninteger number of dimensions.

Strange attractors were developed by Lorenz to describe the fluid dynamics in weather patterns when two air masses of different temperatures converge. Initially, there is turbulence, followed by a new equilibrium state. Small changes in initial conditions can make for large differences in the new state—a phenomenon called the *butterfly effect*. Biological applications of strange attractors include ecological breeding patterns, dynamics of neuron action potentials, and heart rate variability. Fractal dimensions can describe the extent of physiological damage from pulmonary hypertension.

Medical Decision Making

Complexity science may play an important role in medical decision making in the future by adding new descriptors, predictors, and parameters of complex system behavior. At the clinician level, patient care decisions based on clinical judgment,

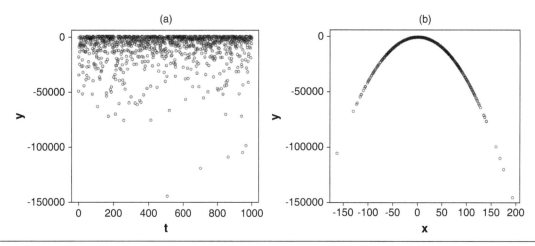

Figure 3   An example of chaos output plotted as (a) a function of time and (b) a function of preceding state

Note: The first plot (a) is the distribution of data as a function of time; the second plot (b) shows the same data plotted as a function of its immediately preceding value.

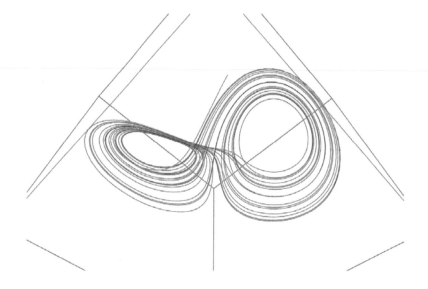

Figure 4   Phase space of the strange attractor

Note: A three-dimensional plot of data converging on a smaller area as they enter a three-dimensional system.

tacit knowledge, and current evidence may be improved by acknowledging limits of conventional clinical trial research but also by recognizing the remarkable successes of conventional research methods. If complexity science improves medical decision making, then system quality, cost, efficiency, efficacy, and safety should measurably improve in the future as more benefit from reduced uncertainty and fewer risks. Ideally, uncertainty would be reduced in the healthcare

system and in clinical practice. Eventually, knowledge added by complexity science may reach some practical limits, to be replaced by other decision-informing tools.

At the policy level, complexity science perhaps also has potential to reduce system uncertainty and improve efficiencies. Even the simple exercise of thinking systemically can be helpful. The notion of time horizons is useful; so is appreciating the fact that systems adapt and that attempting system change often precipitates reorganizing and unanticipated responses. Recognizing the signs of a distressed system expressed as "dissipative structures" may give health and financial decision makers more notice, more control, and the ability to effectively anticipate, adapt to, and manage accelerating change.

J. Michael Menke and Grant H. Skrepnek

See also Chaos Theory; Deterministic Analysis; Managing Variability and Uncertainty; Markov Models; Markov Models, Applications to Medical Decision Making; Markov Models, Cycles; Uncertainty in Medical Decisions

Further Readings

Boulding, K. E. (1956). General systems theory: The skeleton of science. *Management Science, 2,* 197–208.

Emanuel, K. (2008). Retrospective: Edward N. Lorenz (1917–2008). *Science, 320*(5879), 1025.

Liebovitch, L. S. (1998). *Fractals and chaos simplified for the life sciences.* New York: Oxford University Press.

McDaniel, R. R., Jr., & Driebe, D. J. (2001). Complexity science and health care management. In M. D. Fottler, G. T. Savage, & J. D. Blair (Eds.), *Advances in health care management* (pp. 11–36). Oxford, UK: Elsevier Science.

Plsek, P. (2001). Redesigning health care with insights from the science of complex adaptive systems. In *Crossing the quality chasm: A new health system for the 21st century* (pp. 309–317). Washington, DC: Institute of Medicine.

Rickles, D., Hawe, P., & Shiell, A. (2007). A simple guide to chaos and complexity. *Journal of Epidemiology and Community Health, 61*(11), 933–937.

Stacey, R. D., Griffin, D., & Shaw, P. (2000). *Complexity and management: Fad or radical challenge to systems thinking?* (Vol. 1). New York: Routledge.

COMPLICATIONS OR ADVERSE EFFECTS OF TREATMENT

Complications, adverse effects, and adverse outcomes are the downside of disease and treatment. If they occur, they lower the quality of care as experienced from the patients' perspective while increasing cost. The result is worse care at a higher price, the opposite of what we all strive for; better care at a lower price. Thus, complications have lately attracted much attention, and much effort is spent trying to prevent them. By studying them and the mechanisms that underlie them, measures of prevention or reduction may be identified and implemented, thereby improving the quality and cost-effectiveness of care.

Definitions

There are various definitions available on the concepts of "complications" and "adverse effect" in the medical context. Although they may differ on details, common denominators in most definitions are the focus on four elements.

Harm

This element describes the fact that the patient experienced some event or condition that had a negative effect on the patient's health and maybe even resulted in (severe) harm to the patient or in death. It is not clear in all studies how unfavorable an event, outcome, or experience must be with respect to health-related harm to be considered a complication or an adverse effect. If a patient experiences some pain after an operation, does not sleep well, or must stay in the hospital one or two days longer than expected, or if there is a small hematoma, or some wound reddening that disappears in a few days without treatment, most people will agree that this is not really a complication but more an inherent and acceptable consequence of the intervention that was deemed necessary. On the other hand, if a wound abscess or the size of a hematoma and its pressure on the skin necessitate an operation, or if a patient is still in severe pain 6 weeks after discharge and still needs morphine for that, most people will agree that a complication has arisen.

Quality of Care

This element refers to the extent to which the care delivered caused, or contributed to, the harm that was experienced.

Unintentional Harm

This element refers to the fact that the harm was indeed unintentional and not an intentional sacrifice (as, for instance, is quite common in oncological surgery to achieve a radical cancer resection), either as a calculated risk, deemed acceptable in light of an intervention's greater or more likely expected benefit, or as an unpleasant and unexpected surprise to both patient and doctor.

Harm Caused by Substandard Performance

This element addresses the question of the extent to which the harm was (in part) caused by professional substandard performance or even by an obvious error or mistake on the part of a person, group, organization, or other entity. If this is considered to be the case, it will easily lead to the additional questions of whether those substandard elements in the delivery of care *could* have been prevented or *should* have been prevented. From a legal perspective, a positive answer to both the "could" and "should" questions would suggest that some form of compensation might be justified, by a liability procedure or otherwise, depending on the extent of the harm and the extent of the causality.

The worldwide interest in these concepts and in patient safety in general was strongly increased by the Harvard Medical Practice Study (HMPS) and by the report *To Err Is Human* that followed it. In the HMPS, an adverse event was defined as

> an injury that was caused by medical management (rather than the underlying disease) and that prolonged the hospitalization, produced a disability at the time of discharge, or both. (Brennan et al., 2004, p. 145)

The fact that this definition takes element 4, the causality criterion, on board opens it up to the accusation of subjectivity. For many outcomes, the cause may not be entirely clear, or it may be attributed to several risk factors that may even reinforce one another in their causality. The subjective and oversimplified "yes/no somebody's fault" assumption does not often lead to an appropriate representation of causality. The HMPS defined the quality element (negligence) as "care that fell below the standard expected of physicians in their community."

In the current era in which guidelines abound, the "expected standard" is generally reasonably clear. However, at the time of the HMPS, even this may have been less unambiguous.

Complication Registry: An Example

In the Netherlands, around the turn of the century, a nationwide initiative to standardize the prospective registration and analysis of complications took a different approach. Here the issue of causality was intentionally left out of the definition, assuming that at the time a complication or adverse effect is noticed or registered, there will often be insufficient insight into the causality or preventability of the harm inflicted. The Dutch definition of *complication* does include an unambiguous harm threshold, thereby providing a clear-cut criterion for when something is serious enough to be considered a complication. It states,

> An unintended and unwanted event or state occurring during or following medical care, that is so harmful to a patient's health that (adjustment of) treatment is required or that permanent damage results. The adverse outcome may be noted during treatment or in a predefined period after discharge or transfer to another department. The intended results of treatment, the likelihood of the adverse outcome occurring, and the presence or absence of a medical error causing it, are irrelevant in identifying an adverse outcome. (Marang-van de Mheen, van Hanegem, & Kievit, 2005, p. 378)

Thus the assessment of causality is postponed to a later date, when more information is available. This has the advantage of providing the opportunity to standardize or improve the way causality is analyzed, thus providing a clearer answer on epidemiological questions about attributable risk. As a consequence, both judgment subjectivity and interobserver variation should be lower.

As the Dutch complication registry is not confined by a limited set of specified "complications-to-register" at the exclusion of all others, the result is that an essentially unlimited number of different complications could meet the definition. Registering them inevitably may require that free text be used. For analysis purposes, however, free text is useless and must be recoded into a meaningful set of dimensions. Within the Dutch system, a so-called Master Classification has been created that characterizes complications on three main dimensions, and in addition on a severity scale.

The first dimension defines the nature of the complication, answering the "What?" question. Its subcategories have been adapted from the ICD9/10, to better fit the adverse outcome registration purpose, and include types such as bleeding, dysfunction, and infection/inflammation.

The second dimension answers the "Where" question and specifies location, both by organ systems and organs, and by body topography (chest, abdomen, etc.).

In the third dimension, contextual information and (potential) determinants are recorded, while the fourth dimension specifies the harm inflicted on a patient (varying, for the surgical specialties, from full recovery without reoperation, to requiring reoperation, leaving permanent damage, and resulting in death).

The main purpose of the Master Classification is not so much the recoding itself as the facilitation of later data analysis. In combination with a minimum data set, in which elementary patient and context characteristics are recorded, the three-dimensional Master Classification provides maximum analytic flexibility. Sampling and analyzing complications can vary from broad categories such as "all bleeding complications" to very specific subsets such as "all infections in hip replacements leading to death in male patients over 70."

The Dutch approach may not be unique. What is good about it is that the definition and the coding system used, in combination with a minimum data set and the database structure, make it possible to address a wide range of questions without having to return to patient records. That is a crucial characteristic of any online system that aims at monitoring (and improving) the safety of healthcare by analyzing and reducing complications and adverse outcomes.

Causality and Complication Rates

Whether the issue of causality was or was not tackled adequately by the HMPS is still, after all these years, a matter of debate. The treatment of severe, sometimes life-threatening disease may require the weighing of potential benefits and potential harms. Choices will have to be made, and it is not unusual that the higher the goal is, the graver the risks are.

However, unintentional harm does occur to patients on quite a large scale. That in itself is sufficient reason to strive for a reduction of its occurrence or impact. To what extent this harm results from some event totally beyond anyone's control, is the consequence of a calculated risk, or is the consequence of below-standard care may not always be immediately clear, even to insiders.

In the field of patient safety, of complications and adverse effects, simple notions of one-cause-with-one-effect rarely hold. Instead, multiple causes, some within the grasp of doctor or patient, and some totally beyond their control, may combine or even reinforce one another and bring about a single but multicausal complication. Likewise, a single underlying cause may contribute to more than one complication, some less severe and some more so (see Figure 1).

The epidemiologically correct way to deal with the causality of complications would be to calculate the relative risk or odds ratio per determinant, for instance using logistic regression. This, however, does not immediately solve the problem as it requires adequate identification of all relevant covariates. The problem is thus transformed into adequately identifying all potential causal elements, obtaining relevant data of sufficient quality, and correctly analyzing those data using state-of-the-art statistical methods, such as logistic regression or multilevel analysis. Subsequently, relative risks can be used to calculate the attributable risk of one or more particular determinants. An important advantage of this statistically more refined approach, over an assumed simple one-to-one cause-effect relationship, is that such an attributable risk will provide a realistic notion of the health gains that can be expected when this shortcoming is eliminated or reduced, where an inappropriately simple causal relationship will overestimate the health gains of interventions targeting the assumed causes.

Given the definition and other issues, it is not surprising that for many comparable treatments or procedures, there are large differences in published complication rates. The fact that many studies neither provide specific information on the definition used nor have common standards in methodology may explain part of the variation in reported complication rates. In particular, how the definition deals with the issue of causality has been found to

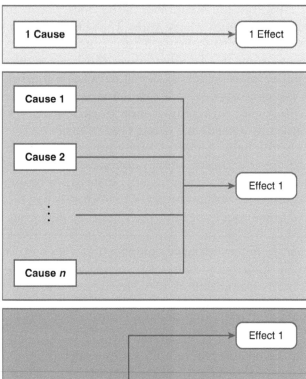

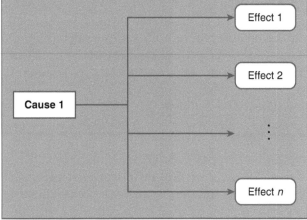

Figure 1 Causal relationships

Note: With respect to complications and adverse effects, one-to-one causality rarely holds. Instead, multiple causes may work together to bring about a single harm, or one cause may lead to several types of harm.

be an important determinant in the differences between complication rates.

Other methodological issues that are related to the reported incidence of complications or adverse outcomes are the type of data collection (prospective or retrospective) and the number of reviewers used. Most important are patient characteristics, which, apart from age, sex, and disease diagnosis, include more subtle determinants such as disease spectrum, comorbidity, the context in which patients are seen, and the type of admissions.

Relevance to Healthcare Providers, Patients, and Medical Decision Making

Complications and adverse effects are, because they compromise quality and increase cost, relevant to many interested parties, not in the least to patients and healthcare providers. For healthcare providers, they are relevant because adequate decision making in medicine requires a weighing of potential harms and benefits. Doctors, when they must make choices on risky interventions for severe diseases, must have a keen insight into the risks of any treatment they consider and into the determinants that define this risk, which may differ between different subgroups of patients.

For patients, information about complications and adverse effects is even more relevant because it is they who bear the consequences. Therefore, patients have a right to know what their risks are and what the consequences are if such a risk materializes and the harm really occurs. It goes without saying that such risk information should not be limited to the risk of mortality but should include morbidity, both less and more severe. Only on the basis of appropriate information can expected benefits and expected harms be adequately weighed.

For the field of medical decision making, complications and adverse outcomes are relevant in more than one way. First, there is the classical threshold approach to medical decision making, which holds that costs (C) and benefits (B) of treatment are weighed in light of an uncertain disease diagnosis. Treatment is the preferred policy if the chance of the disease being present exceeds the treatment threshold, defined by

$$\frac{C}{C+B}.$$

Thus, the higher the cost is (i.e., the risk of adverse effects), the more certain one should be that the disease is indeed present for the benefits to outweigh the harm. Thus, the treatment threshold will be closer to 1. Likewise, the more effective a treatment is, the lower the diagnostic certainty and thus the treatment threshold will be. Or, under the same treatment threshold, the higher the potential risk of harm may be that is deemed acceptable.

Second, modern medical decision making lays great emphasis on shared decision making.

Essential in shared decision making is that patient and caregiver communicate openly about risks and benefits of various choices and decide on the way to go taking into account not only objective evidence, but in addition priorities and preferences of the patient.

Third, a lot of research in the field of medical decision making is on risk perception and on the way that patients, doctors, and others transform an objective chance into a subjective notion of risk. Such research will improve insight into how patients (and doctors) perceive the risks of adverse effects, and weigh them into a final healthcare choice.

J. Kievit and P. J. Marang-van de Mheen

See also Causal Inference in Medical Decision Making; Complexity; Risk Communication

Further Readings

Brennan, T. A., Leape, L. L., Laird, N. M., Hebert, L., Localio, A. R., Lawthers, A. G., et al. (2004). Incidence of adverse events and negligence in hospitalized patients: Results of the Harvard Medical Practice Study I. 1991. *Quality and Safety in Health Care, 13*(2), 145–152.

Edwards, A., & Elwyn, G. (1999). How should effectiveness of risk communication to aid patients' decisions be judged? A review of the literature. *Medical Decision Making, 19*(4), 428–434.

Hayward, R. A., & Hofer, T. P. (2001). Estimating hospital deaths due to medical errors: Preventability is in the eye of the reviewer. *Journal of the American Medical Association, 286*(4), 415–420.

Marang-van de Mheen, P. J., Hollander, E. J., & Kievit, J. (2007). Effects of study methodology on adverse outcome occurrence and mortality. *International Journal for Quality in Health Care, 19*(6), 399–406.

Marang-van de Mheen, P. J., van Hanegem, N., & Kievit, J. (2005). Effectiveness of routine reporting to identify minor and serious adverse outcomes in surgical patients. *Quality and Safety in Health Care, 14*(5), 378–382.

Whitney, S. N., Holmes-Rovner, M., Brody, H., Schneider, C., McCullough, L. B., Volk, R. J., et al. (2008). Beyond shared decision making: An expanded typology of medical decisions. *Medical Decision Making, 28*(5), 699–705.

COMPUTATIONAL LIMITATIONS

There are two aspects to computational limitations in decision making. On the one hand, there is the idea that the human brain is computational and that optimal decisions require lengthy computations but that the human computational capacity is limited, and therefore human decision performance is less than optimal and humans must use alternative strategies (heuristics, etc.) to make decisions.

The second aspect is that computers are limited as well from recommending optimal decisions because the algorithms required, by necessity, take too much time. So computers too must use alternative approaches.

The primary dialectic in decision making pits the *rational-man model,* where decisions are made in accordance with the goal of maximizing utility, against the *natural-man model,* where decisions are made in a way that has been evolutionarily designed to best fit our environment. One engine of this dialectic is the issue of how much computational power is available to the decision maker. Computer scientists have attempted to model both sides in their machines, with results that have important implications for decision makers and those trying to help them. On the other side, psychologists have tried to apply computational models to observed and experimentally induced behavior.

As steam engines provided the motivating analogy in 19th-century science beyond mechanical engineering, computation provides the current leading analogy for many fields, including theories of the mind. Colloquially and even scientifically, authors discuss the brain as if it were a von Neumann computer: We separate thinking memory from storage memory, and we ask what operations our thinking self can perform with how many memory "cells." Research results need to be clear whether they mean computation in its strict sense or in its analogous sense. This entry first addresses machine-based computational limitations and then explores these difficulties in human cognition.

Machines

The field of artificial intelligence is the primary field where computational models of decision making get computer scientists' full attention and where their models get tested. Traditional areas of artificial intelligence—game playing, visual understanding, natural-language processing, expert advice giving, and robotics—each requires processing data taken from the environment to result in a conclusion or action that embodies knowledge and understanding. The nature of "computation" differs in each case. In speech recognition, the current leading methods involve numerical calculation of probabilities. In game-playing, the methods call for deriving and considering many alternative game configurations. For expert systems—beginning with the program MYCIN, whose goal was supporting the management of fever in a hospitalized patient—the computer explores pathways through rules. Thus, the computations involve a mix of quantitative and "symbolic" processing.

In computer science, *computational limitations* refer to two primary resources: time and space. *Space* refers to how much computer memory (generally onboard RAM) is needed to solve a problem. *Time* refers not only to the amount of time needed to solve a problem, in seconds or minutes, but also to the algorithmic complexity of problems. Problems whose solution time doubles if the amount of data input into the solver doubles have linear complexity; problems whose solution quadruples have quadratic complexity. For example, inverting a matrix that may represent transition probabilities in a Markov model of chronic disease has cubic complexity, and sorting a list has between linear and quadratic complexity. These algorithms are said to be *polynomial* (P) in the size of their data inputs. On the other hand, problems whose solution time doubles even if only one more piece of information is added have *exponential complexity*, and their solution takes the longest amount of time (in the worst case). For instance, enumerating by brute force all possible potential strategies for treatment in a specific clinical problem, where order matters, such as the question of which tests should be done in which order (diagnosing of immunological disease being a classic case, with the multitude of tests available), leads to an exponential number of pathways. If a single new test, for instance, becomes available, then every single pathway would have to consider using that test or not, thereby doubling the number of possibilities to be considered. If these strategies are

represented as decision trees, the number of terminal nodes would double.

There is a complexity class between polynomial and exponential called *nonpolynomial* (NP). Most of the interesting problems in decision making have been shown to be in this class, or *NP complete*. For instance, the problem of diagnosis is NP complete, meaning that a general solution could potentially take an unlimited amount of time (for all intents and purposes) of coming up with the best list of diagnoses for a particular patient. A central mystery of computer science is whether an algorithm can be found that would make NP complete algorithms polynomial: Is $P = NP$? If yes, then, with the right programming, the process of diagnosis would *not* take an "unlimited amount of time." However, most computer scientists believe this equation *not* to be the case, that is that $P \neq NP$, and that these time-saving algorithms do not exist. Their belief stems from the fact that it has been shown that, if one NP complete problem can be shown to be solved in polynomial time, then all other NP complete problems can be solved in polynomial time as well. However, so many problems are NP complete and so many people have been looking for solutions for 30 years that it appears unlikely that a solution will be found.

If it is true that $P \neq NP$, then the most important problems for which we want computers to supplement human thought, processing, and decision making will not be able to provide the correct answers in the time in which we need them to do so.

The result in computer science has been the reliance on heuristics that, when used, give good-enough results. The support for this use of reliance was provided by Herbert Simon, who called this primary heuristic *satisficing*.

Heuristic methods were the hallmark of early expert systems that provided decision advice. These were mostly rule-based systems with basically ad hoc methods of adjudicating conflicting rules, such as certainty factors or other measures. Metarules, in particular, were carefully crafted to look "reasonable." Thus, in the case of conflicting rules, a heuristic to be used might be the more "specific" rule (i.e., one where there were more "left-hand side" [antecedent] conditions that were met) over the less specific rule. For instance, a rule that pertained to a specific white blood cell count would be chosen over a rule that simply cited "WBC >

15,000." If costs were represented, the metarule would counsel using the less costly rule (e.g., get a complete blood count rather than biopsy).

Other heuristic systems included *blackboard* systems, where rules or (later) *agents,* with both data-gathering and action-taking capabilities, shared a common data space. The agents reacted relatively autonomously to data available on the common blackboard. Coordination among the agents relied, again, on metarules: More specific agents "won" over less specific ones.

In logic-based systems, the inference systems were based on the soundness and consistency of logical derivation: *modus ponens* (if all men are mortal and Socrates is a man, then Socrates is mortal) and *modus tollens* (if all men are mortal and Thor is not mortal, then Thor is not a man) in predicate logic, or binding and resolution in logic programming, such as is used in Prolog and XSB. However, to deal with uncertainty and apparently conflicting rules, *modal* logics were created that could reason about rules, much as metarules in expert systems were needed to adjudicate among conflicting rules. Some modal logics, for instance, made the implicit assumptions that, unless exceptions were explicitly stated, no exceptions were assumed to be present. While this assumption is reasonable, it may fail in environments where the knowledge base is assembled by experts who do not realize that the system has no idea of what an exception might be or who may be inconsistent in pointing out what exceptions indeed arise.

These disparate efforts converge on a common conclusion: If rational (computer-based) systems want to act rationally in the world, then their metacognition cannot follow straightforward utility-maximization procedures. Satisficing and heuristics will play major roles.

Humans

Researchers in cognitive science address decision making as computational in a number of ways. At the conscious level, they point to the language of decision making: We "weigh" evidence and "balance" pros and cons. At the preconscious level, we make choices based on some sort of psychological version of conscious weighing and balancing—but with the limitations imposed by time and by cognitive boundaries.

A classic limit due to "space" is embodied in the truisms of the *magic number 7*: that our short-term memory (note the computer-like label) can accommodate 7 ± 2 chunks. Since 1956, this limit has become part of social lore. We can remember phone numbers, along with satellite access and secret codes (a potential total of 21 digits), by chunking them into three entities and then recalling each number as 3 chunks (area code, "exchange," number) or 7 digits of access (usually divided into a unit of 3 digits and then 4 remaining digits). Chess masters apparently remember board arrangements because they chunk patterns of many pieces into one pattern, much as expert diagnosticians recall many details about a patient because many findings may be chunked into syndromes that explain the findings or make the findings memorable specifically because they are exceptions to the syndromic rule. For instance, a patient with no crackles in the lung fields but with fever, cough, diminished air entry, infiltrate on an X-ray, and sputum culture positive for pneumococci has pneumococcal pneumonia, notable for the absence of crackles, much like Sherlock Holmes's dog was notable for not barking.

Cognitive scientists have gone further, to opine that the computational limits forced evolution to mold in humans heuristics that are successful precisely because of these limits. Gerd Gigerenzer and Reinhard Selten title their compendium on the subject *Bounded Rationality* as a direct response to Simon and match specific information environments to specific heuristics. Thus, in a noisy but stable information environment, people use the Imitate Others heuristic. Where rational-man theorists see deficiencies in people's abilities to act totally rationally, as defined by the rules of maximizing expected utility, these experimentalists see strength and power in people's abilities to do as well as they can in the limits nature set them.

Thus, the psychologists see people using heuristics in much the way that computer scientists learned to rely on them: for metacognition. In Gary Klein's famous example, firemen, when faced with a new and clearly dangerous situation, rather than calculate all the possibilities and choose the optimal path, use the heuristic of moving to the last safe place ("Take the Last") and consider the options from there. These major heuristics, according to Girgerenzer, fall under the general class of Fast and Frugal—to arrive at a conclusion quickly and with the use of minimal resources is itself a goal.

Other cognitive researchers have gone deeper, delving into the structure of memory that undergirds much decision making. Fuzzy Trace theory points out that memory, beyond short-term and long-term, contains two further types: gist and verbatim. The fuzzy-processing preference is to operate at the least precise level of representation that can be used to accomplish a judgment or decision. This preference is clearly related to the "frugal" aspect of Girgerenzer's conception.

Behavioral-economist researchers, such as Amos Tversky and economics Nobel prize winner Daniel Kahnemann, discovered many biases, discussed elsewhere in this encyclopedia, by comparing human behavior with behavior that maximizing expected utility would dictate. In this sense, the heuristics are *biases* to be corrected. From the cognitive psychologist's perspective, each "bias" reflects a mental mechanism built on a particular strength of the human brain. Thus, people's powerful abilities in pattern matching become the *representativeness* bias; efficient memory retrieval becomes the *availability* bias; the abilities to discern salience and signals become the *anchoring and adjusting biases*.

Synthesis

The demand for decision support delivered by computers in practice forces developers to confront this dialectic. On the one hand, the computer is expected to be correct, evidence-based, and rational. On the other hand, it participates in a real work environment with all the limitations of its users and the time pressures of their jobs. An ideal synthesis would have the knowledge infrastructure of the decision support based on the rational-man model but with a user interface built on principles of bounded rationality and heuristic actions. Current research and practice work toward these ideals on several fronts, although no solution is currently offered. The rational-man-based decision support is reserved for policy recommendations, while frontline decision making depends on heuristics-based decision support that generally does not take human cognitive thinking or relations with the human-computer interface into account.

Hopefully, we shall see proper syntheses in the future.

Harold Lehmann

See also Bounded Rationality and Emotions; Clinical Algorithms and Practice Guidelines; Cognitive Psychology and Processes; Computer-Assisted Decision Making; Expected Utility Theory; Fuzzy-Trace Theory; Heuristics

Further Readings

Cooper, G. F. (1990). The computational complexity of probabilistic inference using Bayesian belief networks. *Artificial Intelligence, 42,* 393–405.

Garey, M. R., & Johnson, D. S. (1979). *Computers and intractability: A guide to the theory of NP-completeness.* New York: Freeman.

Gigerenzer, G., & Selten, R. (Eds.). (2001). *Bounded rationality: The adaptive toolbox.* Cambridge: MIT Press.

Klein, G. (1998). *Sources of power: How people make decisions.* Cambridge: MIT Press.

Miller, G. A. (1956). The magical number seven, plus or minus two: Some limits on our capacity for processing information. *Psychological Review, 63,* 81–97.

Reyna, V. F., & Adam, M. B. (2003). Fuzzy-trace theory, risk communication, and product labeling in sexually transmitted diseases. *Risk Analysis, 23*(2), 325–342.

Simon, H. A. (1985). *The sciences of the artificial* (2nd ed.). Cambridge: MIT Press.

COMPUTER-ASSISTED DECISION MAKING

Computer-based decision support software can assist in arriving at decisions regarding diagnoses and diagnostic workup, therapy choices, and prognoses. Generally, such software systems function by interpreting data about patients using biomedical knowledge that has been encoded into the software. The results of these interpretations are often decision alternatives that are pertinent to the patient under consideration and are presented to the users of the software to assist them in their decision making. The users of the software may be clinicians or patients.

Approaches

A decision support software system has several conceptual components:

1. An inferencing approach typically embodied in an algorithm that enables the system to interpret patient data based on the knowledge available to the system. Examples of such approaches include Bayesian inferencing and production rule evaluation.

2. A knowledge base that comprises the biomedical knowledge available to the system. The knowledge is encoded in a form that corresponds to the inferencing approach being used. For example, a knowledge base for trauma diagnosis might consist of a Bayesian network relating patient symptoms and findings to internal organ injuries.

3. Optional interfaces to other computer systems to obtain data about a patient.

4. A user interface to interact with the user, such as to obtain data, and to present the results from the inferencing.

Based on the mode in which the decision support is invoked, the system may be characterized as one providing solicited advice or one providing unsolicited advice. In the former case, a clinician may seek recommendations from a decision support system to assist with making a differential diagnosis in a patient with an unusual presentation. Such systems usually contain a large knowledge base that spans a domain of clinical interest such as internal medicine or infectious diseases. Unsolicited advice is rendered by systems (a) in response to clinical events that are being monitored, such as the reporting of a critically low value for a serum potassium test, or (b) as a critique of a proposed physician intervention such as prescribing a medication to which the patient is hypersensitive. Decision support systems that offer unsolicited advice, to be able to function, must be integrated with sources of patient data such as an electronic medical record (EMR) system or a computer-based provider order entry (CPOE) system. Systems that offer solicited advice may be integrated with sources of patient data or may be freestanding.

An important aspect of decision support systems for clinical use is how it integrates into the clinical workflow. In other words, the successful use of these systems depends on when and where the system's advice is presented to the clinicians. Thus, various kinds of tools have been created to present advice at particular points in the clinical workflow. For example, reminder systems are used often to advise clinicians in the ambulatory setting about preventive care actions that are applicable to a patient. Electrocardiography (ECG) machines incorporate features to analyze the ECG and print or display the resulting interpretation of the findings with the ECG trace. Rule-based systems critique physician orders and prescriptions in the CPOE application to prevent orders that might have the potential to harm the patient or those that might be ineffective. Such systems also might suggest additional orders called corollary orders: For example, an order for a nephrotoxic medication might lead to a corollary order for performing kidney function tests. Abnormal laboratory test results are highlighted on the screen to draw the attention of the clinician to those values. Furthermore, links to didactic informational resources, also known as infoButtons, can be shown next to the results. These information resources can be used by the clinicians to help interpret the test result and decide on an appropriate action. Treatment planning systems for surgery or radiation therapy are used in a laboratory setting initially to plan the treatment. The outputs of these systems are presented to the clinician during the treatment in the operating room.

Applications and Examples

One of the well-known, early examples of software for computer-assisted medical decision making is MYCIN, developed by Edward Shortliffe at Stanford University. MYCIN provided, on solicitation by physicians, antimicrobial therapy recommendations for patients with bacterial infections. MYCIN was capable of explaining how it arrived at its recommendations.

Internist-1, another early system, assists in diagnostic decision making. It is capable of making multiple diagnoses from patient symptoms and findings in the domain of internal medicine using a very large knowledge base. Internist-1 is available commercially as the Quick Medical Reference

(QMR) system. Over the years, many other computer-based decision support systems have been created to assist with making diagnoses. Among these are the DXplain system for diagnoses in internal medicine, and a Bayesian network-based system for diagnosing the cause of abdominal pain, created by F. T. de Dombal and colleagues.

Computer-assisted decision aids have been used for complex tasks such as radiation therapy treatment planning and surgical planning. In the former case, computer-based tools are used for designing a treatment plan that optimizes the delivery of radiation to a tumor. In the latter case, computer software is used with three-dimensional images of the patient to plan and simulate the surgical procedure.

A separate class of decision-making systems has been investigated to support the need for planning, coordinating, and executing care over extended time periods. The intended use of such systems is often to implement decision support based on clinical practice guidelines. The systems support decision making around the diagnosis, evaluation, and long-term management of a patient. Examples of these systems include the Guideline Interchange Format, ProForma, EON, and Asbru.

Effectiveness and Usage

In clinical studies, clinical decision support (CDS) systems have been shown largely to affect the performance of practitioners in a desirable manner. For example, reminder systems have increased the frequency with which preventive care actions are carried out; diagnostic decision support systems have been shown to help make the correct diagnosis; and CDS embedded in CPOE systems has reduced the ordering of drugs that might cause harm to the patient. Systems that provide unsolicited advice are more likely to affect practitioner performance than are systems that require the practitioner to seek advice. Few studies on computer-assisted decision-making systems have measured the impact of such systems on patient outcomes. Among these studies, relatively few have demonstrated an improvement in patient outcome.

In spite of the beneficial impact of computer-assisted decision-making tools on practitioner performance, these tools are not being used widely yet. One of the challenges in the adoption of CDS systems is the lack of specificity of the decision support, especially for the systems that offer unsolicited advice. These systems must have access to codified patient data. If such data are lacking or are imprecise for a patient, advice is delivered to the practitioner that may not apply to that patient. For example, if there is a record of an allergy to a particular medication, but the severity is not documented for a patient, a decision support system might advise the physician to not order the medication, even though the sensitivity is very mild in this patient and the clinical benefit potentially is large. Another major barrier to the widespread usage of CDS systems is the availability of knowledge bases to cover the different domains of healthcare and of clinical practice. The creation and maintenance of knowledge bases requires much effort from subject matter experts and knowledge engineers. Furthermore, such knowledge bases must be usable in a variety of different host CDS systems and many different practice environments. Financial incentives can also help increase the adoption of computer-assisted decision-making tools. The increasing use of pay-for-performance measures, where providers are reimbursed by payers based on their performance in a range of quality measures, might lead to increases in adoption of tools for decision making.

The use of standards for representing the knowledge and providing patient data to the CDS system will reduce technical barriers for implementing and using CDS systems. The Clinical Decision Support Technical Committee at Health Level Seven (HL7), an organization with international participation that creates standards for healthcare data interchange, is leading the effort for developing knowledge representation standards. HL7 sponsors the Arden Syntax standard for representing rules that are used in a number of commercially available clinical information systems.

Aziz A. Boxwala

See also Bayesian Networks; Clinical Algorithms and
    Practice Guidelines; Decision Rules; Expert Systems

Further Readings

Boxwala, A. A., Peleg, M., Tu, S., Ogunyemi, O., Zeng, Q. T., Wang, D., et al. (2004). GLIF3: A representation format for sharable computer-interpretable clinical practice guidelines. *Journal of Biomedical Informatics, 37*(3), 147–161.

de Clercq, P. A., Blom, J. A., Korsten, H. H., & Hasman, A. (2004). Approaches for creating computer-interpretable guidelines that facilitate decision support. *Artificial Intelligence in Medicine, 31*(1), 1–27.

Garg, A. X., Adhikari, N. K., McDonald, H., Rosas-Arellano, M. P., Devereaux, P. J., Beyene, J., et al. (2005). Effects of computerized clinical decision support systems on practitioner performance and patient outcomes: A systematic review. *Journal of the American Medical Association, 293*(10), 1223–1238.

Greenes, R. A. (Ed.). (2007). *Clinical decision support: The road ahead.* New York: Academic Press.

Hripcsak, G. (1994). Writing Arden Syntax medical logic modules. *Computers in Biology and Medicine, 24*(5), 331–363.

Kawamoto, K., Houlihan, C. A., Balas, E. A., & Lobach, D. F. (2005). Improving clinical practice using clinical decision support systems: A systematic review of trials to identify features critical to success. *British Medical Journal, 330*(7494), 765.

Kuperman, G. J., Teich, J. M., Gandhi, T. K., & Bates, D. W. (2001). Patient safety and computerized medication ordering at Brigham and Women's Hospital. *Joint Commission Journal on Quality Improvement, 27*(10), 509–521.

Maviglia, S. M., Yoon, C. S., Bates, D. W., & Kuperman, G. (2006). KnowledgeLink: Impact of context-sensitive information retrieval on clinicians' information needs. *Journal of the American Medical Informatics Association, 13*(1), 67–73.

Osheroff, J. A., Teich, J. M., Middleton, B. F., Steen, E. B., Wright A., & Detmer, D. E. (2006). *A roadmap for national action on clinical decision support.* Washington, DC: American Medical Informatics Association.

Purdy, J. A. (2007). From new frontiers to new standards of practice: Advances in radiotherapy planning and delivery. *Frontiers of Radiation Therapy and Oncology, 40*, 18–39.

CONDITIONAL INDEPENDENCE

The concept of conditional independence plays an important role in medical decision making. Conditional independence itself concerns whether information about one variable provides incremental information about another variable. The concept is also important in articulating assumptions needed to reason about causality.

Independence and Conditional Independence

The concepts of independence and conditional independence concern whether information about one variable also contains information about another variable. Two variables are said to be independent if information about one gives no information about the other. For example, one might expect that whether an individual is left-handed or right-handed gives no information about the likelihood of developing pneumonia; it would then be said that being left-handed or right-handed is independent of the development of pneumonia. More formally, if $P(Y = y|Z = z)$ is the probability that $Y = y$ given $Z = z$ and if $P(Y = y)$ is the overall probability that $Y = y$, then the variables Y and Z are said to be independent if $P(Y = y|Z = z) = P(Y = y)$; in other words, Y and Z are independent if the information that $Z = z$ gives no information about the distribution of Y; equivalently, Y and Z are independent if $P(Z = z|Y = y) = P(Z = z)$. When two variables X and Y are not independent, they are said to be correlated or to be statistically associated. Independence is also often referred to as "marginal independence" or "unconditional independence" to distinguish it from conditional independence.

The concept of conditional independence is a natural extension of the concept of independence. Conditional independence is similar to independence, except that it involves conditioning on a third variable (or set of variables). Thus suppose that one is interested in the relationship between X and Y within the strata of some third variable C. The two variables, X and Y, are said to be conditionally independent given C if information about X gives no information about Y once one knows the value of C. For example, a positive clinical breast exam is predictive of the presence of breast cancer; that is to say, a positive clinical breast exam and the presence of breast cancer are not independent; they are statistically associated. Suppose, however, that in addition to the results of a clinical breast exam, information is also available on further evaluation procedures such as mammogram and biopsy results. In this case, once one has information on these further evaluation procedures, the results from the clinical breast exam give no additional information about the likelihood of breast cancer beyond the mammogram and biopsy results; that is to say the presence of breast cancer is conditionally independent of the clinical breast exam results given the results from the mammogram and biopsy. More formally, if $P(Y = y|Z = z, C = c)$ is the probability that $Y = y$ given that $Z = z$ and $C = c$ and if $P(Y = y|C = c)$ is the probability that $Y = y$ given that $C = c$, then the variables Y and Z are said to be conditionally independent given C if $P(Y = y|Z = z, C = c) = P(Y = y|C = c)$. When two variables Y and Z are not conditionally independent given C, then they are said to be associated conditionally on C or to be conditionally associated given C. The notation $Y \perp\!\!\!\perp Z|C$ is sometimes used to denote that Y and Z are conditionally independent given C; the notation $Y \perp\!\!\!\perp Z$ is used to denote that Y and Z are unconditionally independent. A. P. Dawid's article "Conditional Independence in Statistical Theory" gives an overview of some of the technical statistical properties concerning conditional independence. The focus here will be the relevance of the idea of conditional independence in medical decision making.

Conditional Independence in Causal Reasoning

For medical decision making, the idea of conditional independence is perhaps most important because of its relation to confounding and the estimation of causal effects. Suppose that a researcher is trying to compare two drugs, Drug A and Drug B, in their effects on depression. Suppose that it has been demonstrated in randomized trials that both drugs result in higher recovery rates than a placebo but that it is unclear whether the recovery rate for Drug A or for Drug B is higher. Suppose that observational data are available to compare Drugs A and B but that no randomized trial has been conducted to make such a comparison. Let X_i be the variable that indicates which treatment individual i in fact received, so that $X_i = 1$ denotes individual i's receiving Drug A and $X_i = 0$ denotes individual i's receiving Drug B. Let Y_i denote whether or not individual i is clinically depressed 1 year after the initiation of drug therapy. For each individual, it might be of interest whether the

individual's depression status would be different under Drug A compared with Drug B. Let $Y_i(1)$ denote individual i's depression status 1 year after the initiation of drug therapy had the individual, possibly contrary to fact, been given Drug A. Let $Y_i(0)$ denote individual i's depression status had the individual, possibly contrary to fact, been given Drug B. The variables $Y_i(1)$ and $Y_i(0)$ are sometimes referred to as counterfactual outcomes or potential outcomes. For any given individual, one only gets to observe one of $Y_i(1)$ or $Y_i(0)$. For individuals who in fact received Drug A, one observes $Y_i(1)$; for individuals who in fact received Drug B, one observes $Y_i(0)$. Because only one of the potential outcomes is observed, it is not possible to calculate the causal effect, $Y_i(1) - Y_i(0)$, for individual i since one of $Y_i(1)$ or $Y_i(0)$ is always unknown.

Although it is not possible to estimate individual causal effects, one can in some contexts, under assumptions articulated below about conditional independence, estimate average causal effects for a particular study population. In what follows, the index i is generally suppressed, and the variables are treated as random, assuming that the subjects in the study are randomly sampled from some study population. One might thus be interested in comparing the average depression rate for the population if the whole study population had been given Drug A, denoted by $E[Y(1)]$, with the average depression rate for the population if the whole study population had been given Drug B, denoted by $E[Y(0)]$. Although it is not possible to observe $Y(1)$ or $Y(0)$ for each individual, one might consider comparing the observed depression rates for the group that in fact received Drug A, denoted by $E[Y|X = 1]$, and the observed depression rates for the group that in fact received Drug B, denoted by $E[Y|X = 0]$. The problem with such an approach is that the group that received Drug A and the group that received Drug B might not be comparable. For example, the group that received Drug A might have had more severe depression or might have consisted of older subjects or might have had worse diets. To attempt to make the groups comparable, control may be made for as many confounding variables as possible, variables that affect both the treatment and the outcome, denoted by C. It is then hoped that within strata of the confounding variables C the group receiving Drug A is comparable with the group receiving Drug B.

More formally, to estimate the average causal effect, $E[Y(1)] - E[Y(0)]$, by control for confounding, it is necessary that the counterfactual variables $Y(1)$ and $Y(0)$ be conditionally independent of the treatment received, X, given the confounding variables C. This conditional independence assumption can be written as $P(Y(1)|X = 1, C = c) = P(Y(1)|X = 0, C = c)$ and $P(Y(0)|X = 1, C = c) = P(Y(0)|X = 0, C = c)$; in other words, within strata of the confounding variables C, what happened to the group that received Drug A is representative of what would have happened to the group that received Drug B if they had in fact received Drug A; and similarly, within strata of the confounding variables C, what happened to the group that received Drug B is representative of what would have happened to the group that received Drug A if they had in fact received Drug B. If this holds, then average causal effects can be estimated using the following formula:

$$E[Y(1)] - E[Y(0)] = \sum_c \{E[Y|X = 1, C = c] - E[Y|X = 0, C = c]\}P(C = c).$$

Average causal effects can be estimated because, within strata of the confounding variables C, the groups that received Drug A and Drug B are comparable. The assumption that the counterfactual variables $Y(1)$ and $Y(0)$ are conditionally independent of the treatment received, X, given the confounding variables C is sometimes referred to as the assumption of "no-unmeasured-confounding" or as "exchangeability" or as "ignorable treatment assignment" or as "selection on observables" or sometimes as simply the "conditional independence" assumption. The assumption plays an important role in causal inference. In practice, data are collected on a sufficiently rich set of variables C so that the assumption that the groups are comparable within strata of C is at least approximately satisfied. Different techniques are available to make adjustment for the covariates C; adjustment can be made by stratification, regression, or propensity score modeling.

In the context of medical decision making, conditional independence is also important for a number of other problems. In many studies subjects drop out of a study before an outcome can be observed. It is not always clear that those subjects that remain in the study are comparable to those that drop out of the study. To make such problems tractable, a certain conditional independence assumption is sometimes made, namely that censoring status is conditionally independent of the potential outcomes $Y(1)$ and $Y(0)$ given the covariates C. In other words, it is assumed that within strata of the covariates C, the groups dropping out of the study are comparable with those who do not drop out; the set C contains all variables that affect both the dropout and the outcome. Conditional independence is also important in the analysis of surrogate outcomes in which some intermediate outcome is taken as a surrogate for the final outcome, which may be more difficult or expensive to collect data on than the surrogate. For example, the Prentice criteria for a valid surrogate outcome consist of the following three conditions: (1) the surrogate outcome, S, must be correlated with the true outcome, Y (i.e., S and Y must not be independent); (2) the surrogate outcome, S, must be affected by the exposure, X; and (3) the exposure, X, and the outcome, Y, should be conditionally independent given the surrogate, S. The third criterion captures the notion that all information about Y contained in the exposure A is in fact also available in the surrogate outcome, S.

Graphical Representation

More recently, graphical models and causal diagrams have been used to reason about independence and conditional independence relations. The technical details concerning such reasoning are beyond the scope of this entry. These diagrams make it clear that statistical association (lack of independence) can arise in a number of ways. The variables X and Y may be associated if X causes Y or if Y causes X. Even if neither X nor Y causes the other, the variables X and Y may be associated if they have some common cause C. In this case, if C contains all the common causes of X and Y, then X and Y will not be marginally independent but will be conditionally independent given C. Finally, if X and Y are independent but if they have some common effect C, then it will in general be the case that X and Y are conditionally associated given the common effect, C, that is, they will not be conditionally independent given C. Another interesting property relating conditional independence to these diagrams can be stated as follows: If the set C contains all variables that are common causes of X and Y and contains no common effects of X and Y, then if neither X nor Y

causes the other, then X and Y must be conditionally independent given C; thus, if X and Y are found not to be conditionally independent given such a set C, then one could conclude that either X has an effect on Y or Y has an effect on X.

These causal diagrams and their relation to conditional independence can also be helpful in understanding different forms of selection bias. Suppose that the occurrence of pneumonia and the level of sugar intake are such that sugar intake has no effect on pneumonia and that sugar intake and pneumonia are completely independent in the population. Sugar intake is however a risk factor for diabetes. Suppose now that all the subjects in a study are taken from a particular hospital. Hospitalization is then a common effect of both pneumonia and of diabetes, which is in turn an effect of sugar intake. By restricting the study to those subjects who are hospitalized one is implicitly conditioning on a common effect of pneumonia and sugar intake/diabetes, namely hospitalization. Thus, in the study it will appear that sugar intake and pneumonia are statistically associated because of the conditioning on the common effect, hospitalization, even though sugar intake has no effect on pneumonia; although sugar intake and pneumonia are marginally independent, they are not conditionally independent given hospitalization. This is an instance of what is often now called Berkson's bias. It is one of several types of selection bias that can be viewed as resulting from conditioning on a common effect and thereby inducing conditional association. See Hernán, Hernández-Diaz, and Robins (2004) for a discussion as to how the ideas of independence and conditional independence, causal diagrams, and the conditioning on a common effect can be used to understand better other forms of selection bias.

Tyler J. VanderWeele

See also Axioms; Causal Inference and Diagrams; Causal Inference in Medical Decision Making; Conditional Probability; Confounding and Effect Modulation; Ordinary Least Squares Regression; Propensity Scores

Further Readings

Berkson, J. (1946). Limitations of the application of fourfold table analysis to hospital data. *Biometrics Bulletin, 2,* 47–53.

Dawid, A. P. (1979). Conditional independence in statistical theory. *Journal of the Royal Statistical Society, Series B, 41,* 1–31.

Greenland, S. (2003). Quantifying biases in causal models: Classical confounding vs collider-stratification bias. *Epidemiology, 14,* 300–306.

Greenland, S., Pearl, J., & Robins, J. M. (1999). Causal diagrams for epidemiologic research. *Epidemiology, 10,* 37–48.

Hernán, M. A., Hernández-Diaz, S., & Robins, J. M. (2004). A structural approach to selection bias. *Epidemiology, 15,* 615–625.

Pearl, J. (1995). Causal diagrams for empirical research. *Biometrika, 82,* 669–688.

Pearl, J. (2000). *Causality: Models, reasoning, and inference.* Cambridge, UK: Cambridge University Press.

Prentice, R. L. (1989). Surrogate endpoints in clinical trials: Definition and operational criteria. *Statistics in Medicine, 8,* 431–440.

VanderWeele, T. J., & Robins, J. M. (2007). Directed acyclic graphs, sufficient causes and the properties of conditioning on a common effect. *American Journal of Epidemiology, 166,* 1096–1104.

CONDITIONAL PROBABILITY

The probability that event E occurs, given that event F has occurred, is called the conditional probability of event E given event F. In probability notation, it is denoted with $p(E|F)$. Conditional probabilities express the probability of an event (or outcome) under the condition that another event (or outcome) has occurred. You could also think of it as the probability within a particular subset, that is, in the subset of patients with event F in their history, the proportion that develop event E.

The conditional probability $p(E|F)$ is the ratio of the *joint probability* of events E and F, which is denoted as $p(E, F)$ or as $p(E$ and $F)$, and the *marginal probability* of event F, denoted with $p(F)$:

$$p(E|F) = \frac{p(E, F)}{p(F)}.$$

If the conditional information ("given event F") makes no difference to the probability of event E, then the two events E and F are said to be *conditionally independent*. For example, if F made no difference to the estimate of the probability of E, that is, if $p(E|F+) = p(E|F-) = p(E)$, then E and F are said to be conditionally independent.

M. G. Myriam Hunink

See also Conditional Independence

Further Readings

Hunink, M. G. M., Glasziou, P. P., Siegel, J. E., Weeks, J. C., Pliskin, J. S., Elstein, A. S., et al. (2001). *Decision making in health and medicine: Integrating evidence and values.* Cambridge, UK: Cambridge University Press.

CONFIDENCE INTERVALS

Any decision in medicine is arrived at through a careful process of examining the evidence and deciding what would be the best course of action. There are many parts to this process, including the gathering of evidence that is of as high a quality as possible, the critical examination of this evidence, and a consideration of the interests of all those likely to be affected by the decision.

This entry concentrates on the process of critically examining the evidence and in particular the importance of confidence intervals to this process. Some key concepts will be defined, before discussing what is meant by statistical and clinical significance and then demonstrating the relevance and importance of confidence limits to medical decision making through examples from the literature.

Key Concepts

In classical statistical inference, the null hypothesis is the hypothesis that is tested. It is assumed to be true and is only rejected if there is a weight of evidence against it. The p value provides evidence in support of the null hypothesis. Technically speaking the p value is the probability of obtaining the study results (or results more extreme) if the null hypothesis is true. Thus a "small" p value indicates that the results obtained are unlikely when the null hypothesis is true and the null hypothesis is rejected in favor of the alternative hypothesis.

Alternatively, if the p value is "large," then the results obtained are likely when the null hypothesis is true and the null hypothesis is not rejected. However, a large p value does not mean that the null hypothesis is correct: Absence of evidence does not equate to evidence of absence. The power of a study refers to the probability that a study will reject the null hypothesis if it is not true. While a nonsignificant p value may be indicative of the null hypothesis being correct, it may also be the result of the study lacking the power to reject the null hypothesis even though it is incorrect.

A result is said to be statistically significant if the p value is below the level set for defining statistical significance. This level is set before a study is undertaken. Conventionally, the cutoff value or two-sided significance level for declaring that a particular result is statistically significant is .05 (or 5%). Thus if the p value is less than this value, the null hypothesis is rejected and the result is said to be statistically significant at the 5% or .05 level.

For example, researchers in Australia (J. B. Dixon and colleagues) recently investigated whether adjustable gastric banding resulted in better glycemic control for type 2 diabetes compared with standard approaches to weight loss. At the end of the study, the 30 patients randomized to gastric band surgery (surgical) weighed, on average, 19.6 kg less than the 30 patients randomized to conventional weight loss therapy (standard), and the p value associated with this difference was less than .001. As this is less than .05, the authors were able to conclude that there was a statistically significant difference in the amount of weight lost between the two therapy groups.

However, a p value is not everything as it gives no information about the likely size of the result or the range of plausible values for it. This additional information is given by calculating a confidence interval for the result. Strictly speaking, a confidence interval represents the limits within which the true population value will lie for a given percentage of possible samples, and it can be calculated for any estimated quantity from the sample, including a mean or mean difference, proportion, or difference between two proportions. In practice, while not strictly speaking correct, it is not unreasonable to interpret; for example, the 95% confidence interval for the mean as being the interval within which the true population mean is likely to lie with 95% certainty, or probability .95. For large samples (say greater than 60), the 95% confidence interval is calculated as

$$\bar{x} - 1.96 \times s/\sqrt{n} \text{ to } \bar{x} + 1.96 \times s/\sqrt{n},$$

where

$\bar{x}$ is the sample mean,

s is the sample standard deviation,

n is the number of observations in the sample, and

1.96 is the two-sided 5% point of the standard normal distribution.

The reason why we can use this simple formula is that, according to the Central Limit Theorem, the mean follows a Normal distribution. The Normal distribution is one of the fundamental distributions of statistics, and it is characterized such that the middle 95% of the data lie within +/- 1.96 standard deviations of its mean value. Conversely, only 5% of the data lie outside of these limits. The sample mean is an unbiased estimator of the true population mean, and while s is the sample standard deviation (for the data collected), the standard deviation of the mean is given by $s/\sqrt{n}$ and is often referred to as the standard error of the mean. Thus 95% of possible values for the true population mean will lie within $1.96 \times s/\sqrt{n}$ of the sample mean.

While the 95% confidence interval is the standard, it is possible to calculate a confidence interval to have greater or lesser coverage, that is, a 90% confidence interval or a 99% confidence interval, and this is done by changing the value of the cutoff point of the standard normal distribution in the expression above. For 90% limits, this changes to 1.64, and for 99% limits, this changes to 2.58.

For the above example, the 95% confidence interval for the mean difference in weight lost was 15.2 to 23.8 kg. Thus, the true mean difference in amount of weight lost between those with surgical intervention and standard therapy lies between 15.2 and 23.8 kg with 95% certainty.

Statistical Versus Clinical Significance

For medical decision making, in addition to statistical significance, it is essential to consider clinical significance, and it is in contributing to this that confidence intervals demonstrate their importance. A clinically significant difference is defined as a difference that is sufficiently large as to make a difference to patients or cause a change in clinical practice. Clinical significance is not a statistical concept, and its level cannot be set by a statistician. It must be arrived at through debate with knowledgeable subject experts, and the value set will depend on context. What is important to patients might be very different from what is considered important by policy makers or clinicians.

Even if a result is statistically significant, it may not be clinically significant, and conversely an estimated difference that is clinically important may not be statistically significant. For example, consider a large study comparing two treatments for high blood pressure; the results suggest that there is a statistically significant difference ($p < .001$) in the amount by which blood pressure is lowered. This p value relates to a difference of 2 mmHg between the two treatments, with a 95% confidence interval of 1.3 to 2.7 mmHg. Although this difference is statistically significant at the .1% level, it is not clinically significant as it represents a very small change in blood pressure and it is unlikely that clinicians and indeed their patients would change to a new treatment for such a marginal effect.

This is not simply a trivial point. Often in research presentations or papers, p values alone are quoted, and inferences about differences between groups are made based on this one statistic. Statistically significant p values may be masking differences that have little clinical importance. Conversely, it may be possible to have a p value greater than the magic 5% but with a genuine difference between groups, which the study did not have enough power to detect. This will be shown by the confidence interval being so large that it not only includes the null difference but also includes a clinically important difference.

There are two sides to clinical significance, depending on whether it is important to demonstrate that two treatments are different from one another (superiority) or whether it is of interest to demonstrate that their effect is the same (equivalence), and confidence intervals have a part to play in both, as outlined below.

Importance in Medical Decision Making

Treatment Superiority

The importance of confidence intervals in studies to demonstrate superiority is best explained by reference to Table 1 and Figure 1. These display the results of seven (theoretical) studies comparing the same two treatments for superiority; that is, the object is to demonstrate that the two treatments are different. The table shows some possible point estimates of the effect size, together with the associated p values.

It is clear from this table that three of the studies are not statistically significant at the 5% level and four are. However, even assuming that a clinically important difference is two units on the measurement scale, it is impossible to tell which of these results are definitely of clinical importance, based on the p values and effect sizes alone. This information can only be obtained by reference to the confidence intervals as these will show the range of plausible values for the effect size, as shown in Figure 1. The left-hand vertical line in the figure represents the value that indicates the two treatments are equivalent and the right-hand line represents the value of a clinically important difference between the two treatments. Looking at Figure 1, it is clear that while four studies are statistically significant (C, D, F, and G), only one, Study G, is definitely clinically significant, as not only is the point estimate of the effect

Table 1   Results of six studies examining the difference between two treatments

Study	Size of Difference	p value
A	0.8	>.05
B	0.8	>.05
C	0.8	<.05[a]
D	1.8	<.05[a]
E	2.5	>.05
F	2.5	<.05[a]
G	2.5	<.05[a]

a. These values are statistically significant.

greater than the clinically significant difference of 2, but also the lower limit for the confidence interval is beyond this value. Of the other six studies, four, including two nonsignificant studies, may possibly be clinically significant as the upper limit of the confidence intervals includes the value set as being clinically important; however, given that the lower limit of the confidence interval is below the limit of clinical significance, clinical significance cannot definitely be inferred.

This examination of the confidence intervals of the effect size is particularly important in the case of studies that do not reach statistical significance, as mentioned above. Even if the p value is greater than .05, it may be that the null hypothesis is genuinely true, or it may be that the study lacked the power to reject the null hypothesis. Looking at Figure 1, Study B represents a case of the former—this result is neither statistically significant nor clinically significant—while Study E is an example of the latter. The point estimate for E is larger than a clinically important difference, but the confidence interval is so large that it includes the null difference.

Treatment Equivalence

Confidence intervals are equally important in studies that examine whether two treatments are equivalent in their effect. For equivalence studies, conclusions will always be based on an examination of the confidence intervals. Before an equivalence trial is carried out the limits of equivalence are agreed on, so that after the trial a decision can be made as to whether the treatments are, to all intents and purposes, the same in their effect. These prespecified limits should be narrow enough to exclude any difference of clinical importance. After the trial, equivalence is usually accepted if the confidence interval for any observed treatment difference falls entirely within the limits of equivalence and includes a value of zero difference. If one of the limits falls outside the limits of equivalence, it would imply that one of the plausible values for the treatment effect was at least as large as a clinically important difference.

A study by I. F. Burgess and colleagues published in 2005 examined whether 4% dimeticone lotion was equivalent to phenothrin, the most commonly used pediculicide, for the treatment of head louse

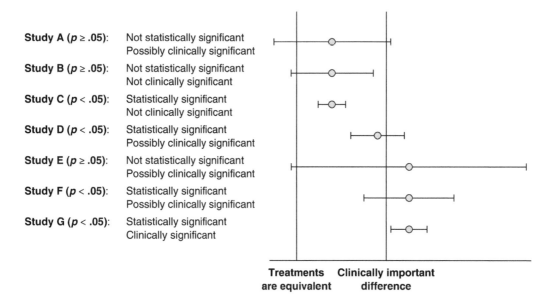

Figure 1   Statistical and clinical significance: Results of seven studies (point estimates together with confidence intervals)

infestation. The main outcome was cure of infestation or reinfestation after cure. Before the study began, it was decided that the two treatments would be declared equivalent if the results were within 20% between treatment groups, based on the 95% confidence intervals, that is, if the upper and lower limits for the 95% confidence interval for the difference between groups were both less than 20% either side of no difference. Of the 127 individuals randomized to receive dimeticone, 89 were either cured or reinfested after cure at follow-up (70%), while 94 of the 125 followed up in the phenothrin group were cured or reinfested after cure (75%). Thus, 5% fewer individuals in the

dimeticone group were cured or reinfested after cure, and the 95% confidence interval for this difference was −16% to 6%. As these 95% limits were within the 20% limits of equivalence set before the study was undertaken, as illustrated by Figure 2, the researchers were able to conclude that the two treatments were equivalent to within 20%.

While a *p* value is a useful starting point, it would be ill advised to make a decision based on this single piece of information, and it is vital to examine the estimate of any effect and its associated confidence interval before making a decision. This will give a range of plausible values for the effect size and will assist one in deciding whether

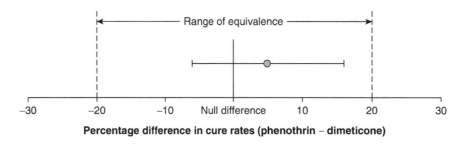

Figure 2   Estimated difference in cure and reinfestation after cure rates between dimeticone and phenothrin, together with the 95% confidence interval for the difference.

any difference found is of clinical importance or whether the study had sufficient power to reject the null hypothesis.

Jenny V. Freeman

See also Effect Size; Hypothesis Testing; Managing Variability and Uncertainty; Sample Size and Power

Further Readings

Altman, D., Machin, D., Bryant, T., & Gardner, S. (2000). *Statistics with confidence.* Oxford, UK: Wiley Blackwell.

Armitage, P., Berry, G., & Matthews, J. N. S. (2001). *Statistical methods in medical research* (4th ed.). New York: Blackwell Science.

Burgess, I. F., Brown, C. M., & Lee, P. N. (2005). Treatment of head louse infestation with 4% dimeticone lotion: Randomised controlled equivalence trial. *British Medical Journal, 330,* 1423–1426.

Campbell, M. J., Machin, D., & Walters, S. J. (2007). *Medical statistics: A textbook for the health sciences.* Chichester, UK: Wiley.

Dixon, J. B., O'Brien, P. E., Playfair, J., Chapman, L., Schachter, L. M., Skinner, S., et al. (2008). Adjustable gastric banding and conventional therapy for type 2 diabetes. *Journal of the American Medical Association, 299*(3), 316–323.

Kirkwood, B. R., & Sterne, J. A. C. (2003). *Essential medical statistics* (2nd ed.). Oxford, UK: Blackwell Science.

Petrie, A., & Sabin, C. (2005). *Medical statistics at a glance* (2nd ed.). Oxford, UK: Blackwell Science.

CONFIRMATION BIAS

Confirmation bias is the tendency for people to search for or interpret information in a manner that favors their current beliefs. This entry communicates psychological research on confirmation bias as it relates to medical decision making. This will help medical professionals, patients, and policy makers consider when it might pose a concern and how to avoid it. The focus is on choosing a test for a simple case of medical diagnosis. The first section discusses how inference and information search ought to take place; the second section discusses confirmation bias and other possible errors;

the final section discusses how to improve inference and information search.

How Should Inference and Information Acquisition Proceed?

No choice of diagnostic tests can cause confirmation bias if the test results are assimilated in a statistically optimal manner. Therefore, this section first discusses how to incorporate test results in a statistically optimal (Bayesian) way. It then discusses various strategies to select informative tests.

Suppose that the base rate of a disease (d) in males is 10% and that a test for this disease is given to males in routine exams. The test has 90% sensitivity (true positive rate): 90% of males who have the disease test positive. Expressed in probabilistic notation, $P(\text{pos}|d) = 90\%$. The test has 80% specificity: $P(\text{neg}|{\sim}d) = 80\%$ (20% false-positive rate), meaning that 80% of males who do not have the disease correctly test negative. Suppose a male has a positive test in routine screening. What is the probability that he has the disease? By Bayes's theorem (see Figure 1, Panel A),

$$P(d|\text{pos}) = P(\text{pos}|d)P(d)/P(\text{pos}),$$

where

$$P(\text{pos}) = P(\text{pos}|d)P(d) + P(\text{pos}|{\sim}d)P({\sim}d).$$

Therefore,

$$
\begin{aligned}
P(d|\text{pos}) \\
= (.90 \times .10)/(.90 \times .10 + .20 \times .90) \\
= .09/.27 = 1/3.
\end{aligned}
$$

Alternately (see Figure 1, Panels B and C), it is possible to count the number of men with the disease and a positive test, and who test positive without having the disease:

$$
\begin{aligned}
P(d|\text{pos}) = \text{num}(d \,\&\, \text{pos})/\text{num}(\text{pos}) \\
= 9/(9 + 18) = 1/3,
\end{aligned}
$$

where

$$\text{num}(\text{pos}) = \text{num}(\text{pos} \,\&\, d) + \text{num}(\text{pos} \,\&\, {\sim}d).$$

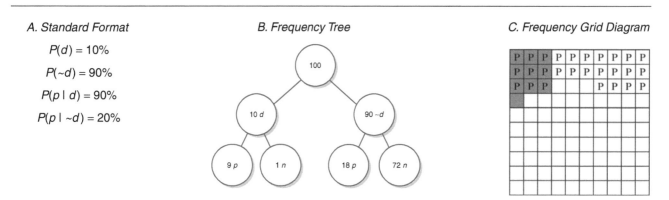

Figure 1   Different formats for presenting probabilistic information

Notes: The means by which probabilistic information is presented have a large impact on how meaningful the information is to people. The standard probability format (Panel A) is complicated for people to work with, although they can be trained to do so. Both the frequency tree (Panel B) and frequency grid diagram (Panel C) provide more meaningful representations of the information. The term "*d*" denotes the disease; "*~d*" absence of the disease; "*p*" denotes a positive test. In Panel C, shaded cells denote presence of the disease.

But how should a diagnostic test be chosen in the first place? The fundamental difficulty is that which test is most useful depends on the particular outcome obtained, and the outcome cannot be known in advance. For instance, the presence of a particular gene might definitively predict a disease, but that gene might occur with only one in a million probability. Another test might never definitively predict the disease but might always offer a high degree of certainty about whether the disease is present or not.

Optimal experimental design ideas provide a reasonable framework for calculating which test, on balance, will be most useful. All these ideas are within the realm of Savage's Bayesian decision theory, which defines the subjective expected usefulness (utility) of a test, before that test is conducted, as the average usefulness of all possible test results, weighting each result according to its probability.

In the case of a test T that can either be positive (pos) or negative (neg), the test's expected utility (eu) would be calculated as follows:

$$eu(T) = P(\text{pos}) \times u(\text{pos}) + P(\text{neg}) \times u(\text{neg}),$$

where u corresponds to utility. Various optimal experimental design ideas quantify, in different ways, the usefulness of particular test outcomes. Suppose one wishes to use improvement in probability of correct diagnosis to quantify the usefulness

of possible diagnostic tests. (This equates to minimizing error.) The probability gain (pg) of a test, with respect to determining whether or not a patient has disease d, is calculated as follows:

$$eu_{pg}(T) = P(\text{pos}) \times [\max(P(d|\text{pos}), P(\sim d|\text{pos}))$$
$$- \max(P(d), P(\sim d))] + P(\text{neg}) \times [\max(P(d|\text{neg}),$$
$$P(\sim d|\text{neg})) - \max(P(d), P(\sim d))].$$

Suppose the goal is to learn whether or not a patient has a disease that occurs in 10% of patients. Test 1 has 95% sensitivity and 85% specificity. Test 2 has 85% sensitivity and 95% specificity. Which test maximizes probability gain? Test 1 has probability gain 0, though Test 2 has probability gain .04. Although Test 1 has high sensitivity, its low specificity is problematic as the base rate of the disease is only 10%. Test 1 does not change the diagnosis of any patient, because, irrespective of whether it is positive or negative, the patient most likely does not have the disease. Test 2's much higher specificity, however, reduces false positives enough so that a majority of people who test positive actually have the disease.

It can be helpful, as an exercise, to consider possible tests' probability gain before ordering a test, in situations where the relevant environmental probabilities are known. In real medical diagnosis, additional factors, such as a test's cost and its potential to harm the patient, should also be taken into account.

Confirmation Bias and Other Errors

Do people typically reason following Bayes's theorem? Do physicians intuitively select useful tests for medical diagnosis? If human cognition and behavior are suboptimal, do they reflect confirmation bias?

From early research on Bayesian reasoning through the present, there has been evidence that people are either too conservative or too aggressive in updating their beliefs. Some research suggests that people make too much use of base rates (the proportion of people with a disease), as opposed to likelihood information (a test result). Other research suggests that people make too little use of base rates, relying on likelihood information too much.

Do these errors lead to systematically overweighting one's working hypothesis (e.g., the most probable disease)? Note that test results can either increase or decrease the probability of a particular disease. Because of this, neither being too conservative nor being too aggressive in updating beliefs in response to test results would consistently give a bias to confirm one's working hypothesis. Thus, while there is plenty of evidence that people (including physicians) sometimes update too much and sometimes too little, that does not necessarily imply confirmation bias.

If people have personal experience with environmental probabilities, their inferences are often quite accurate. In routine diagnostic and treatment scenarios, in which individual practitioners have previously experienced dozens, hundreds, or even thousands of similar cases and have obtained feedback on the patients' outcomes, physicians' intuitions may be well-calibrated to underlying probabilities. Little if any confirmation bias would be expected in these situations. In situations in which relevant data are available but practitioners do not have much personal experience, for instance because rare diseases are involved, intuitions may not as closely approximate Bayes's theorem.

Confirmation Bias in Inference

Apart from the general difficulty in probabilistic reasoning, how might people fall victim to confirmation bias per se? Below, several situations are described that might lead to confirmation bias.

1. If people obtain useless information but think it supports their working hypothesis, that could lead to confirmation bias. Suppose a physician asks a patient about the presence of a symptom that, if present, would support a particular disease diagnosis. Suppose the patient tends to answer "yes" in cases where the question is unclear, so as to cooperate. If the physician does not take the patient's bias to answer "yes" into account when interpreting the answer to the question, the physician could be led, on average, to be excessively confident in his or her diagnosis.

2. Sometimes a test's sensitivity (its true positive rate) is conflated with its positive predictive value (the probability of the disease given a positive result). In situations where the sensitivity is high, but specificity is low or the base rate of the disease is very low, this error can cause confirmation bias. For instance, among people from low-risk populations, a substantial proportion of people with positive HIV test results do not have HIV. Some counselors, however, have wrongly assumed that a positive test means a person has HIV.

3. There are many situations in which people want to reach certain conclusions or maintain certain beliefs, and they are quite good at doing so. Imagine that a physician has diagnosed a patient with a serious illness and started the patient on a series of treatments with serious side effects. The physician might be more likely than, say, an impartial second physician, to discount new evidence indicating that the original diagnosis was wrong and that the patient had needlessly been subjected to harmful treatments.

4. Finally, people sometimes interpret ambiguous evidence in ways that give the benefit of the doubt to their favored hypothesis. This is not necessarily a flaw in inference. If one's current beliefs are based on a great deal of information, then a bit of new information (especially if from an unreliable source) should not change beliefs drastically. Whether a physician interprets a patient's failure to return a smile from across the room as indicating the patient didn't see him or her or as a snub will likely be influenced by whether the patient has previously been friendly or socially distant. Similarly, suppose an unknown researcher e-mails his or her discovery that AIDS is caused by nefarious extraterrestrials. Given the outlandish nature of the claim, and the unknown status of the "researcher," it would be wise to demand a lot of

corroborating evidence before updating beliefs about causation of AIDS at all, given this report. The overriding issue is that one's degree of belief, and amount of change of belief, should correspond to the objective value of the evidence.

Information Acquisition and Confirmation Bias

Do people use statistically justifiable strategies for evidence acquisition, for instance when requesting a test or asking a patient a question? Are people prone to confirmation bias or other errors?

Psychological experiments suggest that people are very sensitive to tests' usefulness when deciding which test to order. Any testing strategy not solely concerned with usefulness will be inefficient. However, if test results are evaluated in a Bayesian way, then although some information acquisition strategies are more efficient than others, none will lead to confirmation bias. Thus, improving probabilistic inference is a first step toward guarding against confirmation bias.

Positivity and extremity are additional factors that may contribute to people's choices of tests. Positivity is the tendency to request tests that are expected to result in a positive result, or a "yes" answer to a question, given that the working hypothesis is true. Extremity is a preference for tests whose outcomes are very likely or very unlikely under the working hypothesis relative to the alternate hypothesis. The evidence substantiating people's use of these particular strategies is somewhat murky. However, use of these testing strategies, together with particular biased inference strategies, could lead to confirmation bias.

Improving Inference and Information Acquisition

Improving Inference

The means by which probabilistic information is presented are important, and evidence suggests that either personal experience or appropriate training can help people meaningfully learn particular probabilities. The literature suggests several strategies to improve Bayesian inference:

1. Present information in a meaningful way. Figure 1, Panels B and C, illustrates two means of presenting equivalent information, in which the

information is presented in terms of the *natural frequencies* of people with (and without) the disease who have a positive or negative test. These formats better facilitate Bayesian reasoning than does the standard probability format (Figure 1, Panel A). Simulating personal experience and providing feedback may be even more effective.

2. Teach Bayesian inference. Although people do not intuitively do very well with standard probability format problems, people can be trained to do better, especially when the training helps people use natural frequency formats for representing the probabilistic information.

3. Obtain feedback. Feedback is critical for learning environmental probabilities, such as base rates of diseases, and distribution of test outcomes for people with and without various diseases. Feedback is also critical for learning when those probabilities change, for instance because of an outbreak of a rare disease. Both individual practitioners and policy makers could think about how to ensure that feedback can be obtained, and patients and citizens should demand that they do so.

Improving Information Acquisition

People are not adept at maximizing either probability gain or individually specified utilities when information is presented in the standard probability format. Taking care to ensure that known statistical information is meaningful may be the single most important way to improve practitioners' capacity for good inference and information acquisition in medical decision making. Use of personal experience and feedback to convey probabilistic information in simulated environments can also facilitate Bayesian performance.

Beyond Confirmation Bias

While confirmation bias in inference and information acquisition may exist, it should be seen in the broader context of statistical illiteracy and misaligned incentives. Those problems may be the root of what can appear to be confirmation bias, rather than any inherent cognitive limitations that people have. For instance, the desire to make a patient feel that he or she is being treated well, and to guard against the possibility of litigation, might lead to ordering a medically unnecessary (and potentially harmful) CT scan following mild head trauma. At the level of basic research, the source of funding can influence the conclusions that are reached. From a policy standpoint, the goal should be to make individual and institutional incentives match public health objectives as closely as possible.

Jonathan D. Nelson and Craig R. M. McKenzie

See also Bayes's Theorem; Biases in Human Prediction; Cognitive Psychology and Processes; Conditional Probability; Deliberation and Choice Processes; Errors in Clinical Reasoning; Evidence Synthesis; Expected Utility Theory; Expected Value of Sample Information, Net Benefit of Sampling; Hypothesis Testing; Probability; Probability Errors; Subjective Expected Utility Theory

Further Readings

Baron, J. (1985). *Rationality and intelligence*. Cambridge, UK: Cambridge University Press.

Baron, J., Beattie, J., & Hershey, J. C. (1988). Heuristics and biases in diagnostic reasoning: II. Congruence, information, and certainty. *Organizational Behavior and Human Decision Processes, 42*, 88–110.

Baron, J., & Hershey, J. C. (1988). Heuristics and biases in diagnostic reasoning: I. Priors, error costs, and test accuracy. *Organizational Behavior and Human Decision Processes, 41*, 259–279.

Gigerenzer, G., Gaissmaier, W., Kurz-Milcke, E., Schwartz, L. M., & Woloshin, S. (2008). Helping doctors and patients make sense of health statistics. *Psychological Science in the Public Interest, 8*(2), 53–96.

Gigerenzer, G., & Hoffrage, U. (1995). How to improve Bayesian reasoning without instruction: Frequency formats. *Psychological Review, 102*(4), 684–704.

Kahneman, D., & Tversky, A. (1972). Subjective probability: A judgment of representativeness. *Cognitive Psychology, 3*(3), 430–454.

Klayman, J. (1995). Varieties of confirmation bias. *Psychology of Learning and Motivation, 32*, 385–418.

Klayman, J., & Ha, Y.-W. (1987). Confirmation, disconfirmation, and information. *Psychological Review, 94*, 211–228.

McKenzie, C. R. M. (2004). Hypothesis testing and evaluation. In D. J. Koehler & N. Harvey (Eds.), *Blackwell handbook of judgment and decision making* (pp. 200–219). Oxford, UK: Blackwell.

McKenzie, C. R. M. (2006). Increased sensitivity to differentially diagnostic answers using familiar materials: Implications for confirmation bias. *Memory and Cognition, 34*, 577–588.

Nelson, J. D. (2005). Finding useful questions: On Bayesian diagnosticity, probability, impact and information gain. *Psychological Review, 112*(4), 979–999.

Nelson, J. D. (2008). Towards a rational theory of human information acquisition. In M. Oaksford & N. Chater (Eds.), *The probabilistic mind: Prospects for rational models of cognition* (pp. 143–163). Oxford, UK: Oxford University Press.

Nickerson, R. S. (1998). Confirmation bias: A ubiquitous phenomenon in many guises. *Review of General Psychology, 2*(2), 175–220.

Oaksford, M., & Chater, N. (2003). Optimal data selection: Revision, review, and reevaluation. *Psychonomic Bulletin & Review, 10*, 289–318.

Savage, L. J. (1954). *The foundations of statistics*. New York: Wiley.

Sedlmeier, P., & Gigerenzer, G. (2001). Teaching Bayesian reasoning in less than two hours. *Journal of Experimental Psychology: General, 130*, 380–400.

Conflicts of Interest and Evidence-Based Clinical Medicine

Physicians' financial interests may have an unconscious influence on their interpretation of the scientific evidence relevant to the treatments they choose for their patients. This indirect determinant of physician behavior has not been extensively studied, but the causal process can be sketched using general principles of cognitive and social psychology and of marketing. The influence of financial interests on clinician knowledge is a distinct topic from their influence on clinician action. The latter topic has been the main concern in discussion of conflicts of interest induced by gifts from pharmaceutical or medical device manufacturers, by managed care or insurance rules, or by payments from interested industries to the directors of nonprofit hospitals or accompanying the intrusion of the commercial management of hospitals and clinics into the doctor-patient relationship.

Ideally, the physician applies medicine's best treatments appropriately for each patient, rationally considering the scientific evidence concerning the treatment's efficacy as well as the patient's unique circumstances. Evidence that would support a treatment generally includes scientific studies proving it works as well as or better than the alternatives, and evidence that the burden of side effects or costs, per unit of health improvement produced, is not excessive. Relevant considerations for the particular patient may include individual characteristics that change the probable success of a treatment, such as being more robust or more fragile than the typical patient. It is also rationally and ethically appropriate to consider the patient's financial or social resources, such as ability to pay for a treatment without bankrupting the family or the capability of adhering to required behavioral changes or medical care demands over the long term. Potential biases in physician judgments of patient resources are not considered further here.

Financial interests may exert an unconscious influence on physicians' interpretation of evidence relevant to the treatment of their patients. An individual clinician's reading of the literature regarding the benefits and costs of patients' treatments can be distorted by the fact that he or she is able to provide some treatments but not others. The same sort of process can sway the production and interpretation of professional association guidelines in a way that promotes the profession, as against the interests of the competing specialties, the patient, or society in general.

Sometimes, financial interests may induce in the physician a kind of psychological blindness that impedes the ability of otherwise ethical people to recognize that the scientific evidence does not support their way of practice. Physicians may not be aware that their judgment is distorted this way even though an objective observer might call their decisions "irrational" with respect to the evidence. In contrast, a physician who consciously chose to use treatments that she or he knew to be ineffective or harmful for the patient because she or he could collect higher fees would be described as "unethical."

Example of Irrational Treatment Decisions Due to Financial Motivation

An orthopedic surgeon opted to simplify his work life by concentrating on only a few types of back surgery, to be able to spend more time with his family. He put out the word seeking referrals and organized the clinic to allow himself to spend as little time in the office and as much in the operating room as possible. During 10 years of this arrangement, evidence accumulated in the literature that back surgery is indicated for a smaller proportion of those who complain of low back pain than had previously been thought and that an elaborate sequence of diagnostic measures and trial treatments can identify patients who likely won't be cured by surgery but may be helped by alternative measures. The physician nonetheless has continued doing the same familiar operations on most patients who come through his door, after only a brief discussion of the surgical options in an initial consultation in the office. There is a compelling financial motivation for the physician to maintain his surgical volume. His family depends on the current level of income, as do the clinic employees, his partners who co-own the clinic with him, and the bank. At this point in his career, doing these procedures is the only skill the physician has that can bring in this much income. However, he has never suggested, even in jest, that he is "just in it for the money," and his friends and coworkers know him to be honestly concerned about his patients. When asked about the studies suggesting more discerning assessment of the patient is required, the physician says they are not applicable to his practice because he is following professional guidelines.

Unconscious Irrationality Due to Conflict of Interest

The physician in the vignette, whose practice is concentrated on a few lucrative surgical procedures, ignored or dismissed the evidence suggesting the procedures are not indicated for many patients. Physicians often experience conflict between the demand for billable activity and their commitment to do what is best for the patient. When they weigh the evidence in resolving this conflict between the competing values, they may give unconscious priority to their own financial interests. It is better for both patient and physician if physicians can be conscious of motivations that may blind them to the scientific evidence.

To promote accurate physician self-awareness, it has been recommended that physicians should disclose their financial interests to patients, as well as the constraints imposed by their employers or the patients' insurance. Thus, the back surgeon could acknowledge that his fee covers his expenses and supports him comfortably, and in exchange he does his best for his patients and makes ongoing efforts to keep up with the state of the art. Talking about what the fees buy—the physician's expert interpretation of the emerging evidence—is as pertinent as discussing the expected efficacy of the treatment and its alternatives, the probabilities of various morbidities, and how other people have adjusted to the outcomes, especially if there is the possibility that patient distrust may undermine adherence. The physician's frank discussion of his interests and his efforts helps the patient engage in informed decision making. Such conversations can also help the physician maintain rationality and integrity: when the motives are acknowledged, the physician is less likely to be unconsciously influenced to recommend a treatment of inferior efficacy just because it is convenient or profitable, or is what others in his subspecialty do. Anticipation of such conversations can motivate the physician to keep up with the evidence so he or she can say in good faith that he or she is offering the patient the best treatments known.

The Role of Professional Organizations in the Interpretation of Scientific Evidence

Physicians associate with similar physicians in professional organizations that provide mutual support, including information on the newest treatment modalities and guidelines on the manner of practice judged to help the members thrive through the appropriate use of their special knowledge and skills to care for patients. Delegating the burden of evaluating treatments in this way can muffle the physician's awareness of the balance of evidence regarding the recommended treatment modalities. As a result of such informational filters, a patient with localized prostate cancer, for example, might be given radiation if he visits almost any radiation oncologist, surgery if he visits any urologist, or expectant management if he visits any general internist. It is not simply that these options are in equipoise for all such patients; these contradictions highlight the impact of professional organizations' shaping of members' views.

Unconscious psychological processes may contribute to this influence at two stages, in the production and the utilization of the guidelines, as illustrated in Figure 1. First, members of professional organizations who have been honored with appointment

to a task force that will produce a guideline statement may experience expectations related to solidarity with the group. The committee may manifest polarization, in which the group's decision may express a more extreme position on a shared value than most of the individuals would hold on their own. Figure 1 shows the relation between the guidelines (B) and the possible treatments consistent with the scientific evidence (A). The effect of polarization is that the guideline highlights only a subset of the supportable interpretations of the scientific literature, and it may extend a little beyond what the general field may find supported. Committees are less likely to produce self-serving guidelines (though it is still possible) when they adopt the discipline of formally meta-analyzing only randomized controlled trials. The competing guidelines authored by Gharib and Surks regarding screening for subclinical hypothyroidism illustrate this point. The second process has to do with the reader's comprehension and recall of the published guidelines. Most guidelines consist of a general recommendation and a list of exceptions or qualifications. When individual practitioners read the guidelines (C in the figure), and again when they recall them at the point of use (D), often the gist is recalled while the detailed exceptions are forgotten. Lines carefully drawn when a guideline statement was composed may be missed or forgotten by the reader.

Beneficial Effects of Financial Motivation

Financial motives do not always interfere with rational patient treatment. Administrative power, including monetary bonuses or penalties contingent on individual or clinicwide performance, is one of the most powerful tools available for changing physicians' behavior. Aligning the rewards with the evidence-based practices can be an effective component of a program to improve medical care. But financial reward schemes can have unintended consequences, distorting physician behavior without benefit to the patient. For example, in the United States, to sustain themselves, the private (e.g., insurance) and public (e.g., Medicaid) systems that pay for medical care impose limits on allowable charges per visit. This has the unintended side effect that low-priority concerns such as prevention may be neglected. To compensate for

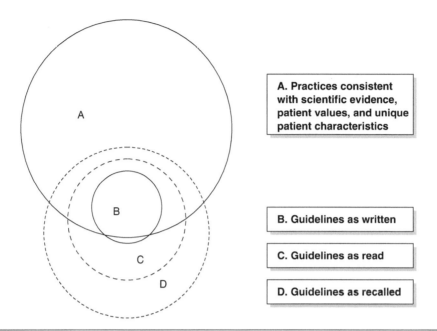

A. Practices consistent with scientific evidence, patient values, and unique patient characteristics

B. Guidelines as written

C. Guidelines as read

D. Guidelines as recalled

Figure 1   Psychological influences on guideline production and utilization

Note: Illustration of psychological influences on the guideline production and utilization process that may bias physician practices. A: the set of possible treatments supported by evidence. B: impact of group polarization on the guideline writers. C and D: impact of gist highlighting processes in comprehension and recall of guidelines.

this, local administrators may advise physicians to deal with just one patient concern during each visit, and schedule additional visits to address other issues. While this stratagem may help a clinic be financially viable, it imposes an additional burden on those patients responsible for co-payment or lacking transportation.

Contributing Factors

Individual clinicians' interpretation of the literature's evidence regarding the benefits and costs of their patients' potential treatments can be unconsciously distorted by how much they can be paid for providing the treatments. The rewards physicians receive for some practices may make it difficult for them to see that they need to give up those practices when a different method of treatment is proven better. Group polarization effects in the production of guidelines, and simplification processes in the comprehension and recall of recommendations, also contribute to the persistence of nonoptimal treatment practices that are financially rewarded.

Robert M. Hamm

See also Bias in Scientific Studies; Clinical Algorithms and Practice Guidelines; Evidence-Based Medicine; Irrational Persistence in Belief; Motivation

Further Readings

Bigos, S., Bowyer, O., Braen, G., Brown, K., Deyo, R., Haldemann, S., et al. (1994). *Acute low back problems in adults: Clinical practice guideline No. 14* (AHCPR Publication No. 95-0642). Rockville, MD: Agency for Health Care Policy and Research, Public Health Service, U.S. Department of Health and Human Services.

Brody, H. (2005). The company we keep: Why physicians should refuse to see pharmaceutical representatives. *Annals of Family Medicine, 3*(1), 82–85.

Bursztajn, H. J., & Brodsky, A. (1999). Captive patients, captive doctors: Clinical dilemmas and interventions in caring for patients in managed health care. *General Hospital Psychiatry, 21*(4), 239–248.

Cain, D. M., & Detsky, A. S. (2008). Everyone's a little bit biased (even physicians). *Journal of the American Medical Association, 299*(24), 2893–2895.

Gharib, H., Tuttle, R. M., Baskin, H. J., Fish, L. H., Singer, P. A., & McDermott, M. T. (2005). Subclinical thyroid dysfunction: A joint statement on management from the American Association of Clinical Endocrinologists, the American Thyroid Association, and the Endocrine Society. *Journal of Clinical Endocrinology & Metabolism, 90*(1), 581–585.

Isenberg, D. J. (1986). Group polarization: A critical review and meta-analysis. *Journal of Personality and Social Psychology, 50,* 1141–1151.

Jones, J. W., & McCullough, L. B. (2007). Are ethics practical when externals impact your clinical judgment? *Journal of Vascular Surgery, 45*(6), 1282–1284.

Rivero-Arias, O., Campbell, H., Gray, A., Fairbank, J., Frost, H., & Wilson-MacDonald, J. (2005). Surgical stabilisation of the spine compared with a programme of intensive rehabilitation for the management of patients with chronic low back pain: Cost utility analysis based on a randomised controlled trial. *British Medical Journal, 330*(7502), 1239.

Smith, W. R. (2000). Evidence for the effectiveness of techniques to change physician behavior. *Chest, 118,* 8S–17S.

Sulmasy, D. P., Bloche, M. G., Mitchell, J. M., & Hadley, J. (2000). Physicians' ethical beliefs about cost-control arrangements. *Archives of Internal Medicine, 160*(5), 649–657.

Surks, M. I., Ortiz, E., Daniels, G. H., Sawin, C. T., Col, N. F., Cobin, R. H., et al. (2004). Subclinical thyroid disease: Scientific review and guidelines for diagnosis and management. *Journal of the American Medical Association, 291*(2), 228–238.

Confounding and Effect Modulation

The relationship between a predictor or study variable and an outcome variable may vary according to the value of a third variable, often called a confounding variable or an effect modulator. This entry clarifies the distinction between confounding and effect modulation (also called moderation or mediation) through the use of path diagrams. The statistical tests for establishing these three relationships are somewhat different (main effects model only for establishing confounding variables; main effects model with interaction term for establishing moderating variables and Sobel-like tests based on a series of regression for establishing mediating variables), so they are discussed separately and their interpretation clarified by example.

Overview

An important feature of a regression model is its ability to include multiple covariates and thereby statistically adjust for possible imbalances in the observed data before making statistical inferences. This process of adjustment has been given various names in different fields of study. In traditional statistical publications, it is sometimes called the *analysis of covariance,* while in clinical and epidemiologic studies it may be called *control for confounding.* Interactions between covariates may also be included in the model and regarded as *effect modifiers* in the sense that the effect on the outcome differs according to the level of the moderator variable. When an outcome is correlated with a study variable but the relationship disappears when adjusted by a third variable, the third variable is often called a mediating variable or mediator. In an epidemiological study of the strength of the association between smoking status and lung cancer, the relationship may be affected by other variables such as the drinking habits, extent of exposure to tobacco smoke, or age of the subject, or other personal or environmental conditions. Variables other than smoking that affect the relationship of smoking and lung cancer are often described as *modulating variables.* Modulating variables are further classified as *confounding variables, effect moderators, effect modifiers,* or *mediating variables* according to their finer properties. Some terms and interpretations used to distinguish different types of modulation are based on statistical definitions and may thus be measured and tested objectively. In other instances, judgments regarding causality will be required, thus introducing concepts not readily amenable to statistical analysis.

Definitions of terms such as *mediation, moderation,* and *confounding* have been questioned because of their implied dependence on the unquantifiable concept of causality. This entry illustrates these through simple statistical modeling and figures, and provides examples of the roles of confounding, mediating, and moderating variables. The first example illustrates the role of "helplessness" as a moderating variable where patients with a "low" helplessness index could have decreasing depression even with an increasing "swollen joint count," whereas patients with a "high" helplessness index have the opposite relationship (increasing depression with an increasing swollen joint count). The second example illustrates the "mediating" role of pain and comorbidities on the association observed between body mass index (BMI) and total unhealthy days (TUD). The association vanishes when the mediating variables are adjusted in the model. The analyses for each of the examples are adjusted for various confounding variables.

Terms and Definitions

The purpose of many epidemiological studies is to determine the effect of a *predictor variable* or *risk factor X* on an *outcome variable Y* while accounting for the effects of another influential variable, denoted by *Z*. To facilitate the discussion, a simple statistical model can be written as

$$Y = a + bX + cZ + dXZ + \varepsilon,$$

where the unknown coefficients *a*, *b*, *c*, and *d* are to be determined by statistical model fitting and ε denotes a random error. The variable *X*, whose effect on *Y* is to be studied, may be called the study, experimental, or condition variable in an experimental study or a risk factor in an observational study. Variable *Z* provides information in addition to the study variable, which may affect the relationship of outcome *Y* to predictor *X*. The variable *Z* is generally described as modulating or modifying the effect of *X* on *Y* but may further be classified as a confounding, moderating, or mediating variable. The relationship of *Y*, *X*, and *Z* is often depicted schematically as in Figures 1, 2, and 3, respectively, for illustrating the three types of relationship.

When either the estimated coefficient of a variable in the model or the relevant (Pearson's) correlation is statistically different from zero (usually at the 5% level), the role of the variable is described as "significant." The variable *Z* may have any of the several different roles that may affect the relationship of *Y* to *X*. These roles are often described in the epidemiological and psychological literature using the following terms and definitions.

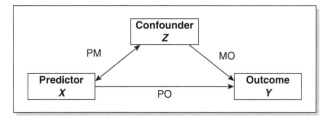

Figure 1   Conceptual model of confounding variable

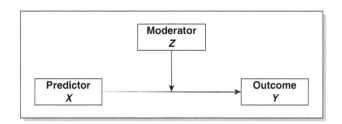

Figure 2   Conceptual model of a moderating variable

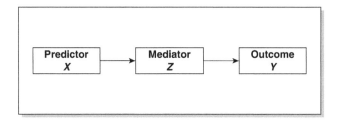

Figure 3   Conceptual model of a moderating variable

Confounding Variable

Variable *Z* is called a *confounding variable* or *confounder* of the effect of *X* on *Y* if *Z* is associated with *Y*, varies over the levels of *X* (with relationship both ways), and is not considered to be a cause of *Y*. This definition requires evaluation of the change in the relationship of *Y* and *X* due to *Z* and a subjective judgment that *Z* does not lie on the causal pathway between *X* and *Y*. A confounding variable may also be called a *lurking variable*. Since the relationship between *X* and *Y* changes with the value of *Z*, uncorrected confounding can result in the effect of *X* on *Y* being inappropriately increased or diminished or even reversed in direction. Confounding may be controlled by matching, stratifying on values of *Z*, or including *Z* in the statistical model.

Moderating Variable or Effect Modifier

Variable Z is called a *moderating variable* or *effect modifier* when its magnitude affects the magnitude or direction of the effect of X on Y and the interaction term XZ is statistically significant.

Mediating Variable

Variable Z is called a *mediating variable* or *mediator* of the effect of X on Y if X significantly affects Z, Z has a significant effect on Y, X affects Y in the absence of Z, and the effect of X on Y is diminished to nonsignificance when Z is added to the model. Some authors also require that Z be considered to be a cause of Y. A mediator is the same as a confounder except for the subjective judgment that the mediator is considered a "cause" of the outcome whereas a confounder is not. A mediator is a variable that is in a causal sequence between two variables, whereas a moderator is not part of a causal sequence between the two variables. The extent to which a variable may be considered a mediator may be assessed statistically by the Sobel-Goodman test. This test requires coefficients estimated from a separate regression fit of the path PM, MO, and PO.

Examples

Example of Mediating Effect

Obesity is an increasingly prevalent public health concern due to the increased risk of mortality associated with excess body fat and the increased risk of developing a variety of diseases such as type 2 diabetes, coronary heart disease, sleep apnea, knee osteoarthritis, and certain cancers. Obesity also has a substantial negative impact on a person's functional capacity and health-related quality of life (QoL). Heo and colleagues attempted to understand to what extent the association between obesity and QoL is mediated by those health problems that often arise in conjunction with obesity such as diabetes, hypertension, and (musculoskeletal) joint pain. In their article "Obesity and Quality of Life: Mediating Effects of Pain and Comorbidities," they hypothesized potential mediating effects of pain and comorbidities on the association between obesity and QoL and tested their hypotheses using data on 154,074 participants from the cross-sectional

survey data from the 1999 Behavioral Risk Factor Surveillance Survey (BRFSS).

The predictor variable of obesity was measured by the BMI. This was calculated from the self-reported weight and height and was classified in six categories (< 18.5 kg/m^2, underweight; 18.5 to 24.9 kg/m^2, desirable weight; 25 to 29.9 kg/m^2, overweight; 30 to 34.9 kg/m^2, Obesity Class I; 35 to 39.9 kg/m^2, Obesity Class II; and ≥ 40 kg/m^2, Obesity Class III). Although they considered four outcome variables, for keeping the illustration simple here, we consider only one outcome variable of TUD dichotomized at 14 days. Potential mediator variables of joint pain (PAIN) were derived from the question "During the past 12 months, have you had pain, aching, stiffness, or swelling in or around a joint?" ($0 = No$, $1 = Yes$) and obesity-related comorbidities (ORCs) were derived from the sum of responses to the nine dichotomous variables arising from questions such as "Have you ever been told by a doctor, nurse, or other health professional that you have high blood pressure?" ($0 = No$, $1 = Yes$). Covariates consisted of the following characteristics: age, sex, marital status (married vs. other), educational attainment ($<$ high school vs. $\geq$ high school), annual income ($< \$25,000$ vs. $\geq \$25,000$), smoking status (current, former, never), and employment status (employed vs. other).

Figure 4 shows the conceptualization of the statistical analysis. To estimate and test the significance of the association between BMI and TUD, the authors ran multiple logistic regressions on the BMI-defined categories on TUD (Path A of Scheme a in Figure 4). To examine mediator effects of PAIN and ORCs on the BMI-TUD association if this association is significant, they followed the guidelines suggested by Baron and Kenny. Specifically, they assessed whether or not (1) BMI effects on PAIN and ORCs (Path B of Scheme b in Figure 4) are significant; (2) the effects of PAIN and ORCs on TUD (Path C of Scheme b in Figure 4) are significant; and (3) the effects of BMI classes on TUD are reduced when Paths B and C (Figure 4) are controlled for, that is, when PAIN and ORCs are added into the model of Path A (Figure 4). If all these conditions are met, the data are consistent with the hypothesis that PAIN and ORCs mediate the relation between BMI and TUD, supporting Scheme b in Figure 4.

Scheme a

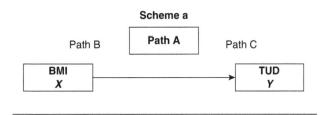

Scheme b

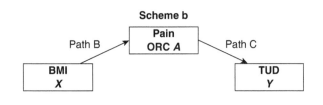

Figure 4   Schema of path diagrams of association between body mass index (BMI) and health-related quality-of-life (HRQOL) outcomes

Source: Heo, Allison, Faith, Zhu, and Fontaine (2003).

Collectively, from all the mediation analyses, the mediator effects of PAIN and ORCs on the relationship between high BMI and TUD are found significant. Moreover, controlling for the putative mediators resulted in nonsignificant effects of all BMI classes on TUD.

Example of Moderating Effect

Naidoo and Pretorius hypothesized that the stress-reducing function of helplessness (Z) has a moderating effect on the relationship between the rheumatoid arthritis (RA) health outcome of depression (Y) and the clinical measurement of the number of swollen joints (X) out of 28 joints in total. A cross-sectional study with 186 patients was undertaken for testing this moderating effect. The moderating variable of "helplessness" (Z) was measured by the Arthritis Helplessness Index (AHI). The AHI is a 15-item self-report inventory based on a 4-point Likert-type format that assesses the extent to which patients believe that they are able to control and cope with arthritis symptoms.

To test the hypotheses that Z moderates the relationship between X and Y, a regression model was fit with "depression" as outcome; swollen joint count (SJC) and helplessness as main effects; and an interaction term of SJC × Helplessness to test for moderation. Potentially confounding variables of age, sex, education, and income were also adjusted. Since the interaction term was found significant, the role of helplessness was established as a moderating variable. The patients with a "low" helplessness index were found to have decreasing depression even with an increasing number of swollen joint counts, whereas patients with a high helplessness index showed an opposite relationship (increasing depression with increasing number of swollen joint counts).

Causality

One of the fundamental goals of statistical design and analysis is to bring evidence based on data toward supporting causality. Understanding confounding and effect modulation are essential parts of getting as close as one can to causality, and separating the ideas of "confounding," "moderation," and "mediation" helps with use of the appropriate level of modeling.

Madhu Mazumdar and Ronald B. Harrist

Authors' note: Madhu Mazumdar was partially supported by the following grants: Center for Education and Research in Therapeutics (CERTs) (AHRQ RFA-HS-05-14), Clinical Translational Science Center (CTSC) (UL1-RR024996), and Collaborative Program in Nutrition and Cancer Prevention (NIGMS R25CA105012).

See also Causal Inference and Diagrams; Causal Inference in Medical Decision Making

Further Readings

Baron, R. M., & Kenny, D. A. (1986). The moderator-mediator variable distinction in social psychological research: Conceptual, strategic, and statistical considerations. *Journal of Personality and Social Psychology, 51,* 1173–1182.

Bennett, J. A. (2000). Mediator and moderator variables in nursing research: Conceptual and statistical differences. *Research in Nursing and Health, 23*(5), 415–420.

Heo, M., Allison, D. B., Faith, M. S., Zhu, S., & Fontaine, K. R. (2003). Obesity and quality of life:

Mediating effects of pain and comorbidities. *Obesity Research, 11*(2), 209–216.

Hill, A. B. (1965). The environment and disease: Association or causation? *Proceedings of the Royal Society of Medicine, 58,* 295–300.

Judd, C. M., & Kenny, D. A. (1981). Process analysis: Estimating mediation in treatment evaluations. *Evaluation Review, 5,* 602–619.

Lipton, R., & Ødegaard, T. (2005). Causal thinking and causal language in epidemiology: It's in the details [Electronic version]. *Epidemiologic Perspectives & Innovations, 2*(8).

MacKinnon, D. P., Fairchild, A. J., & Fritz, M. S. (2007). Mediation analysis. *Annual Review of Psychology, 58,* 593–614.

MacKinnon, D. P., Krull, J. L., & Lockwood, C. M. (2000). Equivalence of the mediation, confounding and suppression effect. *Prevention Science, 1*(4), 173–180.

Murray, D. M. (1998). *Design and analysis for group-randomized trials* (pp. 46–47). New York: Oxford University Press.

Naidoo, P., & Pretorius, T. B. (2006). The moderating role of helplessness in rheumatoid arthritis, a chronic disease. *Social Behavior and Personality, 34*(2), 103–112.

Pearl, J. (1998). *Why there is no statistical test for confounding, why many think there is, and why they are almost right.* UCLA Cognitive Systems Laboratory, Technical Report (R-256). Los Angeles: University of California.

Conjoint Analysis

Conjoint analysis (CA) is a quantitative technique used to elicit preferences. When faced with multiple alternatives, people often make decisions by making trade-offs between the specific features of competing products. CA derives preferences by examining these trade-offs through a series of rating, ranking, or choice tasks. Data generated from CA studies can then be used to determine which combination of features should be most preferred by each respondent.

CA was originally described by Luce and Tukey in 1964 and has since been widely used in market research, in economics, and most recently to examine preferences for competing programs, services, and treatment options in healthcare. This technique is based on three main assumptions. The first is that each product is a composite of different attributes and that each attribute is specified by a number of levels. For example, imagine that you are a researcher interested in eliciting patient preferences for competing pain medications. In this context, attributes might include specific medication characteristics such as route of administration, probability and magnitude of benefit, adverse effects, and out-of-pocket cost. The term *levels* refers to the range of estimates for each attribute. The levels for the attribute "out-of-pocket" costs for an insured population might range from $0 to $30.00 per month.

The second assumption underlying CA is that respondents have unique values, or utilities, for each attribute level. In this context *utility* is a number that represents the value a respondent associates with a particular characteristic, with higher utilities indicating increased value.

The final assumption underlying CA is that a subject's value for a specific product can be calculated by combining the discrete utilities associated with each attribute. Therefore, if the sum of a patient's utilities for the attributes of Medication A is greater than the sum of utilities for the attributes of Medication B, the patient should prefer Medication A to B.

Data generated from a CA study can answer important clinical questions, such as the following: Which attributes most strongly influence preferences? Which treatment is preferred and why? How much risk are patients willing to accept for a specified benefit? If cost is included as an attribute, CA can also estimate patients' willingness to pay.

Steps Involved in Performing a Conjoint Analysis Study

Step 1: Choose the Options, Attributes, and Levels

The investigator must first decide on the set of options to be evaluated. Is the objective to study preferences for all available treatment options for a particular condition or only those options appropriate for a particular subset of patients? Should hypothetical options representing potential future advances be included? If one is examining treatment preferences, are both pharmacologic and nonpharmacologic options to be included?

Once the set of options to be studied are identified, the investigator must choose which attributes and levels to include. Undoubtedly, this is the most difficult step in performing a CA study. Ideally, all the attributes required to choose between competing options should be included in the study. In some cases, the set of attributes is chosen based on data available from published studies. However, whenever possible, obtaining input from relevant stakeholders, via individual interviews or focus groups, is preferred. The estimates, or levels, for each attribute should be based on the best available evidence to date. With computerized programs it is possible to design separate versions of a survey to be able to present patients with individualized information.

Step 2: Choose a Conjoint Analysis Method

There are three main methods of conducting a CA study: full profile, choice-based, and adaptive (ACA, Sawtooth Software). These methods differ primarily in the way respondents are presented with information.

In full profile CA surveys, respondents are presented with complete profiles of hypothetical products that include a specified level for each attribute. Figure 1 describes two profiles from a hypothetical set of profiles examining preferences for pain medications.

Preferences are elicited by asking respondents to rate each profile or to rank a set of profiles. The main advantage of this technique is that it provides respondents with the most realistic descriptions of the products being evaluated. However, respondents tend to employ simplifying tactics to compensate for information overload when presented with full profiles using as few as four attributes, making this technique impractical for complex options.

	Drug 1	Drug 6
Route of administration	Cream	Pill
Probability of benefit	30%	80%
Risk of dyspepsia	10%	30%
Monthly cost ($)	$10	$20

Figure I   Example of profiles used in full-profile conjoint analysis

Choice-based CA (CBC) is currently the most popular method of performing CA studies. As with the full profile approach, traditional CBC studies present respondents with profiles that include all attributes. Respondents are shown a choice set, usually composed of three or four profiles, and asked to indicate which they prefer. An example of a choice task evaluating treatment options for pain using the same attributes as those described above is provide in Figure 2.

CBC is preferred among many researchers because asking patients to perform a choice, rather than a rating or ranking task, is felt to be an easier task and more representative of how people make choices in the real world. In addition, CBC allows the investigator to include a "None" option—which enables respondents to refuse or defer.

ACA (Sawtooth Software, Inc., Sequim, WA) collects and analyzes preference data using an interactive computer program. This method is unique in that it uses individual respondents' answers to update and refine the questionnaire through a series of graded paired comparisons. Because it is interactive, ACA is more efficient than other techniques and allows a large number of attributes to be evaluated without resulting in information overload or respondent fatigue. This is an important advantage, since complex treatment decisions often require multiple trade-offs between competing risks and benefits. ACA surveys begin with a self-explicated set of questions that are followed by a set of paired comparison tasks. Figure 3 provides an example of the latter.

Step 3: Formulate an Experimental Design

The next step in developing a CA survey is to formulate an experimental design to decrease the number of scenarios each respondent evaluates. Imagine a very simple survey evaluating three attributes each having two levels. This small set of attributes and levels yields $2 \times 2 \times 2 = 8$ possible combinations. Increasing the number of levels by only one would yield $3 \times 3 \times 3 = 27$ possible combinations. Since most surveys include more than three attributes, experimental designs are required to identify an efficient subset of the total possible combinations of profiles to enable respondents to evaluate a practical number of scenarios. Fractional-factorial designs

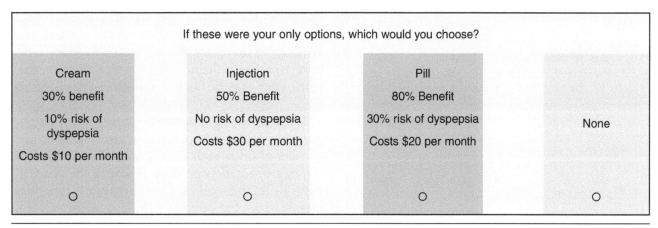

Figure 2 Example of a choice-based conjoint analysis choice task

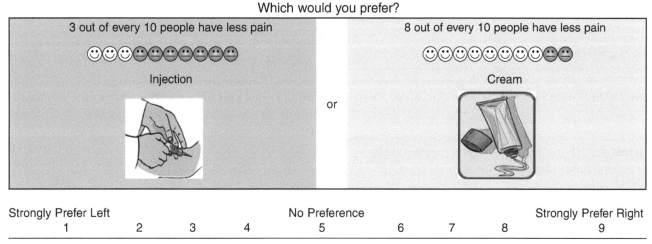

Figure 3 Example of an ACA paired-comparison task

can be generated using software programs, including SAS and Excel. There are also specialized CA software packages such as Sawtooth Software, Inc.

Step 4: Interpreting Conjoint Analysis Data

CA studies generate a utility or part-worth value for each level of each attribute. Part-worths can be calculated using several approaches. One of the most commonly used models is ordinary least squares regression. Recent advances include calculation of part-worths using Hierarchical Bayes Estimation. A full discussion of the models underlying CA is beyond the scope of this entry, however.

CA part-worths are scaled to an arbitrary constant within each attribute and are interval data. A set of hypothetical data are provided in Figure 4. In this example, the constant is the least preferred level of each attribute and is assigned a value of 0.

The significance of the part-worths is found within relative differences between the levels. Because the zero point is arbitrarily set, the absolute value of any specific level has no meaning. Therefore one cannot state that the utility or part-worth assigned to a 1% risk of dyspepsia is the same as that assigned to a $10 monthly cost. Nor can one state that an 80% chance of benefit is three times better than a 50% benefit. However, one can conclude that this respondent prefers pills over creams and that injections are least preferred.

Attribute	Level	Part-Worth
1. Route of administration	Cream	30
	Pill	40
	Injection	0
2. Probability of benefit	30%	0
	50%	30
	80%	90
3. Risk of dyspepsia	1%	20
	10%	5
	25%	0
4. Monthly cost	$5	30
	$10	20
	$30	0

Figure 4   Hypothetical part-worths generated by a conjoint analysis study

One can also conclude that for this respondent the value gained from changing a medication from a cream to a pill (10 additional utility units) is the same as that obtained by decreasing the monthly cost from $10 to $5.

CA surveys also allow the investigator to calculate the relative importance of each attribute. In this context, *relative importance* refers to the amount of importance respondents place on each treatment characteristic and is calculated by dividing the range of each characteristic (difference between levels) by the sum of ranges of all characteristics and multiplying by 100. These values sum to 100 and reflect the extent to which the difference between the levels of each characteristic affects each respondent's preferences. Relative importances are ratio measures and therefore support multiplicative functions. For example, based on the relative importances displayed in Figure 5, the respondent was influenced most by the probability of benefit and felt that route of administration was twice as important as the risk of dyspepsia.

Of note, the relative importances are strongly influenced by the range of the levels chosen. For instance, in this example, one would expect cost to have a greater influence on preference if the maximum cost was $100 per month as opposed to $30.

In CBC studies, it is also possible to gain insight into respondents' preferences by counting the number of times each level was chosen. These data can be presented as proportions (with the denominator being the total number of times the level was presented in the survey). These proportions are ratio data and, unlike part-worths, can be compared within an attribute.

CA studies are most frequently used to predict preferences for available or hypothetical options defined by the researcher. For example, imagine that a researcher is interested in describing preferences for four treatment options for knee pain: capsaicin, acetaminophen, anti-inflammatory drugs, and cortisone injections. Using the attributes defined in Figure 4, the researcher defines each option by assigning an appropriate level to each attribute (see Figure 6).

Respondents' utilities are subsequently entered into a simulation model that yields a preference measure for each product. Sensitivity analyses to estimate the impact of changing specific characteristics on preference can also be performed. For example, using the example above, the investigator could examine how preferences for each of the four options are affected by changing cost, probability of benefit, or risk of toxicity.

Several simulator models are available, such as the first-choice and share-of-preference models. Each model uses different "rules" to estimate preferences. For example, in the first-choice model, the part-worths are summed and the respondent is assumed to choose the product with highest utility. In the share-of-preference model, preferences are calculated by first summing the utilities of the levels corresponding to each option. The utilities are then exponentiated and rescaled so that they sum to 100.

Previous studies of patient treatment preferences have (1) documented significant variability in treatment preferences, (2) found that patient preferences are frequently not aligned with treatment guidelines, and (3) shown that patient preferences may not be concordant with common medical practices. These findings each emphasize the importance of

Attribute	Level	Part-Worth	Range	Relative Importance
Route of administration	Cream	30	40	40/180 × 100 = 22
	Pill	40		
	Injection	0		
Probability of benefit	30%	0	90	90/180 × 100 = 50
	50%	30		
	80%	90		
Risk of dyspepsia	0%	20	20	20/180 × 100 = 11
	10%	5		
	25%	0		
Monthly cost	$5	30	30	30/180 × 100 = 17
	$10	20		
	$30	0		

Figure 5   Example of relative importances generated by a conjoint analysis study

Option	Attribute 1 (Route)	Attribute 2 (Benefit)	Attribute 3 (Dyspepsia)	Attribute 4 (Cost)
Option 1 (Capsaicin)	Level 1	Level 1	Level 1	Level 2
Option 2 (Acetaminophen)	Level 2	Level 1	Level 2	Level 1
Option 3 (Anti-inflammatory)	Level 2	Level 2	Level 3	Level 2
Option 4 (Cortisone injection)	Level 3	Level 2	Level 1	Level 3

Figure 6   Modeling preferences for knee pain

incorporating individual patient preferences into the medical decision-making process.

Important Features

CA has been used increasingly frequently to describe patient preferences for health-related services and treatment options. CA is also a means by which patients' views can be included in setting research priorities, designing trials, and developing policy.

CA has many properties that make it a valuable tool to elicit patient preferences and facilitate medical decision making:

- It can be designed to ensure that patients are made aware of all essential information related to appropriate treatment options and therefore should improve patient knowledge and informed consent.
- It improves the quality of decisions by making the trade-offs between competing options explicit. This is of direct clinical relevance since choices based on explicit trade-offs are less likely to be influenced by heuristics (errors in reasoning), which can lead to poor decisions.
- CA can be used to examine the amount of importance respondents place on specific treatment characteristics. This feature should enable physicians to gain insight into the reasons underlying their patients' preferences, tailor discussions to address individual patients' concerns, and ensure that decisions are made based on accurate expectations.
- It provides simulation capability. This feature allows the investigator to assess the impact of varying specific treatment characteristics on choice. For example, researchers can determine how much benefit patients require before accepting the risk of drug toxicity, whether decreasing the burden or inconveniences of therapy might increase patient acceptance of treatment, or which treatment option fits best with an individual patient's values.

Future Research

A reasonable body of evidence has now shown that CA is a feasible and valuable method of eliciting preferences in healthcare. Future research is now needed to determine if CA can be implemented as a decision support tool to improve informed decision making in medicine at the population as well as the individual patient level.

Liana Fraenkel

See also Utility Assessment Techniques

Further Readings

Kuhfeld, W. H. (2005). *Marketing research methods in SAS: Experimental design, choice, conjoint, and graphical techniques.* Cary, NC: SAS Institute. Retrieved May 15, 2008, from http://support.sas.com/techsup/technote/ts722title.pdf

Luce, D., & Tukey, J. (1964). Simultaneous conjoint measurement: A new type of fundamental measurement. *Journal of Mathematical Psychology, 1,* 1–27.

Orme, B. (n.d.). Hierarchical Bayes regression analysis: Technical paper. *Technical Paper Series.* Retrieved February 13, 2009, from http://www.sawtooth software.com

Sawtooth Software Technical Papers Library: http://www.sawtoothsoftware.com/education/techpap.shtml

Srinivasan, V., & Park, C. S. (1997). Surprising robustness of the self-explicated approach to customer preference structure measurement. *Journal of Marketing Research, 34,* 286–291.

Wright, P. (1975). Consumer choice strategies: Simplifying vs. optimizing. *Journal of Marketing Research, 12,* 60–67.

CONJUNCTION PROBABILITY ERROR

The conjunction rule applies to predictive judgment or forward conditional reasoning. It is a normative rule that states that the probability of any combination of events cannot exceed the probability of constituent events. For example, the probability of picking the queen of spades from a card deck cannot exceed the probability of picking a spade and a queen from the deck. Typically, people can successfully apply the conjunction rule to transparent problems such as the card selection problem. However, there is overwhelming evidence that when problems are less transparent, people often ignore the rule and judge the conjunction of events as more probable than a constituent event, thereby committing the conjunction probability error. Because of the pervasiveness of the conjunction error and its clear violation of normative probability theory, it is important to understand conditions that tend to produce the error, procedures that may reduce its occurrence, and instances where it does not apply.

Conditions That Produce the Conjunction Error

The initial investigation of the conjunction error was conducted within the framework of understanding how heuristic thought processes may produce systematic biases in judgment and choice. In their seminal investigation, Amos Tversky and Daniel Kahneman first explored the conjunction error as resulting from the use of the representativeness heuristic for judging probabilities. According to this heuristic, people judge probabilities for specific outcomes by making a similarity comparison with a model of the population from which the outcomes were sampled. For example, knowing that a person is a member of a particular group, one may use a stereotype of that group as a model to predict behaviors or attributes of the person.

The Linda Problem

An often used example that has been shown to produce robust conjunction errors is the *Linda problem*. As described by Tversky and Kahneman, Linda is 31 years old, single, outspoken, and intelligent. Participants are told that when she was a philosophy major at school, she was concerned with social justice and participated in protests and demonstrations. This background establishes a model of Linda as a sophisticated individual concerned with social issues. After reading the description, participants typically rank the relative likelihoods of predicted occupations and activities that apply to Linda. Three key statements that may be evaluated include the following:

(U) Linda is a bank teller.

(L) Linda is active in the feminist movement.

(U & L) Linda is a bank teller and is active in the feminist movement.

The first statement is unlikely (U) based on the model of Linda and is given a relatively low probability ranking. The second statement is likely (L) based on the model of Linda and is given a relatively high probability ranking. The third statement is the key statement as it conjoins the unlikely and likely events (U & L). As such, it represents a subset of both these events and cannot have a higher probability than either of these. Yet nearly all participants indicate that the conjunction is more probable than the unlikely event. These results are obtained with both statistically naive and statistically sophisticated participants and in situations in which participants are directly assessing the relative likelihoods of the events. Furthermore, a majority of participants still commit the error even when they are asked to bet on these outcomes, implying the effect does not disappear with monetary incentives for correct application of the conjunction rule.

The conjunction error in the Linda problem is constructed by pairing an unlikely outcome from the model with a likely outcome from the model. In the probability calculus, the probability of the combined events can be expressed as follows:

$$\Pr(U \,\&\, L) = \Pr(U)\,\Pr(L|U).$$

This formula makes it explicit that the probability of Linda being a bank teller and active in the feminist movement, $\Pr(U \,\&\, L)$, must be less than or equal to the probability of her being a bank teller, $\Pr(U)$, as the probability of being active in the feminist movement given she is a bank teller, $\Pr(L|U)$, must be less than or equal to 1.0. But according to similarity-based heuristic thinking, combining an outcome that is dissimilar to the model with one that is similar to the model results in an evaluation of moderate similarity for the combined events. If probabilities are then based on such similarity evaluations, the mixed outcome case is judged as more probable than the unlikely constituent outcome, resulting in the conjunction error.

A Second Recipe for Conjunction Errors

The Linda problem used the recipe of combining an unlikely outcome with a likely outcome to produce the conjunction error. A second recipe for creating conjunction errors is to add an outcome that makes the other outcome more likely or plausible. Tversky and Kahneman illustrated this recipe in a health-related example in which participants were told that a health survey had been administered to a large sample of adult males of all ages and occupations. They were then asked to indicate which statement was more likely of a randomly selected person from the survey:

1. This person has had one or more heart attacks.

2. This person has had one or more heart attacks and is over 55 years of age.

The majority of respondents chose the conjunction to be more probable in this instance. The specified age makes it easier for people to imagine this person having had one or more heart attacks. More generally, this type of conjunction error may be attributed to scenario thinking. In the first case, there is no reason to think that the selected individual might have had a heart attack. In the second case, the age-related information fills in some of the causal linkages that make the scenario more plausible and hence seem more probable. This type of scenario-based conjunction error can occur whenever a conjoined outcome provides a causal mechanism for the occurrence of the other outcome.

Application to Medical Decision Making

Tversky and Kahneman also demonstrated the applicability of the conjunction error directly to medical decision making. One of the problems they administered to two different groups of internists indicated that "A 55-year-old woman had pulmonary embolism documented angiographically 10 days after a cholecystectomy." The doctors were asked to rank order the probability that the patient would be experiencing each of a set of conditions. These included "dyspnea and hemiparesis" and "hemiparesis." Across the two samples, 91% indicated that the conjunction of conditions was more likely than the constituent condition. When physicians in an additional sample were confronted with their conjunction errors, they did not try to defend their decisions but simply indicated their surprise and dismay at having made such elementary errors. This last result suggests that the conjunction error is not simply due to misunderstanding how the alternatives are presented in the problem but

instead represents a serious threat to risk assessment that can take place with experts within their own domain of expertise.

Procedures That May Reduce the Conjunction Error

Several criticisms of the work on the conjunction effect have been leveled over the 25 years since it was first reported. These criticisms focus on various features of how the problems are presented. One class of criticisms suggests that the problems may be ambiguously stated so that errors are due to participants misunderstanding what the experimenter is trying to communicate. For example, in several versions of the Linda problem, one simply chooses which is more probable, that "Linda is a bank teller" or that "Linda is a bank teller and is active in the feminist movement." One might argue that the pragmatics of conversation norms lead individuals to interpret the first statement as meaning "Linda is a bank teller and is not active in the feminist movement." Through the years, numerous ways of clarifying the options have been explored. The bottom line, however, is that although some versions may lead to fewer conjunction errors, they generally do not eliminate conjunction errors (i.e., the majority of participants still commit the error even with the reworded statements).

Another criticism has been directed against the normative force of the conjunction error. This argument is based on a strict frequentistic interpretation of probability, which states that it is reasonable to judge probabilities for samples from a population but it is not reasonable to judge probabilities for propensities of unique events. In the Linda problem, either she is or she is not a bank teller, and hence probability is not applicable. Rather than resolve this interpretation at the normative level, researchers have probed whether the conjunction error occurs when people are evaluating probabilities of samples from a population. For example, we can conceive of 100 women fitting Linda's description and estimate the probability that a random sample from this population would have these characteristics. Although some studies have shown a marked reduction of conjunction errors in this case, most have demonstrated very strong conjunction errors still occur. The health survey example discussed above is one case in point.

Related to the issue of interpreting probabilities is the assertion that probabilities are not a natural way of processing frequency information and so people will make errors when forced to consider probabilities rather than frequencies. Several researchers have tested this idea by comparing performance on problems requiring probability assessments versus frequency assessments. Note that the frequency assessment requires that one talk about sampling from a population rather than talk about propensities of individuals. The health survey problem described above has been formulated in frequency terms by asking participants to estimate how many of a sample of 100 individuals from the survey would fit each description. In general, the response format of estimating frequencies sampled from a large population has led to a significant reduction of conjunction errors, with the majority of participants not committing the error. This method would then appear to be a good way to reduce reasoning errors and de-bias judges.

However, a closer look at the pattern of results across numerous studies indicates that it is not the frequency format itself that is strongly reducing conjunction errors; rather, it is the requirement of making estimates that is critical. Numerous studies have shown that choosing which alternative would result in the highest sampled frequency does little to reduce conjunction errors. It is only when estimates must be generated for each option that conjunction errors are dramatically reduced. This occurs even when the estimates are of probabilities rather than of frequencies. This result supports the idea that people have at least two distinct ways to process probability information. One may be more qualitative and heuristic-based and the other more numerical and algorithmic. When the response mode is qualitative in nature, as in ranking and choice, people tend to apply the qualitative heuristic mode of thought and commit conjunction errors. When the response mode requires numerical assessments, people are more inclined to apply the quantitative algorithmic approaches and hence reduce conjunction errors.

Applicability of the Conjunction Rule

It is important to note when the conjunction rule does and does not apply when considering the various tasks associated with assessing probabilities. The conjunction rule applies to predictive judgment or forward conditional reasoning. In this type of reasoning, events are conditioned on a premise represented as a hypothesized model or hypothesized sampling procedure. In the medical decision-making context, it applies to predicting symptoms given a disease or outcomes given a procedure. In these cases, one must be careful to consider whether probability assessments are being inappropriately increased by the consideration of a conjunct that makes a particular outcome easier to envision. It is important to avoid scenario thinking or similarity-based thinking in making these assessments.

The conjunction rule does not apply to diagnostic judgment or backward conditional reasoning. In this kind of reasoning, one is inferring the probability of a hypothesis based on an outcome or a conjunction of outcomes. In medical decision making, this is by far the more common type of assessment. Given a particular set of symptoms one must estimate the likelihood of a given disease as the cause. Here, Bayesian updating applies so that conjoining a diagnostic symptom with a nondiagnostic symptom should lead to an increase in the overall probability of the disease. One possibility is that people commit the conjunction error because they do not correctly differentiate between these two tasks and hence incorrectly apply diagnostic reasoning to a prediction task.

Douglas H. Wedell

See also Bayesian Evidence Synthesis; Biases in Human Prediction; Frequency Estimation; Heuristics; Probability Errors

Further Readings

Gigerenzer, G. (1996). On narrow norms and vague heuristics: A reply to Tversky and Kahneman. *Psychological Review, 103,* 592–596.

Hertwig, R., & Chase, V. M. (1998). Many reasons or just one: How response mode affects reasoning in the conjunction problem. *Thinking and Reasoning, 4,* 319–352.

Sloman, S. A., Over, D., Slovak, L., & Stibel, J. M. (2003). Frequency illusions and other fallacies. *Organizational Behavior and Human Decision Processes, 91,* 296–309.

Tversky, A., & Kahneman, D. (1983). Extensional versus intuitive reasoning: The conjunction fallacy in probability judgment. *Psychological Review, 90,* 293–315.

Wedell, D. H., & Moro, R. (2008). Testing boundary conditions for the conjunction fallacy: Effects of response mode, conceptual focus and problem type. *Cognition, 107,* 105–136.

CONSTRAINT THEORY

Diagnosis—the process by which examination and existing knowledge are used to establish the nature and circumstances of a particular condition—has always been the basis of the practice of medicine. It is the focal point of the doctor-patient relationship. But given rapid advancements in medical science and technology over the past 50 or so years, diagnostic methods have emerged elsewhere across the healthcare system: in all manner of relationships, decision-making processes, management structures, and work in general. Individuals and organizations have, as a consequence, sought new ways to manage these transformations. One such way has been through the application of constraint theory, through which one can organize existing thoughts about complex systems and communicate them through scientific algorithms.

Information Is the Transformation

The basic features, challenges, and opportunities of today's healthcare system are not all-too-different from those of the past. Since the early days of the American republic, there has been plenty of thought about how to integrate a host of general, though interconnected needs related to patients, physicians and other practitioners, government, taxes, insurance, access to and quality of care, and business interests, to name a few.

Yet, in the interim, the vast improvements in science and technology that have been applied to the practice of medicine have produced an increasing amount of data. This has both benefited and swamped the system.

The amount of data available to people throughout the healthcare system, and the capacity to process it, is ever increasing. But for the data to be useful, it must be converted into information; for this to happen, the data must be oriented toward a particular purpose or given some relevance. As medicine becomes more specialized and healthcare more complex, the importance of information and how it flows—whether information is good or not, how people choose to share it, and whether it passes easily between people—makes a difference in the performance of people and organizations throughout the system. In response, a number of models have been developed in an attempt to effectively process data, convert it into information, and capture the flow of that information so that it can be used to make the right decisions.

Quality Improvement Methods

Flawless performance and attention to detail are highly regarded qualities in the medical and healthcare professions. This reality, plus today's economic dimensions and the fact that organizations within healthcare have grown larger and more difficult to manage, has increased the demand for nonmedical professionals who have experience in management techniques that could be applied to improve organizational behavior and, thereby, patient care. High on the list of innovative concepts that have infiltrated the workings of the modern healthcare organization is the implementation of quality improvement programs. Adapted from the engineering and service-outcome approaches that are popular, especially in the business of manufacturing, these programs are highly disciplined, statistically driven methods by which to measure and eliminate any number of "defects" in a production process. In form and function, they require a high level of systematic predictability and a low tolerance for human fallibility. Such programs are intended to be a reliable means by which to use input and output data to achieve the goal of delivering to customers a product or service that satisfies their needs.

A good portion of these programs come out of the Total Quality Management (TQM) philosophy developed in the mid- to late 20th century by, among others, W. Edwards Deming, Joseph Juran, and Kaoru Ishikawa. The TQM movement generally considers that every person and all activities in an organization must be managed toward customer requirements for a product or service. To accomplish as much, especially over the long term, TQM programs begin with four basic assumptions about quality, people, organizations, and management. These assumptions include the beliefs that (a) the production of quality products and services is preferred over compromising quality in an attempt to keep costs low; (b) employees care about the quality of their performance and will work to improve it so long as management pays attention to their ideas, provides them with the means necessary for improvement, and creates a positive work environment; (c) organizations are constituted of interdependent parts that must function as a system; and (d) senior management is responsible for the creation, organization, and direction of the overall system that leads to quality outcomes.

From there, the interventions intended to actually bring about change and improve quality must focus on work processes, analysis of variability and variation in those processes, systematic collection and analysis of data at precise points in the processes, and a commitment to learning and "continuous improvement." Regard for these factors permits the development of new and better methods for performing work, which in turn improves the quality of the product or service being worked on. In all, the outcome relies on giving meaning to an increasing number of variables that must be variously and appropriately integrated into decisions across and through the system.

One of today's acknowledged, though controversial, interventions for service outcome and quality improvement is the theory of constraints, developed by Eliyahu Goldratt. It is grounded in the notion of a "weakest link" in any complex system. That is, at any point in time, there is some phenomenon that limits the function of the system to move beyond its current capacity and closer to achieving its goal. In this cause-and-effect relationship, the phenomenon—the constraint—must be identified and the entire system managed accordingly if the system is to improve. Yet the theory of constraints should not be confused with constraint theory.

Theory of Complexity and Constraint Theory

In complex systems, while the prevailing conditions of a certain environment are stable and predictable, the actions and effects of the elements within it are not. Over the past four decades, with the rise of digital computation and data processing, mathematical proofs have been used to show that complex systems are determined by numberless internal and external factors. These factors are not necessarily statistically significant and, therefore, do not allow prediction in the classical sense. And it may be that one of the statistically insignificant factors turns out to be that which has the greatest impact on the entire system. There have lately emerged across the study of modern mathematics several theorems that clearly identify such factors, including the constraint theory cast by George J. Friedman.

The traditional way to achieve a complete, correct, and consistent method for managing a complex system has been to divide a specific model into submodels that could be refined by specialists and later connected into an aggregate model. But Friedman's contention is that there is no assurance of consistency in the aggregate model even if there is consistency in every submodel. Through the development of constraint theory, he has shown that model structure can be used by cross-functional teams, analysts, and managers to discern inconsistencies in an aggregate model.

Friedman's constraint theory uses the "Four-Fold Way," which is a progressive collection of "views": set theoretic; family of submodels; bipartite graph; and constraint matrix. It separates a given model from computations and chronicles the existence and flow of constraints throughout the model. Each constraint may be tagged and valued as an *overconstraint*—an instance in which more variables exist than the number required for solving a group of equations—or an *underconstraint,* in which fewer variables exist than the amount required for solving a group of equations. The entire operation is typically represented on a bipartite graph (see Figure 1), with a nodes vertex that denotes the relations within the model and a knots vertex that signifies its variables; nodes are represented by squares and knots by circles, and a knot will be connected to a node by an edge if and only if the corresponding variable is present in the corresponding functional relationship of a model. In effect, the nodes are central points, and the knots are points at which the values of the variables pass from one central point to another. The end result is that visualization of the system, before returning to the original group of model equations, can benefit the development of a strategy that ideally would lead to some solution.

The essence of constraint theory is that it enhances the use of computer assistance to bring some level of control to numberless variables in a system. It intends to identify decisive factors, yet does not, as a rule, convey how to eliminate extraneous ones. This, in any case, helps one more accurately analyze the behaviors and performance of the people and forces within the system—and at its various stages, under its various criteria, and with respect to its various needs of integration and design. But for anyone to become proficient—or at least—in the technique of constraint theory requires that one first comprehend the basic concepts of set theory and graph theory, which is more often the domain of mathematicians and engineers than of physicians and healthcare professionals. That is, while they could well have the capacity and knowledge to grasp the particulars of constraint theory, it is more likely that physicians and other healthcare professionals' time, contributions, strengths, and priorities are better invested in the tasks and practices specific to their work.

There is no question that new realities during the mid- to late 20th century—primarily, advances in medical science and technology and the advent of managed care—have necessitated new applications of new knowledge. Nor is there doubt that with such transformations there is a need to incorporate every relative complexity—however overt or subtle, close or remote, old or new—into capable analysis. Being able to understand and act on constraints at a given point in a system is especially imperative today as the healthcare system increasingly relies on the use of knowledge and learning as a basis for skills that allow its highly specialized, productive work to be performed. It therefore needs programs that demand that decision makers be precise in every decision-making capacity, that they know precisely what to do with the available information, and that they are listening to and asking questions that encourage critical thinking and the careful development of ideas. Only then can medical and healthcare professionals tend to the care for and cure of the sick patient.

Lee H. Igel

See also Chaos Theory; Complexity; Computer-Assisted Decision Making

Further Readings

Deming, W. E. (2000). *Out of the crisis.* Cambridge: MIT Press.

Drucker, P. F. (2003). *The new realities.* New Brunswick, NJ: Transaction.

Friedman, G. J. (1976). Constraint theory: An overview. *International Journal of Systems Science, 7*(10), 1113–1151.

Friedman, G. J. (2005). *Constraint theory: Multidimensional mathematical model management.* New York: Springer.

Goldratt, E. M. (1999). *Theory of constraints.* Great Barrington, MA: North River Press.

Goldratt, E. M., & Cox, J. (2004). *The goal: A process of ongoing improvement* (3rd ed.). Great Barrington, MA: North River Press.

Hackman, J. R., & Wageman, R. (1995). Total quality management: Empirical, conceptual, and practical issues. *Administrative Science Quarterly, 40*(2), 309–342.

Ishikawa, K. (1991). *What is total quality control? The Japanese way.* Englewood Cliffs, NJ: Prentice Hall.

Juran, J. M. (1995). *Managerial breakthrough: A new concept of the manager's job* (Rev. ed.). New York: McGraw-Hill.

Warfield, J. N. (2003). A proposal for systems science. *Systems Research and Behavioral Science, 20*(6), 507–520.

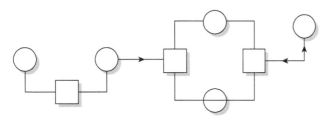

Figure I   Bipartite graph: A nonspecific, simple example (see Friedman, 2005, for specific and complex examples)

CONSTRUCTION OF VALUES

Construction of values refers to the process whereby an individual's preference for a particular health state or more generally, a "good" of any sort, is developed or built (constructed) at the time when that state or good is encountered, either actually or hypothetically. Preference in this context refers to the desirability or undesirability of something, from the subjective perspective of the person assessing or evaluating it. Preferences are the external manifestation of underlying values, and are commonly referred to interchangeably. Value construction occurs in clinical contexts when medical decisions are imminent or in forecasting decision making. In research settings, value construction occurs usually in the consideration of hypothetical choices, such as in preference elicitation surveys or choice experiments. Value construction can be contrasted with value retrieval, in which values already exist and are known to the individual, and are simply retrieved from memory.

Definition

Preferences about goods, health states, or even issues are thought to exist on a continuum, from those that are basic to those that are highly complex. Basic values are easily known and expressed by an individual; these values are quite possibly innate. Complex values require extensive cognitive effort to understand and express and may not be immediately available to an individual. For example, an infant's preference for its mother over another person could be considered a basic, innate preference or value. Similarly, the value one person places on Pepsi versus Coke is basic and known and easy to express. At the other extreme, the value placed on a painful and debilitating yet life-extending therapy might not be known to an individual without the benefit of extensive thought, consideration, and deliberation. The value for this therapy is based on more basic values but is some combination of many considerations and preferences, including trade-offs among conflicting values, resulting in a complex preference. The construction of values refers to this latter process in which an individual uses information and more basic values to construct, or build, the more complex value.

Construction Process

Values are constructed at the time when an individual is faced with a situation that demands knowledge or expression of his or her values. In general, values are called on every time an individual makes a choice or decision, from purchasing one brand versus another to casting a ballot. In the context of health and medicine, values are usually called on when an individual is faced with a decision about a medical intervention or treatment, from something as simple as receiving a flu shot to consenting to surgery. Values are also invoked during surveys and experiments asking about choices and decisions, wherein much of our knowledge about preference construction has been demonstrated.

The construction process generally begins when an individual is faced with a choice or decision that defies basic values. For example, if a person is asked which political party he or she supports, he or she may reply "Democrat" or "Republican." If a person is asked whether she supports Candidate A or Candidate B, she may ask about the candidates' positions on an issue important to her, such as environmental protection. On learning of the candidates' positions, she will choose A or B. If then she is told Candidate A is female and Candidate B is male, and this person prefers to support a female candidate, she will have to consider both the candidates' genders and their positions on environmental protection to make a choice. If the male candidate is a stronger proponent of environmental protection, the person has to weigh the importance of her gender preference against her environmental protection preference to arrive at a decision. This type of choice would be considered to invoke complex values because it is not readily apparent what choice would be dictated from the basic values regarding gender and environmental protection. Values for the candidates hence would be *constructed* from the information and basic values. Value construction occurs when basic values would suffice but information is unknown, when basic values do not exist for the options encountered, or when the complexity of the choice involves combinations of or trade-offs among basic values.

Value construction in medical decision making often involves multiple and conflicting trade-offs, and information is often lacking. Basic values regarding medical decisions can be well-known and accessible, such as the value placed on quality of life or longevity. Yet these values are often encountered in contradiction, making complexity inherent in most medical choices.

Elicitation Process

While value construction occurs implicitly when choices are made, the process becomes more explicit when values or preferences are specifically elicited for decision making or in the context of surveys. Because complex values are based on basic values and potentially information, time and consideration are necessary components of the construction process, though it can be highly person and situation specific. Lacking any of these elements, complex values may be expressed inaccurately as their more basic components, or as entities entirely different from those that would be articulated given sufficient information and consideration. Such occurrences have been demonstrated as preference reversals, which are basically situations in which a person directly contradicts himself or herself in matched choices, or as framing effects, in which the context in which a choice is presented unduly influences the outcome. Such incidents are not adequately described by the theories that underlie decision making and in this context indicate the need for value construction to maximize expression of true preferences, unaffected by context and other external factors. Value elicitation processes should therefore take the necessary elements of value construction into account to produce valid and stable expressions of complex values.

Importance in Medical Decision Making

Acknowledging that values are constructed implies that a process should be followed when decisions are made. Since medical decisions commonly involve complex values and multiple trade-offs, the elements necessary for value construction should be provided to ensure fully informed and formed choices. Complete information and thorough consideration may enable a construction process that leads to decisions that accurately reflect underlying basic values. Understanding of the processes that motivate value formation can provide guidance in eliciting and articulating quality decision making in health and medicine.

Eve Wittenberg

See also Decision Quality; Preference Reversals; Utility Assessment Techniques

Further Readings

Gregory, R., Lichtenstein, S., & Slovic, P. (1993). Valuing environmental resources: A constructive approach. *Journal of Risk and Uncertainty, 7,* 177–197.

Lichtenstein, S., & Slovic, P. (Eds.). (2006). *The construction of preference.* New York: Cambridge University Press.

Payne, J. W., Bettman, J. R., & Schkade, D. A. (1999). Measuring constructed preferences: Towards a building code. *Journal of Risk and Uncertainty, 19,* 1–3, 243–270.

CONSUMER-DIRECTED HEALTH PLANS

Consumer-directed healthcare is an approach to financing healthcare services wherein individuals are given fixed allowances with which they can purchase specified services. Most plans couple this with catastrophic coverage, usually with a high deductible. These plans often receive tax advantages. Variants may be termed *medical savings accounts, health savings accounts,* or *flexible spending accounts.* They have been employed in a number of countries, including the United States, Singapore, South Africa, and China. There are differences in terms of such details as who contributes (employer, employee, or both), the levels of deductibles and co-payments payable, which services can be purchased with these funds, and whether unused contributions can be carried over to subsequent years. Some models employ a "use it or lose it" approach, whereas others allow savings to be accumulated, often tax-free. Consumer-directed models are predicated on the assumption that potential users of care should be the ones making the decisions about what care to receive and from whom.

The Case For

Market Approaches to Allocation

Consumer-based models are based on the premise that, like other commodities, healthcare is a market good and as such its utilization is subject to the predictions of economic theory. In economics, price is the signal that ensures a balance between supply and demand. Economic theorists would thus predict that reducing price would increase demand. In addition, they note that insurance may create what is termed *moral hazard*, a term referring to the prospect that insulating people from risk (a major purpose of insurance) may make them less concerned about the potential negative consequences of that risk than they otherwise might be. For example, those with flood insurance may be more willing to build in flood plains, in the confidence that insurance would cover their losses. Similarly, economic theory would predict that those with health insurance, because they do not have to pay the full cost of any care they receive, would have an incentive to over-use it. Advocates thus argue that consumer-driven models are the best way to achieve cost control because wise consumers will shop around for the best buy, measured in terms of both quality and price. They suggest that an additional benefit of high deductible plans is that insurers will save money by not having to process small claims.

In contrast, other theorists argue that utilization of health services differs from purchases of consumer goods in that it is (or at least should be) based on need rather than demand. Because need is defined by experts rather than by consumers, they further argue that those individuals receiving care are not always in the best position to make treatment decisions, for a number of reasons, including "asymmetric information."

Who Is the Decision Maker?

Consumer-directed models are often presented as an alternative to managed care, which is described as representing control by technocrats, who inhibit innovation, and instead attempt to control costs with "just say no" policies, to the detriment of both patients and providers. Others note that they also represent a rejection of agency models, whereby expert providers are expected to determine what care their patients need, in favor of models wherein the recipients of care act as the decision makers about both what care to purchase and from which providers. Consumer-directed plans are therefore justified as empowering users

of services and being linked to informed decision making. Discussion of these models is thus often associated with language speaking of patient empowerment and of putting patients in control.

Who Pays for What?

In contrast to approaches that pool risks and guarantee coverage for "necessary" services, consumer-directed models try to minimize the extent of cross-subsidization. Consumer-directed care is accordingly associated with a major shift of costs from insurers to consumers, in the form of high deductibles and co-payments; this shift is justified as necessary to make individuals act as informed consumers. In this model, insurance is reserved for catastrophic costs, with the more predictable costs expected to be covered through personal savings. To encourage that transition, governments may define minimum or maximum levels for deductibles and give preferable taxation treatment to the savings account components. Plans may also extend the range of insured benefits if they allow savings to be used for services not traditionally covered by insurance.

The Case Against

Opponents contest most of the aforementioned assumptions.

Impact of Cost Sharing on Utilization

One data source, referred to by both sides of the debate, is the RAND Health Insurance Experiment (HIE), a randomized experiment of various cost-sharing arrangements conducted between 1971 and 1982. The researchers found that cost sharing reduced the use of nearly all health services among study participants (which excluded the elderly and many of those with preexisting serious health conditions). Extrapolating these findings, proponents argue that consumer-directed care will reduce costs and increase efficiency. However, as the RAND group has itself pointed out, this reduced use of services resulted primarily from decisions not to seek out care. Once in the healthcare system, there were only modest effects on the cost of an episode of care. Cost sharing was equally likely to deter appropriate (and effective) care as to deter more marginal (ineffective) visits. In general, the reduction in services did not lead to adverse health outcomes, at least in the short run. However, there were exceptions, particularly for the poorest patients. This evoked concerns that cost sharing might deter preventive and follow-up care and ultimately lead to higher costs and worse outcomes. The experiment did not find any discernible differences in the quality of care, or in how well people took care of themselves. Patient satisfaction tended to be lower in the plans with higher cost sharing. Extrapolating these findings, opponents worry that needed care will not be received. Advocates suggest that certain services (including some preventive care) can be exempted from cost sharing requirements.

Availability of Information for Decision Making

A related set of arguments stresses agency relationships, and the difficulty of individuals attempting to be wise purchasers in areas requiring expertise. Some argue that, left to their own devices, individuals may delay receiving appropriate care. Others respond that this objection is paternalistic and can be overcome if good information is made available about costs and quality.

Adverse Selection

Another set of arguments relates to the highly skewed nature of health expenditures. As studies in the United States and Canada have confirmed, a very small proportion of individuals represent the bulk of health expenditures. The lowest spending 50% account for less than 5% of costs, and similar patterns apply within every age-sex category. Insurers have a strong incentive to avoid those individuals likely to generate high costs, a phenomenon referred to as adverse selection. Similarly, consumer-directed plans are likely to be most attractive to those with better health status. To the extent that risk pooling breaks down, these authors note that there is likely to be a negative impact on the sustainability of an insurance model, with the healthier benefiting from lower premiums, and the sick finding themselves uninsurable.

Choice

Another set of arguments relates to the meaning of patient choice. To the extent that market-based

models assume enough excess capacity to react to increases in demand, choice may be illusory. This may apply where there are not multiple potential providers, including in rural/remote areas, and for certain highly specialized services. It may also apply when individuals do not have sufficient resources to purchase care.

Empirical Results

Consumer-directed plans are relatively recent, and evaluation is therefore limited. The international evidence is mixed, with growing suggestions that they create gaps in access. In the United States, they represent a small proportion of insured individuals (about 3%) but are growing rapidly. The literature suggests a mixed picture. The empirical evidence to date suggests that the bulk of the population—which tends to be healthier—may well reduce use without adverse health effects but that already vulnerable populations (by income, and by health status) may show worse results. Because costs are so highly skewed, the overall savings are likely to be minimal and potentially offset by higher costs among those not receiving necessary care. Premiums are lower, which is to the advantage of those paying for coverage (employers or potential consumers). However, coverage is less, and out-of-pocket costs can be considerable; Bloche estimates that they can exceed $10,000 per year for families. To date, analysts have not yet found impacts on quality of care and have found that few individuals feel confident with the information available to them to date.

The Government Accountability Office Report

A 2006 review by the U.S. Government Accountability Office (GAO) surveyed early experiences with one kind of plan—Health Savings Accounts (HSAs). They found the following:

- The sorts of services covered were similar.
- Those enrolled were much more likely to have higher incomes (51% vs. 18% of all tax filers younger than age 65).
- Costs for enrollees were higher than for those enrolled in traditional (PPO) plans when extensive care was used but lower when use was low to moderate.

- Few participants researched costs before obtaining services; if consumerism were to increase, it "will likely require time, education, and improved decision support tools that provide enrollees with more information about the cost and quality of health care providers and services" (p. 30).
- "Most participants were satisfied with their HSA-eligible plan and would recommend these plans to healthy consumers but not to those who use maintenance medication, have a chronic condition, have children, or may not have the funds to meet the high deductible."

Outlook

Given ongoing problems with both access and cost control in the United States, consumer-directed health plans are likely to play a role. The extent to which they can fulfill their stated goals, however, remains unclear. More evidence is clearly needed, but to date the claims of advocates appear problematic, both in their assumptions about the nature of decision making in healthcare and about the differences between medical care and other consumer goods.

Raisa Deber

See also Decisions Faced by Patients: Primary Care; Patient Rights

Further Readings

Berk, M. L., & Monheit, A. C. (2001). The concentration of health care expenditures, revisited. *Health Affairs, 20*(2), 9–18.

Bloche, M. G. (2006). Consumer-directed health care. *New England Journal of Medicine, 355*(17), 1756–1759.

Davis, K., Doty, M. M., & Ho, A. (2005). *How high is too high? Implications of high-deductible health plans.* New York: Commonwealth Fund.

Deber, R., Forget, E., & Roos, L. (2004, October). Medical savings accounts in a universal system: Wishful thinking meets evidence. *Health Policy, 70*(1), 49–66.

Forget, E. L., Deber, R., & Roos, L. L. (2002). Medical savings accounts: Will they reduce costs? *Canadian Medical Association Journal, 167*(2), 143–147.

Herzlinger, R. E. (Ed.). (2004). *Consumer-driven care: Implications for providers, payers, and policymakers.* San Francisco: Jossey-Bass.

Jost, T. S. (2007). *Health care at risk: A critique of the consumer-driven movement.* Durham, NC: Duke University Press.

Newhouse, J. P., & The Insurance Experiment Group. (1993). *Free for all? Lessons from the RAND health insurance experiment.* Cambridge, MA: Harvard University Press.

Robinson, J. C. (2005). Managed consumerism in health care. *Health Affairs, 24*(6), 1478–1489.

U.S. Government Accountability Office. (2006). *Consumer-directed health plans: Early enrollee experiences with health savings accounts and eligible health plans.* Report to the Ranking Minority Member, Committee on Finance, U.S. Senate, August.

CONTEXT EFFECTS

Normative decision theory is often formulated to assume that decision makers have perfect information, a perfect grasp of their objectives, and the perfect ability to use that information to make uncertain decisions and further their objectives. It is common for psychologists to criticize the use of such strong assumptions as indefensible because they ignore the effects of important situational and contextual factors. In this respect, the term *context* can be defined in two distinct but conceptually related ways: (1) context as the presentation (description), or *framing*, of the decision problem, which determines how the task is conceptualized by the individual, and (2) context as the set of available choice options (e.g., in decision making under risk). Both types of context affect how the decision problem is cognitively represented by the agent, which in turn affects the outcome of the decision making process. Here, these two types of context effects are discussed separately.

Context Effects Caused by Task Framing

In these accounts, the term *context* refers to a set of facts describing a particular situation from a specific point of view. There is evidence that minor changes in the presentation or framing of risky choice problems can have dramatic impacts on choices. Such effects are failures of description invariance because different answers are elicited if decision problems are presented in different but logically equivalent forms, or contexts. A famous example of framing effects is a study by Tversky and Kahneman, in which two groups were presented with an Asian disease story and their choice was between two probabilistically equivalent medical policies—one with a certain outcome and one with a risky outcome having higher potential gain. However, the description for the first group presented the information in terms of lives saved while the information presented to the second group was in terms of lives lost. There was a striking difference in responses to these two presentations: 72% of participants preferred the first policy when it was described as lives saved, while only 22% of participants preferred this option when it was in terms of lives lost. Such failures of description invariance appear to challenge the very idea that choices can, in general, be represented by any single preference function.

Prospect theory was proposed as a psychological account of such framing effects on behavior toward risk. In this theory, choices among prospects are determined by a preference function, in which outcomes are interpreted as gains and losses relative to a reference point (e.g., status quo wealth). Empirical estimates find that losses are weighted about twice as strongly as gains, that is, the utility function is steeper for losses than for gains, which means that the disutility of losing $100 is twice the utility of gaining $100. In the Asian disease problem, when outcomes were framed as lives saved, the majority of choosers were attracted to a sure gain of lives; when framed as losses the majority rejected the sure loss of deaths, which according to the loss function hurts much more, preferring instead to take the more risky policy.

Consistent with prospect theory, the rating of different health states varying in severity is influenced by the perspective of the rater (i.e., his or her own current health relative to the rated health conditions). For example, a mild lung disease scenario and a severe one are rated differently by lung disease patients, whereas healthy nonpatients rate the two scenarios as much more similar. Because patients and nonpatients have a different status quo reference point, they have different perceptions of the same health condition. For a patient suffering from a moderately severe lung disease, a milder case of the same disease would represent a gain in health generating a steep improvement in life quality, whereas a severe case of lung disease would represent a loss in health with a steep cost in quality. In contrast, for a healthy person, both mild and severe cases of lung disease would represent a loss in health.

A similar test of the validity of prospect theory in medical context showed that hospitalization causes a decline in patients' desire for very unpleasant life-sustaining treatment (i.e., individuals express different treatment preferences when they are healthy compared with when they are ill). Thus, direct experience with the discomforts of hospitalization changed patients' attitudes about the value of extending life via aggressive medical treatment. Therefore, the task of divining a patient's "true" end-of-life wishes becomes difficult because decisions to receive life-sustaining treatment stated by healthy individuals may be particularly susceptible to contextual change.

In summary, these recent studies are examples of expanding research questioning the stability of treatment preferences over time and across changes in an individual's health condition, and the general ability of individuals to predict accurately their future feelings and behavioral choices.

Context Effects Caused by the Choice Set

A number of decision experiments have investigated the effect of the context defined in terms of the set of available options. This research draws attention to a general and pervasive feature of human cognition, which is related to how people judge the magnitudes of attributes of choice options such as utilities, payoffs, and probabilities, which are essential ingredients of every decision problem. The basic question is whether there is a cognitive ability to represent absolute cardinal scales on any magnitude, and judgments involving such magnitudes are determined solely by the context. The research is based on evidence from psychophysics and perceptual judgment, which shows that people are not able to represent the absolute magnitudes of the attributes of any stimuli, for example, light, brightness, weight, loudness, happiness, satisfaction, and so on, and instead, they represent such magnitudes on a ordinal scale purely in relation to other magnitudes. For example, people were asked to choose a tone half as loud as a comparison tone. Some people were given a set of candidate tones that included the half-as-loud tone but were mostly quiet. Another group was given a set of tones that also included the half-as-loud tone but were mostly loud. In both groups, people just selected a tone in the middle of the range, so in the quiet group people's estimates of the half loudness were much lower than in the loud group. The conclusion is that people have no real grip on absolute loudness. Other similar findings are consistent with the idea that people are unable to make reliable decontextualized judgments of absolute magnitudes.

A closely related phenomenon indicates that such psychophysical principles carry over to choice. In one study, people choose to trade off risk and return by choosing a gamble (of the form "p chance of x") from a varying range of options that was found to almost completely determine the choice. That is, people chose based not on absolute risk-return level but on the risk-return level relative to the other gamble options available. Parallel work on game playing and financial decisions found similar effects of skew and range, in line with the range-frequency theory of magnitude judgment. This pattern of responses (causing preference reversals) cannot be explained (produced) by any absolute measure of utility or related concepts such as the value-function in prospect theory and rank-dependent utility models.

Similar effects are discovered in medical decision making, in which the context of the rating task was found to influence the way participants distinguish between mild and severe scenarios. In one such study, both patients and nonpatients gave less distinct ratings to the two scenarios when each was presented in isolation than when they were presented alongside other scenarios that provided contextual information about the possible range of severity for lung disease. These results raise continuing concerns about the reliability and validity of subjective quality-of-life ratings, which appear sensitive to the particulars of the rating task. These effects are all predicted by the relativistic (contextual) judgment effects in psychophysics and risky decision making.

An extensive review of the literature also shows that people's judgments about the effectiveness of treatments and the healthcare decisions they make seem to be influenced by the different ways in which evidence from clinical trials can be presented. In particular, three different formats of data presentation have been the focus of a number of research studies: relative risk reduction, absolute risk reduction, and number of people who need to be treated to prevent one adverse event. For example, people gave higher mean ratings of a medical intervention's effectiveness when the benefits were described in terms of a relative risk reduction (34% relative decrease in the incidence of fatal and nonfatal myocardial infarction) rather than as an absolute risk reduction (1.4% decrease in the incidence of fatal and nonfatal myocardial infarction—2.5% vs. 3.9%) or a number-needed-to-treat format (77 persons must be treated for an average of just over 5 years to prevent one fatal or nonfatal myocardial infarction). This tendency is a robust finding across respondents (physicians, health professionals, patients, and the general public) and medical domains. These results can be explained by the relativistic account presented above. Due to a lack of stable underlying scales, people use the lower and upper bounds of 0% (the worst treatment available) and 100% (the best treatment available) of the probability scale as some sort of natural reference scale to map onto when they evaluate the attractiveness of something. Thus, both the relative and absolute risk reductions are evaluated with reference to the same 0% to 100% scale (and usually the former is bigger than the latter as in the example above). The number-needed-to-treat format presents an unbound psychological scale without natural upper limit on that number, and hence 1 out of 77 does not sound as convincing as 34% out of 100%. Similar effects are found in the marketing literature on price perception, where price reductions presented as percentages (save 10%) have stronger effect than amounts (save $3).

Implications

The accumulated evidence suggests that decision making is fundamentally context-dependent and judgments of the value of choice options are context-specific. The implications of this cognitive limit in medicine and public policy are serious, because they strike at the central methodologies used to measure preferences. Popular methods such as functional measurement and conjoint analysis measure trade-offs by asking respondents for attractiveness ratings of stimuli (e.g., policies) consisting of pairs of attributes (e.g., a reduction of x% in the annual risk of death for $y). Ratings of this sort are useful if the trade-offs are independent of what other options are available. Such rationally irrelevant contextual factors are, for example, the range of values on each attribute within the session. Thus, if policy makers judge that a decrease from 20% to 15% in the annual risk of death is worth an expenditure increase from 10% to 30% of the medical (healthcare) budget, then this should be true regardless of whether the range of available expenditure options is from $10 million to $30 million or from $1 million to $100 million. Utility should depend on what happens (i.e., the actual outcomes in terms of 5% risk reduction and $20 million expenditure increase), not what options were considered. However, such independence is often not found and depends on various contextual factors. Therefore, professionals practicing medical decision making should be aware of such context effects to minimize the detrimental impact on clinical outcomes.

Ivo Vlaev

See also Attraction Effect; Bias; Contextual Error; Decision Psychology; Hedonic Prediction and Relativism; Heuristics

Further Readings

Covey, J. (2007). A meta-analysis of the effects of presenting treatment benefits in different formats. *Medical Decision Making, 27*, 638–654.

Ditto, P. H., Jacobson, J. A., Smucker, W. D., Danks, J. H., & Fagerlin, A. (2006). Context changes choices: A prospective study of the effects of hospitalization on life-sustaining treatment preferences. *Medical Decision Making, 26*, 313–332.

Kahneman, D., & Tversky, A. (Eds.). (2000). *Choices, values and frames.* New York: Cambridge University Press.

Lacy, H. P., Fagerlin, A., Loewenstein, G., Smith, D. M., Riis, J., & Ubel, P. A. (2006). It must be awful for them: Perspective and task context affects ratings for health conditions. *Judgment and Decision Making, 1*, 146–152.

Stewart, N., Chater, N., & Brown, G. D. A. (2006). Decision by sampling. *Cognitive Psychology, 53*, 1–26.

CONTEXTUAL ERROR

Overlooking contextual information in the process of medical decision making can have predictable and avoidable adverse effects as significant as those that result from overlooking biomedical signs of a pathophysiologic condition. The failure, for instance, to recognize that a patient is not able to take a medication correctly (e.g., because of cognitive disabilities or cost) may have the same consequences as the failure to prescribe the medication correctly. While the latter type of error has been termed a diagnostic or medication error, the former is designated a *contextual error*.

Contextual Error Versus Biomedical Error

According to the Institute of Medicine (IOM), misguided clinical decision making or care delivery rises to the level of medical error when it results in either a wrong plan to achieve an aim (i.e., error of planning) or the failure of a planned action to be completed as intended (i.e., error of execution). Errors may be due either to failures to elicit essential information during the clinical encounter or, if elicited, to recognize the significance of essential information when formulating or implementing a plan of care.

Medical errors may be classified as contextual when they occur because of inattention to processes expressed outside the boundaries of a patient's skin (i.e., to processes that are part of the context of a patient's illness). They are distinguishable from biomedical errors, which are due to inattention to biomedical processes (i.e., to processes that occur within the patient). For instance, treating poor glucose control in a diabetic with metformin is a biomedical error if the patient has concomitant severe diabetic kidney disease because metformin can cause lactic acidosis in patients with poor renal function. Insulin is an acceptable alternative. On the other hand, prescribing self-administered insulin is a contextual error if the patient's poor control is due to dementia because dementia renders this approach unreliable and unsafe. Note that although dementia has biomedical origins, it is its expression outside the skin in the actions (or inactions) of the patient that are relevant here. It is a part of the context of his or her diabetes management.

Figure 1 presents a framework for comparing contextual error with biomedical error, organized according to failures to elicit or incorporate clinically significant information and to the IOM's classification of medical error. Consider, for instance, examples of mechanisms B1 and C1: Overlooking signs of congestive heart failure in an asthmatic patient who is short of breath, unaware that he or she also has heart disease, is due to "incorrect/incomplete biomedical information." Overlooking medication nonadherence in a patient who is failing to respond to a medical therapy, unaware he or she is uninsured, is due to "incorrect/incomplete contextual information." Although one is a biomedical oversight and the other a contextual one, both cognitive processes lead to errors of planning in the IOM framework.

A typology of error that includes contextual error also illustrates the interdependence of biomedical and contextual information: Note that in mechanisms B2 and C2, biomedical and contextual information each determine whether the other is correctly processed. For example, attributing weakness to a patient's congestive heart failure, unaware that he or she fears exercising after his or her heart attack, represents "overlooking contextual information because of an incorrect biomedical explanation" (C2). Conversely, disregarding signs of dementia in a patient who is not taking his or her medication correctly, assuming he or she is

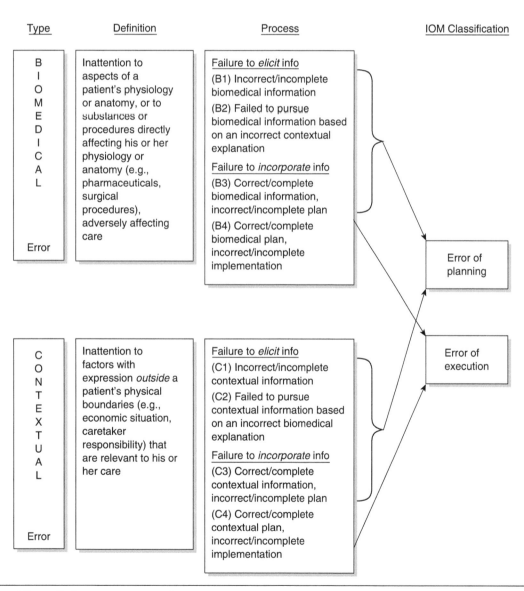

Figure 1   Biomedical versus contextual error

just not interested in complying with the recommended treatment plan, represents "overlooking biomedical information because of an incorrect contextual explanation" (B2).

B3 and C3 errors occur when correctly elicited information (biomedical or contextual) is not incorporated into the care plan. Finally, B4 and C4 pertain to errors in the implementation process. They represent errors of execution, per the IOM definition.

The problems caused by contextual and biomedical errors are remarkably similar. Problems caused by biomedical error have been classified as overuse, misuse, or underuse of medical services. Contextual errors may be classified similarly. For instance, overlooking poor medication adherence leads to overprescribing of additional medication. Sending a patient for elective surgery when he or she is unable to care for himself or herself postoperatively and lacks social support constitutes misuse. And not recognizing when an elder patient warrants evaluation for driving safety results in underuse of services.

Contextual Reasoning and Cognition

Contextualizing care requires cognitive skills distinct from those applied to biomedical decision making. Whereas biomedical reasoning classifies patients into known categories for which there are specific therapies, contextualized decision making explores how they differ from others with similar conditions in ways that require individualized care. Identifying when a diabetic patient with poor glucose control requires the addition of a second medication based on American Diabetes Association guidelines reflects the former; unmasking that the problem is, instead, poor medication adherence related to a diminishing capacity for self-care reflects the latter.

Categorization is generally arrived at through hypothesis testing: During an encounter, the clinician suspects that a patient has a particular condition that requires an accepted approach to care. The hypothesis is tested through clinical or laboratory examination. The process of reducing uncertainty continues until the patient falls into a sufficiently discrete category to prompt initiation of a specific therapy. Such an approach is essentially algorithmic.

The challenge of contextualization is in then discovering from the infinite complexity of the patient's life that which is unique to his or her life situation and relevant to the considered plan of care. As such, it requires moving from a deductive to a theory building approach to clinical reasoning in which unique elements of a patient's life are uncovered and assessed for clinical relevance. It involves a transition from asking "How is this patient similar to others?" to "How are they different?" Having asked and answered the question "Does this patient have diabetes?" one is now asking "Is there anything special about this individual's situation that is relevant to their diabetes management?"

Avoiding contextual errors requires considering contextual factors essential to planning patient care. Broadly these factors have been grouped into 10 categories to consider for each patient: cognitive abilities, emotional state, cultural beliefs, spiritual beliefs, access to care, social support, caretaker responsibilities, attitude toward illness, relationship with healthcare providers, and economic situation. Such factors may or may not have contextual relevance, depending on their relationship to the clinical problem. Simply getting to know a patient is not the objective here; rather, it is understanding how his or her life situation relates to his or her care.

When contextual factors are identified in the course of evaluating a clinical problem, they should prompt further inquiry. For instance, in the setting of deteriorating medication adherence, the clinician might ask of a patient with progressive dementia, "Is she still capable of taking these medications correctly?" If the context is economic, the question could be "Should I choose another medication because of the cost?" For social support, one might ask, "Now that he is weaker, will his wife still be able to care for him at home?" For spiritual beliefs, "Could her minister help her reach a decision?" The goal of these questions is not to place the patient into a predefined category for which there is a preconceived solution. Rather they are to unmask the particulars of a patient's life situation, pointing the way to an individualized plan of care.

Identifying Contextual Errors

The first challenge to identifying contextual errors is defining them. For many medical errors *res ipsa loquitur*, "the thing speaks for itself." If a surgeon operates on the wrong limb or a pediatrician over-looks laboratory evidence of a serious infection in a newborn, there can be little disputing that an error occurred. It may be less clear when a physician's inattention to contextual factors also constitutes a medical error.

A second challenge is finding them. Many medical errors can be discerned from record reviews and incident reports. Contextual errors, however, rarely leave a footprint. The problem is that such errors are, by definition, errors only in a particular context. That context is the patient's life situation, and, if the error occurred, the relevant contextual factors were likely overlooked or their significance unrecognized and undocumented. Hence it is not feasible to identify the presence or absence of contextual errors by examining the medical record. For instance, two patients with a history of atrial fibrillation on warfarin may both meet evidence-based guidelines for anticoagulation; however, one of them may also have contextual contraindications such as transportation difficulties that compromise safe monitoring of the medication, a process that requires frequent blood draws. The clinician who did not attend to the transportation problems is also unlikely to have documented them.

It may not therefore be possible to define and identify contextual errors in clinical practice. An alternative, however, is an experimental rather than observational approach: Rather than looking for errors, one can create simulated situations where errors could occur and then see whether and how often they do. Current research employs incognito or unannounced, standardized patients (USPs) to present as if they are real patients in physician practices with scripted cases embedded with contextual information that is essential to care. If the provider fails to incorporate the contextually relevant factors into the plan of care, he or she will cause a medical error. Since the patient is only an actor, no real harm is done.

A critical component of the method is a protocol for validating each case as an instrument for assessing physician performance at contextualizing care: First a script is drafted based on a real scenario in which contextual factors seem essential to planning appropriate care. Then the narrative is presented to board certified clinicians with content expertise who are randomly assigned to review the text either with or without the critical contextual information. For instance, if the case involves unexplained weight loss in an impoverished homeless man, 10 reviewers are informed that the patient had inadequate access to food and the other 10 are not given this information. Both groups are told that all clinically relevant information has been provided and each clinician is instructed to propose appropriate care. The contextual information (i.e., inadequate access to food) is confirmed as clinically essential when all reviewers with the information propose an alternate plan from those without it. None of the reviewers may confer with one another about the cases. A case is considered validated when the two groups are internally consistent but 100% discordant in their recommended plans of care.

The use of standardized patients and validated cases addresses the challenges of defining and identifying contextual errors outlined above. Such an approach also enables comparison of physician performance across multiple providers in the same discipline. Standardized patients are intrinsically risk-adjusted in that every physician sees the same subject with the same narrative, providing an equivalent and objective standard for comparing practicing physicians.

Preventing Contextual Errors in Medical Decision Making

Considering psychosocial factors in the process of planning care is, of course, not new. In his seminal writing on the biopsychosocial model, George Engel introduced general systems theory as a framework for broadening the biomedical perspective to include social, psychological, and behavioral dimensions. In subsequent writing, he illustrated how perturbations in biomedical and psychosocial systems affect one another. Engel's model has stimulated many projects to define and describe the medical interview in a manner that incorporates psychosocial and biomedical elements into patient care. What has been missing, however, is a benchmark and metric for assessing how well clinicians perform at contextualizing or individualizing care. Contextual error is a discrete phenomenon that reflects the failure of the clinician to adequately integrate psychosocial with biomedical aspects of patient care.

With a metric it becomes possible to identify physician and practice characteristics that are associated with contextual error making and to test interventions that may prevent it. Empirical research is limited but evolving. One recent pilot study of standardized patients and internal medicine residents demonstrated that about two thirds of clinicians in training made contextual errors involving cases with common ambulatory complaints when contextual information was essential to medical decision making. Remarkably, over half were due not to failures to elicit the information but to failures to incorporate it into the plan of care. Obtaining basic knowledge of how and why contextual errors occur should be invaluable to any subsequent effort to prevent their occurrence and ultimately improve patient outcomes.

Saul J. Weiner

See also Clinical Algorithms and Practice Guidelines; Cognitive Psychology and Processes; Medical Errors and Errors in Healthcare Delivery

Further Readings

Engel, G. L. (1977). The need for a new medical model: A challenge for biomedicine. *Science, 196*(4286), 1130.

Kohn, L. T., Corrigan, J. M., & Donaldson, M. S. (Eds.). (2000). *To err is human: Building a safer health system*. Washington, DC: Institute of Medicine, National Academy Press.

Weiner, S. J. (2004). Contextualizing medical decisions to individualize care: Lessons from the qualitative sciences. *Journal of General Internal Medicine, 19,* 281–285.

Weiner, S. J. (2004). From research evidence to context: The challenge of individualizing care. *ACP Journal Club, 141,* A11.

Weiner, S. J., Barnet, B., Cheng, T. L., & Daaleman, T. P. (2005). Processes for effective communication in primary care. *Annals of Internal Medicine, 142,* 709–714.

Weiner, S. J., Schwartz, A., Yudkowsky, R., Schiff, G. D., Weaver, F. M., Goldberg, J., et al. (2007). Evaluating physician performance at individualizing care: A pilot study tracking contextual errors in medical decision making. *Medical Decision Making, 27*(6), 726–734.

CONTINGENT VALUATION

Contingent valuation (CV) is a survey-based method to derive monetary values for the benefits of goods that are not available for purchase in the market. It specifies a hypothetical market whereupon the provision of the good is contingent on the respondent's maximum willingness to pay (WTP) for it (or, in a minority of cases, the minimum compensation they are willing to accept to be deprived of it). A hypothetical market is the construction, specification, and presentation of the imagined scenario on which respondents value the nonmarketed good. Individual values are aggregated to arrive at an overall societal value of the good. This value can then be compared with the societal cost of providing the good, in a cost-benefit analysis.

Why the Interest?

Interest in CV reflects dissatisfaction with other outcome measures, especially quality-adjusted life years (QALYs), in two principal respects. First, QALYs are based on preferences for *health outcomes* only, whereas CV imposes no restriction on which attributes of a program generate value, encompassing (a) health outcomes, including health state, duration, and probability; (b) other attributes, related to the process of care; (c) maintaining the good as an option for future consumption rather than for current consumption (option value); and (d) obtaining satisfaction from others, in addition to or rather than oneself consuming the good (externalities). Second, CV values benefits in the same unit as costs. This is required to assess whether the good represents an overall benefit in absolute terms (allocative efficiency), rather than a benefit relative to another option (technical efficiency). However, the reality is that few CV studies achieve these advantages in practice. Most studies use current patients, so they tend to capture only health outcomes, and few studies use their results to perform a cost-benefit analysis. The theoretical superiority of CV is thus seldom realized in practice.

How Has Contingent Valuation Developed?

CV has been used extensively in transport and environmental economics since the 1960s. It was first applied to healthcare in the mid-1970s, but only a handful of studies were completed before the late 1980s. The development of CV in health economics was led by researchers in the United

States, the United Kingdom, Canada, and Sweden, largely focused on cardiovascular disease. Since 2000, CV studies have been conducted in 35 countries, covering a vast range of diseases and interventions, although the single largest number of applications has been for pharmaceutical interventions (33%). However, CV studies remain rare, with only 265 studies published (as of December 31, 2005) compared with more than 35,000 other forms of economic evaluation on the OHE Health Economic Evaluation database.

Why So Few Studies?

Contingent valuation studies are incredibly complex, difficult, time-consuming, and costly to do well. This is because such studies face a number of methodological issues, for instance, framing effects (how the scenario is described), scale or scope biases (where WTP values are insensitive to the size or range of benefits described), payment vehicle and mode effects (where WTP values are affected by the payment method, e.g., taxation, out-of-pocket payment, or insurance) and payment frequency (e.g., weekly, monthly, or annually), and question order effects (where question order can affect results). These issues can be dealt with through adequate specification and administration of the market so that incentives to answer honestly are maximized. However, the issue of hypothetical bias, where respondents who do not actually have to part with money may state unrealistic valuations, may still be an issue even in a well-designed study since few opportunities exist to test this in practice in healthcare.

The most critical component is the specification and administration of the hypothetical market itself. *Specification* refers to, among other things, detailed information on the health problem, specifying the (attributes of the) good valued, determining the appropriate payment vehicle, how any element of uncertainty will be presented (as individuals are generally not risk-neutral), the relevant time period for valuation (which provides the foundation for the respondent's budget constraint), and the questionnaire format. This last aspect is especially controversial, and there remains considerable debate over the relative benefits of the five principal elicitation formats: (1) *open-ended,* where respondents are asked directly for their maximum

WTP; (2) *bidding,* where respondents who accept or reject a given amount are bid up or down until maximum WTP is achieved; (3) *payment card* (or *categorical scales*), where a specified range of values is presented and respondents are asked to indicate which they would pay; (4) *dichotomous choice,* where respondents are presented with a single WTP value that they either accept or reject; and (5) *multibounded* dichotomous choice, where a single-bound dichotomous-choice question is followed with subsequent questions. The greatest difference is between the former three and latter two formats, where these surveys require different subsamples to be offered different values and logistic regression to be used to estimate the societal WTP.

Values drawn from a CV survey are determined by the characteristics of the hypothetical market specified, as above, as well as the characteristics of the respondent (preferences and income). The key to ensuring that only the latter varies is to undertake behavioral, rather than attitudinal, surveys. Behavioral surveys generate values that, although hypothetical, are substantive rather than formal and require a clearly defined market. This requires researchers to give detailed thought to what and how information is presented to respondents in the survey.

Administration of the hypothetical market refers to the use of face-to-face interview, remote interview (usually by telephone), and self-complete questionnaires (typically postal). In determining the mode of administration to be used, there is a balance to be struck between three factors: (1) the response rate (nonresponse is problematic if the sample not responding is likely to have a significantly different WTP compared with those who did respond); (2) the perceived validity of results (generally that a respondent's WTP will be more valid where respondents are encouraged to consider carefully the questions and their answers); and (3) the cost of the survey. Face-to-face interviews are overwhelmingly recommended to address points 1 and 2 but are very costly, and in health economics other methods are more typically used.

Analysis of results is also complex, particularly ensuring validity and reliability. *Validity* refers to the correspondence between what one wishes to measure and what is actually measured. Ideally validity is determined by comparing the measurement of interest to another measurement that is, a priori, known to be correct (criterion validity)—in this case some form of market value is usually taken to be this external gold standard, reflecting the amount the individual would actually pay. Unfortunately, such a market value with which CV measurements can be compared rarely exists—which is the reason for conducting the CV survey, of course. Research has thus mostly looked to two different approaches to infer validity: construct validity (how well the measurement is predicted by factors that one would expect to be predictive a priori, e.g., that WTP is positively associated with income) and convergent validity (how comparable the values are from two different techniques for the measurement of a phenomenon, such as comparing the implied WTP ranking with ordinal ranking). *Reliability* refers to the reproducibility and stability of a measure. This may be cross-sectional (i.e., results are replicable when administered to independent samples) or temporal (i.e., results are stable when administered to the same sample at two different points in time). The first measure of reliability concerns the reliability of the measurement instrument itself—the instrument obtains the same information on repeated samples. The latter is a measure of the reliability of the WTP values themselves, commonly assessed using the test-retest method, where an initial sample of respondents is later reinterviewed using the same survey instrument. It is the latter that is important for policy purposes.

Although these issues should have been considered throughout the design and development of the study, surprisingly little work has been undertaken in these areas with respect to the use of CV in healthcare.

How Useful Is Contingent Valuation?

The ultimate purpose of conducting CV studies is to assist in medical decision making. However, there is a significant method-policy gap. While studies are increasingly being undertaken, most do not combine CV values with cost, so that a cost-benefit analysis cannot be undertaken. Furthermore, CV values themselves are not comparable due to considerable heterogeneity of methods.

In addition to incorporating cost information with CV studies, an obvious step in tackling the heterogeneity of methods is the development of guidelines. Such an agenda has already been applied in the cost-per-QALY arena, with conventions widely known and used. The closest steps made toward this in CV for health economics have been the five recommendations, made by Richard Smith, that need to be met by good-quality CV studies (response rate, association between WTP and socioeconomic status, sensitivity of WTP to scale and scope of the good, predictive validity, and reliability of elicitation methods), although even if these were met, studies could still fall short of providing the information needed to actually use the values elicited.

An objection to the development of guidelines could be the continued uncertainty around "best practice." However, guidelines for QALY studies were proposed despite methodological uncertainties. While it might be argued that uncertainties surrounding CV studies are larger, and that medical decision-making researchers actually want guidelines for cost-benefit studies rather than CV studies, it would still improve the usefulness of values elicited if methods were common because, relative to another value elicited using the same methods, researchers could infer the degree to which preferences were stronger or weaker. Such an approach need not hinder divergences from the guidelines for further methodological research to be undertaken; guidelines simply impose a constraint to include specific minimum design but do not preclude the use of other approaches or perspectives within the same study.

An alternative viewpoint is that CV is just not up to the job of informing cost-benefit analyses in healthcare (for the reasons mentioned) and therefore should not be used. However, such an opinion might accept the technique as very good at representing the public's intensity of preferences if one accepts the fact that people are familiar with the money metric used. Therefore, while CV should not be used to decide which alternative intervention to provide, it could be used to determine which of the alternative interventions the public really do prefer. Such an approach suggests a very limited and specific role for CV. Proponents of this approach may draw on the fact that results from CV studies are specific to the prevailing income distribution, such that if the current income distribution is not deemed equitable, then the results of CV may well overrepresent the interests of the most affluent in society.

Contingent valuation as applied in health economics is still experimental. Most studies fall far short of the requirements and recommendations in transport and environmental economics, and yet there has been no systematic evaluation of the specific developments that may be required in healthcare to justify such divergences from accepted practice in these other areas. Contingent valuation, and even more so full cost-benefit studies, remain rare in health economics, and their results are not comparable. Without the development of guidelines for the conduct of CV in healthcare, CV holds much unfulfilled promise.

Richard D. Smith and Tracey H. Sach

See also Cost-Benefit Analysis; Cost-Effectiveness Analysis; Cost-Utility Analysis; Discounting; Willingness to Pay

Further Readings

Bateman, I., Carson, R. T., Day, B., Hanemann, W. M., Hanley, N., Hett, T., et al. (2002). *Economic valuation with stated preferences techniques: A manual.* Cheltenham, UK: Edward Elgar.

Drummond, M. F., Sculpher, M. J., Torrance, G. W., O'Brien, B. J., & Stoddart, G. L. (2005). *Methods for the economic evaluation of health care programmes* (3rd ed., chap. 7). Oxford, UK: Oxford University Press.

Olsen, J. A., & Smith, R. D. (2001). Theory versus practice: A review of "willingness-to-pay" in health and health care. *Health Economics, 10,* 39–52.

Sach, T. H., Smith, R. D., & Whynes, D. K. (2007). A "league table" of contingent valuation results for pharmaceutical interventions: A hard pill to swallow? *PharmacoEconomics, 25,* 107–127.

Smith, R. D. (2003). Construction of the contingent valuation market in health care: A critical assessment. *Health Economics, 12,* 609–628.

COST-BENEFIT ANALYSIS

Cost-benefit analysis is a form of economic evaluation that can be used to assess the value in terms of money of healthcare interventions. In contrast with cost-effectiveness analysis and cost-utility analysis, which were developed specifically for the healthcare field, cost-benefit analysis has a long history of use in economics and is particularly linked to the theory of welfare economics. Its link with economic theory has led to some favoring this form of evaluation as the "correct" approach to problems of resource allocation in health systems, although it is worthy of note that other commentators have argued that the cost-utility analysis embodies its own theoretical properties and have coined the term *extrawelfarism* to counter the suggestion that only cost-benefit analysis has a grounding in economic theory.

The characterizing feature of cost-benefit analysis is the measurement of costs and benefits in the same units. In practice, this almost always means that the benefits are measured in monetary terms. For many noneconomists, the concept of placing a monetary value on health, and indeed on life itself, has seemed anathema. Indeed, this apparent aversion to monetary quantification of health outcomes explains the relative infrequency of the use of cost-benefit analysis in health economic evaluation, and the relative popularity of alternative evaluative forms such as cost-effectiveness and cost-utility analysis.

Nevertheless, advocates of the cost-benefit approach have continued to develop methods for the monetary valuation of health outcomes. Many early cost-benefit analyses were based on the human capital approach, which takes the (discounted) stream of lifetime earnings for an individual as a valuation of life. However, this approach implies a zero value for individuals outside formal paid employment and has become less used in recent years. More popular are *stated preference* methods that involve subjects responding to questions concerning their willingness to pay for health outcomes. When subjects are asked to reveal their willingness to pay for health outcomes directly, this is known as the *contingent valuation* approach. As with any method of preference elicitation, how such questions are framed can have important consequences for how a subject responds. However, the problems of framing effects and "protest" responses (where a respondent refuses to answer a question or gives a null value) seem particularly acute in contingent valuation of health outcomes. This may explain why much recent research has been based on using a class of methods known as *discrete choice experiments* that estimate preferences for different attributes at different levels using a series of dichotomous choices across a carefully chosen choice set. When one of the attributes is cost, it is possible to generate indirect estimates of willingness to pay for the other attributes in the experiment. By specifying a profile of levels of the attributes associated with a health state or treatment under consideration it is possible to estimate a monetary value of that health state or treatment.

One of the problems associated with stated preference methods is the danger that respondents overstate their willingness to pay due to the hypothetical nature of the question. That is, if they really had to pay, it is likely that we would observe a lower willingness to pay for the health state or treatment under consideration. In general, *revealed preference,* where willingness to pay is estimated from observed actions in the marketplace, is preferred to stated preference methods. However, the opportunity for revealed preference studies in the healthcare field, where patients rarely pay for their own healthcare, is limited. One example where revealed preference has been used is in studies of behavior regarding radon gas remediation measures taken by households. Radon gas is a naturally occurring phenomenon that is associated with an increased risk of lung cancer and occurs in geographical areas where the geology of the area has a high proportion of granite in the bedrock. Since radon is heavier than air, the simple installation of a sump pump in low-lying areas, such as basements, can reduce the risk of lung cancer. Therefore, the willingness to pay at the household level for such remedial measures can be used to infer the willingness to pay for a reduced risk of lung cancer.

The measurement of both costs and benefits in monetary terms encourages the use of a net-benefit approach to decision making, whereby if a program's benefits exceed its costs, the program should be implemented. Indeed, the ability of cost-benefit analysis to make this comparison is argued by advocates of the approach to be one of its major advantages over other evaluative approaches. Nevertheless, notwithstanding the issues surrounding overestimating in stated preference techniques, many health systems work within a fixed budget for healthcare. In the face of a fixed budgetary constraint, efficient allocation of resources requires the prioritization of programs to be implemented in terms of their cost-benefit ratio rather than simply the condition that benefits exceed costs. From this perspective, the cost-benefit approach to resource allocation is similar to that when *cost-utility analysis* is employed.

Much debate has taken place over whether cost-benefit and cost-utility approaches are formally equivalent, in particular when a monetary value is placed on the quality-adjusted life year (QALY) in cost-utility analysis since this allows net-benefit analysis in monetary terms. The remaining difference between the approaches goes back to the theoretical foundations of cost-benefit analysis in terms of welfare economics. The cost-benefit approach assumes *consumer sovereignty,* that is, the principle that the individual is the best judge of his or her own welfare and it is therefore the individual's values that count. It is reasonable to ask whether this is generally true in healthcare, where there is an asymmetry of information between the physician and the patient regarding the consequences of healthcare intervention. It might be argued, therefore, that cost-benefit analysis in healthcare might work better in those situations where patients have more experience (e.g., visits to the dentist, frequently occurring and more minor problems such as infections and colds, and some chronic conditions such as asthma) and less well for infrequent and more severe problems where patients have little experience (e.g., life-threatening experiences such as cancer treatment).

Andrew H. Briggs

See also Contingent Valuation; Cost-Effectiveness Analysis; Cost-Utility Analysis; Discrete Choice; Economics, Health Economics; Human Capital Approach; Monetary Value; Net Monetary Benefit; Welfare, Welfarism, and Extrawelfarism; Willingness to Pay

Further Readings

Drummond, M. F., Sculpher, M. J., Torrance, G. W., O'Brien, B. J., & Stoddart, G. L. (2005). *Methods for the economic evaluation of health care programmes* (3rd ed.). Oxford, UK: Oxford University Press.

Gold, M. R., Siegel, J. E., Russell, L. B., & Weinstein, M. C. (Eds.). (1996). *Cost-effectiveness in health and medicine.* New York: Oxford University Press.

COST-COMPARISON ANALYSIS

A cost-comparison analysis estimates the total costs of two or more interventions, including downstream costs, and the numbers of individuals affected by each intervention but does not estimate cost-effectiveness ratios relative to health outcomes. This approach was developed in the early 1970s as a method of cost accounting with specific applications to ascertaining the lowest-cost methods of pharmacologic dosing and laboratory testing. An assumption that is usually either explicit or implicit in such analyses is that health outcomes are comparable across interventions. Otherwise, the lowest-cost strategy would not necessarily be desirable.

A cost-comparison analysis, which is also commonly referred to as a cost-consequences analysis, is less demanding to perform because it does not require clinical or epidemiologic data on health outcomes, such as long-term morbidity or mortality, although short-term clinical outcomes or healthcare use are typically reported. This approach is attractive in assessing interventions for which it is difficult to ascertain ultimate health outcomes or to calculate summary measures of health that integrate multiple outcomes. The cost-comparison approach is particularly well-suited to assessing screening and diagnostic-testing strategies. It is typical for such analyses to report summary cost ratios, such as cost per individual tested or cost per case detected, for each strategy, as well as incremental cost ratios for pairwise comparisons.

The time horizon, or the period during which healthcare utilization and costs are included in the analysis, is variable for cost-comparison (or cost-consequences) studies. For analyses of pharmacological or surgical interventions, the time horizon that is used is typically quite short, often 12 months to several years from the time of intervention. On the other hand, cost-comparison analyses of genetic testing strategies typically project the costs of monitoring tested individuals over their remaining lifetimes, which can be 40 years or more.

Most published cost-comparison analyses are conducted from the perspective of a healthcare system and only include direct medical costs. However, it is also valuable to calculate cost-comparison analyses from the societal perspective and to include costs occurring outside the healthcare system. Costs of time spent by patients and family members are important to include for interventions requiring substantial time by individuals and relatives. The exclusion of such costs can make such interventions appear more cost-effective than they are. In particular, if one is interested in comparing the actual costs of clinic-based and home-based therapeutic or rehabilitative strategies from a societal perspective, it is essential to include the costs of unpaid or informal caregiving services.

Prior to the mid-1990s, clear distinctions were generally made between cost-comparison, cost-minimization, and cost-consequence analyses. Since then, differences among these methods have become blurred, and articles using them frequently overlap one another. A given analysis that reports or assumes equivalent outcomes of different interventions might be labeled as a cost-comparison analysis, cost-consequence(s) analysis, cost-minimization analysis, or even cost-effectiveness analysis, depending on the preferences of the authors. Consequently, readers should not assume that the terminology used to describe such studies necessarily corresponds to differences in the analytic methods employed. Originally, cost-comparison analyses reported data only on costs, not on outcomes; cost-minimization analyses reported on costs only after ascertaining that health outcomes were equivalent for the interventions being compared; and cost-consequence analyses reported both costs and health outcomes but did not explicitly compare the two in terms of ratios (to let decision makers decide which information is needed to draw inferences).

Cost-comparison analyses differ from a cost-effectiveness or cost-utility analysis because they do not require a summary measure of health such as QALYs or number of symptom-free days to capture health gains. In addition to requiring less data, comparisons that are restricted to financial measures are often easier for healthcare payers and decision makers to understand and appreciate. If the costs included are restricted to short- or medium-term costs incurred within a single healthcare system or paid by a single payer, such a cost-comparison analysis can also be classified as a budget impact analysis, a business case analysis, or a return on investment analysis.

Many studies that report one intervention to be comparably effective but less costly than another appear to have begun as standard cost-effectiveness or cost-utility analyses. It is likely that after investigators were unable to establish that one intervention was significantly more effective than another in preventing morbidity or mortality, they focused on showing that one particular intervention might be cost-saving. Rather than reflecting an a priori difference in study goals or analytic methods, as is assumed in textbook discussions of cost-consequence analyses, such studies likely indicate an absence of evidence of incremental effectiveness. If one intervention had been found to be more effective, incremental cost-effectiveness ratios would in most cases have been calculated and reported.

A sensitivity analysis allows one to determine the robustness of conclusions with regard to a decision rule. In a cost-comparison analysis that reports that an intervention is cost-saving, a sensitivity analysis can determine the extent to which variation in parameters affects the likelihood of the intervention being cost-saving. Although it is recommended that all economic evaluations include sensitivity analyses, not all cost-comparison analyses do so. This depends on the intended audience and the professional background of the investigators.

Scott D. Grosse

Disclaimer: The findings and conclusions in this entry are those of the author and do not necessarily represent the official position of the Centers for Disease Control and Prevention.

See also Cost-Consequence Analysis; Cost-Minimization Analysis

Further Readings

Bapat, B., Noorani, H., Cohen, Z., Berk, T., Mitri, A., Gallie, B., et al. (1999). Cost comparison of predictive genetic testing versus conventional clinical screening for familial adenomatous polyposis. *Gut, 44,* 698–703.

Koopmanschap, M. A., van Exel, J. N., van den Berg, B., & Brouwer, W. B. (2008). An overview of methods and applications to value informal care in economic evaluations of healthcare. *PharmacoEconomics, 26,* 269–280.

Naslund, M., Eaddy, M. T., Kruep, E. J., & Hogue, S. L. (2008). Cost comparison of finasteride and dutasteride for enlarged prostate in a managed care setting among Medicare-aged men. *American Journal of Managed Care, 14,* S167–S171.

Newman, W. G., Hamilton, S., Ayres, J., Sanghera, N., Smith, A., Gaunt, L., et al. (2007). Array comparative genomic hybridization for diagnosis of developmental delay: An exploratory cost-consequences analysis. *Clinical Genetics, 71,* 254–259.

Papakonstantinou, V. V., Kaitelidou, D., Gkolfinopoulou, K. D., Siskou, O. C., Papapolychroniou, T., Baltopoulos, P., et al. (2008). Extracapsular hip fracture management: Cost-consequences analysis of two alternative operative methods. *International Journal of Technology Assessment in Health Care, 24,* 221–227.

COST-CONSEQUENCE ANALYSIS

A cost-consequence analysis (CCA) requires an estimation of the costs as well as the health consequences and other consequences associated with one intervention compared with an alternative intervention for a health condition; these estimates then are presented in a disaggregated tabular or graphical format. This type of analysis has been described in texts on economic evaluation of new healthcare interventions. However, it is generally mentioned only briefly and categorized as either a formal or an informal variant of a cost-effectiveness analysis (CEA).

Types

When a CCA is performed as a variant of a CEA, it takes an incidence-based perspective and estimates the costs and consequences for an individual or disease cohort for as long as the health condition lasts. However, a CCA also can be performed from a prevalence-based perspective, where the costs and consequences of alternative mixes of interventions can be compared over a 1-year time frame for a population with the condition of interest. This type of analysis is an expanded version of a budget impact analysis (BIA). Health and other consequences of the alternative mixes of interventions are presented annually for the population, as are the costs, which are aggregated by cost category.

Since a single overall number is not generated as a result of a CCA, the perspective does not have to be chosen by the analyst. The perspective of a CCA should be as broad as possible, since the user of the analysis should be able to view a comprehensive listing of the various costs and consequences of alternative interventions. The user then can choose which variables are relevant for their perspective and can ignore the others.

Time Horizon

The time horizon for a CCA should be chosen in the same way as the time horizon for the CEA, the cost-utility analysis (CUA), or the BIA. For an incidence-based CCA, the time horizon will vary, depending on the health condition and the type of intervention, as shown in Figure 1. The duration of the impact of the intervention on the individual with the health condition is the primary determinant of the appropriate time horizon, with acute nonfatal illness requiring a shorter time horizon and chronic or fatal illness requiring up to a lifetime time horizon. Whether or not a healthcare intervention is for prevention or treatment also is a determinant of the appropriate time horizon for the analysis. For a prevalence-based CCA, the chosen time horizon should be relevant to the decision maker. Typically, annualized costs and consequences for 1 to 5 years after a change in treatment patterns is the most relevant time horizon.

Scope

As with other types of economic evaluation, the question of scope of the analysis is important: For example, with interventions that affect life expectancy, should the costs and consequences of alternative interventions include their impact only on condition-related outcomes, or should the impact on healthcare costs and outcomes for other conditions be considered? Generally, costs and consequences for unrelated health conditions are not considered in economic evaluations. Also, which specific costs and consequences should be included is less restricted in a CCA than in a typical CEA or CUA. For a CCA, outcomes may be included that are not typically part of a CEA, a CUA, or a BIA, such as social service costs and dosing convenience. Finally, alternative interventions may have different impacts on different population subsets, and a separate analysis for these different population

subsets is important for all types of economic evaluations, including the CCA.

The following are types of costs that can be included in a CCA: direct healthcare costs; other direct costs, including social service costs and transportation costs; indirect costs, including productivity losses and criminal justice costs; and intangible costs, including costs related to the quality-of-life impact of pain and concern about disease prognosis. Since the goal of the CCA is to give the decision maker as broad a view as possible of the costs of alternative healthcare interventions, all costs that are relevant for the condition of interest should be included. Clearly, the types of costs included will vary with the condition: For example, for an acute illness such as influenza, direct healthcare costs and productivity losses are the most important costs to include. For a chronic psychiatric illness such as schizophrenia, social service costs and criminal justice costs also will be important to include. In addition, intangible costs are important in the analysis of all chronic illnesses.

The following are types of consequences that can be included in a CCA:

- Disease symptoms
- Cure rates
- Mortality rates
- Treatment side effects
- Treatment convenience
- Treatment adherence and persistence
- Patient and family quality of life
- Patient and family overall well-being
- Patient and family satisfaction with treatment

Since the goal of the CCA is to give the decision maker as broad a view as possible of the consequences of the alternative interventions, all aspects of the alternative interventions should be included in the analysis, including convenience and patient and family satisfaction with treatment. These types of consequences generally are not included in CEAs and frequently are not included in CUAs. For example, for influenza, the two neuraminidase inhibitors have different dosing modes: via inhalation (zanamivir) and tablets (oseltamivir). For the treatment of a human immunodeficiency virus infection, many combination treatments are now available that have easier dosing regimens for the patient, which may increase adherence and

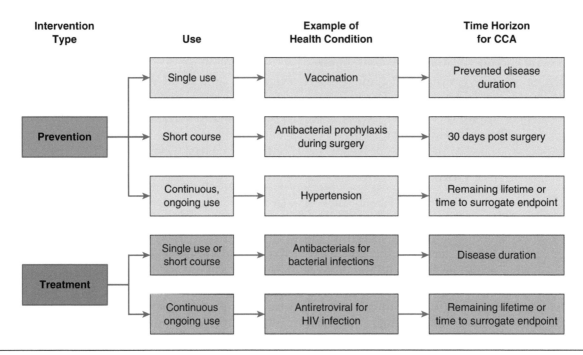

Figure 1   Time horizon for cost-consequence analysis

Source: Adapted from Mauskopf, J. A., Paul, J. E., Grant, D. M., & Stergachis, A. (1998). The role of cost-consequence analysis in healthcare decision making. *PharmacoEconomics, 13,* 277–288.

Note: CCA, cost-consequence analysis; HIV, human immunodeficiency virus.

persistence with treatment and thus increase the effectiveness of the treatment.

As with all economic evaluations, the scope and accuracy of a CCA is limited by the data available. Figure 2 shows the primary data sources for a CCA. Although randomized, controlled clinical trials provide an important data source for CCAs, such trials may have limited external validity because of their generally restrictive inclusion and exclusion criteria. Naturalistic clinical trials or observational data may provide data that more closely approximate the likely costs and consequences in standard clinical practice. Finally, for a chronic illness, the results from a disease progression model can be used to generate estimates of the long-term consequences of alternative interventions when only short-term outcomes data are available.

Sensitivity

Sensitivity analysis is an important component of any economic evaluation because of uncertainty in

the input data as well as the modeling assumptions and other assumptions used to estimate the costs and consequences of the intervention. Thus, the sensitivity of the results of the CCA to changes in the input parameter values and all assumptions should be estimated. One possible way to present this component of the analysis is to use estimates of the ranges of different input parameter values (e.g., 95% confidence intervals for data taken from clinical trial data) to estimate a range of values for each of the costs and consequences estimated.

Presentation

The key distinguishing feature of a CCA is the presentation of the results in a simple, disaggregated format. An example of a CCA presentation is given in Table 1. The cost information should be presented in units (e.g., days in the hospital, physician visits) as well as by cost. The costs also should be presented separately for different cost categories as well as in total. Treatment modes and

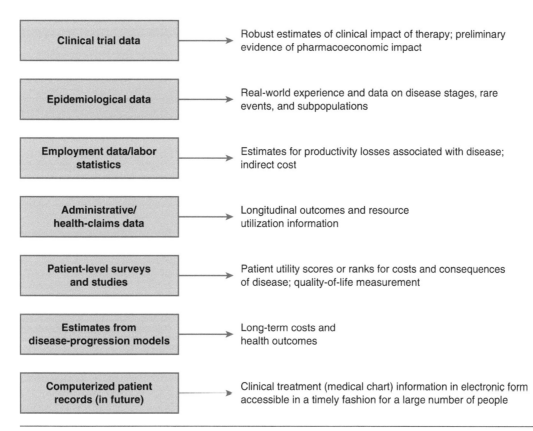

Figure 2   Data sources for cost-consequence analysis

Source: Adapted from Mauskopf, J. A., Paul, J. E., Grant, D. M., & Stergachis, A. (1998). The role of cost-consequence analysis in healthcare decision making. *PharmacoEconomics, 13,* 277–288.

Note: CCA, cost-consequence analysis.

convenience can be included in the tabular listing of the consequences of treatment. In addition to the outcomes for the alternative treatments, a tabular presentation of the results should include two columns showing the difference between the interventions, in units and costs, for each outcome. For an incidence-based CCA, the tabular listing of results applies to one individual or a cohort of individuals over the appropriate time horizon. For a prevalence-based CCA, the tabular listing of results applies to the population of interest to the decision maker and gives annualized results for a 1- to 5-year time horizon.

Advantages and Limitations

There are two types of CCA: An incidence-based CCA can be considered to be a variant of a CEA for a representative individual or for a disease cohort, without the limitation of the consequences to a single outcome and without the calculation of a single ratio of costs to outcomes. The time horizon for an incidence-based CCA is the same as for a CEA, and the data sources will be the same as those for the CEA, with additional sources required for additional cost and consequence measures. A prevalence-based CCA is an extension of a BIA for a prevalent population with the health condition of interest; a prevalence-based CCA includes a broader range of cost categories as well as annualized population estimates of the health and other consequences of a change in the intervention mix.

There are several advantages of a thorough CCA of alternative interventions as an adjunct to other economic value measurements:

- It provides disaggregated information and well-understood measures for a decision maker's review.

Table 1   Example of table of results of cost-consequence analysis for two drugs

Cost Components	Drug A Units	Drug A Costs	Drug B Units	Drug B Costs	Difference (A − B) Units	Difference (A − B) Costs
Direct medical care use and costs						
Drug A or Drug B						
Other drugs						
Physician visits						
Hospital days						
Home care						
Other medical care (e.g., dialysis)						
Direct nonmedical care use and costs						
Transportation						
Social service costs						
Crutches or other equipment						
Paid caregiver time						
Indirect resource use or cost						
Time missed from work for patient						
Time missed from other activities for patient						
Time missed from work for unpaid caregiver						
Time missed from other activities for unpaid caregiver						
Criminal justice costs						
Total direct and indirect costs						
Symptom impact						
Patient distress days						
Patient disability days						
Quality-of-life impact						
Quality-of-life profile scores for patient						
Quality-of-life profile scores for family						
Quality-adjusted life-years decrement for patient						
Quality-adjusted life-years decrement for family						
Patient perception of treatment						
Patient satisfaction scores						
Family satisfaction scores						
Dosing convenience						
Drug adherence						
Drug persistence						

Source: Adapted from Mauskopf, J. A., Paul, J. E., Grant, D. M., & Stergachis, A. (1998). The role of cost-consequence analysis in healthcare decision making. *PharmacoEconomics, 13,* 277–288.

Note: CCA, cost-consequence analysis.

- It allows a decision maker to assign his or her weights to health and other consequences, rather than having an analyst assign weights.
- There is no loss of information when compared with other value measures.
- It can include many consequences that may not be accounted for in other measures, such as dosing, convenience, and patient satisfaction.
- The results can be used as the inputs for a CEA, CUA, or BIA estimate.

There are also some limitations to a CCA:

- Benchmark values and league tables of alternative interventions cannot be developed.
- Direct comparison of value across disease areas is not possible.
- There is no overall quantitative assessment of the value of a new treatment.
- The application of decision-maker weights to the outcome measures may result in decisions based on self-interest rather than on societal value.

Healthcare decision makers need information about the costs and consequences of alternative interventions for different reasons: to determine whether or not to reimburse the different interventions for all the population with the condition of interest or a subset of that population and to determine the extent to which additional healthcare funding will be needed to pay for new interventions for all the population with the condition of interest or a subset of that population. To make these determinations, different national and local healthcare decision makers require information on the costs and consequences of alternative interventions in different formats and with different perspectives, scopes, and time horizons. The CCA can be considered to be a variant of a CEA or an extension of a BIA and can allow the decision maker to choose the combination of costs and consequences that is relevant to him or her and to apply his or her own weights to the consequences.

Because of its limitations in terms of providing overall societal or payer value measures and the associated lack of benchmark values and ability to perform cross-disease comparisons, a CCA will provide the most value when presented together with the results of a CEA, a CUA, and a BIA. Such a package of information will provide a comprehensive assessment of the economic value that can meet all the information requirements of local or national healthcare decision makers.

Josephine Mauskopf

See also Cost-Effectiveness Analysis; Cost-Utility Analysis

Further Readings

Drummond, M. F., O'Brien, B. J., Stoddart, G. L., & Torrance, G. W. (1997). *Methods for the economic evaluation of health care programmes* (2nd ed.). Oxford, UK: Oxford Medical Publications.

Gold, M. R., Siegel, J. E., Russell, L. B., & Weinstein, M. C. (1996). *Cost-effectiveness in health and medicine.* New York: Oxford University Press.

Grant, D. M., Mauskopf, J. A., Bell, L., & Austin, R. (1997). Comparison of valaciclovir and acyclovir for the treatment of herpes zoster in immunocompetent patients over 50 years of age: A cost-consequence model. *Pharmacotherapy, 17,* 333–341.

Kernick, D. (2002). *Getting health economics into practice.* Abingdon, UK: Radcliffe.

Mauskopf, J. A., Paul, J. E., Grant, D. M., & Stergachis, A. (1998). The role of cost-consequence analysis in healthcare decision making. *PharmacoEconomics, 13,* 277–288.

McMurray, J. J. V., Andersson, F. L., Stewart, S., Svensson, K., Solal, A. C., Dietz, R., et al. (2006). Resource utilization and costs in the Candesartan in Heart Failure: Assessment of Reduction in Mortality and Morbidity (CHARM) programme. *European Heart Journal, 27,* 1447–1458.

PausJenssen, A. M., Singer, P. A., & Detsky, A. S. (2003). Ontario's formulary committee: How recommendations are made. *PharmacoEconomics, 21,* 285–294.

Rosner, A. J., Becker, D. L., Wong, A. H., Miller, E., & Conly, J. M. (2004). The costs and consequences of methicillin-resistant *Staphylococcus aureus* infection treatments in Canada. *Canadian Journal of Infectious Diseases and Medical Microbiology, 15,* 213–220.

Straka, R. J., Mamdani, M., Damen, J., Kuntze, C. E. E., Liu, L. Z., Botteman, M. F., et al. (2007). Economic impacts attributable to the early clinical benefit of atorvastatin therapy: A US managed care perspective. *Current Medical Research Opinion, 23,* 1517–1529.

Wang, Z., Salmon, J. W., & Walton, S. M. (2004). Cost-effectiveness analysis and the formulary decision-making process. *Journal of Managed Care Pharmacy, 10,* 48–59.

Cost-Effectiveness Analysis

Cost-effectiveness analysis involves comparison of the additional costs and health benefits of an intervention with those of the available alternative(s). The aim of such an analysis is to determine the value in terms of money of the intervention(s). Within a cost-effectiveness analysis, the health benefits associated with the various interventions are measured in terms of natural units (e.g., survival, life years gained, the number of clinical events avoided). This entry introduces the concept of cost-effectiveness analysis and reviews the key elements, including the incremental cost-effectiveness ratio (ICER), the cost-effectiveness plane, the cost-effectiveness threshold, and the cost-effectiveness frontier.

Concept

The objective of economic evaluation of healthcare interventions is to inform resource allocation decisions in the healthcare sector, through determining whether a proposed intervention is a "good" use of scarce resources. This is assessed through comparison of the additional resources consumed (costs) for the improvement in health benefits generated (e.g., life years gained) associated with one health intervention compared with another. Cost-effectiveness analysis, where the health benefits are measured in terms of a single dimension represented by natural units, is just one type of economic evaluation. It is used to determine which of the alternative interventions provides the most efficient method to achieve a particular outcome (technical efficiency). As such, the units chosen to represent the effect in a cost-effectiveness analysis should be deemed worthwhile (to society or the policy maker), appropriate for measuring the key impact of the intervention, and common across the alternatives to be compared. For example, the cost-effectiveness of a screening test may be established in terms of the cost per case detected, the cost per percent survival at 5 years, the cost per life saved, or the cost per life year gained. Ideally, the measure of effect chosen will relate to a final outcome (e.g., life years gained), but where this is not possible, there should be a way to link it to final effect (e.g., symptom days averted), or it should be

deemed to have value in itself (e.g., cancers detected). Alternative methods for economic evaluation include cost-benefit analysis (where health benefits are measured and valued in monetary terms) and cost-utility analysis (where quality of life is considered alongside quantity of life and health benefits are valued according to patient preferences to construct a composite measure of health outcome, e.g., the quality-adjusted life year or QALY). It should be noted, however, that sometimes the term *cost-effectiveness* is used to cover any of these methods of economic evaluation, where the comparison need not be measured in natural units.

Perspective

The perspective of the analysis determines the extent of the costs and health benefits measured and incorporated. Taking a societal perspective, as advocated by economists, requires the measurement and valuation of all the effects of the intervention(s) irrespective of where, or whom, they affect, including all healthcare costs, all non-healthcare costs, and all costs to the patient, his or her family, and carers. Narrower perspectives restrict the impacts that are included within the analysis, making them more manageable. For example, adopting the commonly used third-party payer perspective for costs would restrict measurement to the costs that fall on the payer (e.g., health insurance company) but would exclude any costs which fall directly on the patient or his or her family and carers. Restricting the perspective for health benefits to the patient would exclude any health benefits received by his or her family, friends, or carers or an altruistic society.

Incremental Cost-Effectiveness Ratio

Cost-effectiveness is assessed by relating the additional costs incurred to provide an intervention to the additional health benefits/effects received as a result of the intervention compared with the available alternative(s). This information is generally reported as an incremental cost-effectiveness ratio (ICER)—a measure of the additional cost per unit of health gain:

$$\text{ICER} = \frac{\text{Cost}_{\text{new intervention}}}{\text{Effect}_{\text{new intervention}}} - \frac{\text{Cost}_{\text{current intervention}}}{\text{Effect}_{\text{current intervention}}}.$$

Incremental cost-effectiveness ratios are only calculated between interventions that address the same patient group with the aim of identifying and selecting the most efficient of these competing (mutually exclusive) interventions. For example, different methods of managing adult women with symptoms of urinary tract infection are mutually exclusive and can be compared within a cost-effectiveness analysis. Cost-effectiveness ratios are not calculated between interventions that address distinct (independent) patient groups. This is because both, or all, the independent interventions may be selected as cost-effective. For example, methods for managing children with symptoms of urinary tract infection should not be compared within a cost-effectiveness analysis with methods for managing men or women. However, once the analysis is done and the ICERs are calculated, independent interventions can (and should) be compared with each other to determine which are funded in a resource-constrained system. This is only plausible where the units of outcomes are measured on the same scale (e.g., life years) for the various interventions or where there is a known common trade-off between the various outcomes.

When determining ICERs for a set of mutually exclusive interventions, the interventions should be ranked in ascending order of effect (or cost) and a ratio calculated for each intervention relative to the next best (more costly) viable intervention by dividing the additional cost by the additional health benefit involved.

Interventions that are both less effective and more costly than other interventions are deemed "dominated" and are not considered viable (Step 2 below). This is because a decision maker should never select an intervention that is both more costly and less effective than an alternative. Interventions that involve larger ICERs than other, more effective, alternatives are deemed "extended dominated" and are also not considered viable (Step 5 below). This is because the intervention would be "dominated" by a program that consisted of a mixture of the next most effective and the next less effective interventions and therefore should not be selected (see Figure 3).

Calculating the ICER: An Example

Consider a situation where there are six mutually exclusive interventions (A to F) that could be adopted. These interventions are characterized by the costs and effects given in the table below.

	Effects	Costs ($)
B	2	211,500
A	10	41,868
D	38	256,731
C	48	879,500
E	68	1,138,000
F	73	1,601,500

(1) Step 1: Rearrange in order of ascending effect.

(2) Step 2: Exclude any interventions where the cost is higher than for an alternative intervention with a greater effect (dominated).

(3) Step 3: Calculate the incremental effect and incremental cost of each intervention in comparison with the prior (less effective) intervention.

	Effects	Costs ($)	Inc. Effect	Inc. Cost ($)
B	2	211,500	Dominated by A	
A	10	41,868	—	—
D	38	256,731	28	214,863
C	48	879,500	10	622,769
E	68	1,138,000	20	258,500
F	73	1,601,500	5	463,500

(4) Step 4: Calculate the incremental cost-effectiveness ratio for each successively more effective intervention, compared with the previous intervention in the list.

	Effects	Costs ($)	Inc. Effect	Inc. Cost ($)	ICER
B	2	211,500	Dominated by A		
A	10	41,868	—	—	—

D	38	256,731	28	214,863	$7,674
C[a]	48	879,500	10	622,769	$62,277[a]
E	68	1,138,000	20	258,500	$12,925
F	73	1,601,500	5	463,500	$92,700

a. Extended dominated.

(5) Step 5: Identify and exclude any interventions that have a higher ICER than more effective interventions (extended dominated), and recalculate the ICERs.

	Effects	Costs	Inc. Effect	Inc. Cost ($)	ICER Recalculated
B	2	211,500	Dominated by A		
A	10	41,868	—	—	—
D	38	256,731	28	214,863	$7,674
C	48	879,500	Extended dominated		
E	68	1,138,000	30	881,269	$29,376
F	73	1,601,500	5	463,500	$92,700

Repeat Step 5 until all dominated interventions are removed and ICERs have been calculated for all nondominated interventions.

Cost-Effectiveness Plane

A cost-effectiveness (CE) plane can be used to provide a visual representation of the results of a cost-effectiveness analysis by plotting the costs against the effects for the various interventions. When comparing just two mutually exclusive interventions, the incremental cost-effectiveness (ICE) plane can be presented as in Figure 1. Here the figure shows a plot of the additional (or incremental) costs and effects of the intervention compared with the alternative (represented by the origin).

The horizontal axis divides the plane according to incremental cost (positive above, negative below), and the vertical axis divides the plane according to incremental effect (positive to the right, negative to the left). This divides the incremental cost-effectiveness plane into four quadrants through the origin. These four quadrants are commonly referenced according to the compass points. The northwest

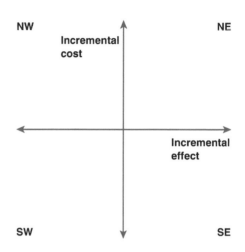

Figure I   Incremental cost-effectiveness plane

(NW) quadrant involves negative incremental effect but positive incremental cost, as such an intervention falling in this quadrant would be "dominated" by the alternative and therefore not be considered cost-effective. The southeast (SE) quadrant involves negative incremental cost but positive incremental effect; an intervention falling in this quadrant would dominate the alternative and therefore be deemed cost-effective. The northeast (NE) quadrant involves positive incremental cost and positive incremental effect, while the southwest (SW) quadrant involves negative incremental cost and negative incremental effect. An intervention falling into either of these quadrants *may* be deemed cost-effective compared with the alternative, depending on the trade-off between costs and effects. Note that the incremental cost-effectiveness ratio associated with an intervention in either the NE or SW quadrant is given by the slope of a line connecting the intervention to the origin.

When comparing more than two mutually exclusive interventions, a cost-effectiveness plane can be plotted, where all interventions appear within the cost and effect space. Alternatively, and more commonly, the interventions can be plotted relative to the least costly, least effective alternative (represented by the origin) on the incremental cost-effectiveness plane (see Figure 2). Note that this requires calculation of the additional costs and effects of each alternative with respect to the same least costly, least effective comparator. In this case, identifying dominant or dominated interventions can be done by systematically dropping a horizontal line and a vertical line through the point representing each comparator. This essentially replicates the process undertaken above for two interventions by making each point in turn the origin. The incremental cost-effectiveness ratio associated with an intervention is determined by the slope of a line connecting it with the next less effective, nondominated, alternative. Steeper slopes represent larger incremental cost-effectiveness ratios.

Plotting an ICE Plane for Multiple Interventions: An Example

Figure 2 illustrates the incremental cost-effectiveness plane for the six mutually exclusive interventions (A to F) under consideration.

The figure clearly indicates that Intervention B is dominated by Intervention A, which involves greater health benefits for a lower cost. In addition, the figure indicates that Intervention C is extended dominated as it involves a higher ICER than a more effective intervention, E (the slope of the line joining D and C is greater than the slope of the line joining C and E). Figure 3 illustrates that a mixed strategy involving programs D and E, represented by any point between M^1 (a strategy with identical health benefits to C that can be achieved at cheaper cost) and M^2 (a strategy involving identical costs to C that involves greater health benefits) dominates Intervention C.

Cost-Effectiveness Frontier

On the cost-effectiveness plane, the cost-effectiveness frontier is established by connecting together progressively more effective, nondominated interventions. This frontier has a gradually increasing slope (ICER), representing the increased price that must be paid for additional effects. The cost-effectiveness frontier for Figure 3 is represented by the line ADEF.

Cost-Effectiveness Threshold: Identifying the Cost-Effective Intervention

Once the dominated interventions have been excluded, the ICERs calculated, and the cost-effectiveness frontier established, one of the remaining (viable) interventions is identified as cost effective and providing value for the money. Traditionally, the cost-effective intervention is identified as the one associated with the largest ICER that falls below a specified monetary threshold (often denoted by λ). This externally set cost-effectiveness threshold represents the maximum amount that the decision or

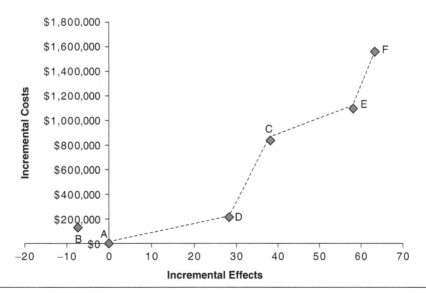

Figure 2   Interventions on the incremental cost-effectiveness plane

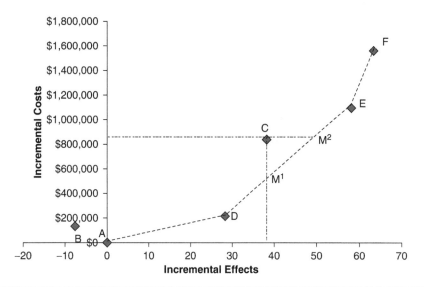

Figure 3   Cost-effectiveness frontier

policy maker is willing to pay for health effects. The threshold can be derived in two ways. The first method involves establishing and fixing the threshold at the maximum price that society is willing to pay for health benefits. The second approach involves deriving the shadow price of health benefits purchased from a fixed budget, that is, the amount by which the health benefits achievable will be improved by relaxing the fixed budget by a small amount. This approach, while theoretically correct, has an enormous informational requirement. Initially it involves selecting interventions onto a list, lowest ICER first, until the budget is expended. During the process, independent interventions are added to the budget while mutually exclusive interventions with higher ICERs replace those with lower ICERs that were included earlier. The following hypothetical example considers a situation where there are three independent programs (cancer screening, management for diabetes, and treatment for heart failure) and each program involves a

choice between four viable mutually exclusive interventions (1 to 4) that could be considered cost-effective. These interventions are characterized by the costs and effects given in the table below.

Assuming a budget of 100,000, the initial budget determination would be as follows:

(6) Step 1: Implement b1 based on lowest ratio of cost to effect.

$$b1 \rightarrow \text{Budget used} = 1,500$$
$$\rightarrow \text{Shadow price} = 1,250$$

(7) Step 2: Add a1 based on ratio of cost to effect.
$$a1 + b1 \rightarrow \text{Budget used} = 6,000$$
$$\rightarrow \text{Shadow price} = 2,813$$

(8) Step 3: Replace b1 with b2 based on ratio of incremental cost to incremental effect.

$$a1 + b2 \rightarrow \text{Budget used} = 6,500$$
$$\rightarrow \text{Shadow price} = 3,846$$

	Cancer Screening (a)			Management of Diabetes (b)			Treatment for Heart Failure (c)		
	Costs	Effects	ICER	Costs	Effects	ICER	Costs	Effects	ICER
1	4,500	1.60	—	1,500	1.20	—	26,000	3.00	—
2	18,000	2.30	19,286	2,000	1.33	3,846	43,000	3.50	34,000
3	27,000	2.69	23,077	7,100	1.67	15,000	65,900	4.10	38,167
4	47,000	3.15	43,478	14,800	1.80	59,231	178,000	5.30	93,417

(9) Step 4: Add c1 based on ratio of cost to effect.

$$a1 + b2 + c1 \rightarrow \text{Budget used} = 32,500$$
$$\rightarrow \text{Shadow price} = 8,667$$

(10) Step 5: Replace b2 with b3 based on ratio of incremental cost to incremental effect.

$$a1 + b3 + c1 \rightarrow \text{Budget used} = 37,600$$
$$\rightarrow \text{Shadow price} = 15,000$$

(11) Step 6: Replace a1 with a2 based on ratio of incremental cost to incremental effect.

$$a2 + b3 + c1 \rightarrow \text{Budget used} = 51,100$$
$$\rightarrow \text{Shadow price} = 19,286$$

(12) Step 7: Replace a2 with a3 based on ratio of incremental cost to incremental effect.

$$a3 + b3 + c1 \rightarrow \text{Budget used} = 60,100$$
$$\rightarrow \text{Shadow price} = 23,077$$

(13) Step 8: Replace c1 with c2 based on ratio of incremental cost to incremental effect.

$$a3 + b3 + c2 \rightarrow \text{Budget used} = 77,100$$
$$\rightarrow \text{Shadow price} = 34,000$$

(14) Step 9: Replace c2 with c3 based on ratio of incremental cost to incremental effect.

$$a3 + b3 + c3 \rightarrow \text{Budget used} = 100,000$$
$$\rightarrow \text{Shadow price} = 38,167$$

Following the initial budget determination, including new interventions (whether independent or mutually exclusive) will involve displacing intervention(s) already included on the list. Thus, when considering a new intervention, the associated ICER is compared with that of the last intervention(s) included in the list that will be displaced by the new program (in the example, this is 38,167). It is the ICER of the displaced intervention that implicitly provides the shadow price for health benefits.

Identifying the Cost-Effective Intervention: An Example

Returning to the example, once the ICERs have been calculated for the nondominated interventions,

they should be compared with the cost effectiveness threshold to establish which intervention provides value for the money.

Assuming a cost-effectiveness threshold of $50,000, Intervention E would be identified as cost-effective as this provides the largest effect at an acceptable "price" (i.e., largest ICER below the cost-effectiveness threshold).

	Effects	Costs ($)	Inc. Effect	Inc. Cost ($)	ICER Recalculated
B	2	211,500	Dominated by A		
A	10	41,868	—	—	—
D	38	256,731	28	214,863	$7,674
C	48	879,500	Extended dominated		
E	68	1,138,000	30	881,269	$29,376
F	73	1,601,500	5	463,500	$92,700

A threshold of $20,000 would mean Intervention D was cost-effective, while a threshold of $100,000 would mean Intervention F was cost-effective.

Elisabeth Fenwick

See also Cost-Benefit Analysis; Cost-Utility Analysis; Dominance; Marginal or Incremental Analysis, Cost-Effectiveness Ratio

Further Readings

Black, W. C. (1990). The CE plane: A graphic representation of cost-effectiveness. *Medical Decision Making, 10,* 212–214.

Cantor, S. B. (1994). Cost-effectiveness analysis, extended dominance, and ethics: A quantitative assessment. *Medical Decision Making, 14*(3), 259–265.

Drummond, M. F., O'Brien, B. J., Stoddart, G. L., & Torrance, G. W. (1997). *Methods for the economic evaluation of health care programmes* (2nd ed.). New York: Oxford University Press.

Johannesson, M., & Meltzer, D. (1998). Some reflections on cost-effectiveness analysis. *Health Economics, 7,* 1–7.

Karlsson, G., & Johannesson, M. (1996). The decision rules of cost-effectiveness analysis. *Pharmaco-Economics, 9,* 113–120.

Weinstein, M. C., & Stason, W. B. (1977). Foundations of cost-effectiveness analysis for health and medical practices. *New England Journal of Medicine, 296*(13), 716–721.

COST-IDENTIFICATION ANALYSIS

Cost-identification analysis is the assignment of a value to healthcare use. The costs of healthcare encounters, treatment episodes, or healthcare interventions are found to consider the economic impact of medical decisions. Cost identification is part of budget impact analysis, cost-minimization analysis, cost-comparison analysis, cost-consequences analysis, cost-effectiveness analysis, cost-utility analysis, and cost-benefit analysis.

Cost-identification analysis is affected by the choice of analytic perspective and time horizon. This choice depends on the type of application and its intended audience. Cost-identification analysis is also affected by simplifying assumptions that may sacrifice comprehensiveness or precision to save research expense.

Standardized Methods

Medical decision models are commonly used to assess the cost-effectiveness of new healthcare interventions. Guidelines for cost-effectiveness analysis (CEA) have been developed so that the cost-effectiveness ratios of different interventions conducted by different analysts may be compared without concern that differences are methodological artifacts. Standardization also enhances the generalizability of study findings, allowing them to be applied to new settings.

Although there are a number of different guidelines for CEA, they largely agree on the principles of cost identification. These guidelines recommend that all relevant costs be included, that resources be valued at their opportunity cost, and that cost be estimated from the societal perspective using a long-term time horizon.

Standards have also been developed for budget impact analysis (BIA). This type of study provides healthcare plans or healthcare providers with information on the total cost of implementation. BIA generally uses a short-term horizon and the perspective of a particular health plan or provider.

Perspective of Analysis

Most studies consider all costs incurred in the healthcare system. Adoption of the societal perspective requires inclusion of costs incurred by patients and their families. These include cost of unpaid caregivers, cost of travel to medical care providers, and the value of time seeking care. A cost-identification analysis sometimes includes the value of wages lost due to illness. In practice, many studies ignore costs incurred by patients and their families. This may result in analyses that are biased in favor of interventions that shift costs from health system to patient.

Time Horizon

The time horizon is the period over which costs are identified. CEA guidelines recommend a long-term perspective, one that includes lifetime costs and outcomes. The use of a short time horizon may result in bias. A short-term horizon may favor an intervention that defers costs to the future or disadvantage one in which benefits are realized after significant delay. A short-term horizon may be appropriate to the immediate concerns of a BIA.

Cost-identification analysis ordinarily expresses the cost of care that spans more than 1 year in real (inflation-adjusted) terms. Future costs are discounted (expressed as the present value) to reflect the lower burden imposed by healthcare costs that will not be incurred until the future. Inflation adjustment and discounting are separate adjustments; both adjustments are needed.

The time horizon has an additional effect on cost-identification analysis; it determines whether fixed costs and development costs are included. In the short run, the decision to provide an additional health service does not increase institutional overhead (e.g., the cost of nonpatient care hospital departments such as human resources, finance, administration, and environmental services). These costs are fixed in the short run. In economic terms, the short-run marginal cost is the cost directly attributable to producing an extra unit of output and does not include the fixed costs of the enterprise.

In the long run, the institution must adjust the size of overhead departments to provide the right amount of services needed by its patient care departments. Additional health services increase institutional overhead over the long run. In economic terms, the long-run marginal cost is equal to the average cost. In other words, the long-run cost of producing an extra unit of output includes the variable cost associated with that output, and a share of the fixed costs of the enterprise.

The difference in time horizon means that BIA ordinarily involves marginal cost and excludes facility overhead. Since guidelines recommend a long-term time horizon, institutional overhead is included in CEA.

The time horizon may also determine whether the cost of developing a new intervention is included. In the short run, the decision maker may regard these as sunk costs, an expenditure that has already been made and is not relevant to subsequent decisions. The long-run horizon requires inclusion of development costs.

The market price of pharmaceuticals must result in sufficient revenue so that over the long run the manufacturer can recoup development costs and earn a return on investment. Managerial and behavioral interventions are often developed as part of a research study, and their development costs are often ignored by analysts. Consistency requires inclusion of the cost of developing these interventions. This cost should be amortized over the expected size of the population of beneficiaries. Failure to include development costs may bias analyses against interventions such as pharmaceuticals and devices, which include development cost as part of their market price.

Methods of Determining Cost

Cost should be representative of the healthcare system where the study will be applied. Cost-identification methods include gross costing, use of data from claims and cost allocation systems, and microcosting. The choice between these methods represents a trade-off between precision and expense. Microcosting is the most accurate method, but it is labor-intensive. Gross costing is less accurate but much easier to employ. Each method has its limits and appropriate use. Multiple methods may be needed within a single study.

Gross Costing

Gross costing requires information on the quantity of each type of health service used and information on unit costs. A count of the resources employed in a particular healthcare strategy may be based on a hypothetical model or expert opinion. Alternatively, actual use may be recorded during the course of a clinical trial. Gathering service use from a study participant involves a trade-off between accuracy and expense. Accuracy can be improved by more frequent surveys and by employing logs and other memory aids. Counts of resources may also be obtained from administrative data of providers or health plans.

The cost of hospitalization may be estimated with different unit costs, including an average daily rate, a specialty-specific daily rate, or a diagnosis-weighted rate. Use of an average daily rate makes the assumption that all days of hospitalization have the same cost. Daily costs vary markedly by diagnosis, however. The accuracy of cost estimates is enhanced if they reflect the effect of diagnosis and the use of surgery and intensive care. Separate rates should be used to estimate the cost of hospitalization in psychiatric and long-term care facilities.

The cost of ambulatory care can be estimated by multiplying a count of visits by a unit cost. Not all ambulatory care visits have the same cost. The accuracy of cost estimates can be improved if they reflect differences in care, such as a hospital clinic or other facility, medical and surgical procedures, emergency room care, or a visit to a specialist or office-based care physician.

Estimates of pharmacy use are often based on patient self-report. The average wholesale price should not be used as the unit cost for pharmacy as healthcare payers receive substantial discounts from this price. Unit cost should also reflect the dispensing fee paid to pharmacies.

It is not desirable to estimate unit costs based on the fee schedule or cost data from a single provider as they may not be representative. Gross costing is not appropriate if the intervention affects the resources employed in care without affecting the units chosen to measure cost.

In the United States, Medicare is the predominant payer, and its payment schedule is often used for unit costs. Physician fee schedules are also available in countries outside the United States. A set of standard unit cost estimates have been offered as part of CEA guidelines used in the Netherlands and Australia. These unit costs have helped standardize estimates of health services costs in CEA studies of new pharmaceuticals. Such standard estimates must be used with care. If a standard estimate for an ambulatory visit includes the cost of associated laboratory tests, it will not capture the incremental effect of an intervention that generates additional laboratory orders.

Gross costing is an important method appropriate for many studies, but the analyst should avoid any analytic assumption that interferes with identification of the effect of intervention on resource use.

Cost Estimates Based on Claims Data

Charges, cost-adjusted charges, and reimbursements from administrative data are widely applied by economic analysts based in the U.S. healthcare system. Administrative data are much less freely available outside the United States. Even within the United States, claims data may not always be available. Managed care organizations are reimbursed according to the number of patients served, and not for the type or quantity of services they provide. As a result, they may not prepare a claim, or they may not be required to provide claims data to the healthcare sponsor.

Claims data provide information on cost from the point of view of the healthcare payer or provider, and this is often the economic cost. Raw charges should not be used as an estimate of the cost of care as they greatly exceed the economic cost.

Charges are cost-adjusted by multiplying by a ratio of cost to charges. This ratio may be determined from data in publicly available cost reports that U.S. hospitals submit to Medicare. Use of cost-adjusted charges makes the strong assumption that the charge for a specific service is proportionate to its economic cost. This assumption is not always warranted. Hospitals may set their charges without knowing the relative cost of different services. There are strategic reasons to overcharge for some services and undercharge for others.

Some analysts have found costing to be more accurate if cost adjustment is done at the department level. A ratio of cost to charges is found for each department in the hospital and applied to the charges incurred in that department. It may be difficult to obtain charges at the department level. Departments may be defined differently in cost reporting and billing systems, making department-level adjustment problematic.

U.S. hospital bills exclude physician charges for inpatient services, and these must be estimated separately. When ambulatory care is provided by a facility, the facility and physician bill separately, and neither cost should be ignored.

Cost information is rarely available to adjust charges for physician services. When charges cannot be cost-adjusted, reimbursement may be a more appropriate estimate of cost. It should include any co-payment made by the patient.

An important limitation to administrative data is their coverage. The analyst must take care not to ignore significant costs not recorded in administrative data.

Activity-Based Costing (ABC) Systems

Activity-based costing (ABC) systems are used in some hospitals in the United States, Taiwan, and Canada. ABC systems are more complex than the cost reports U.S. hospitals submit to the Medicare program to determine reimbursement rates. Costs, services, and products are identified at a much finer level of detail. ABC systems extract databases to determine the quantity of all different services provided. The costs of staff time, supplies, and equipment are assigned to departments. Overhead expenses are distributed to patient care departments. A schedule of relative values is used to find the cost of specific products. The cost of these products is assigned to specific stays or encounters according to products used in providing care.

An important limitation of ABC systems is that they have not been widely adopted. Hospitals may regard ABC estimates as confidential information needed to negotiate contracts. The analyst must consider that hospitals using ABC systems may not have typical costs.

Microcosting

Microcosting is the direct measurement of cost by observation and survey. It is needed when no unit cost is available from fee schedules or claims systems. A common application is to estimate the cost of a novel intervention. Microcosting may be needed when claims data are not sensitive to the effect of an intervention. Since microcosting is too labor-intensive to use for all healthcare, its use must be limited to activities most likely to be affected by the intervention under study.

To find the cost of a treatment innovation, all intervention-related activities must be identified.

When patients must be screened to determine if they are eligible for treatment, this cost is not a research cost but a cost that should be included as it will be incurred when the intervention is replicated in clinical practice.

The cost of labor should not be limited to wage costs. It should also include the employer's share of taxes and benefits. Labor cost is often estimated by determining the number of minutes each worker spends in direct activities involved in providing the service. This effort is measured by direct observation, staff activity logs, supervisor report, or other methods. When the long-run perspective is used, labor costs should include nonpatient care activities: training to maintain credentials, answering the phone, meeting with colleagues, taking vacations, and going on sick leave.

For hospitals and other large institutions, it is not feasible to use microcosting to determine overhead. One approach is to apply the ratio of overhead to direct expense for a similar department in the hospital cost report.

Choice of Cost Method

Guidelines agree that more exact methods should be used to determine the cost of services most affected by the intervention under study. Simpler methods may be employed to avoid spending scarce resources on precise measurement of unimportant services. Each method involves assumptions, and the analyst must review whether these assumptions are appropriate. An important additional concern for CEA studies is the wider applicability of cost estimates and resulting study findings to other providers, health plans, or countries.

Reporting Cost-Identification Analysis

The quality of economic evaluations of healthcare has been studied in a large number of reviews. Some reviews have found modest improvements in the quality of economic analyses since the promulgation of CEA guidelines. Reviews have noted problems with the CEA studies in general and cost-determination methods in particular.

Studies should separately identify the cost of the intervention being evaluated and include all relevant costs. The analyst should identify the cost determination method used, source of cost data,

time horizon, analytic perspective, price index used to adjust for inflation, and discount rate used to express costs in their present value.

Paul G. Barnett

See also Cost-Comparison Analysis; Cost-Consequence Analysis; Cost-Effectiveness Analysis; Cost Measurement Methods; Cost-Minimization Analysis; Costs, Direct Versus Indirect; Costs, Fixed Versus Variable; Costs, Out-of-Pocket; Cost-Utility Analysis; Marginal or Incremental Analysis, Cost-Effectiveness Ratio

Further Readings

Dranove, D. (1995). Measuring costs. In F. A. Sloan (Ed.), *Valuing health care: Costs, benefits, and effectiveness of pharmaceuticals and other medical technologies* (pp. 61–75). Cambridge, UK: Cambridge University Press.

Drummond, M. F., Sculpher, M. J., Torrance, G. W., O'Brien, B. J., & Stoddart, G. L. (2005). *Methods for the economic evaluation of health care programmes* (3rd ed.). Oxford, UK: Oxford University Press.

Luce, B., Manning, W., Siegel, J., & Lipscomb, J. (1996). Estimating costs in cost-effectiveness analysis. In M. R. Gold, J. E. Siegel, L. B. Russell, & M. C. Weinstein (Eds.), *Cost-effectiveness in health and medicine.* New York: Oxford University Press.

Mauskopf, J. A., Sullivan, S. D., Annemans, L., Caro, J., Mullins, C. D., Nuijten, M., et al. (2007). Principles of good practice for budget impact analysis: Report of the ISPOR Task Force on good research practices— budget impact analysis. *Value Health, 10*(5), 336–347.

Ramsey, S., Willke, R., Briggs, A., Brown, R., Buxton, M., Chawla, A., et al. (2005). Good research practices for cost-effectiveness analysis alongside clinical trials: The ISPOR RCT-CEA Task Force report. *Value Health, 8*(5), 521–533.

Smith, M. W., & Barnett, P. G. (2003). Direct measurement of health care costs. *Medical Care Research Review, 60*(3 Suppl.), 74S–91S.

COST MEASUREMENT METHODS

Cost measurement is fundamental to all economic evaluations for healthcare, which have become increasingly important throughout the world in policy decision making concerning new medical interventions. Appropriate cost measurement can contribute to the efficient allocation of resources within the health system. The goal of cost measurement is to assess the costs that are needed to produce or are consequent to the outcomes of the intervention of interest, relative to an alterative intervention such as standard of care.

Cost measurement involves identifying, measuring, and valuing all relevant resource uses that are attributable to the medical interventions, including the resources needed for implementing the interventions and those that are associated with medical and nonmedical outcomes of the interventions. The costs related to a healthcare intervention and its outcomes can include direct medical and nonmedical costs, as well as indirect costs (e.g., work productivity loss).

Generally, cost measurement methods include the following steps: (a) specifying the perspective of the study, (b) identifying relevant resources used, (c) determining the quantity of resources, and (d) valuing these resource items (services, goods, time).

Specification of Study Perspective

Economic evaluation studies can frame decision problems from different perspectives, which will lead to different costs and even the final decision. Therefore, specifying the perspective of the cost analysis plays a crucial role in determining the relevant resources and how they should be measured and valued.

Societal perspective is a standard for cost-effectiveness analysis. From a societal perspective, all resources and their net costs to the society should be taken into account, including patient and unpaid caregivers' time, as well as work productivity loss. A government purchaser may only bear the costs incurred to the government; thus the patient and unpaid caregivers' time would not be included from a government payer perspective. A commercial insurer may only be concerned with the direct medical costs; thus direct medical costs will be included. Therefore, the perspective of the study will determine the relevance of the resources, their quantity, and their costs.

Identification of Relevant Resources

A healthcare intervention has various and far-reaching effects with economic implications.

Ideally, any use of resources that are associated with the alternative healthcare interventions and their effects on health outcomes should be identified. Depending on the study perspective, the nature of the intervention, and health outcomes, many or all of the following resources should be considered in the process of cost measurement: the acquisition and administration of the healthcare intervention (e.g., drug, provider service for the intervention, patient's time involved in the intervention), additional services (e.g., follow-up lab tests) associated with the intervention, change in healthcare resource uses associated with change in health status and outcomes, and change in nonhealthcare resource uses associated with change in health status, such as improved work productivity and reduced unpaid caregivers' time. The study perspective should be considered in determining whether each component should be finally included.

The timelines during which these resources have implications should be considered, which determines the appropriate time horizon of the economic study. An appropriate time horizon should allow inclusion of the full consequences of the intervention.

Though theoretically all relevant resources and costs should be included, the availability of information, resources, and research time are often limited. Some resource items are likely to form the largest components (i.e., cost drivers) of the total and incremental costs. They often involve only a few resource items. These cost drivers should be considered first, especially those resources on which the intervention has a measurable impact. Therefore, the process of resource identification and costing requires scientific rigor as well as researchers' discretion because costing is a methodology for practical purposes.

Measurement of Resource Use

Depending on the list of identified resource uses, the data sources to quantify these resources can include randomized clinical trials (RCTs), an administrative and accounting database, observational studies such as a large national survey and patient registry, the published literature, clinical practice guidelines, and expert opinions. It is common for a variety of data sources to be used in economic modeling studies. The quantification of resources in measurement units also depends on the costing method to be used, such as gross costing or microcosting methods.

It is an increasingly common practice to conduct economic evaluation alongside an RCT, which is often termed a *piggyback evaluation*. Such an evaluation has the advantage of leveraging randomization (thus with good internal validity for incremental costs), and availability of individual patients' data that provide variation and distribution for costs estimation. Some resource use data may be available among those collected for the purposes of the clinical trial. For example, an occurrence of hospitalization is almost always recorded as a serious adverse event because it is a necessary component for reporting in RCTs. Additional resource uses often need to be collected. Patient medical records or patient diaries/interviews can be used. Medical records provide accurate patient-level resource use information without an additional burden on the patients enrolled in the trial, but the records may not include all relevant resources, and the recording method may not be standard across different centers (especially for internal studies). Patient diaries or interviews allow the recording of nonmedical resource uses, such as time (e.g., transportation), that are incurred with the intervention.

In piggyback evaluation, special issues should be noted in resource quantification. In RCTs, extra resources could be consumed due to more frequent lab monitoring, additional scheduled follow-up visits, and better compliance. Such protocol-driven resource use should be excluded to approximate the costs incurred in the real-world practice better. In addition, RCTs often have a short follow-up period, and therefore not all resource use differences between two treatment arms are fully realized. Additional research effort could be expended to overcome such limitations, including conducting an open-label extension study if possible; extrapolating from final endpoints observed in the trial using modeling techniques; and predicting final outcomes from intermediate outcomes based on established models.

Resource Valuation

The assignment of costs to resources, or costing, can be performed from an aggregate (gross) level to a more detailed microlevel. Three basic costing methods are gross costing (top-down costing), unit costing, and microcosting (bottom-up costing).

In gross costing, health services or healthcare interventions are broken down into large components, and these large cost items have to be identified. As a result, gross costing can be simple and transparent. Gross costing estimates an event or diagnosis as a whole. National tariffs are preferably used whenever available, such as diagnosis-related group (DRG) payments in the United States and Australia and health resource group (HRG) payments in Great Britain. These rates are often reliable and standard and allow international comparison.

Unit costing applies costs to each type of resource consumed, such as emergency room visits, inpatient hospitalization stays, physician visits, lab tests and procedures performed, and drugs administered. Unit costs can be obtained from the national payment schedule (e.g., Medicare reimbursement rates), administrative claims database, and published literature.

The microcosting (bottom-up costing) method establishes a very detailed service delivery process (inventory) and identifies the relevant resource items and measures them separately. It is based on direct observation, on an item-by-item basis; thus it could be expensive and time-consuming. Microcosting methods include time-and-motion studies, activity logs, and surveys of patients, providers, and managers. In a piggyback evaluation, microcosting can also be conducted by reviewing medical bills of patients in trials. In the United States, a common method for estimating the economic cost of medical services is to adjust the charges through the use of cost-to-charge ratios to reflect their true economic costs.

A patient can incur loss of time due to time spent in seeking treatment, impaired productivity while at work, and short- or long-term absences from work associated with poor health status. Two methods that are generally used to measure work loss are the human capital method and friction cost method. The human capital method estimates the production cost during the employment period that is lost due to illness. However, the friction method restricts the period of the productivity loss to the period needed to replace the sick employee. So the productivity loss to society is limited to the time before the sick person is replaced.

Special attention should be given to determining drug cost, especially costs of patented drugs. Though the price of the brand drug is often used in economic evaluation, this can overestimate drug cost because the price of the brand drug is not the true market price of the drug with a complex rebate and co-payment system. From a payer perspective, the net drug payment incurred by the payer should be used, which is net of all rebates, co-payments, and other adjustments. From a societal perspective, because the cost transfer from one party to another within the society should be excluded from the costs, the drug price should be greatly discounted for economic evaluation. This is because a portion of the cost is transferred to a pharmaceutical company for rewarding innovation in drugs.

In perfectly competitive markets, the prices of inputs are equal to opportunity costs, but this does not hold for many components in healthcare. Consequently, tariffs and other prices in the healthcare sector should be applied with care, and often other valuation methods are used instead. Ideally, a resource used should be valued at its opportunity cost, that is, the value of its best alternative use. The concept of opportunity costs can help determine the value of those resources.

Incremental costs, instead of total costs, are of central interest because often two or more treatments are compared and evaluated during the decision-making process. Therefore, the cost measurement should focus on the difference in costs between treatments, and common costs that are invariant to treatments should be excluded.

Because costs can be measured in different ways, the choice of cost measurement should depend on the purpose of the study, and it has consequences for the identification of resource items and the measurement of resource use. Some general elements should be clarified in the cost measurement, including the perspective, the list of assumptions, the role of prices, the time horizon, and allocation of overhead costs. The choice of costing method in practice will be highly conditional on the information available, the limited resources available to undertake the analysis, and whether the study involves multiple countries.

Andrew Peng Yu

See also Cost-Comparison Analysis; Cost-Effectiveness Analysis; Cost-Identification Analysis; Costs, Direct Versus Indirect; Costs, Opportunity; Marginal or Incremental Analysis, Cost-Effectiveness Ratio; Time Horizon

Further Readings

Brouwer, W., Rutten, F., & Koopmanschap, M. (2001). Costing in economic evaluations. In M. Drummond & A. McGuire (Eds.), *Economic evaluation in health care: Merging theory with practice* (pp. 68–93). Oxford, UK: Oxford University Press.

Glick, H. A., Doshi, J. A., Sonnad, S. S., & Polsky, D. (2007). *Economic evaluation in clinical trials.* Oxford, UK: Oxford University Press.

Luce, B., Manning, W. G., Siegel, J. E., & Lipscomb, J. (1996). Estimating costs in cost-effectiveness analysis. In M. R. Gold, J. E. Siegel, L. B. Russell, & M. C. Weinstein (Eds.), *Cost-effectiveness in health and medicine* (pp. 200–203). New York: Oxford University Press.

Oostenbrink, J. B., Koopmanschap, M. A., & Rutten, F. F. (2002). Standardisation of costs: The Dutch Manual for Costing in economic evaluations. *PharmacoEconomics, 20,* 443–454.

O'Sullivan, A. K., Thompson, D., & Drummond, M. F. (2005). Collection of health-economic data alongside clinical trials: Is there a future for piggyback evaluations? *Value in Health, 8,* 67–79.

COST-MINIMIZATION ANALYSIS

Cost-minimization analysis is a special form of cost-effectiveness analysis where the health outcomes can be considered to be equivalent between two treatment alternatives and therefore the interest is only on which of the two strategies has the lower cost. Cost-minimization analysis appears to have much to commend it: in particular, it embodies an apparently simplified approach to decision making by looking at only the cost side of the equation. However, there are a number of potential pitfalls that exist in terms of the practical use of cost-minimization analysis.

The first of these represents a problem of definition. Many apparent examples of cost-minimization studies fail to present any justification of the equivalence of health outcomes between two treatments and are therefore more accurately described as cost analysis. A simple cost analysis should not be considered a true cost-minimization study without some form of evidence for the equivalence of health outcomes being presented. Note that these cost analyses are also often incorrectly described as "cost-benefit analyses" due to the net-benefit approach to decision making, particularly in the early health economic evaluation literature.

More recently, as economic evaluation alongside clinical trials has become more common, the problem has become one of interpretation. It is all too common to see "cost-minimization analyses" presented that turn out to be based on the interpretation of lack of significance of an effect measure in a clinical trial as evidence of equivalence. In the clinical trial field, there is a well-known adage that "absence of evidence is not evidence of absence." To interpret the lack of a significance as evidence of no effect is to place the importance of the Type I error (concluding a difference exists when the null hypothesis of no difference is true) above that of the Type II error (concluding that no difference exists when in fact the alternative hypothesis of a difference is true). To properly show that two treatments are no different (within a small margin of error) requires an appropriately designed equivalence study that typically requires a greater sample size to reliably demonstrate equivalence than is recruited to many superiority (difference) trials.

Furthermore, clinical trials typically are powered to detect differences in only a single effect measure (primary trial endpoint). In contrast, health economic analyses are multidimensional, often trading off different effects (risks and benefits) to obtain a composite measure of outcome. It would be very rare indeed for two treatments to be truly equivalent on all measures of outcome and rarer for a clinical trial to be adequately powered to demonstrate such a multidimensional equivalence.

As a consequence of these difficulties, examples of true cost-minimization studies are rare. One of the most popularly cited (though rather old) examples relates to a cost-minimization study of alternative oxygen delivery methods, with the underlying assumption that the treatment (oxygen) is truly equivalent between alternative delivery systems. It is worthy of note that the original analysis (in common with the healthcare perspective of many

economic studies) did not include any convenience to the patient in the analysis.

Although conceptually appealing, due to the simplified approach to decision making, the practical problems associated with cost-minimization analysis have led some commentators to argue the "(near) death of cost-minimization analysis." The appropriate framework for analysis of most studies will be the estimation of cost-effectiveness. It is clear that the use of separate and sequential tests of hypothesis of cost and effect based on superior study designs does not constitute appropriate grounds for using cost-minimization as a decision-making tool.

Andrew H. Briggs

See also Cost-Benefit Analysis; Cost-Effectiveness Analysis; Marginal or Incremental Analysis, Cost-Effectiveness Ratio

Further Readings

Briggs, A. H., & O'Brien, B. J. (2001). The death of cost-minimization analysis? *Health Economics, 10,* 179–184.

Drummond, M. F., Sculpher, M. J., Torrance, G. W., O'Brien, B., & Stoddart, G. L. (2005). *Methods for the economic evaluation of health care programmes* (3rd ed.). Oxford, UK: Oxford University Press.

Gold, M. R., Siegel, J. E., Russell, L. B., & Weinstein, M. C. (1996). *Cost-effectiveness in health and medicine.* New York: Oxford University Press.

COSTS, DIRECT VERSUS INDIRECT

Within economic evaluation, the analysis of costs is meant to provide a valuation of the resources consumed as a result of an intervention. Such an analysis, like that involved in the valuation of outcomes, would result in different answers depending on the perspective of the analyst. The perspective adopted is, in turn, determined by the policy question that the evaluation is seeking to answer. For instance, the health sector perspective generally includes costs of treatment and cost offsets, that is, costs and cost savings to the health sector through, say, differences in hospitalizations associated with differences in outcomes between intervention alternatives. Such a perspective typically includes out-of-pocket payments incurred by patients and charges on other funders of healthcare, including government and health insurers. A narrower perspective on costs might be justified if the evaluation is to address specific funding questions, for instance, to an individual insurer where costs incurred beyond the organization are deemed not to be relevant. Alternatively, a broader societal perspective might be relevant in instances where it is of interest to compare the intervention with options outside the health sector or if the policy in question is concerned with the potential economic impact on patients and their households.

The adoption of the societal perspective generally means the inclusion of indirect costs. These refer to resources incurred outside the health sector, including costs to patients, carers, and firms. Direct costs, in contrast, pertain to the specific resources involved in the delivery of a health intervention, for example, costs of medications, medical consultations, and equipment used in treatment. These terms have very specific definitions in economic evaluation that may differ from their meanings in common parlance. For instance, the term *indirect costs* is sometimes used to refer to the cost of infrastructure such as building and core administrative staff, particularly in the context of university funding.

For purposes here, indirect costs are potentially factored into an economic evaluation in two ways:

1. Time inputs into an intervention such as waiting, treatment, and travel time. Such costs may be incurred by patients, their household, or other parties such as firms that employ patients. These enter into the evaluation specifically as costs.

2. Production gains to the economy resulting from improvements in health to patients. Confusingly, these are generally treated as benefits within an evaluation although it could be argued that such benefits are savings in disease costs that have been brought about by health gains. Again, such benefits are deemed to be to society rather than to any specific party. This approach to valuation is used in cost-benefit analyses and is typically labeled the "human capital approach."

Both aspects of evaluation have in common the problem of how to value a unit of time, whether it is time spent in accessing and receiving treatment or time gained as a result of improved health (through improved survival or improved functioning translating into increased work or leisure time). The issues considered in this entry are thus generally relevant to both aspects of evaluation although the focus will be on Item 1, given that the primary interest is in the assessment of costs.

The Valuation of Time Inputs

Economic theory suggests that any such measure should reflect the opportunity cost of the time input. In practice, this entails first identifying the nature of the displaced activity. Based on such a perspective, it is relevant to consider whether such activity is work or nonwork.

The valuation of the opportunity cost of work time is dependent first on whether output is replaced. In instances where it is not, the opportunity cost is set at the value of the marginal product of labor (e.g., if Fred takes a day off work, then the opportunity cost of that would be measured by his productivity of the previous workday). The value of the marginal product of labor is in turn dependent on a number of macroeconomic variables such as the level of competition in product markets and the presence of income and sales taxes. In general, the full wage rate, which is the gross wage plus other costs to the employer, is a good benchmark estimate for the marginal product of labor since employers will only incur such a cost if the value of additional output exceeds this cost. However, if there is any error caused by imperfect product markets and the presence of taxes, this benchmark will be rendered an underestimate.

Where production is replaced, then the opportunity cost of this time input is best estimated by the marginal cost of labor. This is proxied by the net wage rate (an individual's wage after taxes) and can be seen as an individual's reservation price for selling his or her labor, reflecting the marginal utility (or satisfaction) gained from leisure time balanced against the marginal (dis)amenity of work (the more unpleasant one finds work, the greater the take-home pay an individual would need to be remunerated to forgo leisure). The presence of involuntary unemployment will introduce some error in this estimate, causing the reservation wage to be an overestimate of opportunity cost.

To determine the opportunity cost of nonwork time, a distinction needs to be made first between whether the individual is currently in paid employment or not. For those currently in paid employment, a proxy for this time input is the net wage (in spite of some possible error) since it reflects the marginal valuation of time for that person (for the same reason as stated in the previous paragraph).

For those not in employment and where activity, say housework, is not replaced (for instance, if it means there are certain household chores that ultimately do not get done), then the average wage of a housekeeper is a suitable proxy (the value of the foregone housework). Where it is replaced, that is, done at a later date, then the average net wage across all occupations would be a useful proxy recognizing that there will be some error depending on whether the individual is voluntarily or involuntarily unemployed. Table 1 summarizes the various proxies that are available for valuing the opportunity cost of time.

The friction cost method is an alternative to the valuation of the opportunity cost of time, although its relevance seems only to apply to work time. It essentially values the lost production from time off work by assuming that firms are able to make certain adjustments to absences, in both the short term and the long term, which will to some extent offset potential production losses. In the short term, factors such as the spare capacity within firms and the possibility of workers making up for lost production mean that the value of lost production from short-term absence is less than the marginal cost of labor as reflected in the full wage rate. This contrasts with the usual approach, which values lost production at the full cost to the firm, that is, the wage paid for the entire period of absence. Those advocating the friction cost approach have

estimated that in the short term, the friction cost represents 80% of the full cost of labor. In the longer term, beyond what is known as the friction period, which is based on the average amount of time a particular labor market is able to fill vacancies caused by illness, the costs are deemed to be zero. One criticism of the friction cost approach is that by ignoring leisure time, it implicitly values it at zero. Its advocates have argued that the value of leisure time is instead factored into health outcomes of an economic evaluation (such as quality-adjusted life years) and therefore need not be taken into account in the analysis of costs.

Issues Around the Inclusion of Indirect Costs

The inclusion of indirect costs into an economic evaluation enables a societal perspective, thereby allowing for a complete picture of the resource implications associated with an intervention. A societal perspective is consistent with the notion of social welfare maximization underlying cost-benefit analysis, that is, the maximization of the well-being of individuals within society.

A limitation of narrower perspectives to evaluation is that by definition they do not account for costs that fall outside the organizations or health systems on which they are based and thereby implicitly encourage cost-shifting. For instance, a regulatory agency that evaluates new technologies for public subsidy based strictly on a health sector perspective tends to favor technologies that cost-shift onto households (such as to carers) and other sectors of the economy. Aside from the equity implications of potentially adding to hardships experienced by households already faced with illness, these narrower perspectives can fail to distinguish between new technologies that are genuinely cost-effective and those that simply shift costs away from the health sector.

Table 1   Summary of proxy measures for measuring opportunity cost of time

	Paid Work Time	Nonpaid Work Time
When outputs/activities are replaced	Net wage	Net wage for *employed* individuals Average net wage for *unemployed individuals*
When outputs/activities are not replaced	Gross wage	Wage of housekeeper

The argument against adopting a societal perspective that will enable the inclusion of indirect costs is that such a perspective is often not relevant to decision making in the health sector. Decisions are generally made by organizations geared toward specific secular interests, and therefore evaluation is required to reflect these. For instance, a health sector perspective is often adopted simply because ministries of health are generally not accountable for the downstream implications of healthcare on employment, social services, schooling, and so on. Based on this line of argument, the merits of an evaluation tool ultimately lie simply in the ability of such a tool to match the objectives of those making decisions rather than its comprehensiveness.

One of the difficulties of including indirect costs is the complexities inherent in their measurement and valuation. As highlighted above, the value of time inputs needs to reflect the opportunity cost of that time. The fundamental problem with the empirical analysis of opportunity cost is that it is not directly observable. Ultimately, it needs to be implied from a number of indicators such as employment status of the individual and the nature of the product and employment markets in which the evaluation is taking place. In practice, this opens up certain ambiguities in the methods for estimating time costs, in measuring both the time inputs (e.g., where there is joint production) and their subsequent valuation.

There are also strong equity implications in the way in which indirect costs are generally measured. Because wage rates are used as markers of opportunity cost, the time costs of high-income earners are generally valued more highly than the time costs of low-income earners. This means technologies that benefit the wealthy tend to be favored over those that benefit the poor. This has been used as a further argument for their exclusion from economic evaluation.

The Decision-Making Context and the Inclusion of Indirect Costs

This entry explores the arguments around the inclusion of indirect costs in economic evaluation. Pivotal is the adoption of a societal perspective consistent with the welfare principles underlying cost-benefit analysis. Nevertheless, in healthcare,

such costs often tend to be excluded from analysis, probably because of their lack of relevance to the perspective taken in evaluation and also the equity implications around their valuation. Ultimately, the merits of whether to factor in such costs in evaluation need to be judged pragmatically and based on whether such an approach is consistent with the specific policy questions under consideration.

Stephen Jan

See also Cost-Benefit Analysis; Costs, Opportunity; Costs, Out-of-Pocket

Further Readings

Brouwer, W. B., & Koopmanschap, M. A. (2005). The friction-cost method: Replacement for nothing and leisure for free? *PharmacoEconomics, 23,* 105–111.

Johannesson, M., & Karlsson, G. (1997). The friction cost method: A comment. *Journal of Health Economics, 16,* 249–255 (Discussion pp. 257–259).

Koopmanschap, M. A., Rutten, F. F., van Ineveld, B. M., & van Roijen, L. (1995). The friction cost method for measuring indirect costs of disease. *Journal of Health Economics, 14,* 171–189.

Liljas, B. (1998). How to calculate indirect costs in economic evaluations. *PharmacoEconomics, 13,* 1–7.

Olsen, J. A., & Richardson, J. (1999). Production gains from health care: What should be included in cost-effectiveness analyses? *Social Science and Medicine, 49,* 17–26.

Posnett, J., & Jan, S. (1996). Indirect cost in economic evaluation: The opportunity cost of unpaid inputs. *Health Economics, 5,* 13–23.

Sugden, R., & Williams, A. (1978). *The principles of practical cost-benefit analysis.* Oxford, UK: Oxford University Press.

Costs, Fixed Versus Variable

Costs refer to the economic input required to achieve a certain outcome, that is, the amount one spends to produce a service or a product, or the value imputed to a resource. Costs are distinguished from *charges,* which are the prices of services and do not reflect the actual costs of all inputs. Costs are usually divided into fixed and variable costs. With regard to healthcare, *fixed costs* are expenses that do not vary with physician care decisions or treatment—such as rent, salaries, mortgage payments, and fire insurance—and that do not vary with the level of patient activity, or products, and once sunk, they cannot be easily recovered. They are also called *sunk costs* because they are beyond the control of the entrepreneur. Other types of costs such as wages of production workers or doctors, medical supplies, drugs, electric power to run machines, and bed-days change with the number of patient visits or products offered for sale. These are called *variable costs*.

In a world of limited healthcare resources, medical decision makers must make challenging management decisions. Without a systematic evaluation of benefits of health interventions or programs in relation to their costs, it is difficult to make rational and sound judgments. This entry reviews key elements related to identification, measurement, and valuation of costs.

Identification

By identifying and controlling all relevant costs, healthcare managers are better able to earn a profit and be successful. Fixed costs are those that generally do not vary between payment intervals. Generally, these costs cannot be altered on a short-term basis because of contractual agreements. Variable costs are those that increase with increasing units of service. For example, an increase in the number of patient visits would result in the use of additional materials, extra labor, and wages. One way to determine fixed costs is to consider the expenses that would continue to be incurred if a healthcare facility were to be temporarily closed and no patients were to be treated. In this case, rent, fees, and loan payments would still be due. They generally do not change with increases or decreases in facility activity. It is important to note that fixed costs are unvarying only within a certain range of facility activity. For example, if the facility activity grows enough to require additional space or additional employees, the fixed costs associated with rent or salaries will change as well. Variable costs are those that change as the level of facility activity changes.

Examples of the variable costs within a healthcare facility would be supplies used for each patient visit, and wages for hourly, part-time employees. These costs are driven primarily by the facility's activity and would stop only if the facility were to close for a period of time, such as a month. Once the difference between fixed and variable costs is understood, it is important to know how to distinguish one from the other. For instance, consider a clinic that has fixed costs of $3,800 and variable costs of $7 per patient. To cover its monthly expenses, the clinic would have to earn $3,800 in fees plus $7 per patient treated. If the clinic had only one patient visit per month, it would have to charge $3,807 for that one treatment to cover its fixed and variable costs! If the practice had 1,000 patient visits during the month, its total costs would be $10,800 ($3,800 in fixed costs plus 1,000 patient visits at $7 each). Therefore, this clinic would only have to charge $10.80 per patient visit to cover its fixed and variable costs. This example illustrates that the amount of fixed costs that each patient visit must cover depends on the total number of patient visits across which these fixed costs are to be spread.

For example, for cost control purposes, it is possible to determine a flexible budget using a formula expressed as a linear equation in which the slope is the variable cost per unit (or per direct labor hour). Graphically, this would appear as shown in Figure 1.

By definition, fixed costs do not change with the level of activity. As a result, the budget for cost control purposes would be displayed graphically as shown in Figure 2.

It is important to note that the costs to be included depend on whose perspective is being used and on the question of *whose costs matter?* The view can be that of the healthcare facility, the insurance company, the patient, or society. They are not interchangeable. An action that reduces facility cost, such as early discharge, may increase the cost to the patient or insurance company by, for example, the need to pay for home healthcare or a stay at an extended-care facility. If the societal perspective is adopted, then all costs must be considered. If the perspective is that of the facility, costs such as patient and caregiver time would be excluded since they are not part of the facility's financial responsibility.

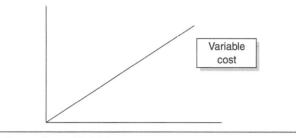

Figure 1   Variable costs

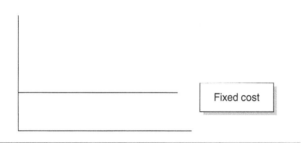

Figure 2   Fixed costs

Measurement

The measurement of costs is similar regardless of the type of analysis being undertaken. Measurement refers to the resource changes included in the analysis. Resources consumed can be divided in a number of different ways. Typically, these will be amounts of labor inputs or outputs but may also include patients' time.

Valuation

The most accurate method of cost estimation is that known as *microcosting,* in which every resource use is identified, measured, and quantified into a unit cost. Microcosting refers to detailed analysis of the changes in resource use due to a particular intervention, like time-and-motion studies. Although many analysts favor microcosting, it tends to be costly. *Gross* or *top-down costing* allocates a total budget to specific services such as hospital stays or doctors' visits. The simplicity of top-down costing may be offset by a lack of sensitivity, which in turn depends on the type of routine data available. The choice between microcosting and gross costing depends on the needs of the analysis. It is common to use substitute proxies for cost, such as Medicare or

Medicaid reimbursement. This method has the advantage of using a nationally relevant estimate as opposed to a single facility's cost. Another popular technique is to start with a facility's charges and then multiply them by an adjustment called the cost-to-charge ratio. Although the cost-to-charge ratio is convenient, it is usually available only for a facility and not for an intervention or diagnosis.

There are two main limitations to conducting a cost study:

1. Costs may vary from one facility to another. They have different purchasing contracts for goods and services. Different staffing levels affect marginal costs and the labor component of variable costs. These may affect the generalizability of the results and may need confirmation before each facility implements changes.

2. The facility may have old costs listed by the accounting system that have not been updated to reflect current market conditions, leading to inaccurate results.

Economic Evaluation

To carry out an economic analysis alongside a study, a researcher can do the following:

- Collect information on the costs and the effectiveness of the alternative interventions from patients in all arms of the trial
- Identify and measure resource volumes, for example, drug quantities for every individual trial patient
- Attach unit costs to each resource item to obtain a mean cost per patient per arm of the trial
- Combine mean patient costs with mean effectiveness measures from the trial to establish the cost-effectiveness of each alternative

Finally, cost studies are typically divided into cost minimization, cost benefit, cost utility, and cost-effectiveness. Cost-minimization studies compare at least two equally effective therapies to find the least expensive. Cost-benefit studies call for converting all outcomes (pain, emesis, renal failure, myocardial infarction, death, etc.) to a monetary value. Cost-utility studies establish the price of a utility metric for each quality-adjusted year of survival. Cost-effectiveness studies decide the cost of avoiding undesirable outcomes (death, ventilation-associated pneumonia, etc.). Suggestions on carrying out cost-effectiveness studies have been disseminated by the U.S. Public Health Service and the European Society of Intensive Care Medicine.

Catherine Kastanioti

See also Cost-Benefit Analysis; Cost-Effectiveness Analysis; Cost-Minimization Analysis; Costs, Direct Versus Indirect; Costs, Semifixed Versus Semivariable; Cost-Utility Analysis

Further Readings

Armstrong, R. A., Brickley, M. R., Shepherd, J. P., & Kay, E. J. (1995). Healthy decision-making: A new approach in health promotion using health state utilities. *Community Dental Health, 12,* 8–11.

Donaldson, C. (1990). The state of the art of costing health care for economic evaluation. *Community Health Studies, 14,* 341–356.

Drummond, M. F., & Davies, L. (1991). Economic analysis alongside clinical trials: Revisiting the methodological issues. *International Journal of Technology Assessment in Health Care, 7,* 561–573.

Drummond, M., & McGuire, A. (2001). *An economic evaluation in health care: Merging theory with practice.* Oxford, UK: Oxford University Press.

Drummond, M., O'Brien, B., Stoddart, G., & Torrance, G. (1997). *Methods for the economic evaluation of health care programmes* (2nd ed.). Oxford, UK: Oxford University Press.

Engoren, M. (2004). Is a charge a cost if nobody pays it? *Chest, 126*(3), 662–664.

Gold, M. R., Gold, S. R., & Weinstein, M. C. (1996). *Cost-effectiveness in health and medicine.* Oxford, UK: Oxford University Press.

Hunink, M., & Glasziou, P. (2001). *Decision making in health and medicine: Integrating evidence and values.* Cambridge, UK: Cambridge University Press.

Meltzer, M. I. (2001). Introduction to health economics for physicians. *Lancet, 358,* 993–998.

Robinson, R. (1993). Costs and cost-minimisation analysis. *British Medical Journal, 307,* 726–728.

Robinson, R. (1993). Economic analysis and health care. What does it mean? *British Medical Journal, 307,* 670–673.

COSTS, INCREMENTAL

See Marginal or Incremental Analysis, Cost-Effectiveness Ratio

COSTS, OPPORTUNITY

The notion of opportunity cost is one of the fundamental concepts of economics. If resources are limited, then there is a choice to be made between desirable, yet mutually exclusive, results. The true or opportunity cost of one alternative is the benefit foregone from not being able to have the next best alternative. The concept has been encapsulated in the truism that "there's no such thing as a free lunch," meaning that things that appear free are always paid for in some way.

The estimation of the opportunity cost of a policy will almost certainly vary depending on the person or persons who are doing the assessing. For example, if a health authority is considering building and staffing a new hospital from public sector funds, the opportunity cost might be the benefit that could have been obtained by increasing or improving facilities and staffing at neighbouring healthcare providers. From this point of view, the choices might be represented as between different policies with the aim of maximizing health, given the funds available to the health authority. However, from the point of view of the public sector as a whole, the opportunity cost might be that this money could have been used to improve the criminal justice system. From this point of view, the choice or trade-off is between improved health and improved criminal justice. From a wider, societal perspective, the evaluation might consider that investment by public services might in some circumstances displace investment by the private sector.

Opportunity cost is a wider concept than accounting or monetary cost. Accounting cost attempts to value the outcomes and resources used in a program or policy at their monetary cost or price. However, not all the outcomes and resources of the policy may have a monetary cost, or there may be no market in the good or service with which to value that outcome, or the price may be thought to omit some important aspect of the benefits or costs of the good or service. If these benefits and costs fall on third parties, they are known as externalities. As an example, consider the use of an intensive care bed after a surgical operation. The monetary value of an hour of care in that bed that is charged to the patient's health insurance or health authority might be calculated as the sum of the hourly salaries of the medical and nursing staff attending the patient, the use of consumables and drugs, and the overheads of the hospital. However, in many hospitals, intensive care facilities are very scarce. The use of this facility by a patient might mean that another patient's planned operation must be postponed until a bed becomes spare, in case it is needed. In these circumstances, the opportunity cost of use of the bed by one patient might be considered in terms of the inconvenience, risks, and costs of cancelling another person's operation. Irrespective of whether resources are allocated to healthcare services by a market mechanism or by a government ministry, they must be valued at their true or opportunity cost if society is to invest its resources efficiently.

One important opportunity cost that is often omitted from decisions about resource allocation in healthcare is the cost of capital. In some countries, public-sector hospitals are owned by one organization, such as a municipality or local government, and managed by another one, such as a health authority. The owner of the facility may consider the cost of the land and building a *sunk cost,* that is, one that has been made in the past and cannot be recovered. This can result in inefficient use of resources (e.g., low bed occupancy rates or underused wards) if the management of the hospital does not pay a rent that appropriately takes account of the alternative use of the land, building, and working capital tied up in the hospital, and this ensures that these costs are reflected in the prices charged to the healthcare purchaser or third-party payer.

People's preference for benefits now rather than in the future is another form of opportunity cost. In this case, the discount rate is a means of adjusting future benefits and costs to current values. Many policies that have an impact on health, especially preventive policies that aim to reduce the risk of future illness, require an immediate investment but might not generate benefits for many years. In these cases, the choice of discount rate can be highly influential in determining whether present-value benefits exceed costs.

The evaluation of the opportunity cost of a policy necessarily implies that all the outcomes of all the feasible alternative policies can be assessed on some common scale. The concept of utility is convenient to measure the relative satisfaction from or desirability of different goods, services, or outcomes. If more than one person is affected by a policy, the utilities of all those persons must be aggregated and compared somehow. An evaluation of alternative health service policies might take into account the effect on health, on work, and on leisure, or the quality of the care provided. These examples illustrate that opportunity cost is a normative concept, that is, it requires an element of subjectivity to decide which benefits and costs to value and the weight that should be given to each type of benefit. A number of conceptual frameworks have been developed to maintain scientific rigour in an evaluation of health technologies. Cost-benefit analysis aims to evaluate all benefits and costs in monetary terms, making use of methods such as contingent valuation or hedonistic pricing to identify people's willingness to pay for each type of benefit, including health. Cost-utility analysis attempts to cut through the debate surrounding the difficulty of valuing different kinds of benefits on a common scale by assuming that health is the only benefit to be valued and that the health of the population is simply the sum of the health of the individuals in it. The Panel on Cost-Effectiveness in Health and Medicine (Gold Report) recommended that all health technology assessments should include a reference case to ensure as far as possible that evaluations by different authors include a common set of outcomes valued by comparable techniques.

The concept of opportunity cost relies on the idea that benefits in one dimension can only be obtained by sacrificing other desirable outcomes. This trade-off implies that the economy is at a point of productive efficiency, that is, it is only possible to produce more of one type of good by diverting resources from the production of another good. However, a principle of Keynesian macroeconomics is that, in some circumstances, there can be underemployed resources. The United

Nations Commission on Macroeconomics and Health assembled considerable evidence that lack of health and education are both a cause and a consequence of enduring poverty. This suggests that policies that tackle the health and education of the poor may be an important lever with which to increase productivity and generate economic growth with benefits for society as a whole.

David Epstein

See also Contingent Valuation; Cost-Benefit Analysis; Cost-Utility Analysis; Discounting; Efficient Frontier; Reference Case; Utility Assessment Techniques; Willingness to Pay

Further Readings

Gold, M. R., Siegel, J. E., Russell, L. B., & Weinstein, M. C. (1996). *Cost effectiveness in health and medicine.* Oxford, UK: Oxford University Press.

WHO Commission on Macroeconomics and Health. (2001). *Macroeconomics and health: Investing in health for economic development.* Geneva: World Health Organization.

COSTS, OUT-OF-POCKET

For most goods and services, the full price is borne by consumers. However, for healthcare services, third-party payers (e.g., government programs or private insurers) typically make partial or full payments on the consumer's behalf. Therefore, the amount paid out-of-pocket (OOP) by consumers represents only a fraction of the full payment received by the providers of services.

The fundamental purpose of imposing cost-sharing requirements on consumers is to control moral hazard (use of services beyond the quantity at which marginal benefit equals marginal cost). Although a risk-averse consumer would prefer full coverage (no OOP obligations) in the first best situation, the first best is generally not attainable because fully insured individuals have an incentive to use care until marginal benefit is zero. These low-benefit services will increase the cost of insurance or the burden on public finance without creating sufficient value to justify the extra cost. Imposing

OOP obligations on consumers trades some risk spreading for the preservation of a partial incentive for the consumer to consider the cost of the chosen services relative to their expected value.

Determinants of Out-of-Pocket Prices

The gap between the total price paid for a service and the OOP price faced by the consumer is a function of the basic provisions with respect to patient obligations contained in the public payment policy or the private health insurance contract under which third-party payments are made. Such provisions are often complex, including deductibles (consumer is fully responsible for the first specified amount of spending during a time period), co-payments (consumer is responsible for a fixed payment for each unit of service received once the deductible has been satisfied) or co-insurance (consumer is responsible for a fixed percentage of the price of each unit of service received once the deductible has been satisfied), and stop-loss (consumer is fully insured for additional services once a prespecified, maximum OOP expenditure has been exceeded during a time period).

In addition to these basic policy provisions, the OOP price to the consumer can also be modified by a number of other factors. Third-party payers often place a variety of restrictions on coverage that can directly or indirectly change consumers' OOP obligations. These include service-specific limits (e.g., maximum number of visits allowed to a certain type of provider during a time period) and overall limits (e.g., lifetime maximum expenditures), after which the consumer will face the full price of additional services. In addition, coverage for some services may be denied if specific requirements are not met (e.g., approval of the service by a "gatekeeper" physician or by a third-party payer's pre-authorization or use review process). Third-party payers also often specify whether or not providers can engage in *balance billing.* Suppose the third-party payment plus the patient's contractual obligation as determined by the provisions discussed above (e.g., co-payments) falls short of the provider's charges. If the provider is allowed to balance bill, the consumer's OOP obligation would increase by the excess of the provider's charges above the amount paid by the third-party payer and the consumer's co-payment obligations. Finally, third-party payers may distinguish between preferred or nonpreferred providers (in-network vs. out-of-network) or treatments (e.g., generic vs. brand name pharmaceuticals) by obligating consumers who elect nonpreferred providers or treatments to pay a higher OOP price. The recent trend toward value-based insurance design operates analogously, identifying classes of patients who may be exempted from OOP obligations for specified services deemed clinically valuable (e.g., diabetes patients may be exempted from insulin co-payments).

Because some of these provisions are based on the use of services over a period of time (e.g., deductibles, service limits), consumer decision making also has an important dynamic aspect. Using an annual deductible for purposes of illustration, the consumer's actual OOP price for any given service can deviate from the rationally anticipated OOP price. Suppose a consumer with a chronic illness knows that he or she has a very high probability of exceeding his or her deductible during the year. Consuming an extra service early in the year will cause the consumer to satisfy his or her deductible sooner, thereby creating an implicit "discount" on a service that will be consumed later in the year. Conversely, a consumer who has not satisfied the deductible late in the year would be unlikely to obtain such an implicit discount by consuming an additional service. More generally, the anticipated OOP price today depends on use earlier in the year, and the anticipated OOP later in the year depends on the use decisions made today.

Richard A. Hirth

See also Dynamic Decision Making; Economics, Health Economics; Pharmacoeconomics; Value-Based Insurance Design; Willingness to Pay

Further Readings

Hirth, R. A., Greer, S. L., Albert, J. M., Young, E. W., & Piette, J. D. (2008). Out-of-pocket spending and medication adherence among dialysis patients in twelve countries. *Health Affairs, 27*(1), 89–102.

Manning, W. G., Newhouse, J. P., Duan, N., Keeler, E. B., Leibowitz, A., & Marquis, M. S. (1987). Health insurance and the demand for medical care. *American Economic Review, 77*(3), 251–277.

COSTS, SEMIFIXED VERSUS SEMIVARIABLE

Consideration of costs is an important factor in medical decisions, including budgeting and planning, pricing for healthcare products or services, operational control, and selection of therapeutic options. Costs may be viewed in different ways. One approach to describe costs is a cost behavior pattern in which a cost is analyzed by its reactions to different levels of activity. Understanding the cost behavior patterns will facilitate medical decision making.

Two common types of cost behavior patterns are fixed and variable costs. Fixed costs remain constant over different levels of activity (e.g., volume, workload). Variable costs vary with changed levels of activity, such as costs for medications and medical supplies, which represent a major part in healthcare. In some cases, neither fixed costs nor variable costs alone can fully describe cost behavior patterns. Semifixed or semivariable costs are conceptually used as other types of cost behavior patterns. Semifixed or semivariable costs contain a portion of fixed costs and another portion of variable costs. Eventually, all costs can be properly explained by different combinations of fixed costs and variable costs. Semifixed and semivariable costs are explained as follows.

Semifixed Costs

Semifixed costs are also called stepped, stepped-fixed, step-variable, step-fixed, or step-function costs. This type of cost remains a constant within a particular range of activity and sharply changes after exceeding the threshold of this range, and then again remains constant during another range of activity. In other words, semifixed costs could be viewed as a combination of multiple fixed costs in which each has a much narrower relevant range. If semifixed costs are plotted against levels of activity, the pattern of semifixed costs looks like steps. Figure 1 illustrates a semifixed cost that increases with increased level of activity. The activity range may be different within each step, and the overall change varies with increased level of activity.

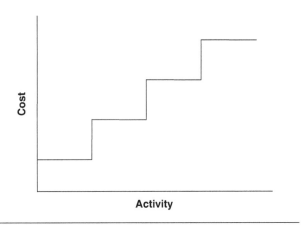

Figure 1   An example of semifixed costs

An example of semifixed costs is the total staff cost for pharmacists. Suppose a pharmacist can handle a maximum of 50 prescriptions per day. Accordingly, a pharmacy needs 10 pharmacists to deal with 451 to 500 prescriptions or 11 pharmacists for 501 to 550 prescriptions. Similar examples include medical or nursing staff costs, administration costs, information technology costs, and equipment maintenance costs.

Semivariable Costs

Semivariable costs are sometimes called mixed costs. This type of cost contains a portion of fixed costs, and the remaining portion varies with an increased level of activity. Semivariable costs can be further classified as linear or nonlinear semivariable costs, and the classification of patterns depends on the relation of the variable portion to the change of activity. Typical figures of semivariable cost patterns are shown in Figure 2. Note that the total cost line does not pass through the origin because there is a fixed cost component.

An example of linear semivariable costs is laboratory costs. For a diagnosis test, the device cost and the annual maintenance cost are fixed, and the total cost of test strips varies with an increased number of tests. A utility cost may be an example of a nonlinear semivariable cost. A basic monthly fee is charged regardless of the amount of the utility used, and an additional charge increases with increased use of the utility; however, the rates may vary with an increased amount of use. Other examples of semivariable costs include car rental (fixed vehicle

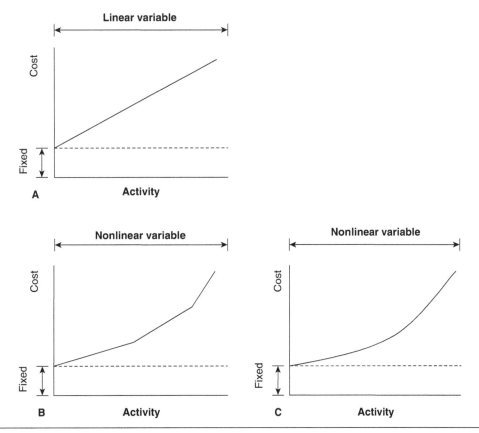

Figure 2   Examples of semivariable costs: linear (A) and nonlinear (B, C)

rental fee plus variable costs for fuel and mileage) and facility costs (fixed rental or maintenance costs plus various total utility costs in general).

Costing Methods

Costs related to medical decisions may evolve in many types of cost behavior patterns, and costs usually require further analysis to provide information for medical decisions. There are at least three methods to analyze cost behavior patterns: top-down, bottom-up, and graph analysis. The top-down method breaks down aggregated cost data into smaller pieces from higher levels (e.g., hospital costs) to lower levels (e.g., departmental costs) based on a principle of allocation. This method is often used for retrospective data, and it is often difficult to break down data to the individual level (e.g., patients). The bottom-up method uses cost data from the individual level and then adds up all costs to the total costs. This method can use either retrospective or prospective data, and patient-level data of use can be further analyzed. Therefore, the bottom-up method is frequently used in economic analyses. However, this method bears several limitations, including difficulty in obtaining sensitive personal data (e.g., payment), so a proxy (e.g., hospital charge) is often used. The graph method is to plot costs against activity levels, as shown in the figures. This method allows investigators to evaluate or present cost behavior patterns in summarized data, but detailed cost information will not be available.

Jun-Yen Yeh

See also Costs, Direct Versus Indirect; Costs, Fixed Versus Variable; Costs, Opportunity; Sunk Costs

Further Readings

Cleverly, W. O. (1997). Cost concepts and decision making. *Essentials of health care finance* (4th ed., pp. 223–227). Gaithersburg, MD: Aspen.

Gyldmark, M. (1995). A review of cost studies of intensive care units: Problems with the cost concept. *Critical Care Medicine, 23*(5), 964–972.

Jegers, M., Edbrooke, D. L., Hibbert, C. L., Chalfin, D. B., & Burchardi, H. (2002). Definitions and methods of cost assessment: An intensivist's guide. *Intensive Care Medicine, 28*(6), 680–685.

Lere, J. C. (2000). Activity-based costing: A powerful tool for pricing. *Journal of Business & Industrial Marketing, 15*(1), 23–33.

Lubasky, D. A. (1995). Understanding cost analyses: Part 1. A practitioner's guide to cost behavior. *Journal of Clinical Anesthesia, 7*(6), 519–521.

COSTS, SPILLOVER

When producing, selling, buying, or consuming a good or service affects people other than those directly involved in the market exchange—for example, when a factory emits smoke that pollutes the air breathed by those in the vicinity—the economic activity is said to "spill over" and impose costs (or confer benefits) on people other than those directly involved in the transaction. Economists call spillover effects *externalities*. The extent of spillover effects in healthcare is one of several features that contribute to the failure of private markets to achieve efficient results and health-related outcomes relative to their costs. Externalities serve as one rationale for public-sector involvement in healthcare.

Spillover effects must be taken into account when evaluating the impact of healthcare services, their financing, and their delivery in cost-benefit or cost-effectiveness analyses and when making decisions about how healthcare resources should be invested. The level and distribution of health status and longevity within a population can also have economic impacts (both financial and in terms of well-being) beyond the individual level.

Classic examples of spillover effects in public health and health services are the transmission and control of communicable diseases and immunization, cases for which untreated disease or services to the individual have costs or benefits for others. Because communicable diseases impose costs (spread of disease to others) beyond those borne by the individual infected, the willingness of the individual to pay for the disease's prevention or treatment may be less than the total value to the community of taking action to prevent the spread of the disease. This circumstance justifies public provision or subsidy of services to prevent disease transmission.

Another spillover effect in healthcare stems from the value individuals place on others' access to and use of needed healthcare. In this case, the rationale for public financing or provision of healthcare is that the welfare of individuals who are taxed or otherwise support health services provided to unrelated others is increased because this subsidy satisfies a moral sentiment of altruism or justice. The provision of healthcare or health coverage to others in a community (local or national) is deemed a "merit good."

The ability to identify and measure spillover effects of an activity or policy depends on what is encompassed by an analysis and the perspective that is adopted in conducting it. A study of the overall use of medical services by Medicare end-stage renal disease (ESRD) patients exemplifies this point. Providers of routine dialysis services receive a capitation payment from Medicare for outpatient services only. The cost of each dialysis treatment depends on its intensity, measured in terms of the rate of urea removal during the procedure. Avi Dor found that less intensive dialysis treatments resulted in higher rates of hospital admissions among Medicare ESRD patients. From the perspective of the outpatient dialysis provider, the cost of lower intensity of outpatient treatments on hospitalization rates accumulates—this cost is manifested by the outpatient provider and is most pronounced in the worse health of patients receiving the less intensive treatment and higher overall Medicare costs for ESRD care. The full impact of the Medicare outpatient ESRD capitation rates and provider treatment decisions can be captured only when a broader analysis is undertaken.

An ethical conundrum that clinicians face is whether they should take costs into account when making treatment choices and recommendations for their patients, given that spending on the care of those with coverage may indirectly make it more difficult politically and fiscally to extend healthcare coverage to those without it. This constitutes a spillover cost of individual doctor-patient transactions. Christine Cassel and Troyen Brennan argue that physicians share a "medical commons" and that they should be accountable for how resources devoted to health services are managed. In prepaid group practices and in fixed-budget national healthcare systems, physicians' ethical duties to individual patients are linked with a shared responsibility for a community's resources. For the larger U.S. healthcare enterprise, however,

the full cost implications of individual treatment choices are not internalized.

Just as the costs of care of people with coverage affect those who are uninsured, uninsurance in a community can affect those who have coverage. The first systematic look at the spillover costs of uninsurance was undertaken by the Institute of Medicine in a study published in 2003. Although healthcare access problems related to lack of coverage are most severe for people who are uninsured, other vulnerable population groups (Medicaid enrollees, low-income inner-city residents, members of racial and ethnic minority groups) who tend to rely on the same care providers (e.g., public clinics, hospital outpatient departments) experience reduced access to care in communities with high uninsurance rates due to crowding and provider instability because of high uncompensated care burdens. Furthermore, communities with higher-than-average uninsurance rates tend to have fewer specialized hospital services such as trauma, psychiatric, or burn units than communities with relatively low rates of uninsurance. This reduced access to a variety of health services experienced across a community is a spillover cost of high uninsurance rates.

As noted by Jeremiah Hurley in his overview of the economics of the health sector, spillover effects have been the subject of much theoretical discussion and far less empirical analysis in the field. Doing a better job of capturing spillover effects will require both a wider-angle lens when focusing on a subject and ingenuity and persistence in acquiring the kinds of data that reveal these effects. The consequence of measuring spillover impacts will be more complete information for policy choices.

Wilhelmine Miller

See also Cost-Benefit Analysis; Cost-Effectiveness Analysis; Economics, Health Economics

Further Readings

Cassel, C. K., & Brennan, T. E. (2007). Managing medical resources: Return to the commons? *Journal of the American Medical Association, 297,* 2518–2521.

Dor, A. (2004). Optimal price rules, administered prices and suboptimal prevention: Evidence from a Medicare program. *Journal of Regulatory Economics, 25,* 81–104.

Hurley, J. (2000). An overview of the normative economics of the health sector. In A. J. Culyer & J. P. Newhouse (Eds.), *Handbook of health economics* (pp. 56–118). Amsterdam: Elsevier.

Institute of Medicine Committee on the Consequences of Uninsurance. (2003). *A shared destiny: Community effects of uninsurance.* Washington, DC: National Academies Press.

Rice, T. (1998). *The economics of health reconsidered.* Chicago: Health Administration Press.

COST-UTILITY ANALYSIS

Cost-utility analysis is a special form of cost-effectiveness analysis where the health outcomes are measured in terms of a preference-based *utility* measure. Like cost-effectiveness analysis, this yields an outcome of the evaluation that is expressed in terms of a cost per unit effect. However, in contrast to cost-effectiveness analysis, provided this measure is considered to be a generic measure of health, then cost-utility analysis is sufficient to efficiently allocate resources from a fixed healthcare budget in terms of maximizing the health achievable from those fixed resources. Of crucial importance is the validity of the preference-based utility measure as a generic measure of health outcome that can be used to compare the allocation of resources across disease areas.

A number of different candidate utility measures have been proposed. Most popular are the disability-adjusted life year (DALY), which has been used extensively by the World Health Organisation (WHO) to compare the burden of disease between countries (particularly in the developing world), and the quality-adjusted life year (QALY), which is widely used in developed countries, such as Australia, Canada, the United Kingdom, and the United States. Other measures, such as the healthy year equivalent (HYE), have not gained widespread acceptance despite apparently addressing some of the acknowledged problems in the other measures.

All the measures have the same fundamental goal—to represent the two dimensions of health, morbidity and mortality, in a single measure that represents the value of the underlying health state in a way that can be validly compared across disease areas. The QALY does this by weighting length of life by a health-related quality-of-life measure. The QALY is simply the area under this quality-adjusted survival curve, and the QALY gained from a treatment under evaluation is estimated as the difference between two quality-adjusted survival profiles representing the treatment under evaluation and the relevant alternative treatment.

The accurate measurement of mortality presents few challenges due to the definitive nature of the health outcome. However, the measurement of health-related quality of life is far more controversial. The health-related quality-of-life measure, to be suitable for quality adjusting life years, must represent a preference for health on a cardinal ratio scale (such that an improvement of 0.2 is twice as good as an improvement of 0.1) that is anchored at the top end by the value of 1 for perfect health and where 0 represents death. Negative values are allowed and represent health states worse than death.

The accurate assessment of health-related quality-of-life utility has become a major research area. Direct utility assessment methods involve asking patients or lay populations to provide a value for a specific health state—often presented to the respondent in the form of a vignette. Popular utility elicitation instruments include the standard gamble, time trade-off, and person trade-off techniques. In recent years, much debate has centered on whether it is patients or lay populations who should form the respondent base for utility assessments. Advocates of the patient-based approach cite the experience of patients as the principal advantage, while advocates of asking lay populations cite the role of the layperson as taxpayer and potential patient in publicly funded systems and suggest that patients may provide strategic responses if they realize that their values are being used to allocate resources. A popular compromise in recent years has been the use of health-related quality-of-life instruments such as the EQ-5D (EuroQol) and Health Utility Index, which are generic descriptive systems for health. These are suitable for use with patients to map into the descriptive system with tariff utility values assigned from large-scale population surveys.

The avoidance of placing a monetary value on health, as is required in cost-benefit analysis, is seen as a practical advantage by many for whom monetary valuation of health is seen as distasteful. Proponents of cost-benefit analysis typically criticize the lack of theoretical foundation for cost-utility analysis, whereas proponents of the approach have claimed it embodies its own justification on the grounds of equitable treatment of health outcomes across individuals, coining the term *extrawelfarism* to describe the ethic embodied in the approach. Nevertheless, monetary valuation in cost-utility analysis cannot be avoided. In the face of a fixed budget constraint, utility maximization requires ranking of interventions by cost-utility ratio with healthcare interventions adopted in order of ascending cost-utility ratio until the budget is exhausted. The cost-utility ratio of the last program funded "reveals" the (shadow) price (willingness to pay) for a unit of health outcome implied by the budget constraint.

A more practical approach to allocating resources has been to consider a "threshold" value of a unit of health output above which a program or treatment would not be funded. Although such an approach has been criticized for failing to recognize the budget constraint (and therefore encouraging uncontrolled healthcare expenditure), the use of arbitrary threshold values as a decision-making rule of thumb is widespread.

The concept of a decision-making threshold has had an important influence on the analysis of cost-utility (and cost-effectiveness) studies by encouraging the use of the net-benefit approach to decision making. By translating health outcome into a monetary value, it is possible to analyze the overall net benefit of a program or intervention conditional on the threshold value. This has led some commentators to question whether there is a practical difference between cost-benefit and cost-effectiveness/utility analyses. Nevertheless, it is important to recognize that in the presence of a fixed budget constraint, net-benefit decision making will not necessarily lead to optimal allocation of resources. This is because the budget may not allow all "net-beneficial" programs to be provided. Where this is the case, the health benefit is only maximized if programs are implemented in order of increasing cost-utility ratio, emphasizing the importance of the continued presentation of the cost-utility ratio.

Andrew H. Briggs

See also Cost-Benefit Analysis; Cost-Effectiveness Analysis; Disability-Adjusted Life Years (DALYs); EuroQol (EQ-5D); Health Utilities Index Mark 2 and 3 (HUI2, HUI3); Healthy Years Equivalents; Net Monetary Benefit; Quality-Adjusted Life Years (QALYs); Utility Assessment Techniques

Further Readings

Drummond, M. F., Sculpher, M. J., Torrance, G. W., O'Brien, B., & Stoddart, G. L. (2005). *Methods for the economic evaluation of health care programmes* (3rd ed.). Oxford, UK: Oxford University Press.

Gold, M. R., Siegel, J. E., Russell, L. B., & Weinstein, M. C. (Eds.). (1996). *Cost-effectiveness in health and medicine*. New York: Oxford University Press.

COUNTERFACTUAL THINKING

Counterfactual thinking in judgment and decision making occurs when the decision maker considers or imagines outcomes of a decision that could have occurred but did not. For example, a patient who experiences a surgical complication that results in disability might easily imagine counterfactual worlds in which his outcome was different. A great deal of theoretical and empirical work on counterfactual thinking in decision making has its genesis in the seminal work of Kahneman and Miller on norm theory.

Types

In most decisions, there are many counterfactual outcomes and several different ways that counterfactual outcomes can be imagined to occur. First, in decisions under uncertainty, chance factors (the "state of the world") could be imagined to have been different. For example, the surgical patient might imagine that his surgery had proceeded without the complication. Second, decisions taken by others could have been different. For example, the surgical patient might imagine that his surgeon had chosen a different procedure that could not lead to the complication. Third, the decision of the decision maker could have been different. For example, the surgical patient might imagine that he had chosen a medical treatment (with a successful outcome) instead. Fourth, the decision maker could imagine himself or herself to be a different person, a so-called social counterfactual. For example, the surgical patient might imagine other people he knows with different health problems.

Each counterfactual can potentially result in a comparison between the actual outcome and the counterfactual outcome. The surgical patient might compare his new life with disability to (a) how he imagines his life might have been if the surgery had been uncomplicated, (b) how he imagines his life might have been if the surgeon had chosen a different surgery, (c) how he imagines his life might have been if he had chosen a medical treatment, or (d) how he imagines the lives of his peers (with different health problems) might compare with his new life.

Ease of Imagining Counterfactuals

Although multiple counterfactuals are nearly always available, the ease with which a particular counterfactual outcome is generated or used in comparisons varies. The psychological literature uses the term *mutability* to refer to the aspects of reality that are most amenable to yielding counterfactuals. For example, exceptional events are more mutable than normal events (so people are more likely to imagine what would have happened if an exception had not occurred than to imagine what would have happened if an exception had occurred). Events under the decision maker's control are typically more mutable than uncontrollable events, actions are more mutable than inactions or omissions, repeatable events are more mutable than one-time events, and effects are more mutable than causes.

Direction and Impact on Postdecision Emotion

Counterfactuals are also referred to by their direction or valence. Upward counterfactuals are alternative outcomes that the decision maker considers superior to the actual outcome. Downward counterfactuals are alternative outcomes that the decision maker considers inferior to the actual outcome. Counterfactual comparisons reliably change the way decision makers feel about their actual decision outcomes (their postdecision affect). Research on counterfactual comparisons has demonstrated that upward counterfactual comparisons, which typically result in lower postdecision satisfaction and more negative postdecision affect, are more common and carry more weight than downward comparisons, which typically result in greater postdecision satisfaction and more positive postdecision affect. In addition, surprising outcomes, which more easily evoke counterfactual alternatives, typically result in more extreme postdecision affect. For example, a rare and surprising recovery is experienced with greater elation than a common and expected return to health.

Functional Impacts

Counterfactual thinking may serve functional purposes. Upward counterfactuals may direct the decision maker to reflect on aspects of the decision process that may have led to a poor outcome and could have been undertaken differently. This reflection may result in an improved decision process if the decision maker is again faced with the same or a similar decision. Downward counterfactuals may reduce postdecision regret by providing the decision maker with a comparison in which the decision outcome can be cast as superior to the counterfactuals.

To the degree to which decision makers actively seek to consider potential alternative outcomes prospectively, they may also anticipate the counterfactual comparisons that are likely to co-occur with particular outcomes. Such anticipated counterfactuals may form the basis for decision-making strategies that seek to, for example, minimize expected regret.

Alan Schwartz

See also Emotion and Choice; Regret

Further Readings

Kahneman, D., & Miller, D. T. (1986). Norm theory: Comparing reality to its alternatives. *Psychological Review, 93,* 136–153.

Mandel, D. R., Hilton, D. J., & Catellani, P. (2005). *The psychology of counterfactual thinking.* New York: Routledge.

Roese, N. J., & Olson, J. M. (Eds.). (1995). *What might have been: The social psychology of counterfactual thinking.* Mahwah, NJ: Lawrence Erlbaum.

Cox Proportional Hazards Regression

In the analysis of survival data, researchers want to ascertain characteristics of the patient that influence patient survival time. The relationship between a single response variable (survival time) and covariates (patient/disease characteristics) is often inferred through the use of a regression model. Typical regression models, such as linear or logistic regression, do not work when the response variable is survival time, since the time to death may not be recorded for all patients at the time of analysis. If a patient is still alive at the time of analysis or has been lost to follow-up, the patient survival time is said to have been right censored (or simply censored) at the time of the last observed follow-up. If the patient has been lost to follow-up, an important assumption in many survival analytic methods is that the reason a patient is lost to follow-up is unrelated to the risk of death.

In survival analysis, when the survival time, T, is possibly right censored, the Cox proportional hazards model is the predominant regression model. The proportional hazards model is written as

$$h(t|X) = h_0(t) \exp[b^T X], \quad (1)$$

where $h(t|X)$ is the hazard function conditional on a set of patient-specific covariates, which is denoted by the vector X, and b represents the vector of regression coefficients that determines the relationship between the covariates and the risk of death. Covariates in the Cox model are handled using standard regression techniques. Thus, categorical factors may be entered into the model using dummy variables, and interactions may be introduced through the multiplication of two covariates. However, due to complications that stem from censored observations, additional methodology, based on what is called the partial likelihood, is needed for estimation of the regression coefficients b.

The conditional hazard $h(t|X)$ provides the patient-specific risk of death over time. The proportional hazards specification, Equation 1, divides the conditional hazard into two components, a baseline hazard function $h_0(t)$ independent of the patient characteristic vector and the patient relative risk function, $\exp[b^T X]$, independent of time;

the relationship between the two components is multiplicative. The baseline hazard function is left unspecified but governs how the patient-specific hazard varies over time. Heuristically, the hazard function is proportional to the probability of death by time t, given the patient has not died prior to time t. For any two patients with characteristics X_1 and X_2, the ratio of their conditional hazards,

$$h(t|X_1)/h(t|X_2) = \exp[b^T(X_1 - X_2)],$$

is independent of time. The term *proportional hazards* refers to the fact that the two conditional hazards are proportional to each other, with the proportionality constant equal to $\exp[b^T(X_1 - X_2)]$.

The widespread popularity of the proportional hazards methodology stems from the interpretation of the regression parameter, b, as a relative risk parameter constant with respect to time, the accuracy of the estimate of the relative risk parameter in the presence of censored data, the development of inferential procedures that are easy to implement with available software, and the efficiency of the regression parameters for a wide range of baseline hazard functions.

An alternative specification of the proportional hazards regression model is through the patient specific (conditional) survival function,

$$S(t|X) = S_0(t)^{\exp[bX]}, \quad (2)$$

where the term $S(t|X)$ represents the probability that a patient with characteristics denoted by the covariate vector X survives beyond time t. This specification of the proportional hazards model enables the regression model to be used for prediction. For example, using Equation 2, the analyst can predict the patient-specific probability of survival beyond 5 years or the median survival time for a given set of patient characteristics. Thus, the proportional hazards model enables a refinement of the Kaplan-Meier estimate of a survival probability by providing an estimate for the probability of survival beyond t years for a patient with characteristics represented by the covariate vector X.

In addition to ascertaining the risk profile of a patient, the proportional hazards model is used to adjust for patient risk in testing the equality of the survival distributions between exposure and treatment groups. This application, often termed the analysis of covariance, has historically been used in the analysis of observational studies. For this application, the proportional hazards model may be written as

$$h(t|Z, X) = \exp[aZ + b^{\mathrm{T}}X],$$

where Z represents the treatment group classification, X represents the vector of potential confounding factors, and the parameter of interest, a, represents the treatment effect on survival time. The analysis of covariance in the setting of survival analysis would test whether $a = 0$, that is, whether there is a treatment effect, after adjusting for potential confounding factors.

An interesting generalization of the proportional hazards model is the incorporation of time-dependent covariates,

$$h(t|X) = \exp[b^{\mathrm{T}}X(t)].$$

Under this generalization, the proportional hazards specification no longer holds, as the relative risk,

$$h(t|X_1(t))/h(t|X_2(t)) = \exp[b^{\mathrm{T}}(X_1(t) - X_2(t))],$$

now changes over time. As a result, the model is often referred to as the time-dependent Cox model rather than the proportional hazard model. The time-dependent Cox model is useful when disease-related patient characteristics change over the course of follow-up. For example, a prostate cancer patient who experiences a prostate-specific antigen (PSA) relapse after receiving a course of therapy is at greater risk of death after relapse than before it. The time-dependent covariate Cox model enables the analyst to recalibrate the risk of death at the point of time during follow-up that the patient experiences the PSA relapse.

Although the proportional hazards model is robust, its application is not universal. The proportional hazards model is termed a semiparametric model because the baseline hazard function, $h_0(t)$, and the baseline survival function, $S_0(t)$, are not specified for the purpose of estimating the relative risk coefficient, b. This provides a robustness quality to this regression model, enabling the proportional hazards regression model to be applied to a wide array of survival data. There are characteristics of the data, however, which need to be compatible with the assumptions implicit in the proportional hazards model, in order for the results of the analysis to be meaningful. For example, in a simplified version of the proportional hazards model with a single binary treatment covariate, the Cox model implies that the survival probability for patients on one treatment dominates the survival probability for the cohort of patients on the other treatment over the entire patient follow-up. If, however, the survival curves cross over time, the proportional hazards assumption does not hold, and the proportional hazards model is not appropriate for data summarization. The validity of the proportional hazards specification is more difficult to diagnose if there are many (possibly continuous) covariates under consideration.

In general, if the proportional hazards assumption is incorrect, application of this model is likely to lead to incorrect conclusions regarding the relationship between the covariates and survival time. In this circumstance, it would behoove the data analyst to consider alternative regression models for survival data. The most common alternative to the proportional hazards model is the accelerated failure time model

$$\log t_i = b^{\mathrm{T}}X_i + e_i,$$

where the e_i represent stochastic errors generated independently from a common but unknown distribution, the vector X denotes the patient-specific covariates, and b is the regression coefficient vector.

An additional assumption in the proportional hazards model is that the relative risk is monotonically increasing or decreasing in the covariates. If some of the important covariates in a particular data set are continuous, such as age or white blood cell count, it is important to assess whether this specification is correct. For example, it is plausible that a patient with either a low or a high white blood count (WBC) is at greater risk of death than a patient with a WBC in the normal range, and thus Equation 1 is inappropriate. An approach to generalizing Equation 1 is based on nonparametric estimation methods, such as spline or kernel estimation, which provide a more flexible approach to specifying the relative risk function.

Finally, like uncensored regression models, individual observations may either provide a poor fit for the model or have undue influence of the estimated regression coefficients. In classical statistical terms, these would be defined as data points with large residuals or high leverage. These data values should be monitored and either downweighted or removed during the course of the data analysis.

Glenn Heller

See also Analysis of Covariance (ANCOVA); Hazard Ratio; Logistic Regression; Nomograms; Prediction Rules and Modeling; Survival Analysis

Further Readings

Collett, D. (1994). *Modelling survival data in medical research.* London: Chapman & Hall.

Cox, D. R. (1972). Regression models and life-tables (with discussion). *Journal of the Royal Statistical Society, Series B, 34,* 187–220.

Fisher, L. D., & Lin, D. Y. (1999). Time dependent covariates in the Cox Proportional Hazards Regression Model. *Annual Review of Public Health, 20,* 145–157.

Harrell, F. E. (2001). *Regression modeling strategies: With applications to linear models, logistic regression, and survival analysis.* New York: Springer-Verlag.

Hosmer, D. W., & Lemeshow, S. (1999). *Applied survival analysis: Regression modeling of time to event data.* New York: Wiley.

CUES

The term *cue* in decision making is a broad one denoting every piece of information outside the decision maker that may help in a decision or judgment under uncertainty. Other personal information such as goals or preferences also influence decisions, but these pieces of information are not called cues. Many ways of integrating cue information exist, called decision rules. Their accuracies crucially depend on the structure of the decision environment, and therefore, statistical models of the decision domain are necessary to derive prescriptions of a good decision strategy.

Cue Values

Cues are variables that can be used to judge, infer, or predict the value of an unknown criterion variable of interest. In a specific decision situation, a cue may take on a certain cue value that is indicative of the value of the to-be-inferred criterion. In medicine, for example, symptoms and laboratory results are cues that are used to infer the underlying disease. Likewise, medical parameters such as blood pressure, smoking habits, and symptom severity may serve as cues to predict the survival time of a patient. Hence, the term *cue* is neutral as to whether it is a cause or an effect of the variable which is inferred. Even a merely statistical relation between cue and criterion (without causation) can render the cue useful for inferences. The inference or prediction can be a classification (categorical variable, e.g., disease), a continuous judgment of a quantity (e.g., expected survival time), or a comparative judgment concerning several options (e.g., which treatment will be most successful?). To be useful for inferences, cues must have a high predictive power or correlation with the criterion variable, called the *ecological cue validity*.

Cue Validity

Like the criterion, cues can be continuous variables (e.g., blood pressure) or categorical variables (e.g., symptoms). Depending on the nature of the cues and criterion, different measures of cue validity may be useful. If cue and criterion are continuous variables, Pearson correlations or partial correlations (if a whole set of correlated cues is used for prediction) measure the predictive power. Likewise, (point-)biserial correlations or different contingency coefficients can be used to express the degree of the statistical relationship between the cues and criterion if one or both variables are categorical or binary. In pairwise comparisons (e.g., "Who of two patients has better survival chances when treated first in the emergency room?") with binary cues (e.g., Symptom X present vs. absent), the validity is often defined as the conditional probability of deciding correctly, given that the cue discriminates between the options. A cue discriminates if it takes on different values for the compared objects. Hence, besides validity, the discrimination rate of a cue is another important aspect of its usefulness for decisions because a cue is only helpful if the values differ between options.

In principle, in a set of statistically related variables, any of these variables can serve as cues for predicting one of the other variables. However, a high cue validity in one inference direction does not imply high validity in the other direction. For instance, there may be a high conditional probability of a symptom given a disease (e.g., fever given pneumonia), whereas the reverse is not necessarily true if the symptom is not specific for the disease. Hence, for using cues in a systematic fashion, their relation to the criterion must be known. If only one valid cue is available for a decision, matters are quite easy since the best bet is to go with the cue. Typically, however, multiple (and potentially contradicting) cues have to be integrated into one judgment or decision that requires conflict resolution and information integration via decision rules. The success of a decision rule depends on its fit to the statistical structure of the environment. For example, if the available cues are highly correlated, it may be worthwhile and time-saving to consider only a small subset of cues because the other information is redundant.

Models of the Environment

The psychologist Egon Brunswik introduced the idea of the lens model, which is an attempt to model the environment, the decision process, and their mutual fit simultaneously. The cues are the "lens" through which the distal criterion variable can only indirectly be perceived. Further developments of the lens model in social judgment theory use a multiple linear regression to predict the criterion on the basis of the cues. This regression informs the investigator how predictable the criterion is given the cues and provides beta weights that measure the contribution of each single cue to a weighted linear prediction of the criterion, hence its ecological validity. On the other side of the lens, one can perform a regression of actual judgments on the cue values as predictors. This can be seen as a model of the decision maker (called policy capturing), and the regression weights measure the influence of the cues on judgments, or cue use. Both regressions can be compared to see if the judgmental cue weighting matches the optimal weighting, that is, if use coefficients match the ecological validities. The use of linear regressions has dominated research for decades, but the idea of analyzing the environmental structure and its match with psychological processes can be applied more

generally, to include nonlinear cue-criterion relationships (e.g., U-shaped or exponential) or nonlinear cue combinations. Optimal decision algorithms can also be identified using machine learning approaches or Bayesian networks, which need a large amount of training in huge databases.

However, the "optimal" rules often need extensive computation to combine cues in sophisticated ways, for example, in Bayesian networks or a weighted additive integration. In many instances, the accuracy of such complex rules can be approximated by simpler algorithms or so-called heuristics. For instance, extensive simulations have shown that linear models often have a *flat maximum*, which means that nonoptimal weighting of cues does not hurt the predictive accuracy very much as long as the direction of the cue-criterion correlation is correctly specified. This is especially the case in environments with many cues that do not differ too extremely regarding their validities. In environments with few available cues of very different predictive power, simple noncompensatory rules such as truncated decision trees or lexicographic rules can approximate the performance of optimal models. In a noncompensatory rule, a bad (or good) value on one cue cannot be compensated for by other cues. For example, if a disease has an obligatory symptom, the missing of this symptom rules out the disease regardless of other symptoms that may be present and fit the diagnosis of the disease. A lexicographic choice rule, for example, would look up the options' values on the most valid cue and ignore other cue information unless the best cue does not discriminate. In this case, the second best cue is searched and so on. The rule is also "noncompensatory" because a choice determined by a better cue cannot be revised by less valid cues. For this simplified rule to work well, one needs an accurate knowledge of the validity hierarchy of cues, that is, which cue is best, second best, and so on.

Models of the Decision Maker

In a research tradition called multiple cue probability learning, psychologists have investigated people's ability to abstract information about cue-criterion correlations from feedback and to use them for prediction. Typically, learning from feedback is not overly successful unless there are only very few cues with simple linear relationships to the criterion. If the situation gets more complex, cognitive feedback or causal models help. Cognitive feedback not only provides outcome feedback after a choice but also gives further information about the direction and the amount of the deviation from the correct judgment or even points to explicit cue-criterion relationships. However, people are generally not successful if cue-criterion relations are nonlinear or cue interactions occur. The judgments can often nevertheless be described by a weighted linear model. In experimental situations with novel tasks and explicit cues, participants sometimes use simplifying noncompensatory strategies, especially under time pressure or when cue acquisition is costly.

On the other hand, experts who have had extensive training and feedback often show remarkable decision accuracy in their domain. For example, weather forecasters are very well-calibrated in predicting the probability of precipitation. Also, pathologists may be very accurate in judging tissue samples as malign or benign although they cannot verbalize how they do it. It is obvious that these experts use effective cues, but neither all the cues used nor the decision rule are accessible to verbalization. In this case, the researcher's challenge is to identify the cues and strategies these experts use. It must be acknowledged, however, that judgments of experienced experts based on multiple explicit verbal cues (e.g., clinical judgments based on personality profiles or symptom patterns) are often outperformed by relatively simple statistical models of the environment.

Arndt Bröder

See also Cognitive Psychology and Processes; Decision Rules; Decision Tree: Introduction; Information Integration Theory; Lens Model; Ordinary Least Squares Regression; Social Judgment Theory

Further Readings

Brehmer, B. (1994). The psychology of linear judgement models. *Acta Psychologica, 87*(2/3), 137–154.
Dawes, R. M. (1979). The robust beauty of improper linear models in decision making. *American Psychologist, 34*(7), 571–582.
Gigerenzer, G., Todd, P. M., & ABC Research Group. (1999). *Simple heuristics that make us smart.* New York: Oxford University Press.
Hammond, K. R., & Stewart, T. R. (Eds.). (2001). *The essential Brunswik.* New York: Oxford University Press.
Martignon, L., & Hoffrage, U. (2002). Fast, frugal, and fit: Simple heuristics for paired comparison. *Theory and Decision, 52,* 29–71.

CULTURAL ISSUES

Culture encompasses the acquired knowledge, beliefs, values, and behavior patterns shared by the members of a particular group of people. Common elements of cultures include language, diet, dress, and religion, among others. In the past, the typical person in any given culture had little if any contact with individuals from other cultures. But marked shifts in economic, social, and political arrangements, including unprecedented worldwide immigration flows, have ended such isolation. Thus, people are constantly interacting with others who embrace customs markedly different from their own; they might even live right next door to them. This creates the real possibility that a person faced with a significant medical issue will be dealing with a healthcare provider from another culture. Such cross-cultural encounters pose challenges to how and how well the required healthcare decisions are made. This entry describes and analyzes some of the most important of those challenges. It also outlines approaches to meeting them.

The Patient–Provider Relationship

The first key challenges bear on the personal relationship between the patient and the provider in a cross-cultural interaction. Specifically, they concern confidence, comfort, and trust.

Confidence

Healthcare providers can serve several distinct decision-making roles vis-à-vis their clients. First, they can be *agents*, making decisions on the patient's behalf, as when the patient says (explicitly or merely implicitly), "I realize that the decision is mine legally, but would you please decide for me? After all, you're the expert, and besides, I'm just too upset by this horrible news to make the decision myself." Second, they can be *co-deciders*, in the spirit of the shared decision-making paradigm. That is, the provider and patient work toward mutual agreement about, say, a workable hypertension management regimen for the patient to follow. Third, providers can be *consultants*, such that the patient reserves the right to decide personally but seeks the provider's opinion as input to the decision process, for instance, in the form of a prostate cancer prognosis or a recommendation for radiation therapy versus radical prostatectomy. Finally, providers can be (and invariably are) *decision managers*, deliberately or inadvertently exerting influence over how the patient chooses by, say, providing literature that favors radiation rather than surgical treatment for the patient's condition. Whether and how the patient allows the provider to assume these roles depends directly on the client's confidence in the provider's competence or expertise. And that confidence can easily be affected by cultural differences.

Impressions of expertise generally, and of decision-making expertise in particular, rest on several considerations. One consideration is *acclamation*, consensus among people one already respects. Such consensus in turn depends on factors such as the person's visibility and regard by one's peers. In the health arena, credentials and accomplishments in contemporary science-based medicine undoubtedly carry great weight even with people who normally have little to do with modern societies. Yet, all else being the same, a provider from a culture different from the patient's own almost necessarily is less well known in that patient's social circles than a provider who shares the patient's own culture and therefore suffers a perceived competence liability. Another consideration is *style of speaking*. People recognized as experts tend to speak with precision and confidence. A provider from a culture different from the patient's is unlikely to be fluent in the patient's native language and thus is incapable of exhibiting the linguistic trappings of expertise. Yet another consideration is *factual knowledge*. People expect true experts to be able to recite extensive facts about the domain in question. And they certainly expect experts to know virtually all the facts they know themselves, and more. As discussed below, cultures often differ in terms of disease prevalence rates as well as common treatments, including folk remedies. A provider from a different culture might well be ignorant of these facts that the patient knows personally, thereby suffering damage to his or her credibility in the patient's eyes.

Comfort

Extensive research (e.g., on the "mere exposure effect") has shown that familiarity generally does not breed contempt but instead fosters at least mild liking. Thus, when a healthcare provider shares cultural customs with a patient, such as language, memories of the same kinds of schools, and similar tastes in entertainment, the patient feels at ease. This comfort can be highly beneficial for managing the stress that naturally accompanies health crises. It also undoubtedly contributes to the success of clinics that cater to immigrant and expatriate communities and which emphasize elements of the pertinent cultures, such as their languages and religious sensitivities. All the common provider decision-making roles—agent, co-decider, consultant, and decision manager—can be enacted more smoothly.

The flip side of the coin is where the greatest challenges lie. When there are significant differences in the cultures of a patient and a provider, those differences often constitute barriers that must be overcome. Studies on decision "bolstering" have shown that, when a person chooses X over Y, in that person's estimation, the appeal of X increases and that of Y diminishes. That person wonders, "How could I have ever even considered Y?" It only stands to reason that, all else being equivalent, people who like and choose Y will be seen as having tastes that are not merely different but in some sense inferior. Thus, in a broader context, it should not be surprising if, when unchecked, other cultures' "choices" are initially regarded somewhat negatively; they are not our own. Their music sounds like "noise," their food tastes too bland or too spicy, and some of their worldviews seem unreasonable. Unaddressed, the resulting discomfort can stand between the patient and provider, even when, ostensibly, the cultural differences in question have nothing to do with medicine.

Trust

Cultural variations are often accompanied by economic and political rivalries. Consider, for instance, the Fleming and Walloon cultures in Belgium or the Malay and Chinese cultures in Malaysia. The resulting antagonisms can fan distrust in all manner of cross-cultural encounters, including medical ones. Initially, at least, patients therefore might easily say things such as the following to themselves concerning a provider from a rival culture: "They usually don't like or respect us, so I wonder if she's that way, too. Will she really give me her best efforts, just like she would one of her own?" Unless and until such fears are dispelled, patients are hesitant about having providers make medical decisions on their behalf.

To address threats to effective cross-cultural patient-provider relationships, particularly concerning comfort and trust, those who seek to promote cultural competency in healthcare offer several recommendations for providers:

- Undertake exercises intended to uncover one's personal feelings about various cultural variations. As suggested previously, these feelings are virtually guaranteed to exist.
- Cultivate respect for customs different from one's own. At minimum, be nonjudgmental about them.
- Avoid stereotyping. A provider should anticipate and prepare for customs that are especially common in a given patient's culture. At the same time, the provider should not lose sight of the extensive individual differences that invariably exist among the members of that culture. Proceeding as if every member of the group is the same invites anger and resentment.

And when the concern is nurturing patient confidence in a provider's competence, there is no substitute for establishing and publicizing a solid track record among patients in a given cultural community. That includes learning more about that culture, especially facts pertaining to medical conditions that are particularly problematic in that community and health practices that are distinctive for the people concerned.

Participation

In many societies, particularly in North America and Western Europe, decisions about medical questions are personal and private affairs, solely between the patient and the physician. Expectations and reality can be markedly different in other societies, particularly ones where collectivism rather than individualism holds sway, for instance, in much of Asia, Africa, and Latin America. By definition, the term *collectivism* refers to an outlook that emphasizes the interdependence of people and the importance of collectives to which they belong. In contrast, *individualism* highlights independence and the relative significance of people's personal interests.

In collectivistic cultures, participation in the medical decision process tends to be broader than in individualistic cultures, with the family often assuming especially prominent roles. For instance, for a long time in Japan, the norm has been not the patient autonomy that is ascendant in the United States but, instead, reliance on the beneficence of the patient's family and physician. Thus, in this alternative arrangement, a physician could disclose to the family that a patient has cancer and the family might choose to withhold that diagnosis from the patient. Prominent roles for families in medical decision making in collectivistic societies are consistent with the high degree of interdependence characteristic of those societies. In those contexts, the reality is that events involving any one member of a family (e.g., a new, high-paying job or a serious illness) often have a much greater impact on the other members than would be the case in an individualistic society where independence is prized. So when one family member becomes sick, prescribed changes in diet for managing chronic conditions such as diabetes must take into account the impacts for numerous individuals besides the person who is ill.

Beyond the family, the traditions in some cultures reserve decision-making roles for others, too. Most notably in some Asian, African, and Native American cultures, these might be people with religious responsibilities, including ones some would call shamans. Other participants might be nonreligious traditional or alternative healers. Patients from cultures that maintain roles for these additional parties sometimes attempt to follow the guidance of these authorities as well as the instructions of their doctors practicing contemporary scientific medicine. Since patients might be reluctant to volunteer such information, it is wise for providers to inquire sensitively about the possibility. When other parties are involved, the provider must, in effect, negotiate a hybrid treatment plan. To do otherwise runs the risk of treatment incompatibilities, perhaps tragic ones.

Language

The complications of patients and providers speaking, reading, and writing different formal languages are apparent. For instance, the provider's misunderstanding of a patient's symptom descriptions could lead to a misdiagnosis and then an ineffective, even harmful, treatment choice. This implicates the need for the services of skilled professional interpreters. (Reliance on bilingual family members and friends is often discouraged because they tend to censor remarks on both sides of a conversation.) But even when a patient and a provider in a cross-cultural encounter use a common formal language, there remain significant risks. Because their life experiences might be so different, so too might be the assumptions they make in a given exchange. That is why it is often advised that clinicians depend especially heavily on open-ended questions and requests (e.g., "Would you please tell me what *you* think led to this?"). Communications can also be compromised by cultural differences in traditions of directness, politeness, and deference to authority or status. Thus, "Yes" in response to a request might not mean "Yes" literally, expressing an intention to comply with that request. The speaker's true meaning might have to be inferred from other aspects of the situation, including nonverbal signals such as facial expressions. Becoming skilled in nonverbal communication is therefore essential although difficult to achieve, especially since the same signal (e.g., a smile) can sometimes carry opposite meanings in different cultures.

Decision Problem Deliberation

The specific decision problems that patients and providers must confront concern acute and chronic conditions as well as health maintenance measures. Effective decision making requires that deciders successfully address certain recurring issues. These include anticipating or recognizing problems that demand decisions (e.g., slowly developing cancers), judging the chances of pertinent events (e.g., that a treatment would work), determining values (e.g., the patient's true feelings about possible outcomes and side effects), and creating or identifying viable options (e.g., crafting effective, doable treatment plans). Specific considerations are likely to affect precisely how these issues are resolved in cross-cultural encounters.

Correlated Health Facts

An especially significant reality of cultural variations is that some of them are correlated with important health facts. Incidence rates are one instance. For genetic reasons, certain diseases are more common in some cultural groups than in others. Sickle cell disease, with relatively high incidence rates among African Americans, provides a ready illustration. The disease has sometimes been misdiagnosed in African American patients because it simply never occurred to their physicians as a possible explanation for their signs and symptoms. That has happened because those doctors had little experience with non-Caucasian patients or, perhaps in a spirit of fair-mindedness, they simply assumed that, physiologically, "people are people." Other incidence rate differences are tied more directly to true cultural variations in behavior. Such is the case for cultural differences in obesity and hypertension traced to customary diets heavy in fats or salt. More generally, if a provider is ignorant of incidence rates that are distinctive for a cultural group, this foreshadows diagnostic errors as well as cases of *blindsiding*. These are cases such as those in which a serious illness is inadvertently allowed to progress to an untreatable state because its actual high-probability presence was never even imagined.

Differential efficacy rates are another health fact sometimes correlated with culture. Treatments that are effective for some cultural groups are less useful for others. For instance, studies have found especially high rates of adverse reactions among East Asian patients for certain antihypertension drugs. The implications of culture-specific efficacy rates for the wisdom of treatment choices are readily apparent. Clearly, when a clinician is called on to serve patients from an unfamiliar culture, a first order of business must be to actively seek out known health fact correlations involving that group.

Explanation and Belief

Cultures sometimes differ in how people explain what they observe. Related to this, cultures can also differ in how people arrive at what they believe or expect to be true. These differences can have implications for the treatment options that occur to patients and providers in cross-cultural encounters as well as for their expectations about the effectiveness of those treatments, if they were to be chosen. For example, in numerous African and Asian cultures, people sometimes believe that a person's illness is punishment for transgressions that the person has committed. Or they suspect that the sick person is the victim of malevolent enemies with spiritual powers that enable them to cast hexes on whomever they wish. These explanations differ sharply from the accounts for sickness that underlie current scientific medicine. And they rationalize radically different treatment alternatives. Whereas scientific explanations point toward treatments that address factors such as pathogens, spiritual or moral explanations implicate actions such as restitution or prayer. A provider who ignores (or worse, belittles) a patient's beliefs in alternative explanations for illness is unlikely to succeed in achieving the patient's cooperation in implementing a purely science-based treatment plan.

In order for a clinician to persuade a patient to undergo a particular treatment, regardless of its character, the clinician must somehow get the patient to conclude that the chances of good outcomes are high. This challenge is conditioned by culture, too. Studies have documented reliable cultural variations in people's probability judgments. Surprisingly for many people, one of the most consistent differences is that the overconfidence implicit in such judgments is stronger among Chinese than among Americans. Further studies have demonstrated that these differences are not a reflection of "ego." Instead, they seem to result from culturally distinct customs for reasoning while arriving at one's conclusions.

Treatment Options and Expectations

If a treatment option goes unrecognized, then neither the patient nor the provider can choose it. On the other hand, they could not disagree and argue about it either. These truisms highlight the importance of cultural variations in the options that come to mind when a medical issue arises. There is good evidence that cultural differences often broaden the pool of alternatives that surface, even

beyond the kinds of scientific and spiritually inspired options suggested previously. For some rural Mexican patients, medical conditions are classified as either "hot" or "cold." Furthermore, to reestablish balance, "hot" conditions are thought to require "cold" treatments, and vice versa. Pregnancy is regarded as a "hot" condition, and thus "hot" treatments would not be on the list of options considered legitimate for a pregnant woman. But vitamins are a hot treatment. And therein lies a conflict that must be worked through since a practitioner of contemporary scientific medicine almost certainly would recommend the regular intake of vitamins to assure the health of the child and the mother. Or consider Japanese family medicine customs. Over time, Japanese patients have developed an expectation that an end result of virtually every visit to the doctor should be a prescription for medicine. There is also an expectation that the patient will be seen again soon, say, in a month. Naturally, then, the treatment plans that experienced, wise, and highly rated physicians craft for patients' consideration conform to these expectations.

The advice implicit in these kinds of scenarios is similar to that articulated earlier with respect to culture-correlated health facts. A provider who anticipates working with patients from a new, unfamiliar culture can at least prepare for the challenges of broader collections of patient-preferred treatment options by studying what the common expectations are within that culture.

Value

The final class of cultural variations that have special significance in deliberations bear on what is perhaps the most fundamental defining characteristic of decision making generally—value. Decision problems are special largely because their solutions are not unique. Since people's ways of valuing things tend to differ, outcomes that are highly pleasing for one patient (e.g., the ebullient personality of the physician's assistant assigned to the patient) can easily be unbearably annoying for another. Cultural variations concerning value are particularly important in the provider's roles as an agent, making decisions on the patient's behalf, and as a co-decider, seeking to reach agreement with the patient about how to proceed in dealing with a medical situation.

There is evidence that physicians can err substantially in their expectations about the values their patients attach to various aspects of medical situations, such as cancer treatment side effects. This should mean that, if a physician is making medical choices for a patient, at least sometimes these value judgment errors should result in the patient being stuck with alternatives that are worse than they could be, in terms of what the patient truly desires. Importantly, these errors are not haphazard; there is evidence for *false consensus*. That is, people tend to believe that others' values are closer to their own than they really are. Suppose that a provider attempts to answer the question, "How would my patient feel about the limited degree of mobility likely to result from this treatment?" The conclusion is essentially, "Pretty much the way I would," and more so than would actually be the case.

There is reason to expect these value assessment errors to be especially large in cross-cultural patient-provider encounters. That is because the values of the patient and provider should differ more than in instances where the parties share a common culture. It is easy to appreciate sizable cross-cultural value differences when the focus is something like tastes in food or music. But the same underlying principles, such as historical isolation of groups of people from one another, should yield similar strong value differences for aspects of health situations. British versus American differences in the appeal of aggressive as opposed to conservative treatments for cancer provide a good example. Relative to Americans, Britons have been more likely to regard the side effects of aggressive treatments to be unacceptably harsh. Heroic and invasive efforts to extend for a few hours the lives of terminally ill patients in Japan constitute another illustration. The justification for some such actions is to provide time for all close relatives to be at their loved one's side at the moment of death, which is extremely important in Japanese society, much more so than elsewhere. Thus, as co-deciders, there would be little disagreement between a Japanese family and their Japanese doctor about undertaking the requested life-extending measures. That might not be so if the

physician were non-Japanese or at least ignorant of Japanese traditions and values.

J. Frank Yates and Laith Alattar

See also Informed Consent; International Differences in Healthcare Systems; Models of Physician-Patient Relationship; Moral Choice and Public Policy; Religious Factors; Worldviews

Further Readings

Fetters, M. D. (1998). The family in medical decision making: Japanese perspectives. *Journal of Clinical Ethics, 9*(2), 132–146.

Hammoud, M. M., White, C. B., & Fetters, M. D. (2005). Opening cultural doors: Providing culturally sensitive healthcare to Arab American and American Muslim patients. *Obstetrics & Gynecology, 193,* 1307–1311.

Juckett, G. (2005). Cross-cultural medicine. *American Family Physician, 72*(11), 2267–2274.

Management Sciences for Health. (n.d.). *The provider's guide to quality and culture.* Retrieved June 7, 2008, from http://erc.msh.org/mainpage.cfm?file=1.0.htm&module=provider&language=English

McDowell, S. E., Coleman, J. J., & Ferner, R. E. (2006). Systematic review and meta-analysis of ethnic differences in risks of adverse reactions to drugs used in cardiovascular medicine. *British Medical Journal, 332,* 1177–1181.

Sequist, T. D., Fitzmaurice, G. M., Marshall, R., Shaykevich, S., Safran, D. G., & Ayanian, J. Z. (2008). Physician performance and racial disparities in diabetes mellitus care. *Archives of Internal Medicine, 168*(11), 1145–1151.

Triandis, H. C., Bontempo, R., Villareal, M. J., Asai, M., & Lucca, N. (1988). Individualism and collectivism: Cross-cultural perspectives on self-ingroup relationships. *Journal of Personality and Social Psychology, 54*(2), 323–338.

Yates, J. F., Lee, J.-W., Sieck, W. R., Choi, I., & Price, P. C. (2002). Probability judgment across cultures. In T. Gilovich, D. Griffin, & D. Kahneman (Eds.), *Heuristics and biases: The psychology of intuitive judgment* (pp. 271–291). New York: Cambridge University Press.

D

DATA QUALITY

Quality data are at the heart of quality healthcare. It is well known that poor data can lead to incorrect diagnoses, prescription errors, or surgical errors with tragic consequences. Similarly, the day-in, day-out consequences of poor data are enormous as well, leading to added time and expense throughout the system. In short, improving data quality is essential.

There are many approaches to defining data. The one that is often used for data quality recognizes that data consist of two interrelated components: data models and data values. *Data models* define *entities*, which are real-world objects or concepts, *attributes*, which are characteristics associated with entities, and *relationships* among them. As an example, each reader is an entity, and his or her employer is interested in attributes such as name, date of birth, and specialty. Relationships may include report manager and subordinates. A *data value* is the specific realization of an attribute/relationship for a specified entity. For example, a member of a medical research team may be assigned the specialty "statistician." Clearly, data, per se, are abstract. *Data records* are the physical manifestations of data in paper files, forms, spreadsheets, databases, and so forth.

Physicians are uniquely positioned to initiate data quality efforts and have much to gain by doing so. However, most are unfamiliar with the thinking that underlies data quality management: As in healthcare, the steps one takes to improve

data quality are rooted in the scientific method. Thus, this entry focuses on physicians. The first part summarizes three key principles of data quality management and the second part offers eight simple prescriptions that physicians can follow to make immediate improvements. These will not, of course, address all the data quality issues that currently afflict healthcare. But they form a solid beginning: the data quality equivalents of the age-old dictum, "First, do no harm."

Principles of Data Quality Management

The "muscle and bone" of data quality are measurement and control. One simply must have the facts and work through the laborious process of formulating and testing hypotheses to search for and eliminate root causes of error. In these ways, data quality management most resembles the scientific method.

If measurement and control are the muscle and bone, then three simple management principles form the head and eyes. The first principle is that data quality is defined not in some strict, technical sense but by customers such as patients, doctors, insurance companies, and billing departments. Specifically, data are of high quality if they meet customers' needs. This is an especially demanding approach because each customer may have different needs and uses for the data. As a consequence, they may rate the quality of data provided differently. For instance, while one patient may understand his or her diagnoses perfectly and take appropriate steps, another may misinterpret the same data and do just the opposite. According to this principle, the same data were of high quality in the first case and of poor quality in the second.

The second principle is that those who create data must be held accountable for its quality. Practically, everyone agrees with this principle in theory, but implementing it is far from trivial. What nurse wants to tell a chief of staff that she cannot read his orders? But experience shows that finding and correcting errors downstream is unreliable, expensive, and time-consuming.

The third principle is that customers and data sources must be tightly coupled if high-quality data are to result. The customer-supplier (C-S) model, depicted in Figure 1, has proven an excellent means of enabling the required communications.

The C-S model features three entities: Customers, as described above, are on the right; suppliers (or data sources) such as laboratories, admissions, and other doctors on the left; and the physician and his or her work processes in the middle. Physicians use data provided by their suppliers to do their work, create new data, and pass relevant data onto their customers. This data flow is illustrated by the left to right arrows in the figure.

More important, the C-S model features four communications channels in the opposite direction from the data flow. These channels help ensure that data needs (i.e., requirements) and feedback, both good and bad, are provided to data sources from customers. Unless physicians seek to actively construct and maintain these channels, they become blocked or noisy. In sum, data sources simply cannot be expected to provide high-quality data without knowing what is expected and understanding how well they are performing.

Prescriptions for Physicians

Assuring data quality can be enormously complex. But data quality can also be quite straightforward. The following are eight prescriptions that physicians can follow to initiate data quality improvement.

1. Treat patients like customers when explaining their diagnoses, courses of treatment, and prognoses. Too often, patients simply do not understand what a physician tells them. Of course, they may be scared and nervous and may not listen well.

And they come from a variety of backgrounds. But the physician must make himself or herself understood, whatever it takes. Use simple words for some people, explain in more complicated terms to others, and draw pictures for still others. Make sure they understand exactly how they can best contribute to their care (e.g., taking their prescriptions). Encourage them to ask questions. And, perhaps most important, say "I don't know" when you don't know the answer.

2. Treat the "next person in the process," whoever it is, as a customer. Patients, and their data surrogates, often get lost in the system. Indeed, this is a systemic problem and cannot be solved by one individual. But treating the next doctor (or clinic) the patient will visit, the technician who must follow the orders, the hospital administrator, and the insurance companies who pay the bills as customers is an effective way to promote a culture that values high-quality data. Talk and listen well to one customer every month (say) and ask them what data they really need from you, what data they actually get, what you're doing that helps, and what you do that slows them down; then make necessary improvements.

3. Become intolerant of simple data errors made by others. One reason for data errors in healthcare is that people tolerate them, even accommodate them, in their work processes. For example, the triage nurse in the emergency room, caregivers, technicians, indeed everyone who sees a patient asks the same questions. This increases the chances of error and is considered by some to be bad practice. Furthermore, when you spot errors, provide feedback to the source of the error, as quickly as you can. Don't blame individuals—most of them are doing their best within an imperfect system. Instead, reach out to managers and ask that they find and eliminate root causes of error. Finally, keep a log of the errors you find. Revisit it from time to time to look for patterns.

4. Become extremely intolerant of simple data errors made by yourself or your team. It only stands to reason that you have to be even more demanding of yourself than you are of others. One way an orthopedist could make sure that he or she was operating on the correct limb would be to ask

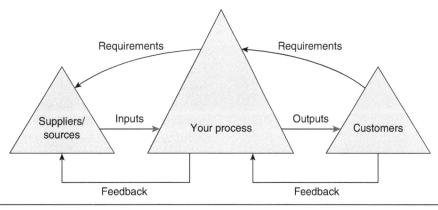

Figure 1   The customer-supplier model

all in the operating theater to concur before starting. Another way could be to write "Not This One" on the left knee when the right is the correct one. Both methods help foolproof the orthopedist's work and that of his or her team. It is an example of a good, proactive way to prevent data errors. Equally important is acknowledging errors when they occur, learning from them, and fixing the root cause to prevent future errors.

5. Make handwriting legible. Much has been written about the frequency and dangers of misread handwriting leading to wrongly filled prescriptions and other errors. As a physician, do whatever you need to do to prevent such error, even typing or learning to print legibly.

6. Put patient records into a computer. So far, healthcare has not yielded much to full automation of patient records. It is a complex technical problem made more complex by not yet fully understood issues such as patient privacy. And automation, in and of itself, is no panacea. But the computer facilitates better record keeping, and better record keeping means better data for making diagnoses, deeper analyses that will improve healthcare, and smoother pathways between all involved. Eventually, all important healthcare data will be digitized and all players interconnected. Physicians can aid the evolution, even if only within their practices and clinics.

7. Learn to distinguish common causes from special causes. If an overtired laboratory technician makes a simple (even if dire) mistake, the solution may be to instruct that person on his or

her responsibilities and the importance of coming to work fully rested (importantly, the root cause of the error may be something else, such as a miscalibrated measurement device). But if seven laboratory technicians make the same mistake over a 6-month period, then a root cause analysis must be conducted—even if each admits that he or she was tired! Perhaps the lab is understaffed, perhaps shifts are too long, perhaps a particular piece of equipment becomes erratic as it heats up late in the day. The prescription is to distinguish "common causes" from "special causes." The analogy is not perfect, but common causes are like chronic conditions. They always exist and are inherent to the process or system. Special causes are like acute conditions. They need to be addressed individually and in different ways. Distinguishing common causes from special causes is not easy. In the example above, the bad lab tests come up one at a time, are discovered by different people, and each may be addressed before the next occurs. So spotting them requires a certain aptitude. But there is no substitute. Telling technicians to get more sleep will simply not cool down an overheating piece of equipment.

8. Lead one improvement project every year. Organizations that put forth reasonably diligent efforts often reap order-of-magnitude improvements to data quality. And they've done so without special investment. The secret is completing improvement projects on a regular basis. Frequently, eliminating a relatively few root causes produces dramatic improvement within a department. So define a problem, assemble a team (and personally

lead it), uncover the root cause, and figure out how to make it go away permanently.

Frank M. Guess, Thomas C. Redman,
and Mahender P. Singh

See also Constraint Theory

Further Readings

Berwick, D. M. (2003). *Escape fire: Designs for the future of health care.* San Francisco: Jossey-Bass.

Berwick, D. M., Godfrey, A. B., & Roessner, J. (2002). *Curing health care: New strategies for quality improvement.* New York: Wiley. (Other publishers have translated earlier versions into Japanese and into Portuguese.)

Halamka, J. (2008). *Vision for hospital's future HIT.* Retrieved May 29, 2008, from http://www.thehealth careblog.com/the_health_care_blog/2008/05/vision-for-hosp.html

Redman, T. (2008). *Data driven: Profiting from your most important business asset* (Chapter 3). Boston: Harvard Business School Press.

DECISIONAL CONFLICT

Every day, people face healthcare decisions involving trade-offs between potential benefits and risks. Which birth control method should I use? Are my symptoms (acne, attention deficit/hyperactivity disorder, hot flashes, chronic pain) bad enough to warrant stronger medication with potentially more serious side effects? Should I have surgery for poorly controlled benign uterine bleeding, back pain, benign prostatic hyperplasia, obesity, osteoarthritis? Should my relative receive care for dementia or terminal illness at home or at a care facility?

Decision making is the process of choosing between alternative courses of action (including inaction). Generally, people choose the option that they perceive will be effective in achieving valued outcomes and in avoiding undesirable outcomes. However, many decisions are *choice dilemmas* or *conflicted decisions*. No alternative will satisfy all personal objectives and none is without its risk of undesirable outcomes.

Among the 2,500 healthcare interventions evaluated by the *Clinical Evidence* group, 13% were classified as "beneficial," 23% as "probably beneficial," 8% as "need to weigh benefits versus risks," 6% as "probably nonbeneficial," 4% as "probably useless or dangerous," and 46%, the largest number, as having insufficient evidence of usefulness. Consequently, patients need help in resolving uncertainty when facing clinical decisions. They may express uncertainty or difficulty in identifying the best alternative due to the risk or uncertainty of outcomes, the need to make value judgments about potential gains versus potential losses, and anticipated regret over the positive aspects of rejected options.

The aim of this entry is to briefly review what has been learned on how patients make difficult decisions by highlighting the value of screening for decisional conflict. The first section summarizes research on patient decisional conflict. It also reviews tools for assessing and addressing decisional needs. The second section reports on the effects of decision support interventions on decisional conflict. The last section highlights the gaps in knowledge and areas needing further research.

Research

Definition of Decisional Conflict

Psychologists Janis and Mann describe decisional conflict as the concurrent opposing tendencies within a person to accept and decline an option. The North American Nursing Diagnosis Association (NANDA) defines decisional conflict as personal uncertainty about which course of action to take when the choice among competing actions involves risk, loss, regret, or challenge to personal life values. Decisional conflict is an intrapersonal psychological construct that is felt by individuals. In lay terms, it refers to one's level of comfort when facing and making a health-related decision.

How Much Do Patients Experience Decisional Conflict?

NANDA defines verbalized uncertainty as the hallmark of decisional conflict (e.g., "I'm not sure which option to choose"). In three large surveys that have been conducted, about half the respondents reported feeling uncertainty about their best course of action. The first is a Canadian national telephone survey in which 59% of respondents reported feeling unsure about what to choose when facing complex decisions regarding medical or surgical treatments or birth control. In the second case, Légaré measured decisional conflict in 923 patients after they were counseled about options in five family practices; 52% of patients had personal uncertainty about common treatment options. In the third case, Bunn and colleagues conducted a household survey of impoverished women in Santiago, Chile, and found that 54% reported personal uncertainty, commonly about decisions around navigating the healthcare system (where, when, and from whom to seek care).

NANDA describes other manifestations of decisional conflict. The aforementioned Canadian survey reported their prevalence as follows: 77% of respondents questioned their personal values, 61% verbalized concern about undesired outcomes, 40% were preoccupied with the decision, 27% wanted to delay the decision, 27% had signs and symptoms of stress or tension, and 26% wavered between choices.

Contributing Factors

Nonmodifiable Factors

The type of decision can influence decisional conflict. In the Canadian survey, higher rates of physical stress were reported by those who had made decisions about placing a relative in an institution (54%) or medical treatment (46%) as compared with those pondering birth control decisions (23%). Decision delay was more common among those deciding about institutionalization (50%), as compared with those making surgical decisions (20%).

Personal characteristics also influence personal uncertainty. In two studies, which controlled for other potential factors, women reported higher decisional conflict than men. A clinical study of patients considering warfarin therapy found that older people had higher decisional conflict scores. In contrast, the Canadian survey found that younger people had higher decisional conflict scores.

Modifiable Factors

According to NANDA, modifiable factors influencing decisional conflict include deficits in (a)

knowledge and expectations (condition, options, benefits, risks, probabilities); (b) clarity of values or priorities (personal desirability or importance of benefits vs. harms); and (c) support and resources (access to advice, support, pressure from others involved in the decision, personal skills, self-confidence, resources). The Canadian survey examined these modifiable factors when controlling for the inherent factors such as type of decision and personal characteristics. More manifestations of decisional conflict were observed with those who had deficits in knowledge as well as support and resources (pressured to select one particular option and unready or unskilled in decision making). When the hallmark of decisional conflict (personal uncertainty about the best course of action) was analyzed separately, those reporting feeling uncertain were also more likely to report problems with the NANDA modifiable factors as compared with those who did not experience uncertainty.

Measuring Decisional Conflict and Modifiable Factors

The Decisional Conflict Scale (DCS) has been developed for research and clinical assessment purposes. It measures personal uncertainty in patients and its modifiable factors such as feeling informed, clear about values, and supported in decision making. This reliable and valid measure shows that greater decisional conflict occurs in those who delay decisions, score lower on knowledge tests, are in the early phases of decision making, and/or have not yet received decision support. High decisional conflict after decision support predicts downstream delay or discontinuance of the chosen option, regret, and the tendency to blame the practitioner for bad outcomes. More recently, the DCS has been adapted for measuring personal uncertainty in health professionals as well.

Decision Support Interventions

Although there are several conceptual frameworks of shared decision making, the Ottawa Decision Support Framework specifically addresses decisional conflict using conceptual definitions and theories from NANDA as well as psychology, social psychology, economics, and social support. The Ottawa framework applies to all participants involved in decision making, including the individual, couple, or family and their health practitioner. The focus here is on patients' needs and the role of the practitioner in supporting them. As illustrated in Figure 1, the framework has three key elements: (1) decisional needs, (2) decision quality, and (3) decision support. The framework asserts that unresolved decisional needs will have adverse effects on decision quality. However, decision support can improve decision quality by addressing unresolved needs with clinical counseling, decision tools, and coaching.

Decisional Needs

Unresolved decisional needs that adversely affect decision quality include the following: decisional

conflict (uncertainty), inadequate knowledge and unrealistic expectations, unclear values, inadequate support or resources, complex decision type, urgent timing, unreceptive stage of decision making, polarized leaning toward an option, and participants' characteristics (e.g., patients' cognitive limitations, poverty, limited education, or physical incapacitation). Therefore, practitioners should be skilled at assessing decision needs by first screening for decisional conflict. A shorter clinical version of the DCS is currently being tested and may hold promising in this regard.

Decision Quality

To help resolve decisional needs, it is important to describe the goal of an intervention. Generally,

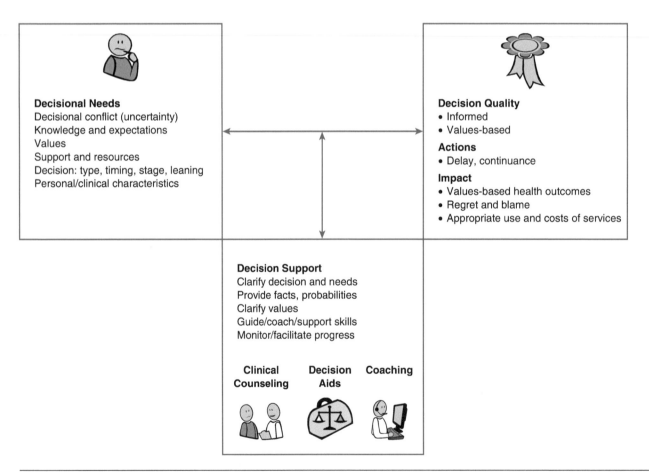

Figure 1   Ottawa decision support framework

Source: O'Connor, A. M. *Ottawa decision support framework to address decisional conflict.* © 2006. Available from http://www.ohri.ca/decisionaid.

medical professionals wish to help people make a "good" decision. However, what is a good decision when there is more than one medically reasonable option and the best choice depends on how a person weighs the known benefits versus harms as well as the scientific uncertainties? Although the issue is not completely resolved, there is emerging consensus that good decisions are ones that are informed and consistent with personal values. Does the person understand the key facts about their condition, options, benefits, and harms? Does the person have realistic expectations (perceptions of chances of benefits and harms)? Is there a match between the option that is chosen and the features of options that matter most to the informed person?

The consequences of decisions are of interest to different groups. For example, behavioral evaluators are often interested in the impact of the decision on behavior. Did a person delay or make a decision? Did the person continue with his or her chosen option? On the other hand, clinicians are interested in the impact of the decision on health outcomes. It is important to note that the types of decisions that create decisional conflict often have no clear best option that has a positive effect on health outcomes. The question the clinician may have to ask is "Did the informed patient achieve the good outcome and avoid the bad outcome that mattered most to him or her?" Health psychologists may find effects on emotions such as regret or blame as most interesting. Health service evaluators and economists often focus on the use of health services and costs.

Decision Support

Decision support is aimed to address a patient's unresolved needs through clinical counseling, decision aids, and coaching. Decision support involves the following: (a) clarifying the decision and the person's needs, (b) providing facts and probabilities, (c) clarifying values, (d) guiding/coaching/supporting in deliberation and communication, and (e) monitoring/facilitating progress.

Health professionals tend to overuse factual information about options and to underuse other strategies. Specific strategies tailored to patients' needs are described in Table 1. Generic and condition-specific decision aids have been developed to assess needs and plan decision support. An example of a generic aid is the Ottawa Personal Decision Guide. It is a framework-based tool to help people and their practitioners structure, record, and communicate decisional needs and plans. The guide incorporates a short version of the decisional conflict scale. It can be self-administered or practitioner-administered. A computer-based 1-page PDF version, as well as a 2-page paper version, is available from the Ottawa Health Research Institute's Web site.

Condition-specific patient decision aids are interventions designed to prepare people for decision making; they do not replace counseling. They help people (a) understand the probable benefits and risks of options, (b) consider the value they place on the benefits versus the risks, and (c) participate actively with their practitioners in deciding about options. According to the International Patient Decision Aids Standards (IPDAS) Collaboration, patient decision aids provide the following: (a) information on the disease/condition, options, benefits, harms, and scientific uncertainties; (b) the probabilities of outcomes tailored to a person's health risk factors; (c) values clarification such as describing outcomes in functional terms, asking patients to consider which benefits and risks matter most to them; and (d) guidance in the steps of decision making and communicating with others. Decision aids may be administered using various media before, during, or after counseling. Most developers are moving toward Web-based materials that can be printed or used online.

Patient decision aids have been developed for a variety of screening, diagnostic, medical, therapeutic, and end-of-life decisions. A list of currently available decision aids is found in the A to Z Inventory of Decision Aids at the Ottawa Health Decision Centre Web site. Reviews of randomized controlled trials of decision aids conclude that they are better than standard care in terms of the following: (a) increasing participation in decision making without increasing anxiety, (b) improving decision quality (improved knowledge of options, benefits, harms), (c) more realistic expectations of the probabilities of benefits and harms, (d) better match between personal values and choices, (e) lowering decisional conflict, and (f) helping undecided people to decide. Patient decision aids may also have a role in addressing underuse and overuse of

Table I   Decision support strategies tailored to decisional needs

Knowledge deficits. Exposure to information about the health condition, options, and outcomes improves knowledge.

- Help the person access information. Balanced presentations of available options and both potential benefits and harms should be presented in sufficient detail for decision making.
- Adapt medium and pace of information delivery to the person's needs (literacy, numeracy, impairments in sight, hearing, cognition).
- Assess the person's comprehension of the information after it is provided; the focus should be on information that is "essential" for decision making.

Unrealistic expectations. Exposure to probabilities of benefits and harms creates realistic expectations.

- Present probabilities in ways that are understandable to patients, for example, event rates using common denominators and time periods and with mixed frames.
- In labs, the chances of outcomes are perceived to be more likely when they are easier to imagine and when you can identify with the people experiencing them. Therefore, in cases where a person overestimates the chances of an outcome occurring, the practitioner may acknowledge the possibility but then describe anecdotes (vivid stories) in which the outcome did not happen. In cases where a person underestimates the chances of an outcome occurring, the practitioner may acknowledge the possibility but then describe anecdotes in which the outcomes did happen. The use of narratives to change patients' expectations has not been evaluated in clinical trials.

Unclear values (personal importance). Values clarification and communication is under active study and debate.

- A person cannot judge the value of unfamiliar outcomes. Therefore, outcomes need to be described in familiar, simple, and experiential terms to help the person judge their personal importance. This means that, rather than providing a label for an outcome (e.g. pain from osteoarthritis), a person is helped to understand how the outcome will affect him or her physically (characteristics of pain, effects on ability to walk, work, and carry on daily activities), emotionally (discouraged), and socially (withdrawn, avoid social activities). Other examples of meaningful outcomes are (a) for depression: You are more likely to answer the phone or go out with your family; (b) for attention deficit disorder: Your child is more likely to read at grade level or to have friends.
- Ask the person to implicitly consider the personal importance of the positive and negative outcomes. Sometimes decision support includes explicit values clarification exercises using numerical approaches (e.g., rating scales (0 = *not at all important* to 10 = *very important*). The relative value of explicit approaches is under investigation.
- A person needs a strategy for communicating his or her values when discussing the options with others. People, including clinicians and family members, are not very good at judging the values of others. It may be helpful to use rating scales or balance scales showing what is important that can be viewed "at a glance."

Unclear or biased perceptions of others' opinions. The optimal method for presenting the experiences of others in the form of narratives is under active investigation.

- Explain available options to broaden personal awareness of alternatives.
- Present examples of others' choices, in a balanced manner, so that a person is aware that people choose different options and there is no "one size fits all" answer.
- Provide statistics on variation in choice (e.g., the percentage of people who choose the different options that are available; the differences in practitioners' opinions; or the differences in practice guidelines). It is also helpful to present the rationales behind the differing opinions. Often, differences in choices reflect scientific uncertainty, or differences in people's circumstances, tolerance for risk or uncertainty, or values.

Social pressures. Conflict resolution approaches may be useful but have not been tested.

- Explore the nature of the pressure, including its source, the areas of agreement and disagreement, and the reasons behind differences in points of view.
- Guide the person to (a) verify his or her perceptions of others' opinions in case there are misconceptions; (b) focus on those whose opinions matter most; and (c) handle relevant sources of pressure.
- Strategies for dealing with people who are exerting pressure include (a) planning how to communicate information and values; (b) inviting others to discuss their perceptions of options, benefits, harms, and values to find areas of agreement and disagreement; (c) mobilizing social support; and (d) identifying a mediator, if needed. Role play and rehearsal of strategies may help.

Lack of support or resources. Help a person access support or resources needed to make the decision. Resources may include health professionals who are personal advocates, family and friends, support groups, or services from voluntary or government sectors. In some cases the practitioner's support is all that is needed to make the decision.

Lack of skills or confidence in decision making. Provide structured guidance, or coaching in the steps of decision making (i.e., deliberating about a decision) and communicating preferences. There is limited evidence that coaching in addition to information improves decision making.

Preferred role in decision making. The type of guidance will depend on the role people prefer to take in decision making. According to Rothert and Talarczyk, the clinicians' expertise lies in providing information about the options available, their outcomes, the associated risk/probability, and the healthcare resources required and available. The patients' expertise includes their preferences or values and personal, social, and available economic resources.

- Degner and colleagues identified three profiles of preference for decisional control: those who want to *keep, share,* or *give away* control of decision making. "Keepers" might guide the deliberation and ask their practitioner for input on the scientific facts. Practitioners might start by providing guidance to "sharers," who would then become actively involved in the decision. A more advisory role might be used by practitioners with those who want to give away control, who would then be asked to provide informed consent. It is important, however, for practitioners not to take preferred roles in decision making completely at face value; providing people with decision support often increases their desire for active participation in decision making. Therefore, people need adequate information about the issues and time to consider which decision-making role they prefer to take.

Decision type, timing, stage, and leaning. Practitioners need to tailor decision support to the type of decision. For example, the approach may differ if the focus is on screening for prostate cancer, treatment of early-stage disease, treatment of recurrence, or end-of-life care. Tailoring support also depends on timing. Short timelines to make big decisions often increases stress, but very long timelines may increase decision delay. In the very early and very late stages of decision making it is important to gauge a person's receptivity to new information and further deliberation. Otherwise, decision support may be irritating or unproductive. The aim of decision support is to help the person progress in his or her stage of decision making, not necessarily "change." Sometimes "maintaining the status quo" is a reasonable option (e.g., forgoing PSA testing, amniocentesis, or hormone therapy).

Personal and clinical characteristics. Decision support should be gender-sensitive and appropriate for an individual's age, developmental stage, education, socioeconomic status, and ethnicity. Adjustments should be made to accommodate a person's physical, emotional, and cognitive capacities. Involving the family or a personal advocate is important when the person's capacities are limited. The characteristics of the practitioner will also influence decision support, based on a person's training, experience, and counseling style.

Monitoring and facilitating progress. Once needs have been addressed, monitor progress in resolving needs, moving through the stages of decision making, and achieving the goal of decision quality (informed, choice matches features that matter most to the informed patient). Decision tools help a patient consider and become committed to taking the next steps.

options. They reduce the uptake of discretionary surgical options that informed people don't value when baseline rates of these procedures are high. They also increase the uptake of colon cancer screening options, which are underused, and lower the rates of prostate cancer screening tests, which are overused.

Gaps in Research

Although decisional conflict is common and decision support interventions can address its modifiable contributing factors, there are three major knowledge gaps. First, most large studies describing people's decisional conflict are from North America. Therefore, more descriptive research is needed on the prevalence of decisional conflict and related factors for the many decisions people face in more diverse populations. Second, the Decisional Conflict Scale elicits people's "overall comfort level" with their knowledge, values, and support. These comfort levels are only modestly correlated with a person's knowledge test scores and their match between their values and the chosen option. Researchers still don't know the relative contribution of each of these variables to downstream behavior. Third, practitioners should be trained to recognize and screen for decisional conflict in their patients so they can refer those who require assistance in resolving their decisional needs. A 4-item clinical version of the Decisional Conflict Scale may hold promise in this regard.

Annette O'Connor and France Légaré

See also Decision Making in Advanced Disease; Patient Decision Aids; Shared Decision Making

Further Readings

Bunn, H., Lange, I., Urrutia, M., Campos, M. S., Campos, S., Jaimovich, S., et al. (2006). Health preferences and decision-making needs of disadvantaged women. *Journal of Advanced Nursing, 56*(3), 247–260.

Carroll-Johnson, R. M., & Paquette, M. (1994). *Classification of nursing diagnoses: Proceedings of the tenth conference.* Philadelphia: Lippincott.

Gattellari, M., & Ward, J. E. (2005). Men's reactions to disclosed and undisclosed opportunistic PSA screening for prostate cancer. *Medical Journal of Australia, 182*(8), 386–389.

Janis, I. L., & Mann, L. (1977). *Decision making.* New York: Free Press.

O'Connor, A. M. (1995). Validation of a decisional conflict scale. *Medical Decision Making, 15*(1), 25–30.

O'Connor, A. M., Drake, E. R., Wells, G. A., Tugwell, P., Laupacis, A., & Elmslie, T. (2003). A survey of the decision-making needs of Canadians faced with complex health decisions. *Health Expectations, 6,* 97–109.

O'Connor, A. M., Stacey, D., Entwistle, V., Llewellyn-Thomas, H., Rovner, D., Holmes-Rovner, M., et al. (2003). Decision aids for people facing health treatment or screening decisions. *Cochrane database of systematic reviews,* 1. Art. No.: CD001431. DOI: 10.1002/14651858.CD001431.

Ottawa Health Decision Centre. (n.d.). *A to Z inventory of decision aids.* Retrieved February 4, 2009, from http://decisionaid.ohri.ca/AZinvent.php

Ottawa Health Research Institute. *Ottawa personal decision guide.* Retrieved February 4, 2009, from http://decisionaid.ohri.ca/decguide.html

Sepucha, K. R., Fowler, F. J., Jr., & Mulley, A. G., Jr. (2004, October 7). Policy support for patient-centered care: The need for measurable improvements in decision quality (Web exclusive). *Health Affairs,* DOI: 10.1377/hlthaff.var.54

Decision Analyses, Common Errors Made in Conducting

Decision analytic modeling (DAM) has been increasingly used within the past 30 years to synthesize clinical and economic evidence and support both clinical and policy-level decision making. Decision models often represent complex decision and synthesize data from a variety of sources, and they may be difficult to validate and interpret. Thus, while DAM can be extremely useful, it is also difficult to do well. Errors are common among neophytes and not uncommon even in published decision analyses. This entry reviews the steps associated with constructing a decision model and describes several of the most common errors in model construction, analysis, and interpretation. It considers both conceptual errors in model construction and errors of computation or calculation. Although DAM is commonly used in economic evaluation, the purview of this entry extends only to model-related aspects of economic evaluation.

Comparators

Every decision analysis compares at least two options. If the decision is a clinical one (e.g., how should localized prostate cancer be treated?) all *feasible* and *practical* options should be considered. These might include doing nothing (or active surveillance), surgery, radiation, brachytherapy, or cryotherapy, and more. If the decision is a policy decision (say, whether a national human papillomavirus vaccination program should be funded), the same criteria apply: Feasible and practical options might include no vaccination, universal vaccination, vaccination targeted at high-risk groups, vaccination targeted at specific age groups, and more. Feasible and practical are clearly subject to interpretation, but the key ideas are that all options that stand a realistic chance of being implemented (feasibility) should be examined, given the resources available to address the problem (practicality).

The decision analysis neophyte often is reluctant to include many options because of concerns that the model will become unmanageably complex. As a result, many models consider only the two or three most intuitively attractive options. Options such as "do nothing" or "supportive care only," or alternate frequencies or intensities of an intervention may be avoided. This is acceptable if the goal is to gain experience in modeling, but it is not acceptable if the goal is to choose the best therapeutic or policy option.

More advanced analysts may also inappropriately constrain the potential options considered. This may be because of a desire to adhere closely to the best quality evidence published in high-impact journals. Or it may be a strategic decision to put a new drug or device in the best possible light by choosing a plausible but weak comparator or by avoiding comparisons across types of interventions (e.g., comparing drugs only to drugs but not to surgery). Regardless of the reason, inappropriately constraining the set of comparators is a common and serious error in modeling.

Model Structure

Decision models represent potential outcomes of alternate strategies using models, which may be simple decision trees, discrete-time state-transition (i.e., Markov) models, discrete-event simulation models, or dynamic infectious disease models. Models may be simple or complex, but should correspond to an underlying theory or biological model of disease.

Underrepresentation

In particular, models must capture important differences across strategies. For example, if two strategies differ mainly in adverse effect profile, the structure of the model must represent adverse effects. An important and common example of underrepresentation is the use of cohort simulation models to represent decision problems in which events within the cohort affect members outside the cohort. For example, vaccination will protect individuals within a cohort, but the herd immunity associated with high rates of coverage will confer benefits beyond the cohort. Failure to represent these additional benefits of vaccination will inaccurately represent the true effect of vaccination on the entire population.

Unclear or Inappropriate Target Population

Neophytes in particular are often unclear about which population is being represented in the model. Models should represent a specific group or population. This includes a value or distribution for age, sex, disease severity, and prevalence and type of comorbid illness.

Perspective

When the perspective of a decision problem extends beyond the individual patient, modeling outcomes only for the patient represents an error. For example, the question of optimal approaches to testing for fetal abnormalities potentially affects the parents, the fetus, and other family members. While appropriate valuation of these outcomes is difficult, constraining the decision problem to one perspective is incorrect, unless the perspective taken is explicitly that of only one individual. Similar errors are often present in models that represent health outcomes of children but ignore families, and models that consider the elderly or disabled, but ignore caregivers.

Time Horizon Bias

Every model represents a limited period of time. The time horizon of the model should extend to or beyond the point at which there are no differences between strategies in life expectancy and quality of life. Neophytes often prefer short time horizons because this reduces model complexity. For example, a model designed to compare computed tomography with abdominal ultrasound imaging for suspected appendicitis in children might focus on short-term events around the abdominal pain, imaging, surgery, and immediate perioperative outcomes. However, one of the main concerns of parents and clinicians is avoiding unnecessary radiation. Thus, representing the long-term cancer risk associated with radiation is an essential aspect to correctly representing this decision problem.

This error is also common among more experienced modelers. For example, decision models often closely follow randomized trials. Because the time horizon of trials is often short, important differences in quality of life and mortality that extend beyond the horizon of the trials may not be represented in models, and bias is therefore introduced. While experienced modelers are often aware of this problem, they may adopt inappropriately short time horizons, in the interest of enhancing the apparent scientific credibility of the model to clinical or policy audiences, by reducing the complexity and the number of assumptions in the model. This is a common and often serious error.

Mortality From Other Causes

While focusing on a particular disease, modelers may neglect to represent competing causes of mortality in a decision model. This means that subjects in the model remain at risk of disease-related adverse events for longer. Differences across strategies may be exaggerated, and error is therefore introduced.

Half-Cycle Correction Problems

As the name suggests, discrete-time cohort simulation models represent risk in discrete time periods. Models represent events as occurring at the beginning or end of discrete time intervals, whereas events can actually occur throughout the interval. Half-cycle correction adjusts for this property of discrete time models by adding (or subtracting) the value (life expectancy, quality-adjusted life expectancy, or cost) associated with half of one cycle length. Neophytes often neglect to introduce a half-cycle correction or assign the incorrect sign to the correction (subtraction instead of addition of a half-cycle or vice versa).

Symmetry

Symmetry refers to consistent representation of model events and outcomes across strategies. Errors of symmetry often occur when modelers use different structural elements (e.g., tree fragments, Markov states) or variable names and expressions across different strategies that represent the same components of the decision problem. Events and outcomes may not be represented or be represented in a different manner when alternate structures are used. Experienced modelers frequently use a common model structure for all strategies to avoid this error.

Model Data

Obtaining, analyzing, and adjusting data for use in decision analytic models represent perhaps the greatest challenge in developing valid models.

Lamppost Bias

The availability of data may constrain and shape the structure of decision models. While some degree of adaptation may be necessary, it is an error to allow the available evidence to play a fundamental role in shaping the structure of the model, just as it is an error to confine a search to the location of the available light. The structure of the model must be shaped primarily by the decision problem, not the availability of evidence. This refers to inclusion of comparators and other aspects of structure, as described above. For example, representing only treatments or adverse effects for which there is strong evidence represents an error.

Rate to Probability Conversion

Transitions between states in Markov models for a discrete time period are commonly expressed using probabilities, referred to as transition probabilities. However, these data are commonly abstracted from the literature in the form of rates. While rates are close to probabilities for very small values, this is less true for larger values. A common neophyte error is to neglect the conversion of rates, as obtained from the literature, into probabilities.

Errors in Value Structure

A complete set of utilities for important health outcomes is rarely available from a single source. Many variables may affect utility values reported in the literature, including source of preferences (patients vs. experts or members of the general public), scaling method, use of direct or indirect utility elicitation, instrument used for indirect utility elicitation (e.g., Health Utilities Index vs. EQ-5D), and computer-assisted versus interview-assisted elicitation, among others. Judgment must therefore be applied when utilities from widely disparate sources are used. In particular, the ordinal relationships among important health outcomes should, in general, be reflected in ordinal scores among utility values used in the model. Uncritical use of published data may result in a model value structure that is not internally consistent or does not correspond with an a priori model of disease. A common error is to overweight the size, quality, or place of publication of a utility study, and underweight consistency and appropriate ordinal relationships among model values.

Adjustment for Age and Comorbidity-Related Utility

As patients age, utility scores for current health status decline. This may be due to acquired comorbidity, age-related decline in functional status, change in preference structure as patients age, or a combination of these. A frequent error in representing the value structure of a model is to assume that the utility of individuals without the disease in question can be assigned a value of 1.0. This assumption results in overestimation of the difference in utility scores between those with and without disease, and correspondingly may overestimate the benefit of treatment or prevention.

A companion error is to adjust for age-related comorbidity among patients without disease but

fail to adjust among patients with disease. For example, if the mean utility for 70-year-old individuals is .90, and the disutility (1 − utility) associated with renal failure is .40, the utility for a 70-year-old with renal failure should reflect the contribution of both factors. A common method of adjustment is to assume that utility is multiplicative, and simply multiply (e.g., .90 × (1 − .40) = .54).

Internal Consistency

Internal consistency refers to the internal mathematical structure of a decision model. Internal consistency is most frequently evaluated using univariate sensitivity analysis. Changes in values of a single variable should have predictable effects on model outputs. A common error is to evaluate inconsistency in a haphazard or unsystematic way. Every variable should be tested across a broad range. Any deviation from predicted behavior represents either a failure of internal consistency (a "bug") or an insight, but more commonly the former. An equally common error is to identify internal consistency problems but fail to correct them because of time or resource constraints.

Murray Krahn and Ava John-Baptiste

See also Cost-Utility Analysis; Decision Tree: Introduction; Decision Trees, Construction; Decision Trees: Sensitivity Analysis, Deterministic; Markov Models; Markov Models, Applications to Medical Decision Making; Markov Models, Cycles

Further Readings

Krahn, M. D., Naglie, G., Naimark, D., Redelmeier, D. A., & Detsky, A. S. (1997). Primer on medical decision analysis: Part 4: Analyzing the model and interpreting the results. *Medical Decision Making, 17,* 142–151.

Philips, Z., Bojke, L., Sculpher, M., Claxton, K., & Golder, S. (2006). Good practice guidelines for decision-analytic modelling in health technology assessment: A review and consolidation of quality assessment. *PharmacoEconomics, 24,* 355–371.

Smith, K. J., Barnato, A. E., & Roberts, M. S. (2006). Teaching medical decision modeling: A qualitative description of student errors and curriculum responses. *Medical Decision Making, 26,* 583–588.

Decision Board

The decision board is a visual aid to help clinicians present information about different courses of action in an efficient and standardized manner. The sole goal of the decision board is to improve communication (i.e., improve information transfer). The decision board can (and has been) successfully modified for other uses: to describe the options to choose between in willingness-to-pay (WTP) surveys and to elicit treatment options of potential patients and patients for policy decision making.

Context

What is the best treatment for an individual patient? It is important to realize that there is often no right or wrong choice. For example, the case of adjuvant chemotherapy for patients with breast cancer presents a situation of choice between potential morbidity and disability now (due to therapy, if chosen) and potential morbidity and inconvenience later (due to recurrence of the disease). The uncertainty of the outcome at the individual level (i.e., there is no way to know in advance what will happen to an individual patient) further complicates the problem and makes the choice a very difficult one. Thus, the question of which course of action to take becomes a preference judgment. However, to make an informed preference judgment one needs to know the relevant courses of action and their potential risks and benefits.

Treatment decision making typically takes place within the context of a doctor-patient encounter. This process is both complex and dynamic and can be done using different approaches (i.e., paternalistic, shared, and informed approaches, with myriad in-between approaches that combine components of different approaches). Besides the paternalistic approach, the vast majority of approaches require that the physician inform the patient about the relevant courses of action and their potential benefits and risks. This is due to the fact that, typically, a doctor is required to determine the diagnosis about the type and severity of the patient's illness, on the basis of which the determination of the available courses of action will be made.

Communication difficulties between doctors and their patients are a well-known problem. It has been argued that doctors and patients talk to each other with different voices. The voice of medicine is characterized by medical terminology, descriptions of medical symptoms, and the classification of these within a reductionist biomedical model. The voice of patients, on the other hand, is characterized by nontechnical discourse about the subjective experience of illness within the context of social relationships and the patient's everyday world. Many studies document that communication misunderstandings experienced by doctors and their patients are common.

Goals and Benefits

The decision board should provide all the relevant clinical information that a patient needs to make a decision or participate in the decision-making process, if he or she wishes to do so. The potential morbidity and mortality effects are described in a probabilistic manner, acknowledging the fact that the final outcome and course of any intervention are uncertain. In other words, there is no way to predict what will happen to an individual patient. Scenarios are constructed to describe the treatment options (e.g., in the case of early-stage breast cancer after surgery, adjuvant chemotherapy vs. no further treatment) and the potential side effects (e.g., in the case of chemotherapy, hair loss, stomach upset, vomiting). Scenarios are also constructed to describe the potential outcome of each treatment option (e.g., in the case of chemotherapy, a cancer-free scenario and a cancer returns scenario).

The decision board can be seen as a specific form of decision aid. Various types of decision aids have been developed over the years designed to help participants in the medical encounter to make treatment decisions. In terms of the goals to be achieved by using a decision aid, different authors have different ideas about what the primary goal should be. Two goals are most commonly cited: (1) to provide patients with information on the potential benefits and risks of different options and (2) to help patients clarify their values so that they will make treatment choices that are consistent with their values. Some other goals mentioned are lowering the cost of care, reduction of decisional conflict, improving patient satisfaction with the decision-making process, encouraging patients to be more involved in the decision-making process, and improving clinical outcomes. While there is agreement on the role of decision aids in information transfer (or knowledge acquisition), there is still debate on whether the other goals are appropriate and feasible.

The sole goal of the decision board is to improve communication (i.e., improve information transfer) about potential courses of action by presenting information simply, using spoken and written language supported by the use of visual aids and relying on repetition. It has been found that when the decision board is administered by the clinician (e.g., doctor), it helps build the relationship between the clinician and the patient. It helps facilitate two-way communication and encourages questions from patients and responses from the clinician. This should be seen as an additional benefit and cannot be assumed to happen every time a decision board is used. In many cases, a relationship between the doctor and the patient already exists (e.g., in the case of a family physician or a specialist treating a chronic condition). In other cases (e.g., a cancer patient meeting his or her oncologist the first time), building the relationship between the patient and his or her doctor might be important.

Format

It is important to emphasize that the decision board does not have a fixed format. It can be seen as a "concept" that leaves "artistic freedom" for its creators to modify according to the special features of the medical problem dealt with. However, within that artistic freedom, a few "rules" should be kept to. For example, after describing all the information about the different courses of action (i.e., the different "pieces of the puzzle"), a visual aid where all these elements are integrated (i.e., a full picture) should be available. This is because it is known that most individuals cannot judge a situation only by valuing the different parts separately. They need to see the full picture to be able to compare the different options. Also, a take-home version should be available for patients, because few decisions are so urgent as to need immediate answers. Where it is feasible, agreeing to defer the decision to allow time for further understanding of the options and for deliberation would be helpful. Finally, the decision

board should be easy to administer, inexpensive to produce, and easily modified to incorporate local variations in practice or new clinical information that becomes available.

The first decision board was developed in 1990 for use in the situation of adjuvant chemotherapy for node-negative breast cancer. The board was made of foamcore, which was found to be both lightweight and more durable than cardboard. With the advent of computer capability, the decision board was computerized, too. The move to a computer-based version has opened new opportunities (e.g., ease of providing more tailored information, ease of supplementing core information on an individual basis, and the ability to present technical information in alternative ways to suit patients' needs) but created other challenges (e.g., difficulties in presenting the full picture due to constraints regarding screen size). Examples of schematic presentations of decision boards can be found in articles mentioned in the Further Readings section.

Research Findings

The decision board was tested in several well-conducted studies (including several randomized controlled trials, where it was compared with current practice). It was found to be clear and understandable, valid, and reliable, and improves information transfer (e.g., knowledge about potential treatment options, their potential benefits and risks). It was also found to be easy to administer and use. It was well accepted by clinicians and patients and is currently being used as part of regular practice in different places. Even though it is not the goal of the decision board, it is interesting to note that it was also found that patient satisfaction with decision making was improved. When tested, it was found that the average time of consultation with the decision board was not increased as compared with the average time of consultation without the board. While it is not the goal of the decision board to maintain (or even reduce) the time of consultation, this is still an interesting finding.

Nonclinical Uses

The decision board can be easily modified to serve as an instrument describing the options to choose between in WTP surveys. In WTP studies, individuals are asked to (a) choose a preferred course of action (or program) and then (b) indicate the maximum amount they are willing to pay to ensure that their preferred option will be available if needed. A weakness that was identified in many WTP questionnaires is the lack of clarity in describing the options compared in terms of their potential benefits and risks. This cast doubts on the validity of the WTP values provided by respondents. The modified decision board was offered as a way to explain the choices to participants in surveys. Because the concept was found to be useful in explaining treatment options to real patients (who are often anxious and confused), it seemed that it would work with healthy people. Indeed, using a modified decision board to explain the different courses of action was shown to be helpful. It was also felt that the use of the decision board can also enhance the credibility of the results among users of information, as it makes explicit the exact question faced by the respondent in the study. However, this point has not been tested yet.

A modification of the decision board is required, because typically subjects in a WTP survey are not patients who suffer from the disease. They should be members of the general population who are typically healthy people. The modification of the decision board depends on whether the WTP question is being asked ex post (i.e., WTP at the point of consumption) or ex ante (i.e., insurance-based approach). For an ex post–type WTP instrument, a preamble is required to describe the medical conditions for which the different courses of action described are required. This helps healthy respondents imagine that they are at the point of consumption of the services described. For an ex ante–type WTP instrument, the preamble should have additional information about the risk of the condition/disease to the individual (or loved ones or other people in the population, depending on the nature of the disease and the question asked). In other words, for an insurance-based question, the respondents need to know the likelihood of their being at the point of consumption.

The decision board can also be used to elicit the preferences about treatment options of potential patients and patients for policy decision making (rather than clinical decision making). An example of such use is a study which attempted to assess if potential patients prefer tissue plasminogen activator (tPA) over streptokinase (SK). In patients with acute myocardial infarction, tPA (compared with SK) has been shown to reduce the 30-day mortality rate at the expense of an increased rate of stroke. The assumption in the literature was that, were it not for cost issues (tPA is much more expensive), all patients presenting with myocardial infarction would choose tPA. A decision board describing the treatment options (without mention of the drug names) was used in face-to-face interviews with individuals at risk for having the event in two hospitals (as it is not possible to ask patients who are experiencing the event). It was found that a substantial proportion of individuals who could potentially require thrombolytic therapy chose SK over tPA. This finding, if found to be consistent, has significant implications for clinical decision making as well as economic and policy implications.

Amiram Gafni

See also Patient Decision Aids; Shared Decision Making; Willingness to Pay

Further Readings

Charles, C., Gafni, A., & Whelan, T. (1999). Decision making in the physician-patient encounter: Revisiting the shared treatment decision making model. *Social Science and Medicine, 49,* 651–661.

Charles, C., Gafni, A., Whelan, T., & O'Brien, M. A. (2005). Treatment decision aids: Conceptual issues and future directions. *Health Expectations, 8,* 114–125.

Gafni, A. (1997). Willingness-to-pay in the context of an economic evaluation of healthcare programs: Theory and practice. *American Journal of Managed Care, 3,* S21–S32.

Heyland, D., Gafni, A., & Levine, M. (2000). Do potential patients prefer tissue plasminogen activator (tPA) over streptokinase (SK)? An evaluation of the risks and benefits from the patient perspective. *Journal of Clinical Epidemiology, 53,* 888–894.

Levine, M. N., Gafni, A., Markham, B., & MacFarlane, D. (1992). A bedside decision instrument to elicit a patient's preference concerning adjuvant chemotherapy for breast cancer. *Annals of Internal Medicine, 117,* 53–58.

Matthews, D., Rocchi, A., & Gafni, A. (2002). Putting your money where your mouth is: Willingness-to-pay for dental gel. *PharmacoEconomics, 20,* 245–255.

Nelson, W. L., Han, P. K. J., Fagerlin, A., Stefanek, M., & Ubel, P. A. (2007). Rethinking the objectives of decision aids: A call for conceptual clarity. *Medical Decision Making, 27,* 609–618.

O'Brien, B., & Gafni, A. (1996). When do the "dollars" make sense? Toward a conceptual framework for contingent valuation studies in health care. *Medical Decision Making, 16,* 288–302.

Whelan, T., Levine, M., Gafni, A., Sanders, K., Willan, A., Mirsky, D., et al. (1999). Mastectomy versus lumpectomy? Helping women make informed choices. *Journal of Clinical Oncology, 17,* 1727–1735.

Whelan, T., Levine, M., Willan, A., Gafni, A., Sanders, K., Mirsky, D., et al. (2004). Effect of a decision aid on knowledge and treatment decision making for breast cancer surgery: A randomized trial. *Journal of the American Medical Association, 292,* 435–441.

Whelan, T. J., Sawka, C., Levine, M., Gafni, A., Reyno, L., Willan, A. R., et al. (2003). Helping patients making informed choices: A randomized trial of a decision aid for adjuvant chemotherapy in node negative breast cancer. *Journal of the National Cancer Institute, 95,* 581–587.

Decision Curve Analysis

Decision curve analysis is a straightforward technique for evaluating diagnostic tests, prediction models, and molecular markers. Unlike traditional biostatistical techniques, it can provide information as to a test's clinical value, but unlike traditional decision analytic techniques, it does not require patient preferences or formal estimation of the health value of various health outcomes: Only a general clinical estimate is required. Differences between biostatistical techniques, decision-analytic techniques, and decision curve analysis are shown in Table 1.

A common clinical problem is when a physician can easily obtain information about T—the result of a diagnostic test, the level of a molecular marker, or a probability from a statistical prediction model—but wants to know $D,$ whether or not a patient has, or will develop, a certain disease state. From a research perspective, the analyst's task is to determine whether doctors should obtain T in order to make decision about $D.$

In this entry's motivating example, D is whether the patient has prostate cancer and is used in decisions about whether or not to conduct a prostate biopsy; T may be the result of a digital rectal examination (normal vs. abnormal) or the level of prostate-specific antigen (PSA), or it may be a prediction model based on multiple factors (such as age, race, and family history). This example is used to discuss drawbacks of the traditional biostatistical and decision analytic approaches to evaluating the value of T, whether a binary diagnostic test, a statistical prediction model, or a molecular marker. Then this entry discusses the novel method of decision curve analysis.

Biostatistical Approaches and Their Drawbacks

Biostatistical analysis of prediction models, diagnostic tests, and molecular markers is largely concerned with accuracy. Such metrics have been criticized by decision analysts as having little clinical value. An accurate test, prediction model, or marker is, in general, more likely to be useful than one less accurate, but it is difficult to know for any specific situation whether the accuracy of a test, prediction model, or marker is high enough to warrant implementation in the clinic. For example, if a new blood marker for prostate cancer increased the area under the curve (AUC) of an established prediction model from .77 to .79, would this be sufficient to justify its clinical use?

Decision Analytic Approaches and Their Drawbacks

Decision analysis formally incorporates the consequences of test results and can therefore be used to determine whether use of a prediction model, diagnostic test, or molecular marker to aid decision making would improve clinical outcome. A typical approach is to construct a decision tree as shown in Figure 1. We denote probabilities and values of each health outcome, respectively, as p_{xy} and as $b_{xy},$ where x is an indicator for the test result and y is the indicator for disease. To determine the optimal decision, the values of each outcome are multiplied by their probability and summed for each decision; the decision with the highest expected value is chosen.

To obtain p_{xy}s for a statistical model or molecular marker, the analyst has to choose a cut point in order to dichotomize results into positive and negative. Different analysts can disagree about the appropriate cut point, entailing that the analysis may need to be run several times for a range of

Table 1   Comparison of decision curve analysis with traditional statistical and decision analysis

	Traditional Statistical Analysis	*Traditional Decision Analysis*	*Decision Curve Analysis*
Mathematics	Simple	Can be complex	Simple
Additional data	Not required	Patient preferences, costs or effectiveness	Informal, general estimates
Endpoints	Binary or continuous	Continuous endpoints problematic	Binary or continuous
Assess clinical value?	No	Yes	Yes

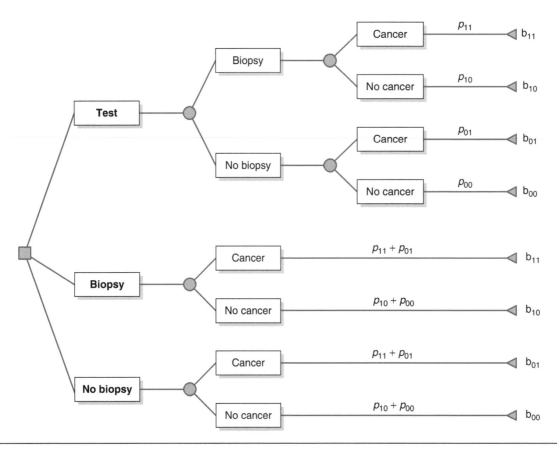

Figure 1   Traditional decision tree to evaluate a test for prostate cancer in men with elevated prostate-specific antigen (PSA)

reasonable alternatives. Choice of b_{xy}s can be even more difficult. A b_{xy} may require data from the literature that can be hard to come by or controversial; moreover, a b_{xy} may require judgments that may reasonably vary from patient to patient. The need for additional data may be one of the reasons why the number of biostatistical evaluations of tests, prediction models, and markers dwarfs the number of decision analyses: In one systematic review of more than 100 papers on cancer markers, researchers failed to find a single decision analysis.

Theoretical Background to Decision Curve Analysis

Traditional decision analysis, unlike biostatistical analyses, can determine the clinical value of a test, prediction model, or marker; however, it requires additional parameters, p_{xy} and b_{xy}, that can be difficult to specify. Decision curve analysis starts by showing that p_{xy}s and b_{xy}s can be related through a simple, clinically interpretable quantity: the threshold probability of disease at which a patient or clinician would opt for further action. The threshold probability of disease is then used to calculate the "net benefit" of different treatment strategies, such as biopsying all men, or biopsying on the basis of a marker. The strategy with the highest net benefit should be used in the clinic.

Threshold Probability of Disease

It is highly unlikely that a man would consent to a prostate biopsy if he was told that his probability of prostate cancer was 1%. Conversely, if the man was told that he had a 99% probability of cancer, there is little doubt as to his course of action. If we were to increase the probability of cancer gradually from 1% to 99%, there would come a point where a man would be unsure of whether or not to be biopsied. We define p_t, the threshold probability of disease for taking some action, such as biopsying a man for prostate cancer: If a patient's estimated probability of disease is greater than p_t, he will opt for biopsy; if it is less than p_t, he will not opt for biopsy. When the probability of disease is equal to the threshold probability p_t, the benefits of opting for biopsy or no biopsy are equal:

$$b_{11} \times p_t + b_{10} \times (1 - p_t) = b_{01} \times p_t + b_{00} \times (1 - p_t),$$

and, therefore,

$$\frac{b_{00} - b_{10}}{b_{11} - b_{01}} = \frac{p_t}{1 - p_t}. \qquad (1)$$

Now $b_{00} - b_{10}$ is the benefit of true negative result compared with a false positive result; in clinical terms, the benefit of avoiding unnecessary treatment such as a negative biopsy. Comparably, $b_{11} - b_{01}$ is the benefit of a true positive result compared with a false negative result; in other words, the benefit of treatment where it is indicated, such

as a biopsy in a man with cancer. Equation 1 therefore tells us that the threshold probability at which a patient will opt for treatment is informative of how a patient weighs the relative benefit of appropriate treatment as compared with the benefit of avoiding unnecessary treatment. As an example, if a man stated that he would opt for biopsy if his risk of prostate cancer were 20% or higher, but not if his risk were less than 20%, we can say that this man thinks that finding a prostate cancer early is worth four times more (i.e., .20 ÷ (1 − .20)) than avoiding the risks, pain, and inconvenience of an unnecessary biopsy.

We can rearrange Equation 1 to obtain

$$-(b_{10} - b_{00}) = (b_{11} - b_{01})\left(\frac{p_t}{1 - p_t}\right). \qquad (2)$$

Net Benefit

The idea of net benefit is similar to that of profit. A business owner choosing between several possible investment opportunities will estimate the expected income and expenditure for each and then choose the option that maximizes the difference between the two.

In medicine, the corollary to income and expenditure is benefit and harm; more specifically, in the case of a diagnostic test, prediction model, or molecular marker, benefit is true cases identified and appropriately treated (T^+, D^+, or true positives); harm is unnecessary treatment (T^+, D^-, or false positives). In our prostate cancer example, we want to biopsy men with prostate cancer (true positives) and avoid unnecessary biopsies of men without cancer (false positives). However, "finding cancer" and "avoiding unnecessary biopsy" are not equivalent in value. Equation 2 gives the number of false positives we would exchange for a true positive in terms of the threshold probability. This becomes our way to convert between "finding cancer" and "avoiding unnecessary biopsy." Where n is the total number of men in the cohort, net benefit is given as

$$\frac{\text{True positives} - \text{False positives} \times \left(\frac{p_t}{1 - p_t}\right)}{n}. \qquad (3)$$

As an illustration, in a cohort of 728 men undergoing biopsy, 202 had cancer; 479 of the men had a risk of cancer of 20% or higher using a prediction model, of whom 163 had cancer. The net benefit at a threshold probability of 20% for biopsying all men is (202 (true positives) − 526 (false positives) × .25) ÷ 728 = .0968; the net benefit of using the prediction model is (163 (true positives) − 316 (false positives) ×.25) ÷ 728 = .1154. Hence, use of the prediction model would lead to a higher net benefit and better clinical outcome.

The unit of net benefit is the number of true positives per patient: It therefore has a maximum at the prevalence, but no minimum. A net benefit has a simple clinical interpretation. For example, a difference in net benefit between two prediction models of .02 could be interpreted as "Using Prediction Model A instead of Prediction Model B is equivalent to a strategy that increased the number of cancers found by 2 per 100 patients, without changing the number of unnecessary biopsies conducted."

Decision Curve Analysis

The threshold probability p_t can be used both to define positive and negative test results and to provide a decision analytic weight. The first stage of decision curve analysis is therefore to use logistic regression to convert the results of the test, marker, or prediction model into a predicted probability of disease $\hat{p}$. Decision curve analysis then consists of the following steps.

1. Choose a threshold probability (p_t) for treatment. Here, "treatment" is defined generally as any further action, such as drug therapy, surgery, further diagnostic work-up, or a change in monitoring, depending on the particular clinical situation.

2. Define patients as test positive if $\hat{p} \geq p_t$ and negative otherwise. For a binary diagnostic test, $\hat{p}$ is 1 for positive and 0 for negative.

3. Calculate net benefit of the test, marker, or prediction model using the formula for net benefit in Equation 3.

4. Calculate clinical net benefit for the strategy of treating all patients. Where π is the prevalence, this simplifies to

$$\pi - (1 - \pi) \times \left(\frac{p_t}{1 - p_t} \right). \qquad (4)$$

5. The net benefit for the strategy of treating no patients is defined as zero.

6. The optimal strategy is that with the highest clinical net benefit.

7. Repeat Steps 1 to 6 for a range of threshold probabilities.

8. Plot the net benefit of each strategy against threshold probabilities.

Interpretation of Decision Curves

To illustrate decision curve analysis, data from men undergoing prostate biopsy in Göteborg, Sweden, as part of a randomized trial of PSA screening for prostate cancer (ERSPC) are used. One of the drawbacks of the PSA test is that it has a positive predictive value in the 20% to 30% range, such that most men with PSA levels above the cut point for biopsy do not have prostate cancer.

Figure 2 shows decision curves for various biopsy strategies in men with elevated PSA in the first round of the ERPSC. These strategies are as follows: biopsy all men (thick grey line); biopsy no man (thick black line); biopsy only those men with an abnormal clinical examination (the digital rectal examination [DRE]; thin grey line); biopsy on the basis of a statistical prediction model incorporating PSA level and DRE (dashed line); biopsy on the basis of a statistical prediction model of PSA, DRE, and an additional molecular marker, the ratio of free-to-total PSA (thin black line). Note that the decision curves are shown only for probability thresholds of 10% to 40%. Only these thresholds are shown because we have asked clinicians about what would constitute a reasonable range: A typical response is that few men would opt for biopsy if they were told they had a risk of prostate cancer less than 10%; on the other hand, it is hard to imagine that a man taking a PSA test would want at least a 50:50 chance of cancer before agreeing to biopsy. The decision curve shows that the statistical prediction model including PSA, DRE, and free-to-total PSA ratio has the highest net benefit across the whole 10% to 40% range. We can therefore conclude that using this prediction model, and the new marker, will improve clinical outcome.

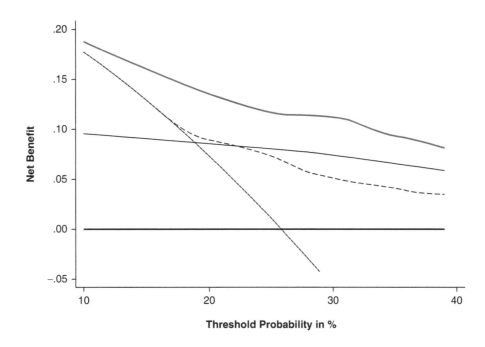

Figure 2   Decision curve analysis for previously unscreened men with elevated PSA

Notes: Biopsy all men (short dashes); biopsy no man (thick black line); biopsy only those men with an abnormal clinical examination (thin grey line); biopsy on the basis of a statistical prediction model incorporating PSA level and DRE (long dashes); biopsy on the basis of a statistical prediction model of PSA, DRE, and free-to-total PSA ratio (thick grey line, top).

It is informative to imagine Figure 2 if it had only shown the decision curve for the PSA and DRE prediction model (the dashed line). The net benefit for this prediction model is only superior to the alternative strategy of biopsying all men for probability thresholds of 20% or higher. We would interpret this as showing that use of the prediction model would help some, but not all men. However, it might also be pointed out that the prediction model only requires data that is routinely collected and is never worse than biopsying all men, so there is little harm in using it, perhaps advising risk-averse men to biopsy irrespective of their risk from the prediction model. If, on the other hand, the prediction model required an additional invasive test or measurement of a novel marker, the decision curve analysis can be described as "equivocal," and it is recommended that a more formal and complex decision analysis be conducted.

Comparison of Decision Curves With Conventional Decision Theory

Figure 2 shows several characteristics of decision curves that are congruent with conventional

decision theory. First, the decision curve for "biopsy all men" crosses both the x and the y axis at the prevalence (26%). If the threshold probability is 0 (i.e., $x = 0$), then false positives have 0 weight, and so net benefit becomes the proportion of true positives, which, in the case of biopsying everyone, is the prevalence. For $y = 0$, imagine that a man had a risk threshold of 26% and asked his risk under the "biopsy all" strategy. He would be told that his risk was the prevalence (26%). When a man's risk threshold is the same as his predicted risk, the net benefit of biopsying and not biopsying are the same. Second, the decision curve for the binary test (DRE) crosses that for "biopsy all men" at 1 − negative predictive value, and again, this is easily explained: The negative predictive value is 81%, so a man with a negative test has a probability of disease of 19%; a man with a threshold probability less than this—for example, a man who would opt for biopsy even if his risk was 15%—should therefore be biopsied even if he was DRE negative. Furthermore, although this cannot be seen in Figure 2, the decision curve for DRE is equivalent to "biopsy no one" at the positive predictive value. This is because for a binary test, a man with a positive test is given a risk at the positive predictive value.

Comparison of Decision Curves With Accuracy Metrics

To illustrate how decision curves and accuracy metrics may diverge, consider the case of a man with elevated PSA after repeat screening. It is reasonable to suppose that different statistical models will be needed for prostate cancer detection, depending on whether a patient has a recent history of screening. Men without recent PSA testing may have an advanced cancer with a high PSA or a localized cancer with a moderately elevated PSA; only the latter is likely for a man undergoing regular screening. Accordingly, both the mean probability of cancer and the relationship between PSA and cancer will differ for previously screened men.

A statistical model for prostate cancer in recently screened men was created using data from rounds 2 to 6 of the ERSPC Göteborg. Differences between prediction models are shown in Table 2. We would expect these different prediction models to have different properties when applied to a data set. Yet when the prediction models are applied to the recently screened men, the predictive accuracies are virtually identical, with AUCs of .6725 and .6732 for the "Round 1" and "Rounds 2 to 6" prediction models, respectively. Figure 3 shows the decision curves for the two prediction models. Although net benefits are close at low threshold probabilities, the "Rounds 2 to 6" prediction model is always superior. An even more extreme case is where we compare a prediction model with just PSA and DRE. The "Round 1" prediction model built on unscreened men has an AUC of .6038 when applied to men with a recent PSA test, again very similar to a prediction model built on this data set (AUC of .6056). However, "Round 1" prediction model has absolutely 0 clinical value with net benefit never higher than those of both "biopsy all" and "biopsy none" (data not shown).

Extensions to Decision Curve Analysis

The formula for net benefit is given in units of true positives but is easily rearranged to give units of false positives.

$$\text{Reduction in False Positives} = \text{Net Benefit} \times \left(\frac{1 - p_t}{p_t}\right)$$

This net benefit can be interpreted as, for example, "Using Prediction Model A instead of Prediction Model B is equivalent to a strategy that reduced the number of biopsies by 10 per 100 patients, without changing the number of cancers found."

Decision curve analysis can also easily incorporate harm, for example, if a test was costly or invasive. The analyst needs to obtain a clinical judgment as follows: "If the test were perfect, how many patients would you submit to the test to find one case?" The reciprocal of this number is the harm and is simply subtracted from the net benefit. For example, if there was an additional test for prostate cancer that was very costly, and clinicians informed us that they would not subject more than 20 patients to the test to find one cancer, the harm of the test would be .05, and the net benefit of any prediction model incorporating the test would be reduced by .05 for all threshold probabilities.

Several other traditional aspects of prediction model evaluation can also be applied to decision curve analysis, including correction for overfit; confidence intervals for net benefit; application to time-to-event data, such as cancer survival; and including competing risks. Simple-to-use R and Stata software for decision curve analysis is available from www.decisioncurveanalysis.org.

Andrew J. Vickers

See also Decision Trees, Construction; Decision Trees, Evaluation; Receiver Operating Characteristic (ROC) Curve; Test-Treatment Threshold

Further Readings

Elkin, E. B., Vickers, A. J., & Kattan, M. W. (2006). Primer: Using decision analysis to improve clinical decision making in urology. *Nature Clinical Practice Urology, 3*(8), 439–448.

Steyerberg, E. W., & Vickers, A. J. (2008). Decision curve analysis: A discussion. *Medical Decision Making, 28*(1), 146–149.

Vickers, A. J., & Elkin, E. B. (2006). Decision curve analysis: A novel method for evaluating prediction models. *Medical Decision Making, 26*(6), 565–574.

Table 2 Differences in prediction comparing men with and without prior screening

	"Round 1 Prediction Model" Created Using Results From Men Without Prior Screening	"Rounds 2 to 6 Prediction Model" Created Using Results From Men With Prior Screening
Prevalence of cancer	25.90%	18.90%
Standardized odds ratio from multivariable prediction model		
PSA	1.56	1.19
DRE	4.67	3.34
Free-to-total PSA ratio	0.37	0.58

Note: Change in odds for a 1-standard-deviation increase in the marker.

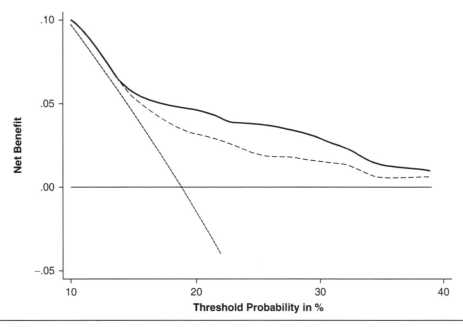

Figure 3   Decision curve analysis for men with elevated PSA on repeat screening

Notes: Biopsy all men (short dashes); biopsy no man (thin black line); biopsy on the basis of a statistical prediction model of PSA, DRE, and free-to-total PSA ratio; prediction model created using data from unscreened men ("Round 1": long dashes); prediction model created using previously screened men ("Rounds 2 to 6": thick line).

DECISION MAKING AND AFFECT

Intuition allows us to make quick decisions in an uncertain environment, not wasting too much time on analyzing possible consequences. Evaluative judgments and decisions are quite often influenced by intuitive feelings rather than analytical conclusions. A doctor in an emergency room, for instance, won't have the time to evaluate the benefits and risks of two similar treatments analytically. The emotion which helps us boost our decision process is called *affect*.

Affect is used as a cue when people define the positive or negative quality of a stimulus; it is experienced as a state and is used whenever quick assignments or attributions are needed to make decisions or judgments. Hence, *affect* is used as an umbrella term referring to states of valence and arousal; it sometimes even includes states of mood, although these are of a more diffuse, low-intensity and long-lasting character. To give an example of experiencing affect, just imagine how fast we associate feelings with words like *cancer* or *emergency*. Thus, some researchers call the reliance on such feelings and their utilization in decision making the *affect heuristic*.

In this entry, a short theoretical background of affective influence in cognition is given, followed by a brief description of psychological models on this topic. Then, various examples according to the affect heuristic and its possible effects in the medical context are examined.

Theoretical Background

Two main attempts can provide a theoretical background for findings on the affect heuristic: First, Epstein's dual-process theory separates "two modes of thinking" into analytical and intuitive, emotional ways of information processing. Secondly, Damasio's theory of "somatic markers" accounts for the importance of affect in decision making.

Epstein's development of the cognitive-experimental self theory introduces a dual process of thinking, assuming two major systems by which people adapt to the world: rational and experimental. Constructs about the self and the world in the rational system refer to beliefs, whereas those in the experimental system refer to implicit beliefs. Neither of the two thinking styles is predominant; they rather function simultaneously. The experimental system is developed through a very long historical evolution and therefore operates more intuitively and automatically. In contrast, the rational system needs more effort to operate; it is mostly used within the medium of language due to its shorter evolutionary history. A wide range of research supports the theory, emphasizing the use of the experimental system in heuristic processing.

Damasio's concept explaining the importance of intuition or affect in decision making was developed by asking the question, "What in the brain allows humans to behave rationally?" His observations led him to the conclusion that human behavior is influenced by "somatic markers" learned in a lifetime. The theory assumes that people mark images with positive or negative feelings, which are directly connected to bodily states. As a result, images can be associated with negative markers that imply an alarming state, or they can be linked to positive markers, meaning a beacon of incentive feeling linked to a bodily state. These assumptions were tested in experiments with patients who had damage to the ventromedial frontal cortices of the brain. Patients with this damage are unable to experience "feelings" and are impaired in their ability to associate affective feelings and anticipated consequences. A gambling game was provided to the participants, where they had to choose cards from any of four card decks. Each chosen card resulted in a gain or loss of a certain amount of money. Patients with the damage to the ventromedial frontal cortices showed their impairment in anticipating future outcomes by their inability to avoid card decks with great outcomes but also great losses. In contrast, "normal" subjects and patients with brain damage outside the prefrontal sections "learned" how to choose the card decks with the lower but continuous payoff. These findings proved that somatic markers increase the accuracy and efficacy of the decision process.

Models of Affective Influence

Psychological models explaining the affective influence on decision making and judgments are often divided by two general categories. One category subsumes associative attempts, when affect is activated in the *semantic memory network* or the *motor network*. Research on semantic memory models analyzes the influence of affective states on the encoding, retrieval, and interpretation of new information. Experiments on affective congruency are derived from this attempt, stating that individuals in a happy mood are more likely to interpret ambiguous information in a positive and more generalized way. For instance, a patient in a good mood might be too positive in describing his or her symptoms, which could complicate the assessment of the right diagnosis. Findings concerning the motor network focus on approaching and avoiding movements depending on the positive or negative affect, respectively. Therefore, positive valence could be especially useful in stimulating motor action.

A second category refers to inferential models. These are based on the influence inferred by current or anticipated absence or presence of an affective experience. On the one hand, affect can serve *as information*, using a shortcut to decisions and judgment when no alternative explanation is available—as explained in the following examples about the affect heuristic. On the other hand, the influence of affect can occur due to the *intended regulation* or maintenance of an emotional state and therefore lead to accordant decisions. Following this attempt, individuals are not only intending a mood-congruency due to their affective state, but also seek to modulate their mood depending on the contextual needs. Hence, the good mood of the patient could be "adjusted" when telling the risks of a possible disease—and might lead to an adequate description of experienced symptoms.

The Affect Heuristic

A wide range of research is done referring to the affect heuristic, mostly associated with the affect-as-information model—using affective states as useful tools when no other information is available. Findings due to this affect heuristic have various aspects and may interfere with decisions in the medical context. Each of these aspects is described, followed by examples of the effects affect might have on medical decision making.

Preference

Early research already proved that the repetitive presentation of objects leads to positive attitudes and affect toward these objects—independently of any cognitive evaluation. Even more, adding positive or negative meaning to objects guides evaluative judgments, respectively. People therefore are much more susceptible to the affective meaning, albeit any cognitive scrutiny. For instance, the preference of certain drugs and other medical treatments might stem from familiarity or iterated application without taking into account other possibilities. Therefore, medical staff has to be cautious, not wearing blinders or ignoring alternative treatments.

Proportion

Another source of affective influence could be observed by experiments dealing with people's willingness to save a stated number or proportion of lives. Although not rationally comprehensible, the preference of a life-saving intervention is rather evaluated by the proportion than by the numbers of lives that could be rescued. This tendency only changed when two or more interventions could be compared—then the number of lives became more important. Similar findings revealed a study on the support for airport safety. To evaluate benefits of treatments, health professionals are often provided with numbers and statistics—it might be advantageous for them to be aware of the fallacies followed by presented proportions and to always compare different sources of information.

The Evaluation of Risk

A further example in using affect rather than analytical thought concerns the correlation of risks and benefits. Although there is a positive relation in the world, people perceive a negative relation when it comes to everyday decisions: If the benefit is perceived as high, risk is perceived as low and vice versa. Examples can be found in the use of drugs (which are perceived to have a low benefit and a high risk potential) and also medical treatments (e.g., X-rays or antibiotics) that are perceived to have a high benefit and a low risk.

Moreover, despite rational knowledge or evaluation, people often respond rather emotionally in considering dangerous stimuli. For instance, fear can much easier be experienced when people are confronted with dangerous stimuli that evolution has prepared us for (e.g., spiders, snakes, or heights), even when they are cognitively harmless. In contrast, stimuli without an evolutionary history tend to evoke little fear (e.g., guns, smoking)—although they can actually harm us. In the same vein, addictive behaviors tend to be underestimated. Thereby, the strength of a positive or negative affect guides the perception of risks and benefits of an activity.

Numeracy Formats

Quite often, people make a nonoptional choice by "feeling" that this would be the better option. Hence, numeracy is found to have a positive influence in comprehending probability numbers. In a study analyzing the accuracy in decision making of forensic psychologists and psychiatrists, they were asked to determine whether a patient would commit an act of violence in the following 6 months. As an orientation, clinicians were provided with an assessment of another expert that was either given in terms of relative frequency (e.g., "of every 100 patients similar to Mr. Jones, 10 are estimated to commit violence to others") or statistical probability (e.g., "10% of patients similar to Mr. Jones are estimated to commit violence to others"). Although both probabilities were similar, Mr. Jones was evaluated to be more dangerous when clinicians were informed in terms of relative frequency. Consequently, experts are not resistant against their affective influence on decision making. However, also patients run the risk of misinterpreting information when seeking healthcare decisions (e.g., cancer screening).

Communication of Medical Risk

Risks and benefits of medical treatments are of high relevance for the care seeker. However, as decision options in the medical context are mostly unfamiliar to the patient, "affective cues" could assess meaning to the provided information. In a study analyzing people's ability to perceive the quality of healthcare information, positive and negative affective attributes were included to a presented health plan. Findings showed that participants preferred the health plan more often when positive affective categories were added. Furthermore, the risk of a certain disease is influenced by people's experienced worry rather than actual numbers of deaths from this disease. Therefore, it is important to communicate risks and benefits of illnesses and treatment options to give patients an adequate opportunity to make their right choice.

Stephanie Müller and Rocio Garcia-Retamero

See also Emotion and Choice; Errors in Clinical
    Reasoning; Mood Effects; Numeracy; Risk Perception

Further Readings

Alhakami, A. S., & Slovic, P. (1994). A psychological study of the inverse relationship between perceived

risk and perceived benefit. *Risk Analysis, 14*(6), 1085–1096.

Damasio, A. R. (1994). *Descartes' error: Emotion, reason, and the human brain.* New York: Avon.

Fetherstonhaugh, D., Slovic, P., Johnson, S. M., & Friedrich, J. (1997). Insensitivity to the value of human life: A study of psychophysical numbing. *Journal of Risk and Uncertainty, 14*(3), 282–300.

Loewenstein, G. F., Weber, E. U., Hsee, C. K., & Welch, E. S. (2001). Risk as feelings. *Psychological Bulletin, 127,* 267–286.

Peters, E., Hibbard, J., Slovic, P., & Dieckmann, N. (2007). Numeracy skill and the communication, comprehension, and use of risk-benefit information. *Health Affairs, 26*(3), 741–748.

Peters, E., Lipkus, I., & Diefenbach, M. A. (2006). The functions of affect in health communications and in the construction of health preferences. *Journal of Communication, 56,* S140–S162.

Slovic, P., Finucane, M. L., Peters, E., & MacGregor, D. G. (2004). Risk analysis and risk as feelings: Some thoughts about affect, reason, risk and rationality. *Risk Analysis, 24*(2), 311–322.

Slovic, P., Peters, E., Finucane, M. L., & MacGregor, D. G. (2005). Affect, risk, and decision making. *Health Psychology, 24,* S35–S40.

Winkielmann, P., Knutson, B., Paulus, M., & Trujillo, J. L. (2007). Affective influence on judgments and decisions: Moving towards core mechanisms. *Review of General Psychology, 11*(2), 179–192.

DECISION-MAKING COMPETENCE, AGING AND MENTAL STATUS

The term *competence* in decision making is often linked to the phrase *legal competence*. Here, for example, a judge may go by a patient's bedside to determine if the patient is legally competent to make a medical decision on his or her own behalf. The term *decisional capacity* and notions related to the assessment of decisional capacity belong to the realm of physicians in two areas: (1) assessing the capabilities of patients to make medical decisions in medical care and (2) assessing the capabilities of individuals to make decisions on whether to participate in human research studies as study volunteers. This entry provides an overview of decisional capacity; addresses the role of physicians in assessing decisional capacity of patients; discusses various assessment procedures for patients, including aging patients and patients with compromised mental states; and closes with a brief look at the implications for future research.

Overview

Decisional capacity is often phrased as being a question of whether a particular individual has the ability to make choices on his or her own behalf. It has been argued that decisional capacity itself has many components, including but not limited to cognition, memory, mood, emotion, and valuation, among others, which can be affected by age and/or mental status. But the above definition overstates the concept of decisional capacity because—even if all components are intact in an individual—in reality very few individuals make decisions solely on their own behalf.

In reality, individuals come to and make choices after considering opinions from others and make decisions of accepting or rejecting alternatives offered to them from a set of options on the basis of the opinions of others in any number of areas: on what to base a decision, on how to choose among a set of alternatives, and on how much to value a benefit in the context of related harms. And all this information is received and processed into a decision where it is virtually impossible to ensure that all intentional or nonintentional attempts to manipulate the information are able to be identified and extracted from the information and the decision. This extraction of manipulated information is essential in any decision that is worth making.

Physician Assessment

Medical Decision Making

In medical decision making—in absence of an emergency where the individual needs to be acted upon medically to save his or her life, with that emergency further characterized as lacking an advance directive developed and signed by this patient at some time before the emergent event—an individual has three options open to him or her when offered a medical opinion. First, the individual can accept the proffered opinion. Second, the individual can reject the proffered opinion.

Third, the individual can elect to delay choice until a later time in the hope that something will be developed scientifically (or that more understanding will be gained scientifically) before the medical condition or disease under consideration takes the upper hand in the individual and before that medical condition reaches a state where it can no longer be reasonably eliminated, slowed, or otherwise managed medically no matter what attempts are made to do so.

The phrase *decisional capacity* is used in a much more basic sense in medical decision making than in other arenas of competency of judgment. Issues of rejecting physician-recommended medical interventions may mean that the patient will die from a medical condition or disease process that is otherwise medically considered to be curable, eliminable, eradicable, treatable, or at least manageable by the physician.

Human Subjects Research

Physicians also have to assess the decisional capacity of individuals volunteering their services for research. As noted in the U.S. Code of Federal Regulations, because the goal of human subjects research is to possibly develop scientific knowledge for use in future generations, participation in a research study may not guarantee benefit to the individual study volunteer. Given this, the individual study volunteer may be asked to bear considerable risk of morbidity and mortality in the name of the advancement of scientific knowledge for future generations. To what extent an individual with mental health conditions, such as severe schizophrenia, understands that research is not aimed at helping the individual patient is an active research question.

Assessment Procedures

The question of how decisional capacity is best assessed is also an active research question. Assessment procedures may be unstructured or structured. Structured approaches to decisional capacity may be by a computer-generated tool, by a handheld device, or by a paper-and-pencil assessment. The issues regarding assessment of decisional capacity are not related to not having the instruments to record responses to questions. There is a wide range of tools to record the answers to assessment questions. Rather, what is missing in the assessment of decisional capacity in medical care and medical research is an answer to the following question: What are the questions that should be asked in the assessment of decisional capacity both in medical care and research on human subjects?

Decisional capacity can be assessed as a changing (evolving) state over time across different choices; on a choice-by-choice basis; or on a hierarchy of choice, where an individual is able to make a choice at a very basic level but yet incapable of choosing at a more complex level where choices have to be made.

Hierarchical Choice

The most basic question in decisional capacity in medical care of patients is the following: Do you want to live or die? For example, if a patient with symptomatic valvular heart disease is asked, "Do you agree to having the doctor perform surgery on your valve?" The patient may respond, "No, I do not want surgery on my heart." The question here is, what is the missing piece in the discussion? If the patient does not understand that the doctor not performing the valvular surgery means that the patient will die, then the patient has not understood the surgery question being posed. Two questions remain: First, has the surgeon given the patient enough information to understand that the present choice, to accept or reject the valve operation, has the consequence the patient will die, or die sooner without the surgery than if he or she had elected to have the surgery and made it through the surgery without dying? Second, does the patient have the decisional capacity to accept or reject the surgical intervention, a surgical operation on his or her heart valve, on his or her own behalf?

Surrogate Decision Making

There is a third underlying question: How would the surgeon respond, regarding his or her operating on a patient, if the patient did not have decisional capacity but the patient's designated surrogate decision maker wanted the surgery to be done on the patient's behalf? This question about surrogate decision making and the response of the surrogate decision maker does not stand alone but again

begets a set of questions: What if the patient grimaced each time the surgeon asked the patient directly if he or she wanted to have the operation, would the surgeon still be willing to operate? What if the patient screamed at the surgeon every time the surgeon asked the patient directly whether he or she wanted to have the operation and only screamed at the surgeon when the surgeon broached the issue of the operation, would the surgeon still be willing to operate? What if the patient grimaced, screamed, and attempted to grab and hold onto anything the patient could grab onto each time an attempt was made to place the patient on a gurney to take the patient anywhere outside of the patient's room, would the surgeon still be willing to operate?

This illustrates that there may be definite circumstances in which the surgeon may object to performing a medical procedure on a decisionally impaired patient even if the procedure was necessary to save the patient's life (as in severe valvular heart disease) and even if the patient's designated surrogate agreed to the operation (such as valvular heart repair) on the patient's behalf.

Advance Directives

A final question comes up when a patient begins to lose decisional capacity, recognizes such, and then develops advance directives in clinical care and in research specifying what he or she would be willing to have done in the clinical and research arenas in a variety of circumstances. Here again, simply the placement of a preference in a written and signed advance directive does not necessarily mean that the preference will be carried out or acted on in any way. The carrying out of a decision in an advance directive assumes that those physicians responsible for caring for the patient (or principal investigators and researchers involved in recruitment of patients into studies and their institutional review boards) also agree with what is to be done as specified in the advance directive.

Advance directives that specify nonaction (e.g., do not resuscitate, do not intubate, do not place a feeding tube, do not treat an infection with antibiotics) are more likely to be respected than are certain types of advance directive that may specify action (e.g., do take me to surgery for valvular heart repair should I need it in the future, or do involve me in all invasive research studies in schizophrenia, which is a disease that I possess, even if I do not have decisional capacity to make the statement of my willingness to participate). One of the problematic characteristics of neurodegenerative disease is the change in personality that can accompany the neurodegenerative process. Here the patient who led a very mild life of careful decision making may become an irascible person quick to anger, and the question can be legitimately asked, is the irascible patient now present in the room with his or her physician or surgeon or with a research principal investigator the "same person" as the patient who signed the advance directive at an earlier time in either a clinical or a research context?

While the phrase *decisional capacity* often connotes the cognitive realm, one of the human mind's key features related to decision making involves not only cognition but memory. Without memory of past and present events, philosophers have argued that there isn't a thread of holding the "same person" together as one unified whole who is to be counted as the person who is the decision maker choosing among sets of options on his or her own behalf.

There is much that is not known about decisional capacity in medicine. For example, depression has in many mental health circles been considered a disorder of mood, yet severe depression is also a disorder affecting cognition and memory, where the severely depressed individual may pay little attention to consideration of any option in his or her care while in the severely depressed state.

In addition to considering issues related to what constitutes the "same person" in the area of advancing neurodegenerative disease, consideration should also be given to patients who face similar issues with other neurologic conditions (e.g., memory problems due to traumatic brain injury) and mental health conditions (e.g., alternating states of severe mania and severe depression). Is the patient in a state of severe mania the same person as the patient in the state of severe depression? Here, the body may be the same but the mental states may be dramatically different.

In addition, memory is no longer viewed in terms of the presence or absence of short- versus long-term memories. Contemporary research on memory includes descriptions of gist versus verbatim memory in normal persons. Individuals volunteering their participation in research studies have helped

the acquisition of further scientific delineations of memory including episodic memory; semantic memory; the distinction between implicit and explicit memory; recollection in anterograde and retrograde amnesia; autobiographical memory and autonoetic consciousness; long-term memory following transient global amnesia; the prospect of new learning in amnesia; and the fate of recent and remote memory for autobiographical and public events, people, and spatial locations.

Implications for Future Research

The development of the notion of substitute consent (advance directives and surrogate decision makers) is essential for future scientific research in all medical conditions that break down the person beyond what he or she was in terms of memory and thinking. Yet there is much research to be done in identifying what are the key questions that humans need to be approached with to determine their capacity for decision making at a given time and over time to ensure that they are protected from intrusions that they not only prefer not to have, but that they outright object to as humans.

Dennis J. Mazur

See also Decisions Faced by Institutional Review Boards; Informed Consent

Further Readings

Bravo, G., Duguet, A. M., Dubois, M. F., Delpierre, C., & Vellas, B. (2008). Substitute consent for research involving the elderly: A comparison between Quebec and France. *Journal of Cross-Cultural Gerontology,* 23(3), 239–253.

Dunn, L. B., Nowrangi, M. A., Palmer, B. W., Jeste D. V., & Saks, E. R. (2006). Assessing decisional capacity for clinical research or treatment: A review of instruments [review of the current status of decisional capacity assessment tools]. *American Journal of Psychiatry,* 163, 1323–1334.

Dunn, L. B., Palmer, B. W., Appelbaum, P. S., Saks, E. R., Aarons, G. A., & Jeste, D. V. (2007). Prevalence and correlates of adequate performance on a measure of abilities related to decisional capacity: Differences among three standards for the MacCAT-CR in patients with schizophrenia. *Schizophrenia Research,* 89, 110–118.

Guillery-Girard, B., Quinette, P., Desgranges, B., Piolino, P., Viader, F., de la Sayette, V., et al. (2006). Long-term memory following transient global amnesia: An investigation of episodic and semantic memory. *Acta Neurologica Scandinavica, 114,* 329–333.

Jefferson, A. L., Lambe, S., Moser, D. J., Byerly, L. K., Ozonoff, A., & Karlawish, J. H. (2008). Decisional capacity for research participation in individuals with mild cognitive impairment. *Journal of American Geriatric Society, 56*(7), 1236–1243.

Piolino, P., Desgranges, B., Belliard, S., Matuszewski, V., Lalevée, C., de la Sayette, V., et al. (2003). Autobiographical memory and autonoetic consciousness: Triple dissociation in neurodegenerative diseases. *Brain, 126*(Pt. 10), 2203–2219.

Reyna, V. F., & Hamilton, A. J. (2001). The importance of memory in informed consent for surgical risk [gist vs. verbatim memory]. *Medical Decision Making, 21,* 152–155.

Rosenbaum, R. S., Köhler, S., Schacter, D. L., Moscovitch, M., Westmacott, R., Black, S. E., et al. (2005). The case of K.C.: Contributions of a memory-impaired person to memory theory. *Neuropsychologia, 43,* 989–1021.

Saks, E. R., Dunn, L. B., Wimer, J., Gonzales, M., & Kim, S. (2008). Proxy consent to research: The legal landscape. *Yale Journal of Health Policy, Law, and Ethics, 8,* 37–92.

U.S. Code of Federal Regulations. (2007). 45.46.102.d.

DECISION MAKING IN ADVANCED DISEASE

Decision making in advanced disease is complex and challenging. Decisions are emotional and often have irreversible outcomes (e.g., death). For many, the desire to live longer is strong, but unrealistic, when faced with advanced illness, and goals must be realigned toward comfort and quality of life. Some medical interventions are invasive and detract from quality of life without lengthening life. Decision makers include professionals, patients, their families, and external parties (institutions, insurers, governments). These decision makers may have diverse goals, priorities, values, and cultural backgrounds, affecting their beliefs about care near the end of life. Prognostication and communication are critical to good decision making. In advanced disease, preferences for decision-making style are individual, often unstated, and change over the illness course. Advance directives involve decisions about theoretical future events. Near the end of life, many people lose capacity to make decisions and this responsibility falls to their families. This is often at a time of great stress and influenced by emotions, grieving, and caregiving burdens. Sometimes a time-limited trial of therapy is used to facilitate decision making in these difficult situations.

Why Is Decision Making Needed in Advanced Disease?

Patients with advanced disease are faced with complex treatment options (disease-focused or supportive therapy, hospice, clinical trials) and choices about commencement, continuation, or withdrawal of interventions such as artificial hydration and nutrition, blood transfusion, cardiopulmonary resuscitation, circulatory support, dialysis, and invasive ventilation.

Studies of quality of death in America have found that death frequently occurs in hospitals and is accompanied by the use of highly technical interventions (e.g., invasive ventilation, cardiopulmonary resuscitation) and significant pain and distress. Invasive medical interventions close to death are not associated with better outcomes and are sometimes against the expressed wishes of patients. Trials of interventions to improve quality of care at the end of life (the SUPPORT study) have so far been unsuccessful.

When Are Decisions Needed?

Decision making in advanced disease requires recognition (usually by the clinician) that a decision needs to be made. Even not making a decision may be a decision itself. Timing of the decision requires recognition and communication of the following: incurable disease, limited prognosis, potential future-course and alternative-management options. Decision making may be impaired by the assumption that only one option is available (e.g., active treatment is pursued due to failure to recognize supportive care as a valid treatment option).

In many advanced illnesses, especially neurological illnesses, ability to communicate is lost as disease progresses. Decision-making capacity may also be lost due to an acute crisis requiring intubation or sedation or to delirium, which commonly occurs close to death. Ideally, patients with advanced illness are able to express their treatment preferences, write advance directives, and appoint a surrogate decision maker (medical power of attorney) before they lose capacity.

Prognostication

Decision making in advanced disease relies on prediction of prognosis: the expected duration and quality of life, and likely future course of the disease. Advanced cancer is often characterized by a short decline in function toward death. Advanced nonmalignant diseases (chronic organ failure) have a more gradual decline worsened by recurrent exacerbations. Death is the result of an acute exacerbation that fails to respond to treatment, thus timing is less predictable. Chronic frailty or dementia follows a slow, drawn-out decline. Instruments are available to predict prognosis based on type and stage of disease, symptoms, physical function (performance status), and test results. These instruments predict chances of being alive at a certain point or give a median survival for a similar group of patients; they cannot predict how long an individual will live. Physician predictions of individual prognosis are often inaccurate and tend to be overly optimistic. Physicians are reluctant both to make prognostic estimates and to communicate them to patients. Patients' estimates of their own prognosis are also often inaccurate. These failures of prognostication and communication hinder decision making.

Communication

Physicians may be reluctant to initiate discussions about end-of-life care for fear of removing hope. However, patients often do prefer to receive prognostic information, and denying them this knowledge may impair preparation for death. Patients are willing to discuss preferences but rarely initiate these conversations; thus clinicians need to be proactive. Communication goals include eliciting preferences (for information, decision making, and treatment), understanding values and beliefs, and establishing goals of care—priorities (for quality or quantity of life), hopes, and legacies. Patients

may have specific wishes to fulfill, events to live for, and preparations to make (financial, practical, or legal). Clinicians also must provide information about diagnosis, prognosis, and treatment options. A majority of patients in English-speaking countries want detailed information, while patients in other countries may prefer less information. When presenting treatment options, clinicians have an obligation to be realistic. Rather than present a laundry list of all possible treatments, only options that are feasible given the circumstances should be discussed.

Decision-Making Styles

The prevailing attitude in Western medicine is respect for individual autonomy, and thus shared or autonomous decision making is preferred. However, patients express a range of preferences, with between 30% and 60% preferring shared decision making. Age, gender, and ethnicity may influence preferences, but inconsistently; thus, individual preferences need to be elicited. Preferences may alter with each decision and with disease course; patients closer to death are more likely to delegate responsibility to their physician. Decision style also varies with the magnitude of the decision and the certainty of the outcome. For example, a decision about which antibiotic to prescribe for pneumonia is usually made by a physician based on established medical knowledge. These unilateral decisions are usually communicated to the patient, who then may choose to accept or reject the recommendation.

While Western culture highly values autonomy, other cultures value family decision-making styles. Such families may request that information regarding diagnosis, prognosis, and treatment be withheld from the patient. This can cause conflict with a clinical team focused on individual autonomy; however, autonomy includes the right to defer decision making to one's family. These issues can be addressed by eliciting cultural beliefs about truth telling and decision making of patients and their families.

Surrogate decision making is required if patients lose decision-making capacity. It is most often performed by a close family member. Ideally surrogate decisions are based on substituted judgment (what the patient would want in this circumstance) and best interest (what is thought to be best for the patient at this time). Substituted judgment is best derived from previous conversations or statements; however, patients infrequently express their wishes to family members. Families are often inaccurate in predicting patients' treatment preferences. They also consider factors such as quality of life, emotions, and their own values when making decisions. Caregiver anxiety or depression may also influence surrogate decisions. Surrogate decision making can be burdensome for families if they are asked to make decisions without information, assistance, and recommendations from clinicians. They may feel guilt or responsibility for their relative's death. Surrogate decision making can also be a source of conflict if clinicians consider further aggressive treatment futile and families insist that it continue.

Perspectives of Decision Makers in Advanced Disease

Clinicians

Models of care for advanced disease promote multidisciplinary teams; thus, multiple clinicians may be involved in decision making. These clinicians may have diverse backgrounds and training (e.g., physicians, nurses, social workers, psychologists, and chaplains) and thus diverse views on care in advanced disease.

Treatment recommendations may be influenced by specialist training and practice location. Clinicians untrained in principles of palliative care may not feel confident in offering this option. Conventional medical teaching (e.g., antibiotics for pneumonia) may not always be the best option for a person close to death. Clinicians have a professional responsibility to provide recommendations rather than abdicating all decisional responsibility to the patient. Recommendations should be based on both medical knowledge and the priorities and values of the patient and family.

Clinicians are also influenced by real and perceived ethical dilemmas. Consensus supports the ethical nature of treatment withdrawal and withholding artificial nutrition and hydration in terminal illness, surrogate decision making, and the principle of double effect (unintentional hastening of death with treatment aimed at comfort). Physician-assisted suicide and euthanasia are illegal in most countries and American states, exceptions being the Netherlands, Switzerland, Washington, and Oregon.

Physicians sometimes use futility to facilitate treatment decisions in advanced disease. This principle holds that physicians are not obliged to provide treatment considered futile. The definition of futility is controversial and lacks consensus. Futility definitions may be quantitative—the treatment won't work (e.g., cardiopulmonary resuscitation in advanced disease), or they may be qualitative—treatment will only prolong a state of poor quality of life (e.g., persistent vegetative state). Definitions of futility are subject to value judgments; thus, a process of communication and negotiation is recommended when futility issues arise.

Patients

Patients faced with life-threatening illness are more willing to accept aggressive and toxic treatment, with minimal chance of benefit, than their clinicians and healthy people. Decision making is influenced by values and priorities (for quantity or quality of life), past experiences, family, friends, and presence of children. Patients' perception of their prognosis (which is often inaccurate) influences their treatment choices. Access to and availability of services may influence treatment decisions (e.g., geographic access to radiotherapy is often limited). Patient priorities near the end of life may include pain and symptom management, sense of control, avoiding prolonged dying, relieving families' burden, strengthening relationships, and preparation, including financial and funeral arrangements. Concerns may include treatment toxicity, burden (appointments, tests, side effects), and financial costs.

Family

Families of people with advanced illnesses may be hoping for cure or prolongation of life while also experiencing anticipatory grief. Caregiving is often characterized by loss of employment and financial security and stresses of maintaining family function and their own health. Information needs of families may be different from those of patients, especially as disease progresses. Families may not be in close proximity and thus may be faced with difficult decisions of timing travel to be with their family member. Surrogate decision making places additional burden on families, and preexisting conflicts are likely to be escalated by decision-making responsibilities. Family conferences are often used in advanced disease, especially in the intensive and palliative care units. These meetings usually involve at least two clinicians (often physician and social worker) and all family members (including friends or other caregivers) relevant to the patient.

External

External organizational, cultural, and political factors influence decision making in advanced disease. These factors may not be evident on an individual level but influence the experiences of groups. For example, the number of regional hospital beds is a stronger predictor of place of death than patient preference. Availability of hospice services reduces hospital deaths.

Health insurers and reimbursement options also influence decisions. In the United States, the Medicare Hospice Benefit is available to patients with an estimated prognosis of less than 6 months. Because of difficulties in prognosticating for nonmalignant diseases, these patients are underserved by hospice. Patients often need to forgo disease-modifying treatments to be eligible for hospice. This condition causes some people to delay hospice until terminal stages of illness.

Decision-Making Processes

Six Thinking Hats

This model was developed by Edward de Bono to promote parallel thinking in group decisions. Decision makers consider issues from one perspective simultaneously and then move on to the next. Principles of this strategy can also be applied to advanced disease.

Information (White Hat)

Information needed includes prognosis, options available, and likely outcomes of each option. Often, information gathering and provision is the role of the clinician. Different styles of presenting and framing information influence patients' decisions. Patients and their families are increasingly accessing Internet sources, which may lead to misinformation. Cancer Web sites frequently discuss treatment options and side effects but rarely prognosis. In advanced disease there may be limited evidence, thus uncertainty and probabilities play a large role. A treatment-response rate may be small, but who responds or experiences side effects is largely unpredictable.

Emotion and Intuition (Red Hat)

Patients' and families' emotions may include denial, hope, anger, or a sense of abandonment. Patients may be concerned about being a burden to others, loss of control, and dignity. Both patients and clinicians are influenced by spiritual, religious, and cultural beliefs about death. Patients and families may also have emotional reactions to the decision-making process itself, for example, feelings of anger and resentment toward the process or clinical team.

Caution (Black Hat) and Optimism (Yellow Hat)

Consequences of each option (positive and negative) need to be considered. While active treatments may extend life, supportive therapy also has positives of symptom control and quality of life. Costs may include treatment burden, side effects, caregiving burden, and financial costs. Patients and their families may hold false hopes for prolongation of life or cure. Hope may need to be redirected toward comfort and quality of life.

Creativity (Green Hat)

Creative solutions in advanced disease may include flexibility of decisions (e.g., pursue Plan A with Plan B if unsuccessful), or two options simultaneously (supportive care and active treatment). Second opinions and advice from colleagues may also suggest creative options.

Process Control (Blue Hat)

The clinician's role is to summarize, conclude, and make plans for follow-up. Retention of information in times of stress is poor, and questions are often thought of after conversations. Time may be needed to consider options and make a decision.

Decision Aids

Question prompt lists are available for advanced cancer or those seeing a palliative care team to help patients gather information. Decision aids are available for early-stage cancer, but few are available for advanced disease. Guidelines, care plans, and hospital policies can be used to facilitate decision making, but few have been published.

Practical Decision Making: Issues to Consider

In clinical practice, certain practical considerations may facilitate treatment decisions. These include the following:

- What is the performance status and extent of disease? These may make aggressive treatment unrealistic.
- Is the condition reversible or treatable?
- What are the possible complications or worst outcome, and are these acceptable to the patient?
- Does treatment contribute to patient comfort and/or safety?
- Is it logical, appropriate, and humane?
- Does it make good medical and common sense?
- What are the costs?
- What do the patient and family want?

Conflict

Conflict may arise between patient and family and clinician (e.g., wanting to continue treatment that clinician considers futile), between members of the treating team, or between various family members. Conflict may be avoided by clear communication about prognosis, expected outcomes, and goals of care. Communication can be facilitated by family or team meetings. Approaches to conflict resolution include ethics or palliative care consultation or independent mediation. If conflict cannot be resolved, strategies involve a time-limited treatment trial (with explicit outcome measures), or transfer of care to another clinician. Unfortunately, some conflicts have ended in legal and public disputes.

Katherine Hauser and Declan Walsh

See also Advance Directives and End-of-Life Decision Making; Decision-Making Competence, Aging and Mental Status; Decisions Faced by Surrogates or Proxies for the Patient; Physician Estimates of Prognosis

Further Readings

Back, A. L., & Arnold, R. M. (2005). Dealing with conflict in caring for the seriously ill. "It was just out of the question." *Journal of the American Medical Association, 293,* 1374–1381.

Council on Ethical and Judicial Affairs, American Medical Association. (1992). Decisions near the end of life. *Journal of the American Medical Association, 267*(16), 2229–2233.

Council on Ethical and Judicial Affairs, American Medical Association. (1999). Medical futility in end-of-life care: Report of the Council on Ethical and Judicial Affairs. *Journal of the American Medical Association, 281*(10), 937–941.

Covinsky, K. E., Fuller, J. D., Yaffe, K., Johnston, C. B., Hamel, M. B., Lynn, J., et al. (2000). Communication and decision-making in seriously ill patients: Findings of the SUPPORT project (The Study to Understand Prognoses and Preferences for Outcomes and Risks of Treatments). *Journal of the American Geriatrics Society, 48*(Suppl. 5), S187–S193.

de Bono, E. (1999). *Six thinking hats.* Boston: Back Bay Books.

Matsuyama, R., Reddy, S., & Smith, T. J. (2006). Why do patients choose chemotherapy near the end of life? A review of the perspective of those facing death from cancer. *Journal of Clinical Oncology, 24*(21), 3490–3496.

Meisel, A., Snyder, L., Quill, T., & American College of Physicians-American Society of Internal Medicine End-of-Life Care Consensus Panel. (2000). Seven legal barriers to end-of-life care: Myths, realities, and grains of truth. *Journal of the American Medical Association, 284*(19), 2495–2501.

Parker, S. M., Clayton, J. M., Hancock, K., Walder, S., Butow, P. N., Carrick, S., et al. (2007). A systematic review of prognostic/end-of-life communication with adults in the advanced stages of a life-limiting illness: Patient/caregiver preferences for the content, style, and timing of information. *Journal of Pain and Symptom Management, 34*(1), 81–93.

Quill, T. E., & Brody, H. (1996). Physician recommendations and patient autonomy: Finding a balance between physician power and patient choice. *Annals of Internal Medicine, 125,* 763–769.

Stagno, S. J., Zhukovsky, D. S., & Walsh, D. (2000). Bioethics: Communication and decision making in advanced disease. *Seminars in Oncology, 27,* 94–100.

Weissman, D. E. (2004). Decision making at a time of crisis near the end of life. *Journal of the American Medical Association, 292*(14), 1738–1743.

DECISION MODES

A decision is a commitment to a course of action that is intended to serve the interests and values of particular people, which often differ sharply from one person to the next. A good example is a patient's choice of radical mastectomy over lumpectomy as a treatment for breast cancer, where the patient seeks to do what is best for both herself and her family, especially her young children. There is considerable variability in not only *what* different people (and even the same person on different occasions) decide when facing the same dilemmas, but also in *how* they decide. The term *decision modes* is used to characterize such qualitatively distinct means by which people reach their decisions. This entry describes and reviews several of the major decision modes that have been acknowledged. It also discusses their conceptual and practical significance, particularly in medicine.

A Big Picture

There are myriad decision modes. But almost all of them can be classified into a small number of categories defined according to several metadecisions that are made, consciously or otherwise, in virtually every decision situation. Here the expression *metadecision* refers to a decision about how to decide. The decision mode tree in Figure 1 provides a big-picture view of the decision modes that result from these metadecisions. The discussion proceeds from the "Responsibility" node near the top of the tree down to the bottom.

Responsibility

In every decision situation, someone—either an individual person or a collective—must assume responsibility for making the decision in question. Thus, for example, in the contemporary United States, it is understood that the patient herself has the responsibility—or "right," "privilege," "authority," "obligation," "burden," even "duty"—for deciding how her breast cancer will be treated. Usually, on a local basis, at least, assumptions about decision-making responsibility are so broadly accepted, so "natural," that the issue never crosses people's minds. Discussions of responsibility do not

occur except under extraordinary circumstances, such as when the assumptions are contested. Only then do people realize that responsibility typically has been established via earlier metadecisions made by others, including society, as suggested by the "Prior metadecisions" node in the decision mode tree. For instance, many Americans are first spurred to think about responsibility for cancer treatment decisions when they learn that Japanese responsibility customs are different from their own. They are surprised to learn that in some long-standing Japanese traditions, a cancer patient might not even be told by her physician and her family that she has the disease. Or take the case of end-of-life decisions. When the patient is incapacitated, as in the Terri Schiavo case in Florida, which ended on Schiavo's death in 2005, who has the right to decide—the patient's spouse, the patient's parents, the state legislature, Congress, or the courts? Many people had never pondered such knotty questions until media coverage of the Schiavo case forced them to do so.

Digression: Adequacy of Mode Metadecisions

Part of the full scientific story of human decision behavior is an understanding of how and why people make the mode metadecisions that they do. But there is a practical side, too. Suppose that, at some metadecision choice point in the mode tree, the decider goes down one path rather than some other. Furthermore, suppose that this increases the odds that the eventual decision will be effective. Then it is legitimate to say that that metadecision is better than it would have been otherwise. The following discussion briefly addresses adequacy concerns as well as questions about how particular metadecisions are reached.

Choice Point ❶: Reauthorization

The first metadecision facing the responsible or recognized decider—one person or several—is about whether and how to shift at least some of that responsibility to others, authorizing them to take part in the decision process. At one extreme, the recognized decider might do nothing, *retaining* full responsibility. For instance, a heart disease patient might declare, "Whether I receive

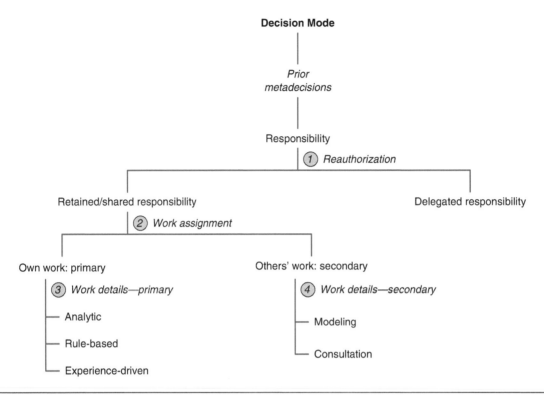

Figure 1   Decision mode tree

angioplasty is my decision and mine alone." At the opposite extreme, responsibility is *delegated* or relinquished entirely, a circumstance sometimes described as "agency," as when a patient says to his doctor, "I'm no expert, but you are, so would you please decide for me, as if you were choosing for your own father?" Between those extremes, the recognized decider might elect to bring others into the picture to *share* decision-making responsibility. That is, the decision process becomes a (more) collective one, as in the shared medical decision-making paradigm, where the patient and the physician assume joint responsibility for choosing medical treatments.

There are several reasons that recognized deciders sometimes favor either retaining or relinquishing some or all of the responsibility they inherit. Especially significant among those reasons are prevailing customs or even laws. A good illustration is provided by socially (and sometimes legally) sanctioned personal autonomy principles that encourage patients to lean toward making their own treatment decisions. Other motivations as well as consequences of authorization choices are sketched presently.

Retaining Responsibility

Two aims are common for those choosing to retain full decision-making responsibility. The first is preserving the perquisites of decision-making authority. People who have such authority cannot help using it to serve their own, personal interests, it seems. Thus, relinquishing that authority, or even sharing it, poses a significant risk. This is part of the rationale for patient autonomy principles such as those embodied in informed consent requirements: Empowered patients will not knowingly choose treatments that harm them. A second common goal in holding onto decision-making responsibility consists of short-term time constraints. If a decision needs to be made in a hurry (e.g., triage in an emergency room), all else being the same, the fewer people there are who must reach agreement, the better things are.

Cast against the sought-after aims of retaining extant decision-making authority are several threats to decision effectiveness. There is evidence that people often overestimate their own skills. Such overconfidence would induce deciders to believe that they can perform essential decision-making tasks better than others whose true expertise is actually superior. Such overconfidence is not universal, however. It appears weakly if at all when there is unambiguous evidence of one's incompetence. Thus, although a trained physician might overestimate his ability to make decisions better than those of his peers, similar overestimation should be less common among naïve patients. A second major drawback of retaining decision-making authority is related to the first—excessive workload. Suppose that a physician refuses to delegate decision tasks because she incorrectly believes that no one else can make those decisions as well as she can. Then, in short order, she is likely to be so overwhelmed that all her decisions suffer and so does her personal well-being.

Sharing Responsibility

The most compelling motivation for a decider choosing to share decision-making responsibility is embodied in the adage, "Two (or more) heads are better than one." That is, sharing decision-making responsibilities seems to promise better decisions because of the energy and also the specialized knowledge that other people bring to the table. "Political" benefits beckon, too. The people brought into the decision process are more likely to accept instead of resist the resulting decisions, since people rarely protest against themselves. Similarly, sharing partly shields the originally recognized decider from the blame that often spews forth when decisions turn out badly (e.g., the wrath of a family whose loved one dies in a surgical procedure chosen solely by a physician).

The anticipated rewards of sharing decision-making responsibility sometimes go unrealized or are overshadowed by the costs of sharing. One threat to the effectiveness of sharing is free-riding, the tendency for members of a group to do less than their fair share of the work, partly because they expect that others will pick up the slack for them. Another is the documented phenomenon whereby information that is possessed by every participant in a meeting tends to be overly represented among the topics actually discussed. This means that knowledge possessed uniquely by individual discussants is neglected. This defeats a primary aim for broadening participation in the decision-making process in the first place, the

exploitation of specialized expertise (e.g., the unique insights that an endocrinologist, an oncologist, and a gynecologist can bring to a case conference). And then, of course, there are the increased coordination costs demanded by the sharing of decision-making responsibility (e.g., the hassles of finding mutually suitable meeting times for all participants in the decision process, to say nothing of the time spent in the meetings themselves).

Delegating Responsibility

The advantages envisioned for delegating decision-making responsibility to others are partly the same as those for sharing (e.g., taking advantage of specialized knowledge). But the prospects of lower costs are especially alluring. After all, the originally recognized decider is freed entirely (although typically for a fee, broadly defined) from having to work through the decision problem in question; that problem would belong to someone else altogether.

Yet delegation carries with it burdens and risks that are easy to overlook. First off, to delegate properly, a recognized decider must understand decision processes as well as the current decision problem in sufficient detail to know what kinds of expertise are required to solve that problem effectively. Consider, for example, the challenge of determining whether the training of a physician's assistant is sufficient to allow her to decide whether to send home patients who do not need further attention. Furthermore, the decider must know how to appraise others' expertise (e.g., "Is this *particular* assistant up to the task?"). Ample research indicates that our ability to evaluate expertise is less than ideal, being vulnerable to numerous potentially misleading indicators, such as candidates' skills at mimicking the speaking style of recognized authorities. An especially important challenge is assuring *incentive alignment*. This means that those to whom decision-making authority is delegated would gain no benefit from making decisions that are contrary to the interests and values of the people the decisions are supposed to serve. That is, they have no conflicts of interest. Incentive alignment is at the heart of controversies about physicians' dual responsibilities to patients and insurers.

Choice Point ❷: Work Assignment

Once responsibility for making a decision is settled, the actual work of reaching that decision must be carried out. There are two alternatives for who performs particular aspects of that work—the recognized deciders or someone else. When those deciders execute the required tasks themselves, the modes are referred to as *primary*; otherwise they are *secondary*. Decision making typically encompasses a wide variety of chores. Therefore, work assignment for a given decision problem can easily involve both primary and secondary modes for different elements of the overall effort. The problem of determining whether a decision task should be assigned to a secondary mode is largely the same as that of determining whether to delegate an entire decision problem to someone else. Thus, the same principles apply.

Choice Point ❸: Work Details—Primary

As indicated in the decision mode tree, there are three major classes of primary modes: analytic, rule-based, and experience-driven.

Analytic Decision Making

The essential, distinguishing feature of *analytic* decision making is that the decider reasons through what makes sense as a solution to the decision problem at hand, with no constraints on the inference process. When most people hear and use the term *decision making,* this is what they have in mind. There are two principal variants of analytic decision making, substantive and formal.

In *substantive* analytic decision making, the decider reasons according to a conception of how nature (broadly conceived) works, that is, how one event or action leads to another, which in turn yields other occurrences, and so on. Effectively, the decider relies heavily on mental simulations of the chains of events that plausibly might ensue if various alternative actions were chosen. Then the decider pursues the option whose simulation turns out best in the decider's eyes. Consider, for example, how a physician might reason through the sequences of potential biological consequences if she were to recommend alternative drug therapies for a patient experiencing both hypertension and diabetes. If the sequence for one particular therapy includes a highly probable severe drug interaction, the physician backs away from that course of action.

The defining characteristic of *formal* analytic decision making is that significant elements of the decider's reasoning entail operations on symbolic representations of key elements of the decision situation. These operations might be carried out in the decider's head or perhaps via a computer. As an example, consider a decision analysis in which a kidney patient's utilities for various health states are, via expected utility formulas, aggregated with probability assessments for potential outcomes, to yield treatment recommendations.

Rule-Based Decision Making

Rule-based decision making relies on decision rules of this form: *If Conditions C1, C2, C3, . . . hold, then pursue Action A.* Sometimes deciders develop such rules on their own, summarizing personal observations and arguments (e.g., when a physician says, "Over the years, I have noticed that . . ."). But some rules are provided by experts, as in the case of the National Comprehensive Cancer Network's practice guidelines for treating osteosarcoma. Rule-based decision making is not as simple as it might seem. For instance, it requires a prior decision about whether to accept a particular decision rule, say, on the basis of its developers' reputations. And applying that rule often demands a tough judgment as to whether the current situation matches the rule's preconditions sufficiently closely.

Experience-Driven Decision Making

The word *experience* is used in two distinct but related senses in the expression *experience-driven decision making.* The first sense implicates decision making that is nearly the antithesis of analytic decision making in that it does not entail breaking decision problems down into their components, such as utilities versus probabilities. Instead, the decider has an undifferentiated psychological experience that somehow pushes the decider toward one potential action rather than its competitors. Furthermore, the decider typically cannot explain the decision process and it may well be nonconscious. Instead, those asserting a reliance on such nondeliberative, "intuitive," "recognition-primed," or "System 1" decision making often say things such as "For some reason, it just felt like the right thing to do." One prominent line of scholarship on such decision making is commonly identified with the somatic marker hypothesis for risk taking. According to this theory, over repeated experiences, people gradually develop biologically mediated associations with high-risk alternatives, associations that compel them to shy away from those alternatives even before they can offer reasons for why they feel the way they do. Significantly, individuals with damage to the medial prefrontal cortex, who are notorious for poor decision making, do not develop these risk-repelling associations.

The second sense of *experience* in some kinds of experience-driven decision making refers more directly to the decider's past cognitive activities. The core idea is that, as the decider repeatedly encounters—experiences—a particular situation, the decider learns, in the broad sense of the term. Imagine a teenager who chooses to light up a cigarette for the first time in a certain type of situation, as in the presence of particular friends. If this scenario is repeated over and over, eventually the teenager no longer deliberately and reflectively "chooses" to smoke. Nevertheless, he routinely finds himself smoking in that scenario. What was once an analytic decision has evolved into an automatic, experience-based one. More generally, automatic decision making is such that *If Conditions C1, C2, C3, . . . present themselves, then the decider* will *pursue Action A.* Furthermore, the process has the usual characteristics of automaticity: The decider has no control over the process, the process is virtually effortless, and the decider has minimal awareness of it.

Considerations

In a given situation, the primary modes are likely to be attempted in this order: experience-driven, rule-based, analytic. By its nature, experience-driven decision making, particularly the automatic, habitual variety, just pops out when the given routine has been established and when the triggering conditions are encountered. Otherwise, the decider has no choice but to seek an applicable decision rule or, if that fails, make the decision analytically. The latter is a last resort since it is so labor-intensive. But there may very well be no choice since, although decision rules are indeed common, they do not fit or exist for every situation (e.g., not every patient situation matches an available practice guideline).

It is important to recognize that in a given decision episode, more than one primary mode might be invoked. However, because they "run" so rapidly and effortlessly, if they are available, experience-driven modes are likely to exert inordinate influence as compared with more deliberative analytic and rule-based modes. This can be worrisome since the arbitrariness of the events giving rise to experience-driven modes (e.g., chance peer encounters that nurture smoking habits) provides no assurance that these modes yield effective decisions. Similar considerations apply to the problem of improving decision-making practices. Clearly, approaches that work for reshaping analytic decision-making practices would be useless for experience-driven ones.

Choice Point ❹: Work Details—Secondary

For the most part, secondary decision modes can be viewed as tools for assisting analytic decision making. That is, in the process of reaching a decision analytically, the decider draws on the efforts of other people (or devices) as special resources.

Modeling

The *modeling* mode is deceptively simple. The decider identifies another decider who has faced the same dilemma and just mimics that person's decision, allowing that model to do all the work of thinking through what is reasonable to do. Although seldom discussed, modeling occurs often, as when a patient chooses as his own physician the same one he learns was selected by the boss he admires at work. More generally, modeling is the mode implicit in herding behavior, which is observed among both lower animals in stampedes and humans in financial markets. Modeling is unquestionably easy, but it is beset by significant risks, too. Simply observing the model's decision without also learning whether it was effective for the model is one risk. Another is assuming that the model's interests and values are identical to the decider's own, an assumption that is often highly suspect, as when choosing doctors.

Consultation

In the *consultation* mode, the decider acquires advice about the decision problem from either a real person or a device, such as a computer program—advice that the decider is free to accept or reject. The advice might be a "bottom line" recommendation as to the action the decider should pursue. Such is the case when a patient asks for a second opinion: "Should I have the proposed surgery or shouldn't I?" (Note that the consultant might have arrived at a recommendation via any of the primary decision modes distinguished previously, e.g., analytic, rule-based, or experience-driven.) Alternatively, the advice could pertain to some specific element of the decision problem, as when a patient asks, "What are the available treatments for my condition, and what can go wrong with each of them?"

In principle, consultation seems almost perfect as a complement to analytic decision making. After all, it allows for the application of specialized expertise to every critical aspect of the decision problem. But therein lies perhaps the greatest hazard: assessing such expertise. Ideally, deciders' conclusions about the expertise of their potential consultants should be based on the track records of the candidates; that is, they should be evidence based. Studies have shown, however, that conclusions are strongly affected by factors that easily can have nothing to do with track records (e.g., an authoritative manner). They have also demonstrated that, left to their own devices, people often fail to seek such records and are confused about how to best use them when they are available.

J. Frank Yates

See also Automatic Thinking; Intuition Versus Analysis; Judgment Modes; Shared Decision Making

Further Readings

Bechara, A., Damasio, H., Tranel, D., & Damasio, A. R. (1997). Deciding advantageously before knowing the advantageous strategy. *Science, 275,* 1293–1295.

Christensen, C., Larson, J. R., Jr., Abbott, A., Ardolino, A., Franz, T., & Pfeiffer, C. (2000). Decision making of clinical teams: Communication patterns and diagnostic error. *Medical Decision Making, 20,* 45–50.

Evans, J. St. B. T. (2008). Dual-processing accounts of reasoning, judgment, and social cognition. *Annual Review of Psychology, 59,* 255–278.

Helfand, M. (2007). Shared decision making, decision aids, and risk communication. *Medical Decision Making, 27*(5), 516–517.

Klein, G. A. (1998). *Sources of power: How people make decisions.* Cambridge: MIT Press.

Yates, J. F. (1990). *Judgment and decision making.* Englewood Cliffs, NJ: Prentice Hall.

Yates, J. F. (2003). *Decision management.* San Francisco: Jossey-Bass.

Yates, J. F., Price, P. C., Lee, J.-W., & Ramirez, J. (1996). Good probabilistic forecasters: The "consumer's" perspective. *International Journal of Forecasting, 12,* 41–56.

DECISION PSYCHOLOGY

Decision psychology is a scientific discipline with two main dimensions: choice and values underlying choice. Decision psychology can be undertaken to describe how humans make decisions; how humans should make decisions; what humans can do if they would like to change the way they make decisions; how much an individual understands about a decision; how much risk an individual is willing to take in an uncertain decision; how to influence the decision making of others; how to control or prevent unwanted influences by others on decision making; if and when to implement surrogacy decision making (the individual or someone on behalf of the individual deciding to give over decision making to another); whose beliefs and preferences should be incorporated in a decision; and how that process of incorporation of beliefs and preferences into a decision should be carried out.

The psychology of medical decision making can focus on individuals making decisions on their own; doctors and patients making decisions together; competent patients giving over decision-making authority to others; patients who today are fighting to preserve their decision-making abilities against progressive neurodegenerative diseases or other mental-impairing conditions that if continue unabated will eventually lead to those patients being characterized as being without decisional capacity; and finally, patients who are now without decisional capacity and for whom decisions need to be made.

Types of Decision Making

Descriptive Versus Normative

In all types of research on the psychology of decision making, including medical decision making, the question arises whether the researcher is interested in describing how decisions are actually made by individuals confronted with a decision-making task (descriptive decision making) or whether the researcher is interested in describing how decisions that are actually made by individuals compare with a model or framework of how decisions should be made (normative decision making).

Population Versus the Individual

The basic distinction with medical decision making is whether the decision making under consideration is decision making regarding the population as a whole (or at least sizeable groups within that population) versus the individual patient. The difference between these types of decision making can be seen in the arena of immunization against disease, where the population may benefit by the immunization program but the individual may bear the brunt of death or severe morbidity from the adverse outcomes associated with the vaccine.

Studies of Decision-Making Psychology

Subjects

The subjects of studies of decision-making psychology may include hypotheses about choices, judgments, or other types of reasoning and include as study participants citizens, patients, healthcare providers (physicians and nurses), and other members of the healthcare team (social workers, chaplains, among others) and associated administrative teams (for example, information technologists), as well as students or trainees in all of these areas and more.

Psychological Models

When normative models are tested in the psychology of decision making, these models may include expected utility theory or game theory as well as psychological models, such as prospect theory.

These normative models do not exhaust the models of decision-making psychology, which also include preference theories, emotive theories, and ethical and moral theories.

Decision Making Under Risk

The classic decision-making situation is one that is common in all models of decision-making psychology: having to choose between alternatives, each of which is characterized by an estimated risk. The classic examples of medical decision-making psychology are characterized by psychologists Amos Tversky and Daniel Kahneman as embodying a form of decision making under risk.

The fact that patients do not necessarily think solely in terms of risk in decision making has also been noted, primarily in ethical perspectives on decision making. However, the focus on risk has perhaps been singled out because of the overattention that is often paid to discussions of benefits. This point was noted by Barbara J. McNeil and colleagues in one of the earliest patient-preference papers in the medical literature, published in the *New England Journal of Medicine*. In this scientific paper, McNeil and colleagues identify the fact that the very data that physicians use in published research papers in the area of oncology is the "5-year survival curve," which sets forth the best treatment as the treatment that offers the best 5-year survival. But in their study, McNeil and colleagues note that some study participants preferred not to take the short-term risks of a treatment that are often necessary to achieve this 5-year survival and would rather go with a treatment that had a better chance of short-term survival and forgo the better chances of long-term survival offered by the rival treatment.

Risky Versus Riskless Choices

The basic decision study in medical decision making is typically between a gamble (trade-off) and a sure thing. Do patients and physicians go for the gamble or do they prefer the sure thing? Risky choice, as noted by Kahneman and Tversky, is undertaken in a circumstance where there is no future knowledge about consequences. In addition, in medical decision making, the risky choice is made on the basis of data where it may not be clear how the individual fits into the published, peer-reviewed medical literature related to the decision. Indeed, here, it is assumed that peer-reviewed medical literature associated with the medical condition or disease process that the patient has can shed light on the diagnostic or therapeutic decisions. In the real world of decision making, many times there is no published, peer-reviewed medical literature that fits the patient's case, and medical decision making thus depends highly on physician clinical experience and opinion.

Elicitation Versus Construction of Preferences

One of the key areas of research in the psychology of decision making is in the very basic notion that underlies its research: Are preferences about risky versus riskless choices actually involving preferences that are being elicited from study participants who already have formulated their preference (regarding the point about which a preference is being elicited) in the past and—as much research has assumed—are now just retrieving their previously constructed preference in response to a question being asked by the researcher? Or are the study participants actually formulating (constructing) the preferences they are offering to the researchers at the time they are being asked the question?

Future Research Areas

Jerome P. Kassirer, former editor of the *New England Journal of Medicine*, offers the following questions that need to be asked as future research areas in the psychology of decision making: First, have most of the subjects in the published medical literature to date experienced the outcomes they were asked to assess? Second, have most of the subjects undergone a preference elicitation procedure before in their life when they agree to the researcher's request to participate in the researcher's study? Third, what is to be done about the fact that preferences may well change over time? Fourth, what is to be done if different preference procedures lead to different results in the same subject? Fifth, what is to be done when the same subjects reports that he or she places the same value on a state of morbidity associated with a medical condition or disease process as on being in a state of perfect health?

To Kassirer's questions can be added two others: How do aspects such as a patient's emotions, which are present or actually elicited during the preference elicitation procedure, to be accounted for in the psychology of decision making? How are patients with strong belief and value systems to be approached by such procedures and methodologies of assessing preferences when they object to the taking of gambles?

Continued research in the psychology of decision making is needed to better understand how humans make decisions now and in what sense these same humans may want to change the way they make decisions and opt for another framework to achieve in some sense a better decision.

Defective Decision Making

Psychophysiologic correlates of defective decision making are most often discussed in relation to the dementias, yet contemporary researchers study those seemingly healthy older adults who seem to be free of obvious neurologic or psychiatric disease, but have deficits in reasoning and decision making. We will first consider decision making in the dementias and then decision making in apparently normal aging.

Decision Making and Dementia

The impact of dementias on cognitive processes and the psychology of decision making often includes a fluctuating cognition with variations in attention, alertness, and visual-perceptual problems with complex (well-formed and often detailed) visual hallucinations. Contemporary research in aging, neuropsychology, imaging, and neurophysiology are attempting to distinguish early versus later stages of dementia of various types (e.g., Alzheimer's disease, Lewy body dementias, dementia of Parkinson's disease) to aid in research on prevention of dementia. Yet contemporary research is still trying to distinguish dementias from what otherwise seem to be apparent changes of normal aging in various groups of people.

Decision Making and Apparently Normal Aging

Natalie L. Denburg and colleagues are interested in defining the psychophysiologic correlates of defective decision making in normal aging. These researchers investigated the scientific hypothesis that some seemingly normal older persons have deficits in reasoning and decision making due to dysfunction in a neural system. The authors argued that this hypothesis (a) is relevant to the comprehensive study of aging and (b) addresses the question of why so many older adults fall prey to fraud.

The authors (in a series of three studies) investigated a cross-sectional sample of community-dwelling participants and argue that they demonstrated that a subset of older adults (approximately 35%–40%) do not perform well and appear to be working with a disadvantage on a laboratory measure of decision making that closely mimics everyday life by the manner in which it attempts to factor in reward, punishment, risk, and ambiguity.

The authors found that the same poor decision makers may also display defective autonomic responses such as those previously established in patients with acquired prefrontal lesions.

Finally, the authors present data demonstrating that poor decision makers are more likely to become the victims of deceptive strategies such as deceptive advertising. Examples of such deceit may include fraud but may also include misrepresentations encountered in other daily activities, including television broadcast advertising designed to motivate the sale of prescription medicines within the broadcast. Here, we see that the intricacies of decision making—initially described by Daniel Bernoulli in 1738 in his work on the exposition of a new theory on the measurement of risk and built by Kahneman and Tversky in the 1970s—are in turn affected by the processes of normal aging on the human brain; that is, these normal aging processes affect the very activities described above as the psychology of decision and decision making. Clearly, the psychology of decision making has to be better understood in terms of the contemporary research on normal and abnormal processes of aging and the way these affect risk and benefit consideration by humans.

Decisional Capacity

Far away from the universities where university students served as study participants in the work of Tversky and Kahneman, the concept of decisional capacity began to be developed. The notion

of decisional capacity—that is, the capacity to make a decision—is often raised in two arenas: clinical care and research on human subjects.

1. In the *clinical setting*, the question is raised whether that individual has the capacity to consent to or reject the medical intervention being offered.

2. In the *research setting*, the question is raised whether that individual has the capacity to consent to or reject participation as a study volunteer in a research study to which he or she is being asked by a principal investigator.

The issue of decisional capacity is appropriately raised in areas of cognitive decline or cognitive problems, such as dementia; confusion or delirium; and mental-health cognitive biases and disease processes. The issue of decisional capacity can also be raised in the case of adults with symptomatic or asymptomatic medical conditions and disease states in intensive care units or simply in hospital wards.

Decision making in both clinical care and research on humans is complex, whether the individual is declared to have decisional capacity or not. Let us consider each domain separately.

Clinical Care

In the clinical setting, if the patient is in the hospital and declared to have decisional capacity, the question is: How long will that capacity be manifest in that individual?

In the clinical setting, if the patient is in the hospital—without an advance directive and without that individual declaring at some prior time a family member or significant other to serve as his or her surrogate decision maker—and is declared not to have decisional capacity, the question becomes: What form of substituted judgment will be used on the patient's behalf?

Research on Humans

In the research setting, if the individual has come to a hospital emergency room for care, or is admitted to the hospital for care, or is transferred from the medical ward to the intensive care unit for care, how is decisional capacity to be assessed in each of these areas? The areas of an "advance research directive" to be prescribed by individuals before they lose decisional capacity are also open areas for research on human study volunteers.

The domains of substituted judgment in clinical care or in research on humans, as yet, have only been minimally explored by medical decision makers, with plenty of opportunities for research as our population ages and these issues multiply.

Future Research

All research underlying the psychology of decision making, from Tversky and Kahneman to Denburg and colleagues, depends heavily on questionnaire studies. The accuracy of future research depends heavily on the development of the best questionnaires to diagnose and follow individuals with cognitive and decision-making decline to make certain accurate diagnoses are made at each point in development and aging. The evaluation of patient response to therapy will also depend on treatment versus treatment comparison, which in turn will depend on optimal questionnaire studies to demonstrate the efficacy between therapies used to prevent, manage, and ideally treat, slow, and cure these conditions.

Dennis J. Mazur

See also Human Cognitive Systems; Risk Attitude; Unreliability of Memory

Further Readings

Bechara, A., Damasio, H., & Damasio, A. R. (2000). Emotion, decision making and the orbitofrontal cortex. *Cerebral Cortex, 10,* 295–307.

Bechara, A., Damasio, H., & Damasio, A. R. (2003). Role of the amygdala in decision-making. *Annals of the New York Academy of Sciences, 985,* 356–369.

Bechara, A., Damasio, H., Tranel, D., & Damasio, A. R. (2005). The Iowa Gambling Task and the somatic marker hypothesis: Some questions and answers. *Trends in Cognitive Sciences 9,* 159–162, Discussion 162–164.

Collerton, D., Burn, D., McKeith, I., & O'Brien, J. (2003). Systematic review and meta-analysis show that dementia with Lewy bodies is a visual-perceptual and attentional-executive dementia. *Dementia and Geriatric Cognitive Disorders, 16,* 229–237.

Denburg, N. L., Cole, C. A., Hernandez, M., Yamada, T. H., Tranel, D., Bechara, A., et al. (2007). The orbitofrontal cortex, real-world decision making, and normal aging. *Annals of the New York Academy of Sciences, 1121,* 480–498.

Ernst, M., Bolla, K., Mouratidis, M., Contoreggi, C., Matochik, J. A., Kurian, V., et al. (2002). Decision-making in a risk-taking task: A PET study. *Neuropsychopharmacology, 26,* 682–691.

Eslinger, P. J., & Damasio, A. R. (1985). Severe disturbance of higher cognition after bilateral frontal lobe ablation: Patient EVR. *Neurology, 35,* 1731–1741.

Grober, E., Hall, C. B., Lipton, R. B., Zonderman, A. B., Resnick, S. M., & Kawas, C. (2008). Memory impairment, executive dysfunction, and intellectual decline in preclinical Alzheimer's disease. *Journal of the International Neuropsychological Society, 14,* 266–278.

Mazur, D. J. (2007). *Evaluating the science and ethics of research on humans: A guide for IRB members.* Baltimore: Johns Hopkins University Press.

Terry, A. V., Jr., Buccafusco, J. J., & Wilson, C. (2008). Cognitive dysfunction in neuropsychiatric disorders: Selected serotonin receptor subtypes as therapeutic targets. *Behavioural Brain Research, 195*(1), 30–38.

DECISION QUALITY

In its landmark report, *Crossing the Quality Chasm,* the Institute of Medicine set out six aims for high-quality medical care: that care should be effective, efficient, equitable, safe, timely, and patient-centered. A significant part of the quality of medical care is determined by the large and small decisions that doctors and patients make every day about seeking care, having tests, starting treatments, and stopping treatments. It is important to know to what extent decisions contribute to or detract from quality of care. To a great extent, the quality of a decision depends on the decision situation, on the perspective of the person who is judging the quality, and on what is being judged (e.g., whether it is the decision or the decision maker that is the unit of analysis). Careful attention to these issues is important to create valid and reliable assessments of decision quality.

Decision Situation

The decision situation plays a big role in determining the quality of a medical decision. There are situations in medicine where a treatment or approach has considerable evidence of a significant benefit with considerable evidence of minimal harm. Most clinical guideline committees, such as the U.S. Preventive Services Task Force (USPSTF), set out explicit criteria for grading the clinical evidence for the benefits and harms of different tests and treatments. When the benefits are determined to outweigh the harms, there is a "right" answer that can be termed *effective care*. For example, the use of beta blockers following a heart attack fit the criteria for effective care. Most patients have a strong desire to reduce the risk of repeat heart attacks and death, and most feel the modest side effects of the medicines are worth the benefit. As a result, high-quality decisions in these situations are about efficiently delivering proven, effective care to all those who may benefit. Decision quality can be inferred by the percentage of eligible patients who receive the proved treatment, or the percentage of care that is "consistent" with the guidelines.

Not all situations in medicine are examples of effective care. In fact, a surprising number of decisions do not have sufficient evidence of benefit for one option over another, or have evidence of equivalence of two or more options, or have evidence of substantial harm that accompanies the benefit. In these situations, often called *preference-sensitive decisions,* there is not a clearly superior approach, and the preferences of individual patients are critical to selecting the "best" choice. Simply examining treatment rates will not provide enough information to determine the quality of decisions—a more sophisticated approach is needed.

Many different stakeholders have recognized this complexity and have called for attention to this challenge. The Institute of Medicine has defined patient-centered care as "healthcare that establishes a partnership among practitioners, patients and their families (when appropriate) to ensure that decisions reflect patients' wants, needs and preferences and that patients have the education and support they need to make decisions and participate in their own care" (p. 7). Researchers in the field of medical decision making have also focused on two themes that are in this definition— that patients are informed and that choices for tests and treatments reflect patients' goals and preferences. In an international consensus process, researchers, providers, policy makers, and patients

overwhelmingly supported a definition of decision quality as the extent to which a decision reflects the considered preferences of a well-informed patient, and is implemented.

To assess decision quality in preference-sensitive decision situations requires assessing the extent to which patients are informed, for example, through a set of multiple-choice knowledge items. It also requires assessing patients' *considered* preferences for the potential health outcomes, their risk attitudes, and their willingness to make trade-offs over time. And finally, it requires assessing the treatment implemented. The patient's preferences would then be used to calculate value concordance, or the amount of association between their preferences and the treatments received. One approach is to aggregate over a group of patients, controlling for other factors that may influence treatments, to determine the extent to which the variation in treatments is explained by variation in patients' preferences. This could be used to compare different hospitals or providers. For example, those who are consistently able to inform their patients about the key facts of the situation, and those who are able to document that patients' preferences for key health outcomes are significantly associated with their treatment rates would be able to demonstrate higher decision quality than those who cannot inform their patients and who are not able to show any consistent association between patients' preferences and treatments.

Conceptual Framework

This definition reflects the commitments of normative decision theory, which holds that a decision should be judged by the process by which an alternative was selected rather than by the outcomes that resulted from the decision. Most normative theories make the assumption that individuals are self-interested and goal-directed in their behavior. Actual behavior shows that people make decisions that are not consistent with self-interest, as people often pay attention to irrelevant factors and make suboptimal decisions. Many normative theorists ascribe these gaps to inattention, ignorance, or lack of adequate elicitation of preferences. Others use these as a starting point for research into the heuristics that people use and how they attempt to simplify complex decision situations so as to minimize cognitive load, conflict, and other issues. These prescriptive approaches still assume a fairly analytic mode of processing, although recognizing boundaries and limits.

An alternate view of decision making emphasizes a very different cognitive mode of information processing. Intuitive modes are fast, unconscious, and rely on heuristics and rules of thumb. The processing is tacit and is colloquially referred to as "going with your gut" or "sleeping on it." Studies in the laboratory and in real life have found that consumers view some choices more favorably when made in the absence of attentive deliberation. In these studies, the "quality" of the decision was evaluated by the consumers' satisfaction or happiness with their choice. Whether consumers' views (e.g., happiness with their selection) are an appropriate proxy for the quality of medical decisions has been debated.

The focus on process does not mean that outcomes are not important in the evaluation of decisions. In fact, over multiple decisions, it is assumed that this type of logical process will achieve better outcomes. In financial or economic decisions where money is used to measure the "value" or outcome, it is fairly easy to evaluate or compare groups of decisions (e.g., return on a stock portfolio using a dartboard to pick stocks as compared with using a more logical process that incorporates information and preferences). For healthcare, however, there is not a fungible outcome measure that is universally valued. Time is not fungible; it cannot be bought or sold, and neither can health. Many might assume that survival could be a clear outcome measure to compare treatments or decision protocols; however, many studies have documented variable tolerance to trading length of life and quality of life. Evaluating medical decisions by whether they produce better outcomes is difficult—in large part because there is no fungible measure.

That does not mean that the appropriate approach is to ignore outcomes. Studies have shown that the laypeople often view the outcomes as more important than the process used to get there. An oft-cited example is that most patients and family members would not be likely to agree that a decision to undergo surgery was good when the patient died during the procedure. Thus, quality of the decision depends greatly on the perspective through which it is being judged and may be evaluated differently on an individual basis than when combined as a group of events. In this same case, the provider, who has a broader context from which to evaluate decisions, may recognize that for the majority of times it has been used, the procedure has helped and that this was a good decision that had a bad outcome.

Policy Makers

Policy makers are important stakeholders in medical decision making, although their influence is often opaque to patients and sometimes to providers as well. Through decisions about benefits, coverage, access, accreditation, accounting, and financing of care, policy makers and administrators enable and constrain the options that providers may offer and that patients may accept, the amount of time they have to discuss choices, and the cost to the patient of various alternatives. For policy makers, medical decisions are statistical groupings that have economic and health implications. The tension between making decisions that benefit an individual and decisions that benefit a group are real and challenging. The quality of decisions from their perspective may not be evaluated on the extent to which individuals get what they want, but on whether, on average, the group gets better outcomes at the same or lower costs. Policies may negatively affect a minority of people for the benefit of the majority. Also, instead of individualization, they may favor stability and eliminating variation.

Karen R. Sepucha

See also Informed Decision Making; Shared Decision Making; Utility Assessment Techniques

Further Readings

Bell, D., Raiffa, H., & Tversky, A. (1988). Descriptive, normative and prescriptive interactions in decision making. In D. Bell, H. Raiffa, & A. Tversky (Eds.), *Decision making: descriptive, normative, and prescriptive interactions* (pp. 9–30). Cambridge, UK: Cambridge University Press.

Elwyn, G., O'Connor, A., Stacey, D., Volk, R., Edwards, A., Coulter, A., et al. (2006). Developing a quality criteria framework for patient decision aids: Online international Delphi consensus process. *British Medical Journal, 333,* 417.

Institute of Medicine. (2001). *Envisioning the National Health Care Quality Report* (M. P. Hurtado, E. K. Swift, & J. M. Corrigan, Eds.). Washington, DC: National Academy Press.

Klein, G. (1998). *Sources of power: How people make decisions.* Cambridge: MIT Press.

Mulley, A. G. (1989). Assessing patients' utilities: Can the ends justify the means? *Medical Care, 27,* S269–S281.

Redelmeier, D. A., Rozin, P., & Kahneman, D. (1993). Understanding patients' decisions. Cognitive and emotional perspectives. *Journal of the American Medical Association, 270,* 72–76.

Sepucha, K. R., Fowler, F. J., Jr., & Mulley, A. G., Jr. (2004). Policy support for patient-centered care: The need for measurable improvements in decision quality. *Health Affairs* (Web Exclusive): DOI: 10.1377/hlthaff.var.54.

DECISION RULES

A decision rule is a decision-making tool combining fixed history and physical examination items and/or a simple diagnostic test used for explicit application to a clinical decision. Although many decisions about management of patients are accurately made on the basis of clinical judgment, some decision making can be improved through application of a standardized decision rule that has been developed and tested through a rigorous evidence-based process. Implementation of a rule can bring greater certainty to the clinician about the course of action to follow given a particular patient presentation, or it may lead to an improved ability to predict the probability of disease.

A decision rule is developed in a systematic process, using prospective studies often involving large numbers of patients, to meet an outcome determined to be clinically important and necessary for improved healthcare. The three stages of rule development are those of derivation, validation, and implementation. Derivation involves identifying decision items of the rule and ensuring that items are clearly defined and have demonstrated reliability. Validation requires analysis of whether the rule is accurate and reliable and meets the intended outcome; is acceptable to clinicians; can be used by different health professionals; and is suitable for application to diverse patient populations. The

final stage of rule development involves analysis of the impact of implementation of a rule on patient management and healthcare.

Course of Action

A decision regarding referral or not for further testing is frequently required in clinical assessment. Referral may be to low-cost tests, as in the case of plain radiographs for identification of fracture, or to more expensive tests such as dual-energy X-ray absorptiometry to assess bone mineral density for osteoporosis screening. Clinical decision rules have demonstrated advantages over clinical judgment in these decisions. Further useful applications of clinical decision rules include guiding referral for cranial computed tomography for minor head injury and venous ultrasonography for lower-limb deep vein thrombosis.

Ankle and knee decision rules are examples of rules designed to explicitly suggest when to refer for radiography. The ankle and knee rules were developed to inform referral to radiography of patients with acute injury and potential fracture in primary care and emergency department settings. Impetus for development of ankle and knee decision rules arose from recognition that plain radiographs were commonly ordered for patients following ankle and knee blunt trauma from blows and falls, in the absence of fracture. High healthcare costs of unnecessary radiographs and patient time spent having the procedure were identified. Although the plain radiograph is relatively low cost, ankle and knee trauma are common, resulting in high volumes of ankle and knee radiographs and therefore substantial healthcare costs. Implementation of ankle and knee rules was intended to impact on these costs and lead to healthcare savings.

Concern of the clinician or, in some cases, the patient that a fracture may be missed can influence clinical decisions. Justification for these concerns is that if radiography is not ordered for a patient with a fracture, there could be serious consequences. Delayed or overlooked diagnosis of fracture can affect clinical outcome and may result in increased healthcare costs and lost productivity. A clinician who misses an ankle or knee fracture may be subject to claims of malpractice. For these reasons, acceptance of a rule by clinicians requires a guarantee that a rule will identify clinically important fractures.

Ottawa Knee Rule

Although other ankle and knee decision rules exist, the Ottawa ankle and knee rules are credible, with well-documented evidence of rule development in different countries with some studies conducted independent of the developers of the rule. The example used to illustrate rule development is the Ottawa knee rule.

Five history and physical examination items form the basis for decision making in the Ottawa knee rule. Rule items are age 55 years or older, tenderness at head of fibula, isolated tenderness of patella (no bone tenderness of knee other than patella), inability to flex to 90°, and inability to bear weight both immediately and in the emergency department for four steps (unable to transfer weight twice onto each limb regardless of limping). Radiographic examination is suggested for patients with acute knee injuries with any one or more than one of the decision items. Rule items were derived in initial prospective investigation from 23 standardized variables on the basis of interassessor reliability, high correlation with fracture, and mathematical analysis.

Numerous studies have investigated the validity of the Ottawa knee rule in adult patients older than 18 years. Different analyses of sensitivity and specificity of the rule have shown similar results. Sensitivity is the proportion of patients with fracture for whom the results of the rule indicate radiography. Specificity is the proportion of patients without fracture for whom the results of the rule do not indicate radiography. The Ottawa knee rule has high sensitivity with extremely low to zero false negative rates, an important factor in acceptability of the rule to clinicians, whose main concern is not to miss a fracture. Low specificity tends to accompany high sensitivity, and this is true of the Ottawa knee rule. This could mean that healthcare costs would not be reduced as much as anticipated by rule implementation, as some patients would be inaccurately selected for radiographs. Interassessor reliability of physician interpretation of the rule is excellent. Examination of the validity and reliability of the rule in very small patient samples has shown less positive support for use

of the rule by triage nurses in emergency departments.

Implementation of the Ottawa knee rule as compared with clinical judgment alone brings significant societal cost savings due to decreased use of knee radiography and, for those patients discharged promptly as a consequence of no radiography, less time spent in the clinic. Economic analysis has also considered estimates of the value of missed fracture in terms of damages awarded for delayed diagnosis of knee fracture in the event of compensation. Although very small change in sensitivity from 1.0 would result in missed fractures, studies consistently report sensitivity of 1.0, and therefore economic analysis finds negligible impact of missed fracture with implementation of the rule. The rule does have exclusion criteria, and any benefits identified of rule implementation may not apply to patients younger than 18 years and all cases where circumstances may make it difficult to obtain reliable information from the patient, such as serious communication problems for whatever reason. The success of implementation of Ottawa knee rules and also Ottawa ankle rules has led to further proposals of decision rules for other regions, with the same intent of assisting decision making regarding referral to further testing in cases of blunt trauma.

Prediction of Probability of Disease

Prediction of potentially life-threatening disease can be problematic as observed in cases of serious illness, including acute myocardial infarction, cancer, and pulmonary embolism. Decision rules are one of the approaches used to improve management of these patients.

Development of decision rules for pulmonary embolism, for example, occurred in response to worrying evidence that this potentially fatal condition frequently goes undiagnosed. Without a decision rule, difficulties in accurate separation of those with and without pulmonary embolism have been demonstrated even when clinical assessment is accompanied by a range of sophisticated and expensive tests. As well as the problem of a potentially fatal missed diagnosis, patients incorrectly diagnosed with pulmonary embolism will receive anticoagulant therapy, which they do not need, with possibility of serious side effects.

Wells Rule

The decision rule developed by Wells and colleagues for pretest probability estimate of pulmonary embolism has been thoroughly investigated and is widely recognized. The seven decision items of the Wells rule and the scoring system were derived from 40 initial items through mathematical analysis. Rule items are clinical signs and symptoms of deep vein thrombosis (leg swelling and pain with palpation of the deep veins); an alternative diagnosis is less likely than pulmonary embolism; heart rate >100 beats per minute; immobilization (bed rest, except to access the bathroom, for at least 3 consecutive days) or surgery in the previous 4 weeks; previous objectively diagnosed deep vein thrombosis or pulmonary embolism; hemoptysis; and malignancy (treatment that is ongoing, within the past 6 months, or palliative). The rule assigns points of 3.00 to the first two items, 1.5 to the next three items and 1.0 to the last two items. Patients are categorized according to their score as low probability if <2; moderate probability if 2 to 6; and high probability if >6. The Wells rule has demonstrated moderate or better interassessor reliability.

In early stages of rule development, it was decided that combining the Wells rule with the D-dimer blood test could bring benefit in identifying those without pulmonary embolism and therefore those with no need for imaging tests. A diagnostic algorithm was created, including Wells rule and D-dimer test, which has validated accuracy for identifying those patients in whom pulmonary embolism can be safely ruled out. A decision regarding probability of pulmonary embolism is made first on the basis of the Wells rule. Low, moderate and high probability groups all then undergo D-dimer test to assess for D-dimer fragments present in pulmonary embolism but also present in many other conditions. On application of the rule and D-dimer test, patients with low probability who also have a negative D-dimer test are separated out as without pulmonary embolism, and anticoagulant therapy is withheld from these patients. On prospective investigation, no low-probability patients in whom pulmonary embolism was excluded on the basis of the diagnostic algorithm subsequently died of pulmonary embolism. Using the algorithm, patients with moderate and high probability on the basis of the Wells rule are D-dimer tested and then are investigated with pulmonary angiography or ventilation perfusion scanning, both of which have demonstrated limitations.

Subsequent refinement has resulted in a diagnostic algorithm with two categories—the simple Wells rule (as compared with the original Wells rule, with three categories). The simple Wells rule categorizes patients as pulmonary embolism–unlikely in a case of a score <4 and pulmonary embolism–likely if the score is >4. Computed tomography is the preferred imaging technique in the algorithm for exclusion or confirmation of pulmonary embolism in patients with a score >4. Those with a score <4 and unlikely to have pulmonary embolism have a D-dimer test as in the original algorithm and, if this is negative, are excluded from diagnosis of pulmonary embolism; if the D-dimer is positive then patients have computed tomography. Prospective investigation has validated the safety of the algorithm. There is low risk for incorrectly diagnosing a patient who subsequently goes on to have pulmonary embolism and enhanced potential for correctly excluding diagnosis of pulmonary embolism with application of this algorithm. Wells scores, original and simple, have acceptable reliability.

Mathematical Techniques in Rule Development

Decision items of a rule are derived from a number of variables selected in a transparent process of review of the literature and consultation with relevant experts. A methodologically sound approach is to evaluate all items with possible relevance to the rule prospectively to assess association with rule outcomes. Investigation of potential rule variables involves univariate and multivariate techniques and estimates of reliability.

An accepted exemplar for rule development is the Ottawa ankle rule. The two rule outcomes are no fracture or insignificant fracture (defined as avulsions 3 mm or less across) or clinically significant fracture. In the preliminary screen of 32 clinical variables, chosen on the basis of evidence and clinical experience of investigators, univariate association and reliability of each variable were assessed. Variables with moderate or better reliability (kappa value > .6) and found to be strongly associated with a significant fracture in univariate logistic regression analysis were then analyzed with multivariate techniques of multiple logistic regression analysis and recursive partitioning analysis.

Univariate logistic analyses, chi-square test for categorical data, and unpaired t test for continuous data compared one variable at a time with the outcome. Although these analyses have the advantage of simplicity, a limitation lies in the inability to demonstrate relationships between the variables. Swelling and tenderness over the medial malleolus were both initially associated with fracture in univariate analyses. However, swelling was excluded on the basis of subsequent multiple regression analyses because of finding of high correlation of swelling with tenderness and superior interassessor reliability of tenderness. Only tenderness was retained in the rule.

Initial multivariate analyses of stepwise logistic regression based on logarithmic equations resulted in a model that missed more than half the ankle fractures. Logistic regression analysis seeks overall accuracy rather than an emphasis on sensitivity and thus provided an unacceptable model. It had been determined that for clinician acceptance the ankle rule had to have 100% sensitivity for detecting clinically significant fracture. Recursive partitioning methods create branches of smaller and smaller subpopulations of patients, and this analysis yielded the accepted ankle rule, with 100% sensitivity though low specificity and the smallest number of variables. Reliability of the combination of rule items was good, kappa = .72.

Accuracy statistics differ depending on the purpose of the decision rule and are not limited to reports of sensitivity and specificity. Confidence intervals (CI) indicate the range of variability associated with rule application and should be reported with results of diagnostic accuracy. The Ottawa knee rule, for example, reported sensitivity of 1.0 (95% CI, .94–1.0) and specificity of .48 (95% CI, .45–.51). The Wells rule for pulmonary embolism, as a further example, reported in terms of probability of the disease for the different categories as follows: low pretest probability (3.4%; 95% CI, 2.2%–5%); moderate pretest probability (28%; 95% CI, 23.4%–32.2%); and high pretest probability (78%; 95% CI, 69.2%–86.0%). Likelihood ratios indicate how much an individual decision item or a rule will raise or lower the pretest probability that a patient has the outcome of interest and can be calculated from sensitivity and specificity

data. A nomogram proposed by Fagan presents pretest probability, likelihood ratio, and posttest probability scales in diagrammatic form, allowing simple estimation of posttest probability with the use of a ruler if the other values are known.

Use of Decision Rules

A number of potential barriers to clinical uptake of a rule exist related to clinician knowledge, attitude, and behavior. Acquisition and retention of rule knowledge can be problematic. The volume of new evidence can be overwhelming, and clinicians may have difficulty in selecting out valuable information critical to improving their clinical practice. Application of a decision rule requires precise recall of the rule plus calculations where specified, and this may be difficult without pocket prompt cards or computer assistance aids. Clinicians may have doubts about the quality of a rule, the time it will take to implement it in practice, and uncertainty regarding what the rule may deliver for them and their patient. It may feel better to the clinician to continue to make decisions in the same way as they have always made them.

An important advantage of decision rules is certainty of an accurate decision irrespective of clinician experience. Despite this and other advantages of rule use, widespread clinical implementation does not automatically follow their development, even if the evidence is strongly supportive. Investigation of the clinical uptake of the Ottawa ankle rules has demonstrated this, with unsatisfactory reports that the rule has not been as widely used as anticipated even by informed clinicians. Inadequate use of the rule has now directed interest to barriers to uptake. Healthcare benefits of decision rules will only be fully realized when barriers to their clinical uptake are addressed.

Kate Haswell, John Gilmour, and Barbara Moore

See also Clinical Algorithms and Practice Guidelines; Diagnostic Tests; Logistic Regression; Nomograms

Further Readings

Guyatt, G., Walter, S., Shannon, H., Cook, D., Jaeschke, R., & Heddle, N. (1995). Basic statistics for clinicians: Correlation and regression. *Canadian Medical Association Journal, 152,* 497–504.

Lang, E. S., Wyer, P. C., & Haynes, R. B. (2007). Knowledge translation: Closing the evidence-to-practice gap. *Annals of Emergency Medicine, 49,* 355–363.

Laupacis, A., Sekar, N., & Stiell, I. G. (1997). Clinical prediction rules. A review and suggested modifications of methodological standards. *Journal of the American Medical Association, 277,* 488–494.

McGinn, T. G., Guyatt, G. H., Wyer, P. C., Naylor, C. D., Stiell, I. G., & Richardson, W. S. (2000). Users' guides to the medical literature XX11: How to use articles about clinical decision rules. *Journal of the American Medical Association, 284,* 79–84.

Nichol, G., Stiell, I. G., Wells, G. A., Juergensen, L. S., & Laupacis, A. (1999). An economic analysis of the Ottawa knee rule. *Annals of Emergency Medicine, 34,* 438–447.

Stiell, I. G., Greenberg, G. H., Wells, G. A., McDowell, I., Cwinn, A. A., Smith, N. A., et al. (1996). Prospective validation of a decision rule for use of radiography in acute knee injuries. *Journal of the American Medical Association, 275,* 611–615.

Stiell, I. G., Wells, G. A., Hoag, R. H., Sivilotti, M. L. A., Cacciotti, T. F., Verbeek, R., et al. (1997). Implementation of the Ottawa knee rule for use of radiography in acute knee injuries. *Journal of the American Medical Association, 278,* 2075–2079.

Wells, P. S., Anderson, D. R., Rodger, M., Stiell, I., Dreyer, J. F., Barnes, D., et al. (2001). Excluding pulmonary embolism at the bedside without diagnostic imaging: Management of patients with suspected pulmonary embolism presenting to the emergency department by using a simple clinical model and D-Dimer. *Annals of Internal Medicine, 135,* 98–107.

Wolf, S., McCubbin, T. R., Feldhaus, K. M., Faragher, J. P., & Adcock, D. M. (2004). Prospective validation of Wells criteria in the evaluation of patients with suspected pulmonary embolism. *Annals of Internal Medicine, 44,* 503–510.

Writing Group for the Christopher Study Investigators. (2006). Effectiveness of managing suspected pulmonary embolism using an algorithm combining clinical probability, D-dimer testing, and computed tomography. *Journal of the American Medical Association, 295,* 172–179.

DECISIONS FACED BY HOSPITAL ETHICS COMMITTEES

Hospital ethics committees (HECs) are relatively new bodies in the field of healthcare. They are multidisciplinary hospital groups that assemble for the purposes of ethics education, case consultation, and policy development. A minority of HECs pursue research activities, typically about effectiveness of case consultations and policy review. Ethics committees may advise healthcare professionals, patients, and family members about dealing with troubling cases, ethical conflicts or dilemmas, and ought to provide a nonthreatening forum that allows for the airing of different opinions, and discussion of the moral justifications for choosing one course of action over another.

Ethics committees may facilitate the decision-making process. Common reasons for consultations are questions about treatment limitations, and/or who ought to be included in the decision-making process. Recommendations from HECs are typically advisory in nature and not binding, but in some jurisdictions ethics committee recommendations may have legal weight.

History

Current HECs are derived and expanded from decision-making groups from the past. In the 1950s, some Catholic hospitals formed "medico-moral" committees, to ensure that Catholic teaching on such matters as contraception, sterilization, and abortion were followed.

In the 1960s, some pioneering hospitals developed committees to choose which patients ought to receive experimental dialysis, treatment with an artificial kidney for kidney failure. Shana Alexander's article in *Life* magazine in 1962 describes a typical meeting of the Seattle Artificial Kidney Committee, comprised of a lawyer, a minister, a banker, a housewife, an official of state government, a labor leader, and a surgeon. The article, titled "They Decide Who Lives, Who Dies," describes a re-creation of the discussion about which of several patients ought to receive life-saving dialysis. The members discussed such topics as the patients' education, employment status, financial status, marital status, how often they went to church, etc. Some have called this type of committee the "God Squad," having the power to choose who would live or die, and many believe the social criteria that were addressed by this committee were unfair and inadequate. Nevertheless, this article highlighted the need for the development of decision-making bodies that could reflect on the ethical problems posed by new technologies, and that such committees ought to have wide representation.

In 1975, pediatrician Karen Teel suggested that hospital ethics committees be established to help physicians and parents make decisions for impaired newborns, to "provide a regular forum for more input and dialogue in individual situations and to allow the responsibility for these judgments to be shared." Her recommendation was that hospital ethics committees composed of "physicians, social workers, attorneys, and theologians" might help in reviewing difficult cases. Her article was cited by the New Jersey Supreme Court in its decision in the *Quinlan* case.

Karen Ann Quinlan was 21 years old in 1975, when she stopped breathing after taking recreational drugs with alcohol. She was placed on an artificial breathing machine, but had sustained severe brain damage, and remained in a coma. Eventually, her parents asked to have her taken off the ventilator. Prior to that time, the American Medical Association held that withdrawing a ventilator to allow death to occur was unethical. The Court's *Quinlan* decision in 1976 authorized the removal of the respirator, and recognized that HECs, as described by Teel, might be useful in the review of difficult cases, and might possibly keep such cases out of the judicial system. Still, HECs did not become common in the 1970s, although that is the era that Institutional Review Boards (IRBs) were begun, to more closely regulate human experimentation in medicine.

After a series of court cases, "Baby Doe" regulations were devised in the 1980s, in response to parents who chose to refuse medical therapy for infants born with abnormalities. In turn, these cases stimulated some centers to form Infant Care Review Committees, to review which treatments made sense for impaired newborns, and to ensure that treatments were not withheld without careful review.

Despite the sporadic and ad hoc formation of all these ethics committee forebears, by 1983, only 1% of U.S. hospitals had developed HECs. That same year, the President's Commission published the guide *Deciding to Forego Life-Sustaining Treatment* and, as an appendix to this publication, described a recommendation for roles and composition of HECs.

After the Baby Doe cases, and the President's Commission report, HECs became much more common. Finally, in 1992, the Joint Commission on Accreditation of Health Care Organizations (JCAHO) added a requirement that hospitals have procedures for dealing with ethical issues. For a hospital to remain accredited it is required to have an ethics committee or some process that could provide for the functions of an ethics committee; HECs are now found in almost all hospitals.

Hospital Ethics Committee Functions

Ethics committees typically address three main responsibilities: education, policy development, and case consultation. A small minority of ethics committees, usually at larger academic centers, may also be involved in research activities.

Ethics committees typically are composed of physicians, nurses, social workers, and clergy as members. Some committees also have lawyers, hospital administrators, community representatives, and, if available, may have specialists from psychiatry, palliative care, neurology, pediatrics, transplantation, intensive care units, and/or allied health services, such as physical therapy. Larger committees are typically found at academic medical centers. It is critical that committee membership be diverse, to facilitate broad discussion from those of different backgrounds. Committee composition can be widely variable, depending on the size and resources of the hospital.

Education

The first task of an HEC is education of its own members. Members should be willing to attend regular meetings and share in the education of the group. Education may include review of previous ethics consultations, hospital policies, and relevant state laws, as well as reports from various authoritative bodies and ethics commissions. Members may share ethical problems from their discipline, or areas of expertise.

Some committee members may also plan educational activities, such as regular hospital rounds to help identify cases of concern, and conferences to educate hospital staff members and trainees. Ethics presentations, such as *How to Fill out an Advance Directive,* or *How to Select a Health Care Proxy,* may be offered to educate the community. HEC members may review troubling cases in retrospect, to explore justifications for the actions taken, and may consider whether policy changes are necessary if multiple cases identify a common problem in the hospital.

Policy Development

HECs also help develop or review hospital policies. For example, HECs commonly write or review policies on topics such as informed consent, surrogate decision making, how to enact a do not resuscitate (DNR) order, brain death, blood transfusion and Jehovah's Witnesses, utilization of scarce resources, organ donation after cardiac death, and the hospital's code of ethics, and some may even review business contracts as part of JCAHO's requirement for organizational ethics.

Case Consultation

Not all members of HECs are prepared or trained to perform case consultation, and it can certainly be intimidating for a family member to be asked to meet with a dozen strangers to discuss difficult medical decisions for their loved ones. Instead, most clinical ethics case consultations are performed by small teams or individuals who have undergone more extensive training in bioethics and mediation. The consultant or team of consultants may review the cases later with the larger committee, or a subgroup dedicated to the consultation process. In some centers, particularly smaller hospitals, where the committee may be smaller, the entire committee may review cases. More than 81% of U.S. hospitals now have an ethics consultation service of some kind. In 1998, the American Society for Bioethics and Humanities (ASBH) published *Core Competencies for Health Care Ethics Consultation,* a guide to knowledge areas and skills useful for ethics consultation, which has been followed up by the publication of several books and series of ethics cases by clinical ethics consultants.

Although ethics consultations may be requested for a wide variety of specific problems, there are common underlying themes of conflict. The conflict may be between the patient and the healthcare team, the family and the healthcare team, different specialists within in the healthcare team, or the family and the patient. Generally, conflicts arc about two major questions. These general questions are

What is the right or best thing to do in this situation? And, because there may be different choices or opinions about what is the best course of action,

Who gets to decide?

So the first category of questions above asks about treatment options or limitations. More specific examples include the following: Should we take this elderly lady off the breathing machine, and allow her to die? Should we put her on multiple machines to keep her alive as long as her heart is beating? Are we allowed to turn off her pacemaker? Should we provide dialysis, now that her kidneys have failed, even though she is unconscious? Should we feed her through a tube into her stomach, since she can no longer eat? Should we attempt resuscitation efforts if her heart stops beating? How long will it take before we can know if she will improve or recover? Can we treat her with natural herbs instead?

The second category of questions asks who ought to make decisions when there are differences of opinions about the best course of action. Specific examples include the following: Does this patient have the capacity to make choices herself? That is, can she express an understanding of risks, benefits, and alternatives to the treatment offered and make an informed choice? If she is too sick to make a choice, did she leave an Advance Directive or Living Will that serves as a written expression of her wishes? Did she name someone to make healthcare decisions for her if she is unable? How do we know what she would want? Did she ever make statements about what types of treatments she would or would not want? Does the whole family have to agree with the treatment option offered? What role does her distant relative have, who hasn't seen her in many years but demands that *everything* be done to keep her alive?

A third category of questions that commonly lead to ethics consults are not truly ethics questions, but are questions about communication, policy clarification, or support. Large hospitals are busy places, and the healthcare system is fragmented. Sometimes, it is hard to know "what to do" or "who gets to decide" because there are communication difficulties. Ethics consultants can help identify and bring the right people together who need to share in the decision-making process. Consultants often facilitate family meetings, to get family members and key members of the treating healthcare team together at one time to clarify the situation. The following are some examples: What is the prognosis? How ought we decide what to do when one doctor tells us one thing, but another doctor tells us something else? Would a consultation from a specialty service such as neurology clarify the prognosis? Is physician-assisted suicide allowed in this state? What does the hospital policy say about making an order for DNR if the family objects?

Often, a healthcare professional will offer a treatment choice but may want extra support or agreement from other knowledgeable but neutral third parties that the choice offered was reasonable, and the ethics consult service can assist the patient, family, and healthcare professionals about evaluating justifications for making that choice. Ethics consultants must be careful to decide whether the consults they receive are appropriate for themselves to handle, or whether they should be more appropriately directed to a psychiatrist, the hospital lawyer, palliative care team, or chaplain.

Sample Process for Ethics Case Analysis

Ethics consultants must be practical, because solutions need to be found for problems involving real patients, rather than mere theoretical concerns. No one theory of ethics may be sufficient to adequately address all the questions an HEC may encounter.

Many committees use some form of casuistry for case review. In casuistry, there are no absolute moral rules. Casuistry is a method of reasoning that examines known example cases where there is general agreement that certain paradigm cases should be treated in certain ways. The case at hand is then compared with the paradigm cases, to assess the similarities and differences from them to determine an appropriate moral response. Casuistry starts with paradigmatic cases in which principles clearly apply and moves to complex or ambiguous cases.

The more similar a case is to a paradigm, the more clear the recommendation may be, and the better moral justification for a recommendation. A question often asked is, "Are there morally relevant differences why we should treat this case differently than another case?" State and federal laws, hospital policies, and the results of prior well-known cases may set limitations on possible recommendations. It is the specific details of the case in question that determines the final recommendation.

A number of approaches to case review using an underpinning of casuistry have been developed. These approaches are ways of organizing the information of a particular case that may allow for comparison with other cases. One well-known approach has been called the Four Topic method, described by Albert Jonsen, Mark Siegler, and William Winslade. For each case, details must be evaluated in each of four main areas: Medical Indications, Patient Preferences, Quality of Life, and Contextual Features.

Another more recent approach developed by the National Center for Ethics in Health Care of the Veterans Health Administration uses the acronym CASES. The CASES approach recommends the following steps: Clarify the consultation request, Assemble the relevant information, Synthesize the information, Explain the synthesis, Support the consultation process. More details of this method can be found on the National Center for Ethics Web pages.

Authority of Ethics Consultants

In most instances, the role of the ethics consultants is to facilitate the decision-making process, not to make decisions themselves. Decision making in healthcare is properly left between the physician who has knowledge of the treatment options and the patient who has to undergo some treatment or his or her appropriate representative.

Although the ethics consultant may offer a recommendation, the final decisions are often left to those who will be most affected by the decision. Ethics consults are most often advisory in nature, and not binding. However, some jurisdictions allow ethics committees to have more legal weight.

One of the most common reasons physicians request ethics consultation is when they believe the therapy they are providing is futile or nonbeneficial, but the patient or his or her representative asks to continue treatment, even though the chance of meaningful recovery is exceedingly low. Physicians and ethicists tried to better define "futile" treatment in the 1990s, but were unable to come to an agreed-on definition. In 1999, Texas was the first state to adopt a law regulating end-of-life decisions, providing a due process mechanism for resolving futility disputes. This law, signed by then Governor George W. Bush, has been tested in the courts. The Texas Advance Directives Act directs if an attending physician refuses to honor a patient's or family's request for continued treatment, the refusal shall be reviewed by an ethics committee. If the ethics committee determines that the life-sustaining treatment is medically inappropriate, the family may attempt to transfer the patient to another physician or another facility. If no facility agrees to accept the patient in 10 days, then the life-sustaining treatment can be withdrawn, even over the family's objections. The first case that received national attention was that of Baby Sun Hudson, who was taken off a ventilator in March 2005, after a court reviewed the process followed by the hospital. The Hudson infant had a condition that would not allow his lungs to grow. No other state has enacted such a process yet, but under the support of this law, multidisciplinary ethics consultation has helped families accept treatment limitations in many of the cases brought for review by the ethics committees in larger Texas hospitals.

How ethics committees ought to reach a conclusion is not stated in the Advance Directive Act. There is no regulation that notes whether there needs to be unanimous consensus or simply a majority vote of the ethics committee. Ethical decision making is not typically the result of democratic activities such as voting, it is about determining appropriate justification for individual actions; that is one reason why most ethics committee decisions are advisory in nature.

Common Topics

Common topics addressed by HECs or consultants include decision-making capacity, informed consent, surrogate decision making, advance directives, end-of-life decision making, privacy and confidentiality, reproduction and perinatal issues, failure to cooperate with medical recommendations, decision making for minors, critically ill infants, discharge dilemmas, quality-of-life issues, allocation of scarce resources, and genetic testing

and gene therapy. Some HECs may tackle topics and policies on human research, but intensive review of research activities is accomplished by IRBs, which are more closely regulated by federal policy. Finally, decisions about whether a patient meets criteria for listing for organ transplantation is usually addressed by transplantation committees, which may request the presence of an ethics consultant for review of a case or policy development, but is handled much differently than the dialysis committee God Squads of the 1960s.

Richard A. Demme

See also Advance Directives and End-of-Life Decision Making; Bioethics; Decisions Faced by Institutional Review Boards; Decisions Faced by Surrogates or Proxies for the Patient; Law and Court Decision Making; Shared Decision Making

Further Readings

Alexander, S. (1962). They decide who lives, who dies. *Life, 53,* 102–125.

ASBH Task Force on Standards for Bioethics Consultation. (1998). *Core competencies for health care ethics consultation.* Oakbrook, IL: American Society for Bioethics and Humanities.

In re Quinlan (1976) 70 N.J. 10, 355 A. 2d. 647.

Jonsen, A., Siegler, M., & Winslade, W. (2006). *Clinical ethics: A practical approach to ethical decisions in clinical medicine* (6th ed.). New York: McGraw-Hill.

Lo, B. (2005). *Resolving ethical dilemmas: A guide for clinicians* (3rd ed.). Baltimore: Lippincott Williams & Wilkins.

National Center for Ethics in Health Care: http://www.ethics.va.gov

President's Commission for the Study of Ethical Problems in Medicine and Biomedical and Behavioral Research. (1983). *Hospital ethics committees: Proposed statute and national survey. Deciding to forego life-sustaining treatment* (Appendix F, pp. 439–557). Washington, DC: Government Printing Office.

DECISIONS FACED BY INSTITUTIONAL REVIEW BOARDS

Institutional review boards (IRBs) are part of the main committees within institutions authorized to provide independent scientific and ethical review and evaluation of research studies on humans. Their tasks are to optimally protect human study participants by the review and evaluation of the risks and benefits of a research study from scientific and ethical perspectives in the context of making as certain as possible that the study is aimed at developing appropriate scientific knowledge for use by future generations of humans. IRBs accomplish these tasks by carrying out their own systematic review and evaluation of the science and the ethics of the study from the primary perspective of protecting human research study participants.

While regional IRBs and private IRBs exist, most IRBs are local to allow for the recognition of and sensitivity to local issues in the consideration of research on humans. Historically, review boards evaluated research by peer review, review by the principal investigator's peers in good standing. Today, U.S. federal regulations require IRBs to be composed of a more representative community membership—including members of vulnerable populations or those knowledgeable about and familiar with the research the IRB is charged with evaluating with respect to vulnerable subjects—in the attempt to bring multiple perspectives into the scientific and ethical review and evaluation of research studies.

Vulnerable subjects include the following:

- children, pregnant women, prisoners, and individuals who are permanently or temporarily challenged or disabled physically, mentally, or emotionally;
- individuals who because of the temporary states when exacerbations of their medical, psychological, or psychiatric conditions occur will have impaired capacity to make medical decisions; and
- individuals who are challenged by their educational level or social status, with regard to their capacity to enter into the discussions entailed in understanding the nature of research on humans and the implications of their participation in research.

While the importance of decisional capacity is essential to the participation of anyone in a research study, IRBs lack precise criteria defining "decisional capacity." This entry reviews key elements related to understanding the nature of voluntary research participation and an IRB's responsibilities relating to research involving human subjects.

Research Participation

Research as defined by the *U.S. Code of Federal Regulations* is a "systematic investigation including . . . development, testing, and evaluation, designed to develop or contribute to generalizable knowledge" (38 *CFR* 16.102 d and 45 *CFR* 46.102 d). Any development of innovative therapies in clinical care needs to be formulated into a research study as soon as feasible. For example, a radiologist may devise a stent for a patient with an abdominal aortic aneurysm where the patient has a variant anatomy that will not allow use of a regular-sized and regular-shaped stent in an emergency. But the concept that a different form of stent for repair of abdominal aortic aneurysms can be designed and developed that better meets the various anatomical requirements of variously sized and shaped human beings is a research hypothesis that needs to be submitted to regulators as a new research medical device and subsequently reviewed by an IRB as a research study with a well-developed scientific protocol and well-developed informed consent form for consideration of approval as a research study within an institution or set of institutions.

Research studies are designed to attempt to develop general knowledge for use by future populations by recruiting study participants to serve as human subject volunteers who will bear risks of study participation even though they may not benefit in any way from their research participation and who may be reversibly or irreversibly mentally, physically, or emotionally harmed by their participation in a research study.

Therapeutic Misconception

Although a survey has found that individuals volunteering their participation in a research study prefer to be referred to as *study participants,* the term *human subject* is often used in an attempt to make certain that study volunteers do not misinterpret that they are involved in research, not clinical care. The term *therapeutic misconception* has been used in the peer-reviewed medical literature to identify the phenomenon of study participants mis-understanding what they are getting involved with when they volunteer for a research study. Some study participants may mistakenly assume research participation is a form of clinical care.

Clinical Care

Participating in a research study is not clinical care. In clinical care, in absence of emergency, a patient presents himself or herself to a physician for care which typically involves diagnosis (history, physical examination, laboratory testing of bodily fluids, imaging of various parts of the body) to identify the medical cause of a patient's symptoms. Once a clinical diagnosis is made, the physician then develops a management and treatment plan to cure, manage, or alleviate the patient's symptoms. Diagnosis, management, and treatment may be the results (end products) of previous research on humans, but they do not constitute research.

The peer-reviewed medical literature postulates a set of reasons why research can be mistaken for clinical care: (a) Research on humans is conducted in the same clinical environment as patients see their clinicians and within which the patients receive their care, (b) research is conducted by the same physicians who care for the patient for their clinical medical conditions, and (c) research is conducted by the same medical providers who the patient sees assisting in or providing their clinical care.

In 1978, the National Commission for the Protection of Human Subjects of Biomedical and Behavioral Research pointed out in the *Belmont Report* that research is not clinical care because the patient seeing a medical provider is expecting to benefit from the medical opinions and recommendations of that provider. In contrast, research is conducted in those circumstances where there is no answer as to what is the best way to help or benefit a patient or a group of patients with specific medical complaints or condition. Therefore, research is conducted to attempt to get better answers to the medical questions that are not understood in terms of the best way to diagnose, manage, or treat a patient; for example, how a treatment will compare with a placebo (placebo-controlled trial) or how one treatment (Treatment 1) will compare with another treatment (Treatment 2). There is no certainty in the outcome of any research study.

Also, research is not clinical care because the primary goal of the research team is to observe and evaluate potential participants at $time_0$ (the time before any research activities have been started) until $time_n$ (where n = the time of study closure or a time after study closure). The key to the majority of research studies is to determine by observation and measurement whether and to what extent the research intervention causes a change in the study participant. A study intervention may be an exposure to a newly developed medical product (device or prescription medicine), instrument, or intervention (invasive or noninvasive) used to screen (identify disease in asymptomatic individuals), diagnose (identify disease or medical conditions in symptomatic individuals), manage, or treat disease.

The purpose of the research study in the above cases is to determine if the newly developed medical product, instrument, or intervention compares in terms of benefits and risks with the study placebo, product, or intervention to which it is being compared in the research study. These comparisons are done by techniques used to observe, measure, and compare the newly developed research entity with the entity now used in the standard practice of care.

Obligations of an Institutional Review Board

The obligation of an IRB is to best protect human study volunteers. This is accomplished by the thorough systematical review and evaluation of the research study, its scientific objectives and its scientific goals, and the scientific methods selected by the principal investigator and the study sponsor to achieve those objectives and goals. The IRB meets its obligation by reviewing and evaluating each research study in terms of its science and its ethics.

Science and Ethics Evaluation

The IRB has a dual role in review of proposed research studies. First, the IRB must be certain that it fully understands the science that is being undertaken. Second, after fully understanding the science, the IRB must fully explore the ethical issues surrounding that science. While one may argue that in particular research studies, the evaluation of the science and ethics can go on simultaneously, this is not always true. In the evaluation of some research study proposals, if the IRB does not understand the science that is being proposed, it cannot understand the ethical issues surrounding that science.

The evaluation of the science and ethics of a submitted research study is done to achieve the best possible science to both minimize risks to study volunteers and to generate the best possible scientific knowledge. To begin to achieve the above goals, the principal investigator and study sponsor submit to the IRB for review and evaluation a study protocol and an informed consent form.

Scientific Protocol

The scientific protocol describes the research question (study objective), the scientific methodology that will be used to answer the research question, the composition and qualification of the research team, and the surveillance practices that will be put into place to identify any potential harm to a study participant. The ongoing observation of all study participants to look for any harm occurring related to study participation is an ongoing obligation of the principal investigator, research team, and study sponsor. The aim is to identify a harm and begin the chain of communication that will result in that harm being minimized and the research subject being treated as soon as that harm is identified.

There are three ongoing chains of obligations. The first chain of obligation is to attempt to make sure that no harms befall a study participant. The second chain of obligation is the obligation to recognize the occurrence of a harm to a study participant as soon as possible after that harm occurs. The third chain of obligation is to contact the study participant regarding the harm as soon as possible so that the extent of the harm can be minimized, if possible, through management and treatment. Part of this third chain of obligation is for the research team to contact those who will be responsible for the care of the participant until that harm is optimally treated and managed until resolution. It is the primary obligation of the principal investigator and study sponsor to include explicit descriptions of all three chains (prevention, recognition, and communication and

care) in the study protocol and informed consent form and to ensure research team members are trained in prevention, early recognition, early communication, and early establishment of care for the injured study participant.

Informed Consent Form

The informed consent form is a form that is given to the individual considering research study participation that specifies in language that is accessible to nonscientists the study objectives, the risks of the study, alternatives available in clinical care that could be opted for instead of participating in the research study, who is funding the study, who are the members of the study team who are responsible for the conduct of the study, and the chains of obligation of recognition, communication, and care related to any harm that might befall a study participant. The informed consent form also specifies the study participant's rights should an adverse outcome happen to him or her during study participation.

Identification of Conflicts of Interest

Within the overall tasks of review and evaluation of research studies in their ethical and scientific dimensions, the IRB is responsible for identifying any and all conflicts of interest that are present in the research study and in its review. There may be conflicts of interest present in relationships on an IRB with respect to a particular study being evaluated. These conflicts of interest may be financial or nonmonetary. A financial conflict of interest would be illustrated by stock ownership of an IRB member in a company that is the study sponsor of the research study being submitted to the IRB for review. A nonfinancial conflict of interest may be a work relationship between an IRB member and the principal investigator. For example, the principal investigator of a study being submitted to an IRB may be the direct supervisor of the IRB member in question. All conflicts of interest on an IRB with regard to a particular study must be eliminated. Elimination of conflict of interest is the recusal of the IRB member from any participation in the review and evaluation of the particular study in question.

Time-Appropriate Continuing Review

The IRB is also responsible for the identification of time-appropriate continuing review points whereby the IRB rereviews and reevaluates the research study for the development of new risks, excessive risk borne by study volunteers, and prevalence and types of adverse outcomes. When an IRB, after careful systematic review, decides to approve a study it then assigns a date to review that study.

For example, any research study involving new prescription medicines that have new mechanisms of action will require early review of adverse outcome occurrence by the IRB to determine whether new risks are occurring in study participants. Here, the IRB receives, reviews, and evaluates all new risks that are occurring in study participants at all sites where the study is being conducted. The IRB reviews all new risks to make certain that the research team is handling the risks, that the study participants are notified about the adverse outcome that has occurred, and that optimal care is being provided to the injured study participant. Optimal care is provided by making all appropriate contacts with the study participants and the study participants' physicians, ensuring transparent communication about the adverse outcomes and that the study participants receive appropriate care, management, and treatment.

If problems do occur, the IRB makes certain that the study is suspended until the study is modified to minimize any subsequent occurrence of the adverse outcomes in other study participants and to make certain that all study participants are willing to continue in the research study after these new risks are identified. This latter point may require that all study participants reconsent regarding their willingness to continue in the research study with the new identified risks reported. If there is unwillingness on the part of the principal investigator or study sponsor to follow IRB recommendations regarding the safety of the study volunteers, the IRB must terminate the study and notify appropriate regulators and authorities.

Communication of Risks

The IRB ensures that the principal investigator and study sponsor have correctly and clearly identified and communicated all known risks and that reasonably estimated risks are clearly described in the study protocol and in the informed consent form. For example, there must be a true conceptual search for what risks a new prescription medicine with a new mechanism of action might reasonably have. This may demand consultation with experts in the field. And at minimum, the IRB conducts its own searches of the peer-reviewed medical and scientific literature to ensure that all risks are being recognized and stated clearly in the informed consent form.

Patients' Understanding of Rights

The IRB ensures that the informed consent form does not attempt to mislead study volunteers about their rights regarding research participation. Rights here include the right to terminate participation in the research study at any time when they can do so safely. The inclusion of the point of safely terminating research participation is crucial because, for example, in the study of a prescription medicine, it must be recognized by the participant (and made clear in the informed consent form at study entry) that some study prescription medicines (e.g., beta blockers) cannot simply be stopped at any time, but rather must be tapered off safely under a physician's supervision to minimize adverse outcomes.

Another example where a research study cannot simply be stopped is that of a medical device requiring surgical placement. In these cases, an operation must be scheduled to surgically remove the device. Again, it is necessary that all study volunteers understand these points at their entry into the study and all points must be transparently disclosed in the study's informed consent form.

Decision-Making Tasks

The IRB's main decision-making tasks involve protection of human subjects. These tasks at minimum are dependent on the IRB making as certain as possible that (a) it has all known information related to the research study and (b) the information in the informed consent form is translated into nonscientific language and its exposition and presentation are as clear as possible to the study participant.

Relevant Information

Before the IRB can begin to protect study participants, it must have all relevant information from principal investigators and study sponsors regarding what is known about the research entity to be studied. The IRB then on its own systematically rechecks the peer-reviewed medical literature and calls on experts to make certain that the information provided by the principal investigator and study sponsor is consistent with what is medically known and scientifically understood about the research entity being studied, including all risks that are reasonably foreseeable. The concept of what it means for a risk to be "reasonably foreseeable" must be explored by the IRB because a precise operational definition is open to debate. Securing a wide range of expert opinion and the IRB's own thorough exploration of the peer-reviewed medical and scientific literature are good places to start in determining reasonably foreseeable risks.

Scientific and Legal Information

The IRB must be certain that the language used in the scientific protocol and informed consent form is not being used to hide information. For example, it is not sufficient to simply say to the study volunteer considering study participation (or to state in an informed consent form) that there are "unknown risks" when those unknown risks are in fact known risks that can be specified. The principal investigator and study sponsor's obligations are to disclose risks, not to hide risk from disclosure. In addition, medical terms need to be translated into nonscientific language, and legal terms need to be translated into nonlegal language.

From the scientific perspective, while it is possible that any new research entity may possess unknown risks, including risks of severe adverse outcomes or increasing risk factors for other disease or medical conditions, the IRB needs to fully explore all foreseeable risks related to the research entity being studied and independently verify if the estimates provided by principal investigators and study sponsors are declared and fully described to each study participant as he or she considers whether to volunteer participation in a study.

From the legal perspective, there should be no use of language that attempts to minimize the liability of study sponsors, research institutions, and principal investigators. There must also be a full disclosure of participants' rights to seek court opinion in specific areas of liability.

Dennis J. Mazur

See also Informed Consent

Further Readings

Appelbaum, P. S. (1997). Rethinking the conduct of psychiatric research. *Archives of General Psychiatry, 54,* 117–120.

Bonnie, R. J. (1997). Research with cognitively impaired subjects: Unfinished business in the regulation of human research. *Archives of General Psychiatry, 54,* 105–111.

Code of Federal Regulations: http://www.gpoaccess.gov/cfr/index.html

Elliott, C. (1997). Caring about risks: Are severely depressed patients competent to consent to research? *Archives of General Psychiatry, 54,* 113–116.

Lavery, J. V., Grady, C., Wahl, E. R., & Emanuel, E. J. (Eds.). (2007). *Ethical issues in international biomedical research: A casebook.* New York: Oxford University Press.

Manson, N. C., & O'Neill, O. (2007). *Rethinking informed consent in bioethics.* Cambridge, UK: Cambridge University Press.

Mazur, D. J. (2007). *Evaluating the science and ethics of research on humans: A guide for IRB members.* Baltimore: Johns Hopkins University Press.

Mazur, D. J., & Hickam, D. H. (1993). Patient interpretations of terms connoting low probabilities when communicating about surgical risk. *Theoretical Surgery, 8,* 143–145.

National Commission for the Protection of Human Subjects of Biomedical and Behavioral Research. (1979). *The Belmont report* (DHEW Publication No. (OS) 78-0012). Washington, DC: Government Printing Office.

Office of Civil Rights, Department of Health and Human Services. (2002). Standards for privacy of individually identifiable health information: Final rules. *Federal Register, 67,* 53182–53273.

Rosen, C., Grossman, L. S., Sharma, R. P., Bell, C. C., Mullner, R., & Dove, H. W. (2007). Subjective evaluations of research participation by persons with mental illness. *Journal of Nervous and Mental Disease, 195,* 430–435.

DECISIONS FACED BY NONGOVERNMENT PAYERS OF HEALTHCARE: INDEMNITY PRODUCTS

See Decisions Faced by Nongovernment Payers of Healthcare: Managed Care

DECISIONS FACED BY NONGOVERNMENT PAYERS OF HEALTHCARE: MANAGED CARE

The concept of private indemnity insurance in healthcare refers to a fee-for-service plan where beneficiaries are compensated for their out-of-pocket costs, up to the limiting amount of the insurance policy. Unlike managed care organizations (MCOs), which overlay tools to control the utilization and cost of services, private indemnity insurance policies allow beneficiaries unrestricted provider choice and reimburse providers on a fee-for-service basis. Many indemnity plans are offered with deductibles, where the beneficiary will be required to pay copays (generally determined with percentages) for additional services required above the deductible amount.

When a private indemnity plan begins to control costs by restricting the choice of providers, it is typically referred to as an MCO. It is useful to think of MCOs on a continuum of loosely to more heavily managed products and from highest to lowest patient cost-sharing, beginning with private indemnity plans on the loosest end, progressing to preferred provider organizations (PPOs), open panel health maintenance organizations (HMOs), and finally closed panel HMOs with the tightest control over cost combined with the lowest patient cost sharing. In general, physicians are most affected in their medical decision-making ability in dealing with the most tightly managed MCOs.

Introduction to Managed Care

Managed care refers to the systematic method of reducing healthcare costs while attempting to improve the quality of patient care. A managed care organization uses these methods to finance and deliver healthcare to people enrolled in the organization's plan. Prompted by the Health Maintenance Organization Act of 1973, which provided grants and loans to assist in the startup of health maintenance organizations, today's managed care environment consists of a variety of private health benefit programs. Widely credited with restraining the runaway medical cost inflation of the late 1980s, managed care has come under attack in recent years by those who say it focuses on efficiency at the expense of patient care. Despite criticism, managed care has become an entrenched foundation of today's national healthcare system, with roughly 90% of insured Americans enrolled in plans with some form of managed care.

Characteristics of Managed Care Organizations

Managed care organizations typically provide a panel or network of healthcare professionals who deliver a comprehensive assortment of healthcare services to enrollees. MCOs usually have specific standards for selecting the providers in the network and for establishing formal quality improvement and utilization review programs. In addition, they tend to focus on preventive care and to offer economic incentives that encourage enrollees to use care efficiently.

MCOs employ a number of techniques to reduce costs and make the delivery of services more efficient while ensuring high quality standards. These may include the following:

- Financial incentives for physicians and patients to select more efficient forms of care from providers who are in the panel
- Mechanisms for reviewing the medical necessity of services
- Beneficiary cost sharing
- Restrictions on inpatient hospital admissions and length of stay
- Selective contracting with healthcare providers
- Rigorous management of the most costly healthcare cases

Additionally, MCOs often cut expenses by negotiating favorable fees from their panel of healthcare providers, choosing cost-effective providers, and offering economic incentives for providers to practice more efficiently. MCOs may also rely on disease management, case management, wellness incentives, patient education, utilization management, and utilization reviews as indirect ways of lowering costs.

On the surface, there appears to be a conflict between the goals of an MCO and the goals of a physician, with the MCO focusing on cost and efficiency and the physician focusing on quality of care and the best care for the patient. However, when managed care works as intended, the final outcome is the most appropriate evidence-based care delivered by providers and producing the highest-quality, best value outcomes for the patient.

Contracting With Health Plans

The contracts that physicians develop with health plans can have a major impact on their medical decision making. The following are key factors in selecting contracts.

The scope of the plan's network. This affects a physician's ability to refer patients to the healthcare providers they want.

Carve-out networks. These are specialty-specific and ancillary health networks with which the plan has subcontracted to provide services—such as behavioral health, laboratory work and imaging—that either fall outside of the medical insurance benefit (e.g., vision and dental care) or that traditionally represent a high-cost service.

The plan's medical director. A good rapport with the plan's medical director can be helpful when navigating the health plan rules and appeals processes for noncovered services, such as additional testing and extended lengths of stay for inpatients.

Clinical guidelines. Physician decision making can be affected by the clinical guidelines that health plans follow. Most plans adhere to industry standards, such as those found in *Milliman Care Guidelines*. Such guidelines are typically updated annually with evidence-based authorization criteria that encourage high-quality care through tools such as care pathways, flagged quality measures, and integrated medical evidence.

Premium physician networks and rating systems. Some plans sell their subscribers "premium networks," which are groups of physicians who have demonstrated a high volume of successful outcomes. Certain plans even rate their physicians and publish this information to members. These plans usually provide regular feedback to physicians regarding their performance, with the goal of improving quality and efficiency. A low rating may be cause for removing a physician from the plan's premium network.

Pay-for-performance programs. These programs base provider reimbursement on high-quality results and appropriate decision making. Consequently, pay-for-performance programs tend to encourage physicians to make the most appropriate medical decisions to achieve optimal patient outcomes.

Following Health Plan Rules

Physicians who contract with a health plan are obligated to follow the rules of that plan. These directives will directly affect the physician's medical decisions and may vary from plan to plan. Health plan rules may include the following.

Precertification. Since a lack of precertification may result in the denial of payment, physicians may avoid ordering specific medical treatments or procedures that they know will be denied.

Referrals. Physician referral patterns are affected by the plan's provider network, as patients receive their maximum benefit level when referrals are made within the network.

Disease management programs. This is the process of using integrated care to reduce healthcare costs and improve the quality of life for people with chronic disease, such as coronary heart disease, cancer, hypertension, and diabetes. In the United States, disease management has become a big business, with more than half of all employer-sponsored health plans offering disease management programs. Effective disease management can reduce labor costs by cutting down on absenteeism and insurance expenses. Many disease management vendors even offer a return on investment for their programs. Disease management programs generally have their own sets of evidence-based rules. When a plan employs disease management programs, physicians will support the care management guidelines of the program for the benefit of the patient.

Medical management. This refers to the activities, such as utilization management and quality assurance, that MCOs employ to control the cost and quality of healthcare services provided to their members. A plan's medical management guidelines may affect the physician's decision making as the plan manages resource utilization to contain costs while promoting high-quality care.

Pharmacy formularies. As established by a health plan, a formulary is a list of approved drugs that physicians may prescribe and that pharmacies may dispense. Health plan formularies are continually evaluated by groups of experts working together in committees that are commonly called "pharmacy and therapeutics" (P&T) committees. Health plans often use formularies as a managed care mechanism for controlling inventories and promoting the use of the most cost-effective products that are safe and beneficial to patients. Formularies can differ from plan to plan, and this will affect the physician's decision making when it comes to prescribing medications for patients.

Denials and appeals. In case payment or a certain treatment is denied, it is helpful if physicians and practice administrators understand the appeals process, so that they can assist patients.

Legal issues. Medical decision making is also affected in general by laws and regulations that govern the healthcare, insurance, and other related industries. These may include federal regulations such as the Health Insurance Portability and Accountability Act (HIPAA), compliance, antitrust, antikickback, and Stark laws, and Medicare fraud and abuse laws. With respect to medical decision making, ethics dictates and laws uphold that physicians should base their medical decisions on what is right for the patient rather than on payments or benefits the physician will receive as a consequence of a medical decision.

Conversations With Patients

When developing treatment plans and discussing medical options with patients, it is helpful if physicians are familiar with the basics of the patient's health insurance coverage. These details will affect the physician's decisions for each patient and may include the following:

- *Health plan and product*, including whether or not the patient is in a high-deductible or consumer-directed health plan that may generate high out-of-pocket costs due to the benefit design
- *Benefits coverage*, including noncovered services and the patient's financial responsibility for treatment
- *Coverage of drug formularies*, which may be limited to a list of preferred drugs or to generics for certain medications
- *Referral network*, keeping in mind that patients appreciate referrals to healthcare providers that are within their network

A physician who is familiar with the main elements of the market's major health plans will be on the same page with many of his or her patients.

Physician Perspectives on Managed Care

Attitudes of healthcare professionals regarding how managed care affects medical decisions may vary, depending on their affiliation and the experiences they have had. While many advocate that measures be taken to reduce unnecessary costs, a large number of physicians are understandably negative about managed care techniques that appear to take medical decision-making capabilities out of the hands of medical professionals.

Managed care has been successful in reining in costs and promoting quality in recent years; however, there is still a way to go in terms of easing the administrative burden that the MCO cost-cutting techniques place on physician practice. Such "hassle factor" issues may include the following.

Requirements regarding drugs. It is a challenge for physicians to keep current on the different plan formularies, recognizing that the patient's financial responsibility will change depending on what drug is prescribed. In addition, some managed care organizations require preauthorizations for certain medications.

Medical testing. Managed care can reduce unnecessary or inappropriate medical tests and procedures. This is a cost-saving technique that can improve patient care, but it also means that physicians who want to order medical tests are required to share clinical information with the patient's health plan. Establishing and managing this process can be resource-intensive.

Medical case management. Most health plans have a medical management function that coordinates the efforts of all healthcare providers and facilitates recommended treatment plans to ensure that appropriate medical protocols are followed and that patients achieve medical rehabilitation. Medical case management can reduce unnecessary costs while streamlining patient care, leading to faster, more successful recoveries. This process can sometimes create an adversarial relationship between physicians and health plans—with physicians wanting patients to stay in hospitals longer, on the one hand, and insurance companies seeking to keep costs low, on the other. As a result, hospitals have had to set up denial databases and invest significant resources to track down and get reimbursed for claims that were initially denied by the health plans.

Advocacy and Stewardship

In general, nonprofit hospitals and other healthcare organizations exist to serve the community by providing healthcare services that the population needs, as well as outreach programs, such as health education and wellness programs. Consequently, most physicians and other individuals who are affiliated with hospitals have a sense of stewardship in regard to the community.

A number of physician leaders urge other doctors to speak up and actively work for what they believe is right for patients and for the healthcare system in general. Through their involvement in legislative reform, the formation of physician and consumer groups, and other activities, physicians can bring about change and protect the interests of themselves, their patients, their communities, and the hospitals they serve.

Michael McMillan and Wendy Kornbluth

See also Government Perspective, General Healthcare; Government Perspective, Public Health Issues

Further Readings

Austrin, M. S. (1999). *Managed health care simplified: A glossary of terms.* Clifton Park, NY: Delmar Thomson Learning.

Blakely, S. (1998, July). The backlash against managed care. *Nation's Business.* Retrieved October 5, 2007, from http://findarticles.com/p/articles/mi_m1154/is_n7_v86/ai_20797610/pg_1?tag=artBody;col1

Cairns, K. D. (2002). *Contemporary managed care issues for physicians* (2nd ed.). Newtown, PA: Handbooks in Health Care.

Harris, D. M. (1999). *Healthcare law and ethics: Issues for the age of managed care.* Washington, DC: AUPHA Press.

The Henry J. Kaiser Family Foundation. (2004). *Kaiser public opinion spotlight: The public, managed care, and consumer protections.* Retrieved October 5, 2007, from http://www.kff.org/spotlight/managedcare/index.cfm

Kaiser Family Foundation Health Care Marketplace Project. (2007). *Health care costs: A primer.* Retrieved October 5, 2007, from http://www.kff.org/insurance/upload/7670.pdf

Kaiser Family Foundation Health Care Marketplace Project. (2007). *Trends in health care costs and spending.* Retrieved October 5, 2007, from http://www.kff.org/insurance/7692.cfm

Kongstvedt, P. R. (2001). *The managed health care handbook* (4th ed.). New York: Aspen.

Price Waterhouse Coopers for America's Health Insurance Plans. (2006). *The factors fueling rising healthcare costs 2006.* Retrieved October 5, 2007, from http://www.ahipbelieves.com/media/The%20Factors%20Fueling%20Rising%20Healthcare%20Costs.pdf

Reschovsky, J. D., Kemper, P., & Tu, H. (2000). Does type of health insurance affect health care use and assessments of care among the privately insured? *Health Services Research, 35*(1, Pt. 2), 219–237.

Tindall, W. N. (2000). *A guide to managed care medicine.* Sudbury, MA: Jones & Bartlett.

DECISIONS FACED BY PATIENTS: PRIMARY CARE

Primary care is defined as the level of the healthcare system that provides individuals with (a) the gateway into the system for all their needs and problems; (b) care focused on the individual and his or her context (not disease-oriented); (c) care for all but very uncommon or unusual conditions; (d) continuity of care; and (e) the coordination or integration of the care provided by other levels of the system or by other professionals. Thus, primary care is defined by a series of functions which, in combination, are unique at this level. Countries with a strong primary care component have better health outcomes and are better at keeping costs under control.

In the United States, the ecology model of medical care reveals that on average each month, out of 1,000 individuals, 800 experience symptoms, of whom 327 will consider seeking medical care. Of those, only 217 will visit a physician in the office (113 visit a primary care physician and 104 visit other specialists). Of those visiting a physician, 21 will visit a hospital-based outpatient clinic, and of these, 8 will be hospitalized. Although it is essential to ensure quality of care at every level of the healthcare system, it is apparent that opportunities are being missed by limiting quality and safety programs to hospitals when the largest proportion of individuals seeking medical advice are doing so in primary care. Consequently, it is important to study communication and decision making in primary care because of the potential beneficial impact on the quality of care for a large number of individuals.

This entry reviews the characteristics and nature of decisions faced by patients in the context of primary care. The first part explores the characteristics and nature of decisions that are most frequently encountered in primary care. The second part outlines some examples of interventions that address the specific challenges that patients face when making decisions in this clinical context. The last section of the entry summarizes the lessons learned from these initiatives.

Characteristics and Nature of the Decisions

The National Ambulatory Medical Care Survey estimated that in 2004, a total of 910.9 million visits were made to physician offices in the United States. Although 58.9% of visits were to physicians in the specialties of general and family practice, internal medicine, pediatrics, and obstetrics and gynecology, 87.2% of all preventive care visits were covered by primary care physicians. The

leading illness-related primary diagnoses were essential hypertension, malignant neoplasms, acute upper respiratory infection, and diabetes mellitus. In a large comparative study of 115,692 visits in primary care in Australia, New Zealand, and the United States, in each country, primary care physicians managed an average of 1.4 morbidity-related problems per visit. The relative frequency of health problems managed was similar across the three countries, with the five most frequent health problems covering the following clinical areas: musculoskeletal, cardiovascular, ear/nose/throat, skin, and psychosocial.

Results from cross-sectional studies of decision making also provide valuable insight into the characteristics and nature of decisions that are most frequently faced by patients in primary care. For example, in a study of 1,057 audiotaped encounters of routine office visits to both primary care physicians and surgeons, the authors observed that a total of 3,552 clinical decisions were made. However, only 9.0% of these decisions met the definition of completeness for informed decision making. In another study of family physicians' views on difficult decisions faced by their patients, participants identified the five most frequent decisions as follows: cancer therapy, antidepressant drug therapy, level of care, lifestyle issues, and screening tests. In a third study of 212 video-recorded doctor-patient consultations for routine appointments in 12 general practice surgeries in the United Kingdom, it was observed that in addition to those involving medical treatment, there was a range of decision-making opportunities that were not dealt with satisfactorily. More important, it was also observed that most decisions were made by physicians with little effort on their part to foster active participation of their patients in decisions.

Taken together, results from these studies suggest that decision making in primary care is influenced by the following principal characteristics: (a) Many problems and decisions are experienced in one single clinical encounter; (b) decisions are more likely to be about chronic conditions, preventive care, and lifestyle issues; and (c) primary care providers rarely foster active participation of their patients in decisions, which in turn might partly explain the low prevalence of informed decision making.

Interventions

In population-based surveys, individuals facing health-related decisions indicate that their preferred method for obtaining information remains the counseling offered by their physician. Patients facing decisions in primary care are no exception. Therefore, most patients expect their physician to have the necessary skills to give them adequate support for making informed decisions. Given their systematic approach to evidence, clinical practice guidelines—defined as systematically developed statements to assist practitioners and patients with decisions about appropriate healthcare for specific circumstances—have been very popular with medical organizations. However, most studies that aim at improving adherence of clinicians to recommendations of clinical practice guidelines have met with very little success.

In recent years, growing concerns regarding the absence of evidence about patient preferences in clinical practice guidelines have fostered an international interest in patient decision aids. Patient decision aids are tools designed to help patients participate in clinical decision making. They provide information on the options and help patients clarify and communicate the personal values they associate with different features of an option. When compared with usual care or simple information leaflets, patient decision aids improve decision quality and the measures of feeling informed and clear about values during the decision process.

Single Clinical Encounter

A promising initiative that may help primary care providers and their patients access a wide variety of patient decision aids consists of the implementation of call centers staffed by nurses coupled with a database of patient decision aids made available online. A second strategy that might assist decision making when many problems and many decisions are encountered in one single clinical encounter is to train healthcare providers in a generic manner so that they can improve their own decision-making process, recognize decisional conflict in their patients, and then foster better decisions.

Chronic Conditions, Preventive Care, and Lifestyles Issues

Ongoing intervention initiatives suggest that it is feasible to implement patient decision aids for chronic conditions in primary care. Indeed, many trials of patient decision aids have already focused on chronic conditions such as type 2 diabetes, osteoporosis, benign prostatic hyperplasia, or mental conditions and showed beneficial impact on patients and physicians. Interestingly, in the case of chronic conditions, patient decision aids have the potential to foster quality decision-making processes across time, places, and healthcare providers. The underlying hypothesis is that the decision aid will ensure that all healthcare providers involved in the pharmaceutical care of the patient will use the same evidence-based information to improve the quality of care. Notwithstanding when and where the patient receives care for his or her specific condition and who provides this care, a common procedure to support informed decisions by patients in primary care is being used.

Patient decision aids also reduce overuse of controversial medical procedures such as prostate cancer screening tests and lessen the underuse of beneficial public health measures such as childhood vaccination. Therefore, promoting the use of such aids in the context of primary care has the potential of improving the quality of the decision-making process of patients regarding lifestyle issues and public health recommendations. However, addressing lifestyle issues with patients in primary care contexts will require involving other healthcare professionals and extending the concept of high-quality health-related decision making from the medical office into the mainstream. Thus, in the years to come, it is expected that there will be more initiatives applying an interprofessional approach to decision making in primary care.

Active Participation of Patients

In a review of optimal matches of patient preferences for information, decision making, and interpersonal behavior, findings from 14 studies showed that a substantial portion of patients (26% to 95% with a median of 52%) was dissatisfied with the information given (in all aspects) and reported a desire for more information. Nonetheless, in the context of primary care, although patients and doctors agree that more information needs to be made available to patients to help them make difficult decisions, they do not agree about patients' acceptance of decision aids or patients' willingness to participate actively in decision making. This is congruent with the existing literature indicating that the current level of participation of patients in decisions in clinical contexts is low. Results from a systematic review of 28 studies on the barriers and facilitators to fostering participation of patients in decisions as perceived by health professionals suggest that health professionals may be screening, a priori, which patients they believe are competent to participate in decisions. This is of some concern because physicians may misjudge patients' desire for active involvement in decision making. Therefore, interventions directed at patients and the system will be needed for patients to have direct access to the needed information.

Lessons Learned

Ensuring quality of care is dependent on ensuring the quality of the decision-making processes in clinical settings at every level of the healthcare system. This entry briefly reviewed the characteristics and challenges of decision making in primary care. It also highlighted how some intervention initiatives have addressed these specific challenges. Although several gaps in knowledge remain, there are signs that the agenda is beginning to focus on improving the quality of primary care patients' decision making by providing them with innovative decision support interventions. In turn, the impact of these interventions should translate into improved patient and population health outcomes, the ultimate goal of improved clinical decision making.

France Légaré

See also Decision Making in Advanced Disease; Patient Decision Aids; Shared Decision Making

Further Readings

Bindman, A. B., Forrest, C. B., Britt, H., Crampton, P., & Majeed, A. (2007). Diagnostic scope of and exposure to primary care physicians in Australia, New Zealand, and the United States: Cross sectional analysis of results from three national surveys. *British Medical Journal, 334*(7606), 1261.

Braddock, C. H., Edwards, K. A., Hasenberg, N. M., Laidley, T. L., & Levinson, W. (1999). Informed decision making in outpatient practice: Time to get back to basics. *Journal of the American Medical Association, 282*(24), 2313–2320.

Ford, S., Schofield, T., & Hope, T. (2006). Observing decision-making in the general practice consultation: Who makes which decisions? *Health Expectation, 9*(2), 130–137.

Gravel, K., Légaré, F., & Graham, I. D. (2006). Barriers and facilitators to implementing shared decision-making in clinical practice: A systematic review of health professionals' perceptions. *Implement Science, 1*(1), 16.

Green, L. A., Fryer, G. E., Jr., Yawn, B. P., Lanier, D., & Dovey, S. M. (2001). The ecology of medical care revisited. *New England Journal of Medicine, 344*(26), 2021–2025.

Hing, E., Cherry, D. K., & Woodwell, D. A. (2006). National ambulatory medical care survey: 2004 summary. *Advanced Data,* (374), 1–33.

Kiesler, D. J., & Auerbach, S. M. (2006). Optimal matches of patient preferences for information, decision-making and interpersonal behavior: Evidence, models and interventions. *Patient Education and Counseling, 61*(3), 319–341.

Légaré, F., O'Connor, A. C., Graham, I., Saucier, D., Cote, L., Cauchon, M., et al. (2006). Supporting patients facing difficult health care decisions: Use of the Ottawa Decision Support Framework. *Canadian Family Physician, 52,* 476–477.

O'Connor, A. M., Bennett, C., Stacey, D., Barry, M. J., Col, N. F., Eden, K. B., et al. (in press). Do patient decision aids meet effectiveness criteria of the international patient decision aid standards collaboration? A systematic review and meta-analysis. *Medical Decision Making.*

Starfield, B. (1998). *Primary care: Balancing health needs, services, and technology.* Oxford, UK: Oxford University Press.

Wennberg, J. E. (2004). Practice variations and health care reform: Connecting the dots. *Health Affairs* (Web Exclusive), DOI: 10.1377/hlthaff.var.140.

DECISIONS FACED BY SURROGATES OR PROXIES FOR THE PATIENT, DURABLE POWER OF ATTORNEY

Ideally, medical decisions are made collaboratively by the patient and the healthcare provider.

However, when patients cannot fully participate in their own decisions, an alternative decision-making model must be implemented. Surrogates may be required for medical decision making regarding issues of morbidity, mortality, hospital discharge, and research participation. Physicians are faced with the challenge of evaluating decisions made by surrogates. Patients who are unable to contribute to their medical decisions include children and adults who lack capacity, because they either lost or never attained capacity. Adults may lose capacity temporarily or permanently. Temporary loss of capacity may be due to a psychiatric or acute illness, while permanent loss may be the result of an acute event such as brain trauma or a degenerative condition such as Alzheimer's disease. When patients are unable to fully participate in medical decisions, healthcare professionals look to a surrogate or proxy to make decisions on behalf of patients. The issues that surrogates and healthcare professionals face, as well as controversies around the role of the surrogate as representative of patient values, are discussed in this entry. Although some details of these issues may be culturally specific, the broad ethical challenges can be found throughout all of Western medicine. For this entry, the context of American healthcare is used to illustrate these challenges.

Patients may appoint a surrogate in advance by using legal forms such as a Durable Power of Attorney for Healthcare. In the absence of such an advance directive, state laws and customs usually dictate who may act as a surrogate. These may be family members, close friends, or legal guardians appointed by the court. To make appropriate medical decisions, the surrogates should have knowledge of the patient's values and be able to adequately represent those values; it is helpful if the surrogate has specific knowledge about the patient's wishes. Most important, the surrogate should understand the role: to decide in the manner in which he or she believes the patient would decide and not based on the surrogate's own wishes in the situation. This standard is usually referred to as *substituted judgment*. When a surrogate does not sufficiently know the patient's wishes or values, the decision should be made based on the patient's best interests. Important cultural aspects of decision making may require increased communication and consideration by the healthcare professional. Decision-making considerations for surrogates vary depending on the nature of the choice, life and death, quality of life, research participation, or a discharge planning decision. A discussion of these areas would be incomplete without highlighting the contemporary controversies involved in the utilization of surrogates in healthcare settings.

Life and Death Decisions

Decisions about life and death include a variety of medical treatment choices, such as the use of dialysis, pressors, antibiotics, chemotherapy, ventilators, and artificial nutrition. Healthcare professionals should be aware of the law in the state in which they practice because the legal scope of the surrogate's role varies greatly among states and regions. For example, the surrogate's decision making may be limited only by the requirement to act consistently with the patient's best interests. However, some states, such as Missouri, New Jersey, and New York, use the *clear and convincing* evidence standard, which requires clear and convincing evidence of the patient's wishes regarding withdrawal of life-sustaining treatment. The U.S. Supreme Court validated this standard in the landmark case of *Cruzan v. Director, Missouri Department of Health*, 497 U.S. 261 (1990). Furthermore, some states place additional limitations on the power of the surrogate. For example, the New York Health Care Proxy Law places decisions regarding artificial nutrition and hydration outside the scope of a surrogate's authority unless a written advance directive specifically grants the surrogate such decision-making power. Healthcare professionals should understand the patient's values and local laws regarding life and death decisions to properly facilitate a surrogate decision maker's role.

Decisions about life and death, whether made in an intensive care unit, on a regular patient ward, or while receiving care at home, may be emotionally burdensome for some surrogates, while it provides a positive opportunity to interact with the patient for others. Although emotions play fundamental roles in good decision making, they also may obscure the decision-making process. The role of deciding for someone else may lead surrogates to second-guess decisions to the extent that they become emotionally paralyzed and incapable of making good, reasoned medical decisions. Surrogates may mistakenly believe that they alone are responsible for deciding whether and when the patient will die. The residual impact of these emotions may be significant on both individuals and families. Emotions need to be recognized and, when appropriate, either affirmed or redirected. Identifying the emotions overlaying a decision may lead to better decision making by increasing the surrogate's awareness of the impact of his or her emotions on decision making.

Healthcare professionals may lessen the burden on surrogates by providing accurate information as well as clear treatment recommendations. The plan should be goal centered as defined by known patient values. For example, it would be inconsistent for a patient or surrogate who has chosen a pure hospice goal to insist on certain resuscitative measures. A goal-centered plan entails a coherent set of medical choices. It is the responsibility of the healthcare professionals to explain the role of the surrogate and continue to focus the discussion on the patient's global wishes and moral values. This usually includes advising the surrogate to use all sources of information and support, including the patient's friends, family, and spiritual advisors. This collaborative approach has the added benefit of distributing the sense of responsibility for choices that the patient may have wanted but that surrogates find morally troubling.

Research Participation

When medical decisions include the enrollment of a patient into research, issues of surrogate consent become more complex. Research exposes the patient to additional procedures beyond those performed only for the patient's benefit within a preferred treatment regimen established by a clinician. It is unclear in which circumstances a surrogate has the right to enter the patient into a research trial. Controversial instances in which even surrogate consent is waived to conduct research highlight concerns in this area. For example, the study of an artificial blood substitute, PolyHeme, challenges whether patients who lack capacity to consent can be ethically enrolled in any research. In general, enrollment of decisionally incapacitated patients in research where the risks are greater than minimal can only be undertaken when the patient might benefit directly and there are appropriate safeguards. In these cases, the level of justification for enrollment by a surrogate decision maker must meet a higher standard due to the increased degree of uncertainty of harm.

Advance directives for research constitutes one proposal to provide guidance to surrogates and healthcare providers about whether to enroll someone in clinical research. In such directives, a patient agrees to participate in research in general while they have decision-making capacity and before a decision must be made. Despite the attempt by the National Institutes of Health to use these documents, they are very rare and often offer little help in making particular decisions about unique, unanticipatable circumstances. In the end, the decision concerning whether to enroll an incapacitated patient into research falls to the healthcare provider and healthcare surrogate. In rare instances, states have prohibited this type of enrollment in an effort to provide protection from abuse to vulnerable populations. This protection may actually harm patients by not allowing them access to potential therapies in situations without a good treatment standard.

The protections for vulnerable populations were developed in the historical context of significant abuses and a recognition that the clinician researcher may have conflicting motivations. In cases of high-abuse potential or significant harms, a surrogate decision maker may be augmented by a patient advocate or a special independent review committee. A third-party moderator provides a perspective less entangled by the emotional responsibility to the particular person when assessing the level of acceptable risk. These third parties generally have the power to exclude patients from research participation but cannot demand their inclusion.

Controversies

Controversies in surrogate consent include fluctuations in patient capacity, retention of some capacity, evaluation of surrogates for capacity, and variations of standards by country and culture. For some illnesses, a patient's capacity to understand fluctuates over time. In these cases, a patient may have the ability to participate at one point but not at another. For example, a patient may understand the situation in the morning but not later the same day or the next day. Except in emergency cases, capacity assessments should be performed over a length of time before the utilization of a surrogate for decision making. In cases where capacity may soon be lost, every effort should be made to consent a patient during a lucid time for anticipatable events. It is illegitimate to rely on a surrogate out of simple ease when direct consent can be attained.

Although most literature on surrogate cases describes unconscious patients as the paradigm for discussion, there are many instances where patients retain (or develop) degrees of capacity. In these cases, the surrogate and healthcare providers should allow degrees of patient participation. For instance, a normal teenager who requires a surrogate for legal reasons should still be included in the discussion about healthcare matters. Similarly, a mildly demented patient may still be able to provide broad input on values and pleasures. These cases create increasingly complicated situations for interpreting whether patient expressions are appropriate for consideration in the particular decision.

When a surrogate decision maker is identified, he or she is assumed to have decision-making capacity. However, this assumption may be challenged when inconsistent decision making arises. The healthcare provider must grapple with how to assure that good decision making occurs, while respecting the surrogate. Since the surrogate is not a patient, there may be a limited ability to formally evaluate the surrogate for cognitive capacity. In removing a surrogate from the decision-making role, the healthcare provider must articulate clear reasons for doing so beyond a simple disagreement of choice.

Finally, the way in which surrogates act may vary considerably by region and culture. This becomes most trying when there are mismatched expectations of surrogate decision making between patients and the generally accepted model within the region in which they are being treated. For instance, in the United States, competent patients are fully informed and make their own decisions. However, there are cultures in which healthcare decisions are deferred to a surrogate, often a husband, father, or eldest son. The healthcare provider must adjudicate when the patient has opted out of a cultural background and the degree to which the tradition might be considered unjust. Healthcare providers should carefully account for these various complexities when relying on surrogates.

Conclusion

A surrogate decision maker may be called on to make a variety of difficult decisions. Although only research and life and death decisions have been discussed, a similar set of issues may be applied to choices of quality of life, which may include where to send patients to reside for their best healthcare and social benefit. Because of the general value of patient participation in decision making, there is always a preference to avoid the need for surrogate decision making. However, when there are no better alternatives, the surrogate has an obligation to decide carefully, and the healthcare provider has an obligation to confirm that the surrogate enacts the role properly.

Margot M. Eves and Paul J. Ford

See also Advance Directives and End-of-Life Decision Making; Bioethics

Further Readings

Hyun, I. (2002). Waiver of informed consent, cultural sensitivity, and the problem of unjust families and traditions. *The Hastings Center Report, 32*(5), 14–22.

Kim, S. Y., Appelbaum, P. S., Jeste, D. V., & Olin, J. T. (2004). Proxy and surrogate consent in geriatric neuropsychiatric research: Update and recommendations. *American Journal of Psychiatry, 161*(5), 797–806.

Muthappan, P., Forster, H., & Wendler, D. (2005). Research advance directives: Protection or obstacle? *American Journal of Psychiatry, 162*(12), 2389–2391.

Rabow, M. W., Hauser, J. M., & Adams, J. (2004). Supporting family caregivers at the end of life: "They don't know what they don't know." *Journal of the American Medical Association, 291*(4), 483–491.

Stocking, C. B., Hougham, G. W., Danner, D. D., Patterson, M. B., Whitehouse, P. J., & Sachs, G. A. (2006). Speaking of research advance directives: Planning for future research participation. *Neurology, 66*(9), 1361–1366.

Tulsky, J. A. (2005). Beyond advance directives, importance of communication skills and the end of life. *Journal of the American Medical Association, 294*(3), 359–366.

Decision Tree: Introduction

A decision tree is a powerful method for classification and prediction and for facilitating decision making in sequential decision problems. This entry considers three types of decision trees in some detail. The first is an algorithm for a recommended course of action based on a sequence of information nodes; the second is classification and regression trees; and the third is survival trees.

Decision Trees

Often the medical decision maker will be faced with a sequential decision problem involving decisions that lead to different outcomes depending on chance. If the decision process involves many sequential decisions, then the decision problem becomes difficult to visualize and to implement. Decision trees are indispensable graphical tools in such settings. They allow for intuitive understanding of the problem and can aid in decision making.

A decision tree is a graphical model describing decisions and their possible outcomes. Decision trees consist of three types of nodes (see Figure 1):

1. *Decision node:* Often represented by squares showing decisions that can be made. Lines emanating from a square show all distinct options available at a node.

2. *Chance node:* Often represented by circles showing chance outcomes. Chance outcomes are events that can occur but are outside the ability of the decision maker to control.

3. *Terminal node:* Often represented by triangles or by lines having no further decision nodes or chance nodes. Terminal nodes depict the final outcomes of the decision making process.

For example, a hospital performing esophagectomies (surgical removal of all or part of the esophagus) for patients with esophageal cancer wishes to define a protocol for what constitutes an adequate lymphadenectomy in terms of total number of regional lymph nodes removed at surgery. The hospital believes that such a protocol should be guided by pathology (available to the surgeon prior to surgery). This information should include histopathologic cell type (squamous cell carcinoma or adenocarcinoma); histopathologic grade (a crude indicator of tumor biology); and depth of tumor invasion (PT classification). It is believed that number of nodes to be removed should increase with more deeply invasive tumors when histopathologic grade is poorly differentiated and that number of nodes differs by cell type.

The decision tree in this case is composed predominantly of chance outcomes, these being the results from pathology (cell type, grade, and tumor depth). The surgeon's only decision is whether to perform the esophagectomy. If the decision is made to operate, then the surgeon follows this decision line on the graph, moving from left to right, using pathology data to eventually determine the terminal node. The terminal node, or final outcome, is number of lymph nodes to be removed.

Decision trees can in some instances be used to make optimal decisions. To do so, the terminal nodes in the decision tree must be assigned terminal values (sometimes called payoff values or endpoint values). For example, one approach is to assign values to each decision branch and chance branch and define a terminal value as the sum of branch values leading to it. Once terminal values are assigned, tree values are calculated by following terminal values from right to left. To calculate the value of chance outcomes, multiply by their probability. The total for a chance node is the total of these values. To determine the value of a decision node, the cost of each option along each decision line is subtracted from the cost already calculated. This value represents the benefit of the decision.

Classification Trees

In many medical settings, the medical decision maker may not know what the decision rule is. Rather, he or she would like to discover the decision rule by using data. In such settings, decision trees are often referred to as classification trees. Classification trees apply to data where the *y*-value (outcome) is a classification label, such as the disease status of a patient, and the medical decision maker would like to construct a decision rule that predicts the outcome using *x*-variables (dependent variables) available in the data. Because the data set available is just one sample of the underlying

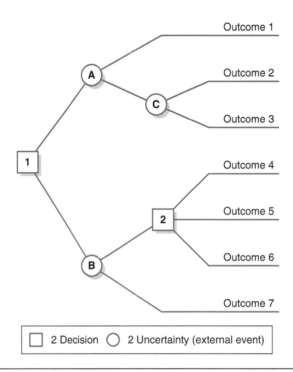

Figure 1   Decision trees are graphical models for describing sequential decision problems.

population, it is desirable to construct a decision rule that is accurate not only for the data at hand but over external data as well (i.e., the decision rule should have good prediction performance). At the same time, it is helpful to have a decision rule that is understandable. That is, it should not be so complex that the decision maker is left with a black box. Decision trees offer a reasonable way to resolve these two conflicting needs.

Background

The use of tree methods for classification has a history that dates back at least 40 years. Much of the early work emanated from the area of social sciences, starting in the late 1960s, and computational algorithms for automatic construction of classification trees began as early as the 1970s. Algorithms such as the THAID program developed at the Institute for Social Research, University of Michigan, laid the groundwork for recursive partitioning algorithms, the predominate algorithm used by modern-day tree classifiers, such as Classification and Regression Tree (CART).

An Example

Classification trees are decision trees derived using recursive partitioning data algorithms that classify each incoming x-data point (case) into one of the class labels for the outcome. A classification tree consists of three types of nodes (see Figure 2):

1. *Root node:* The top node of the tree comprising all the data.

2. *Splitting node:* A node that assigns data to a subgroup.

3. *Terminal node:* Final decision (outcome).

Figure 2 is a CART tree constructed using the breast cancer databases obtained from the University of Wisconsin Hospitals, Madison (available from http://archive.ics.uci.edu/ml). In total, the data comprise 699 patients classified as having either benign or malignant breast cancer. The goal here is to predict true disease status based on nine different variables collected from biopsy.

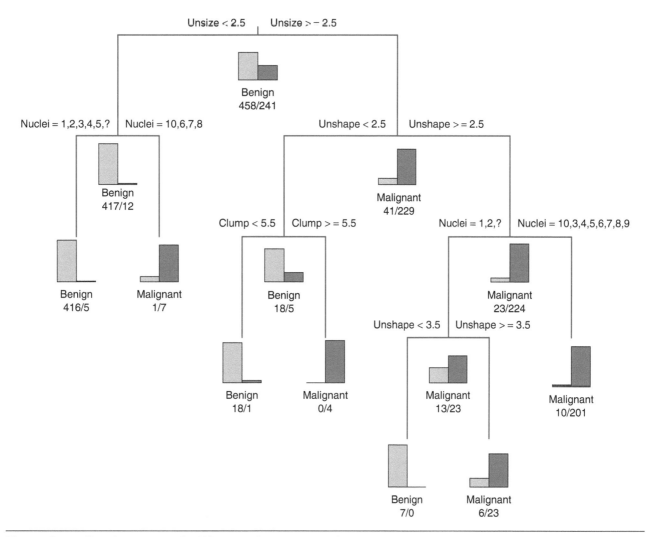

Figure 2   Classification tree for Wisconsin breast cancer data

Note: Light-shaded and dark-shaded barplots show frequency of data at each node for the two classes: benign (light shaded); malignant (dark shaded). Terminal nodes are classified by majority voting (i.e., assignment is made to the class label having the largest frequency). Labels in black given above a splitting node show how data are split depending on a given variable. In some cases, there are missing data, which are indicated by a question mark.

The first split of the tree (at the root node) is on the variable "unsize," measuring uniformity of cell size. All patients having values less than 2.5 for this variable are assigned to the left node (the left daughter node); otherwise they are assigned to the right node (right daughter node). The left and right daughter nodes are then split (in this case, on the variable "unshape" for the right daughter node and on the variable "nuclei" for the left daughter node), and patients are assigned to subgroups defined by these splits. These nodes are then split, and the process is repeated recursively in a procedure called recursive partitioning. When the tree construction is completed, terminal nodes are assigned class labels by majority voting (the class label with the largest frequency). Each patient in a given terminal node is assigned the predicted class label for that terminal node. For example, the leftmost terminal node in Figure 2 is assigned the class label "benign" because 416 of the 421 cases in the node have that label. Looking at Figure 2, one can see that voting heavily favors one class over the other for all terminal nodes, showing that the decision tree is accurately classifying the data. However, it is important to assess accuracy using external data sets or by using cross-validation as well.

Recursive Partitioning

In general, recursive partitioning works as follows. The classification tree is grown starting at the root node, which is the top node of the tree, comprising all the data. The root node is split into two daughter nodes: a left and a right daughter node. In turn, each daughter node is split, with each split giving rise to left and right daughters. The process is repeated in a recursive fashion until the tree cannot be partitioned further due to lack of data or some stopping criterion is reached, resulting in a collection of terminal nodes. The terminal nodes represent a partition of the predictor space into a collection of rectangular regions that do not overlap. It should be noted, though, that this partition may be quite different than what might be found by exhaustively searching over all partitions corresponding to the same number of terminal nodes. However, for many problems, exhaustive searches for globally optimal partitions (in the sense of producing the most homogeneous leaves) are not computationally feasible, and recursive partitioning represents an effective way of undertaking this task by using a one-step procedure instead.

A classification tree as described above is referred to as a *binary recursive partitioned tree*. Another type of recursively partitioned tree is multiway recursive partitioned tree. Rather than splitting the parent node into two daughter nodes, such trees use multiway splits that define multiple daughter nodes. However, there is little evidence that multiway splits produce better classifiers, and for this reason, as well as for their simplicity, binary recursive partitioned trees are often favored.

Splitting Rules

The success of CART as a classifier can be largely attributed to the manner in which splits are formed in the tree construction. To define a good split, CART uses an impurity function to measure the decrease in tree impurity for a split. The purity of a tree is a measure of how similar observations in the leaves are to one another. The best split for a node is found by searching over all possible variables and all possible split values and choosing that variable and split that reduces impurity the most. Reduction of tree impurity is a good principle because it encourages the tree to push dissimilar cases apart. Eventually, as the number of nodes increases, and dissimilar cases become separated into daughter nodes, each node in the tree becomes homogeneous and is populated by cases with similar outcomes (recall Figure 2).

There are several impurity functions used. These include the twoing criterion, the entropy criterion, and the gini index. The gini index is arguably the most popular. When the outcome has two class labels (the so-called two-class problem), the gini index corresponds to the variance of the outcome if the class labels are recoded as being 0 and 1.

Stopping Rules

The size of the tree is crucial to the accuracy of the classifier. If the tree is too shallow, terminal nodes will not be pure (outcomes will be heterogeneous), and the accuracy of the classifier will suffer. If the tree is too deep (too many splits), then the number of cases within a terminal node will be small, and the predicted class label will have high variance—again undermining the accuracy of the classifier.

To strike a proper balance, pruning is employed in methodologies such as CART. To determine the optimal size of a tree, the tree is grown to full size (i.e., until all data are spent) and then pruned back. The optimal size is determined using a complexity measure that balances the accuracy of the tree as measured by cost complexity and by the size of the tree.

Regression Trees

Decision trees can also be used to analyze data when the y-outcome is a continuous measurement (such as age, blood pressure, ejection fraction for the heart, etc.). Such trees are called regression trees. Regression trees can be constructed using recursive partitioning similar to classification trees. Impurity is measured using mean-square error. The terminal node values in a regression tree are defined as the mean value (average) of outcomes for patients within the terminal node. This is the predicted value for the outcome.

Survival Trees

Time-to-event data are often encountered in the medical sciences. For such data, the analysis focuses on understanding how time-to-event varies in terms of different variables that might be collected for a patient. Time-to-event can be time to death from a certain disease, time until recurrence (for cancer), time until first occurrence of a symptom, or simple all-cause mortality.

The analysis of time-to-event data is often complicated by the presence of censoring. Generally speaking, this means that the event times for some individuals in a study are not observed exactly and are only known to fall within certain time intervals. Right censoring is one of the most common types of censoring encountered. This occurs when the event of interest is observed only if it occurs prior to some prespecified time. For example, a patient might be monitored for 2 weeks without occurrence of a symptom and then released from a hospital. Such a patient is said to be right censored because the time-to-event must exceed 2 weeks, but the exact event time is unknown. Another example of right censoring occurs when patients enter a study at different times and the study is predetermined to end by a certain time. Then, all patients who do not experience an event within the study period are right censored.

Decision trees can be used to analyze right-censored survival data. Such trees are referred to as survival trees. Survival trees can be constructed using recursive partitioning. The measure of impurity plays a key role, as in CART, and this can be defined in many ways. One popular approach is to

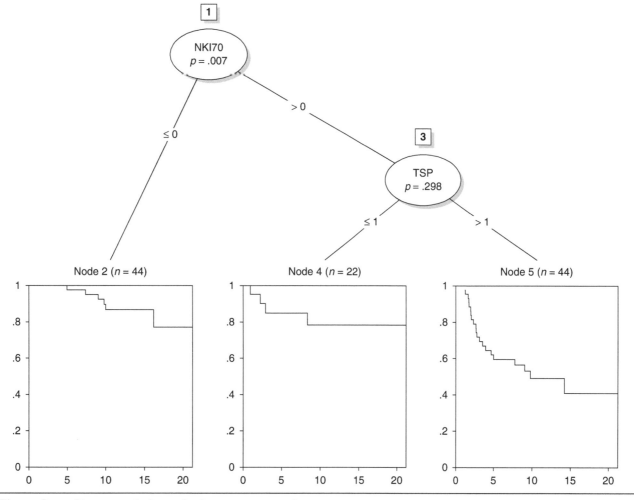

Figure 3   Binary survival tree for breast cancer patients

Note: Dependent variables NKI70 and TSP are gene signatures. For example, extreme right terminal node (Node 5) corresponds to presence of both the NKI70 and TSP gene signatures. Underneath each terminal node are Kaplan-Meier survival curves for patients within that node.

define impurity using the log-rank test. As in CART, growing a tree by reducing impurity ensures that terminal nodes are populated by individuals with similar behavior. In the case of a survival tree, terminal nodes are composed of patients with similar survival. The terminal node value in a survival tree is the survival function and is estimated using those patients within the terminal node. This differs from classification and regression trees, where terminal node values are a single value (the estimated class label or predicted value for the response, respectively). Figure 3 shows an example of a survival tree.

Hemant Ishwaran and J. Sunil Rao

See also Decision Trees, Advanced Techniques in Constructing; Recursive Partitioning

Further Readings

Breiman, L., Friedman, J. H., Olshen, R. A., & Stone, C. J. (1984). *Classification and regression trees.* Belmont, CA: Wadsworth.

LeBlanc, M., & Crowley, J. (1993). Survival trees by goodness of split. *Journal of the American Statistical Association, 88,* 457–467.

Segal, M. R. (1988). Regression trees for censored data. *Biometrics, 44,* 35–47.

Stone, M. (1974). Cross-validatory choice and assessment of statistical predictions. *Journal of the Royal Statistical Society, Series B, 36,* 111–147.

DECISION TREES, ADVANCED TECHNIQUES IN CONSTRUCTING

Decision trees such as classification, regression, and survival trees offer the medical decision maker a comprehensive way to calculate predictors and decision rules in a variety of commonly encountered data settings. However, performance of decision trees on external data sets can sometimes be poor. Aggregating decision trees is a simple way to improve performance—and in some instances, aggregated tree predictors can exhibit state-of-the-art performance.

Decision Boundary

Decision trees, by their very nature, are simple and intuitive to understand. For example, a binary classification tree assigns data by dropping a data point (case) down the tree and moving either left or right through nodes depending on the value of a given variable. The nature of a binary tree ensures that each case is assigned to a unique terminal node. The value for the terminal node (the predicted outcome) defines how the case is classified. By following the path as a case moves down the tree to its terminal node, the *decision rule* for that case can be read directly off the tree. Such a rule is simple to understand, as it is nothing more than a sequence of simple rules strung together.

The *decision boundary*, on the other hand, is a more abstract concept. Decision boundaries are estimated by a collection of decision rules for cases taken together—or, in the case of decision trees, the boundary produced in the predictor space between classes by the decision tree. Unlike decision rules, decision boundaries are difficult to visualize and interpret for data involving more than one or two variables. However, when the data involve only a few variables, the decision boundary is a powerful way to visualize a classifier and to study its performance.

Consider Figure 1. On the left-hand side is the classification tree for a prostate data set. Here, the outcome is presence or absence of prostate cancer and the independent variables are prostate-specific antigen (PSA) and tumor volume, both having been transformed on the log scale. Each case in the data is classified uniquely depending on the value of these two variables. For example, the leftmost terminal node in Figure 1 is composed of those patients with tumor volumes less than 7.851 and PSA levels less than 2.549 (on the log scale). Terminal node values are assigned by majority voting (i.e., the predicted outcome is the class label with the largest frequency). For this node, there are 54 nondiseased patients and 16 diseased patients, and thus, the predicted class label is nondiseased.

The right-hand side of Figure 1 displays the decision boundary for the tree. The dark-shaded region is the space of all values for PSA and tumor volume that would be classified as nondiseased, whereas the light-shaded regions are those values classified as diseased. Superimposed on the figure,

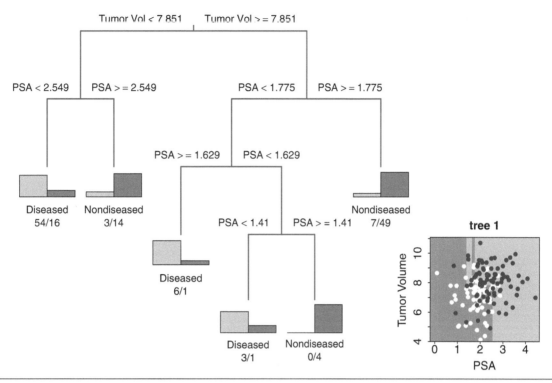

Figure 1   Decision tree (left-hand side) and decision boundary (right-hand side) for prostate cancer data with prostate-specific antigen (PSA) and tumor volume as independent variables (both transformed on the log scale)

Note: Barplots under terminal nodes of the decision tree indicate proportion of cases classified as diseased or nondiseased, with the predicted class label determined by majority voting. Decision boundary shows how the tree classifies a new patient based on PSA and tumor volume. Gray-shaded points identify diseased patients, and white points identify nondiseased patients from the data.

using white and light-gray dots, are the observed data points from the original data. Light-gray points are truly diseased patients, whereas white points are truly nondiseased patients. Most of the light-gray points fall in the light-shaded region of the decision space and, likewise, most of the white points fall in the dark-shaded region of the decision space, thus showing that the classifier is classifying a large fraction of the data correctly. Some data points are misclassified, though. For example, there are several light-gray points in the center of the plot falling in the dark-shaded region. As well, there are four light-gray points with small tumor volumes and PSA values falling in the dark-shaded region. The misclassified data points in the center of the decision space are especially troublesome. These points are being misclassified because the decision space for the tree is rectangular. If the decision boundary were smoother, then these points would not be misclassified. The nonsmooth

nature of the decision boundary is a well-known deficiency of classification trees and can seriously degrade performance, especially in complex decision problems involving many variables.

Instability of Decision Trees

Decision trees, such as classification trees, are known to be unstable. That is, if the original data set is changed (perturbed) in some way, then the classifier constructed from the altered data can be surprisingly different from the original classifier. This is an undesirable property, especially if small perturbations to the data lead to substantial differences.

This property can be demonstrated using the prostate data set of Figure 1. However, to show this, it is important to first agree on a method for perturbing the data. One technique that can be used is to employ bootstrap resampling. A bootstrap sample is a special type of resampling procedure. A data point is randomly selected from the data and then returned. This process is repeated *n* times, where *n* is the sample size. The resulting bootstrap sample consists of *n* data points but will contain replicated data. On average, a bootstrap sample draws only approximately 63% of the original data.

A total of 1,000 different bootstrap samples of the prostate data were drawn. A classification tree was calculated for each of these 1,000 samples. The top panel of plots in Figure 2 shows decision boundaries for four of these trees (bootstrap samples 2, 5, 25, and 1,000; note that Tree 1 is the classification tree from Figure 1 based on the original data). One can see clearly that the decision spaces differ quite substantially—thus providing clear evidence of the instability.

It is also interesting to note how some of the trees have better decision spaces than the original tree (recall Figure 1; also see Tree 1 in Figure 2). For example, Trees 2, 5, 25, and 1,000 identify some or all of the four problematic light-gray points appearing within the lower quadrant of the dark-shaded region of the original decision space. As well, Trees 5, 25, and, 1,000 identify some of the problematic green points appearing within the center of the original decision space.

An important lesson that emerges from this example is not only that decision trees can be unstable but also that trees constructed from different perturbations of the original data can produce decision boundaries that in some instances have better behavior than the original decision space (over certain regions). Thus, it stands to reason that, if one could combine many such trees, the classifier formed by aggregating the trees might have better overall performance. In other words, *the whole may be greater than the sum of the parts* and one may be able to capitalize on the inherent instability using aggregation to produce more accurate classifiers.

Bagging

This idea in fact is the basis for a powerful method referred to as "bootstrap aggregation," or simply "bagging." Bagging can be used for many kinds of predictors, not just decision trees. The basic premise for bagging is that, if the underlying predictor is unstable, then aggregating the predictor over multiple bootstrap samples will produce a more accurate, and more stable, procedure.

To bag a classification tree, the procedure is as follows (bagging can be applied to regression trees and survival trees in a similar fashion):

1. Draw a bootstrap sample of the original data.

2. Construct a classification tree using data from Step 1.

3. Repeat Steps 1 and 2 many times, independently.

4. Calculate an aggregated classifier using the trees formed in Steps 1 to 3. Use majority voting to classify a case. Thus, to determine the predicted outcome for a case, take the majority vote over the predicted outcomes from each tree in Steps 1 to 3.

The bottom panel of plots in Figure 2 shows the decision boundary for the bagged classifier as a function of number of trees (based on the same prostate data as before). The first plot is the original classifier based on all the data (Tree 1). The second plot is the bagged classifier composed of Tree 1 and the bootstrap tree derived using the first bootstrap sample. The third plot is the bagged classifier using Tree 1 and the first four bootstrapped trees, and so forth. As number of trees increases, the bagged classifier becomes more refined. Even the decision boundary for the bagged classifier using only five trees (third plot) is substantially smoother than the original classifier and is able to better classify problematic cases. By 1,000 trees (last plot), the bagged classifier's decision boundary is fully defined. The accuracy of the bagged classifier is substantially better than any single bootstrapped tree. Table 1 records the misclassification (error) rate for the bagged predictor against the averaged error rate for the 1,000 bootstrapped trees. The first column is the overall error rate, the second column is the error rate for diseased patients, and the third column is the error rate for nondiseased patients. Error rates were calculated using out-of-bag data. Recall that each bootstrap sample uses on average 67% of the original data. The remaining 33% of the data is called out-of-bag and serves as test data, as it is not used in constructing the tree. Table 1 shows that

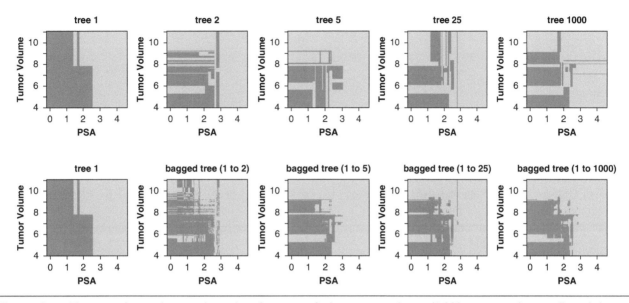

Figure 2   Top row shows decision boundary for a specific bootstrapped tree (1,000 trees used in total), and the bottom plot shows different aggregated (bagged) decision trees

Note: Bagged trees are more robust to noise (stable) because they utilize information from more than one tree. The most stable bagged tree is the one on the extreme right-hand side and shows decision boundary using 1,000 trees.

the bagged classifier is substantially more accurate than any given tree.

Random Forests

"Random forests" is a refinement of bagging that can yield even more accurate predictors. The method works like bagging by using bootstrapping and aggregation but includes an additional step that is designed to encourage independence of trees. This effect is often most pronounced when the data contain many variables.

To create a random forest classifier, the procedure is as follows (regression forests and random survival forests can be constructed using the same principle):

1. Draw a bootstrap sample of the original data.

2. Construct a classification tree using data from Step 1. For each node in the tree, determine the optimal split for the node using M randomly selected dependent variables.

3. Repeat Steps 1 and 2 many times, independently.

4. Calculate an aggregated classifier using the trees formed in Steps 1 to 3. Use majority voting to

classify a case. Thus, to determine the predicted outcome for a case, take the majority vote over the predicted outcomes from each tree in Steps 1 to 3.

Step 2 is the crucial step distinguishing forests from bagging. Unlike bagging, each bootstrapped tree is constructed using different variables, and not all variables are used (at most M are used at each node in the tree growing process). Considerable empirical evidence has shown that forests can be substantially more accurate because of this feature.

Boosting

Boosting is another related technique that has some similarities to bagging although its connection is not as direct. It too can produce accurate

Table 1   Misclassification error rate (in percentage) for bagged classifier (1,000 trees) and single tree classifier

Classifier	All	Diseased	Nondiseased
Bagged tree	27.2	28.8	25.9
Single tree	34.9	36.7	33.0

classifiers through a combination of reweighting and aggregation. To create a boosted tree classifier, the following procedure can be used (although other methods are also available in the literature):

1. Draw a bootstrap sample from the original data giving each observation equal chance (i.e., weight) of appearing in the sample.

2. Build a classification tree using the bootstrap data and classify each of the observations, keeping track of which ones are classified incorrectly or correctly.

3. For those observations that were incorrectly classified, increase their weight and correspondingly decrease the weight assigned to observations that were correctly classified.

4. Draw another bootstrap sample using the newly updated observation weights (i.e., those observations that were previously incorrectly classified will have a greater chance of appearing in the next bootstrap sample).

5. Repeat Steps 2 to 4 many times.

6. Calculate an aggregated classifier using the trees formed in Steps 1 to 5. Use majority voting to classify a case. Thus, to determine the predicted outcome for a case, take the majority vote over the predicted outcomes from each tree in Steps 1 to 5.

The idea of reweighting observations adaptively is a key to boosting's performance gains. In a sense, the algorithm tends to focus more and more on observations that are difficult to classify. There has been much work in the literature on studying the operating characteristics of boosting, primarily motivated by the fact that the approach can produce significant gains in prediction accuracy over a single tree classifier. Again, as with bagging, boosting is a general algorithm that can be applied to more than tree-based classifiers. While these aggregation algorithms were initially thought to destroy the simple interpretable structure (topology) produced by a single tree classifier, recent work has shown that, in fact, treelike structures (with respect to the decision boundary) are often maintained, and interpretable structure about how

the predictors interact with one another can still be gleaned.

Hemant Ishwaran and J. Sunil Rao

See also Decision Tree: Introduction; Recursive Partitioning

Further Readings

Breiman, L. (1996). Bagging predictors. *Machine Learning, 26,* 123–140.

Breiman, L. (2001). Random forests. *Machine Learning, 45,* 5–32.

Breiman, L., Friedman, J. H., Olshen, R. A., & Stone, C. J. (1984). *Classification and regression trees.* Belmont, CA: Wadsworth.

Efron, B. (1982). *The jackknife, the bootstrap and other resampling plans* (Society for Industrial and Applied Mathematics CBMS-NSF Monographs, No. 38). Philadelphia: SIAM.

Freund, Y., & Shapire, R. E. (1996). Experiments with a new boosting algorithm. In *Machine Learning: Proceedings of the 13th International Conference* (pp. 148–156). San Francisco: Morgan Kaufman.

Ishwaran, H., Kogalur, U. B., Blackstone, E. H., & Lauer, M. S. (2008). Random survival forests. *Annals of Applied Statistics, 2*(3), 841–860.

Rao, J. S., & Potts, W. J. E. (1997). Visualizing bagged decision trees. In *Proceedings of the 3rd International Conference on Knowledge Discovery and Data Mining* (pp. 243–246). Newport Beach, CA: AAAI Press.

DECISION TREES, CONSTRUCTION

A decision model is a mathematical formulation of a decision problem that compares alternative choices in a formal process by calculating their expected outcome. The decision tree is a graphical representation of a decision model that represents the basic elements of the model. The key elements of the model are the possible *choices, information* about chance events, and *preferences* of the decision maker. The choices are the alternatives being compared in the decision model. The information consists of an enumeration of the events that may occur consequent to the choice and the probabilities of each of their outcomes. Preferences are captured by assessing utilities of each outcome that measure the desirability of each outcome. In addition to a utility, each outcome may be associated with a financial cost.

The decision tree is a convenient method, analogous to a high-level graphical language, of specifying the elements of the decision model in a way that leads naturally to a method for quantitatively evaluating the alternative choices, in a process known as averaging out and folding back the tree.

Formulating the Problem

Decision tree construction requires a properly formulated *decision problem*.

Decision Context

The first step is determining the context of the decision. This consists, at a minimum, of the clinical problem (e.g., chest pain), the healthcare setting (e.g., a hospital emergency room), and any characteristics of the patient to which the analysis is restricted (e.g., the age range, gender, or existing comorbid conditions). The context also specifies the timeframe being considered.

Specific Question

The second step is formulating a specific question that is to be answered by the decision analysis. It must be a comparison of specific alternative actions that are available to the decision maker. In healthcare decision making, choices generally involve diagnostic tests and treatments. An example of a clearly formulated decision is whether a patient with a suspected condition should be observed without treatment, given a diagnostic test, or treated empirically. Each choice must be unique. Choices may also contain combinations of actions with later decisions contingent on results of tests or outcomes of observation. These combinations of choices are referred to as *policies*. Typically, decision models involve multiple successive choices, which, in combinations, correspond to alternate policies. These combinations may differ according to the specific elements (e.g., one test or treatment as compared with another) or according to how these elements are applied (e.g., using differing rules for responding to the outcome of a diagnostic test or varying the amount of time before contingent action is taken). For these reasons, the number of decision alternatives that can be considered in a decision model can become very large as the number of combinations of the various factors increases.

Node Types

Standard decision trees contain three basic types of nodes. Decision nodes are typically represented by an open square, chance nodes by an open circle, and terminal nodes by rectangular boxes. Branches are represented as straight lines connecting nodes.

Overall Tree Structure

A simple decision tree is shown in Figure 1. By convention, the root of the tree is a decision node and is represented at the left of the figure, and the terminal nodes (referred to as the "leaves" of the tree) are at the right. According to conventions for drawing decision models that are published in the journal *Medical Decision Making* in the first issue of each year, lines representing branches of the same node are parallel and vertically aligned. *Medical Decision Making* also specifies that the branches should be attached to lines at right angles to nodes, as in Figure 1, but a common variation uses a fan of angled lines from each node leading directly to branches, as in Figure 2.

There can be any number of branches of a decision node as long as they represent distinct alternatives. The branches of a chance node must represent a *mutually exclusive* and *collectively exhaustive* set of events. In other words, the branches must all represent distinct events, and the set of branches must cover all possible outcomes at the chance node. Consequently, the probabilities of the branches must sum to exactly 1. There is no universal convention for the order in which the branches of a node appear. Branches of decision nodes are specified in an order that makes clinical sense to the analyst, keeping in mind that this order will determine the order in which the expected value of each branch is displayed after evaluation. When there are many choices, they may be arranged so that groups of similar strategies are adjacent. Branches of chance nodes are usually arranged so that if there are branches

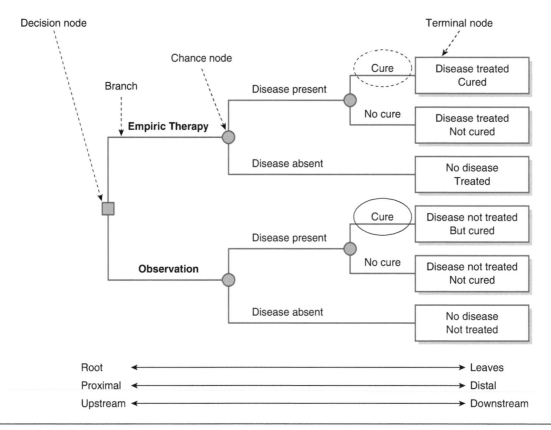

Figure 1   Example decision tree

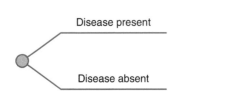

Figure 2   Alternate format for branches

representing occurrence of specific events, they appear on top, and the branch representing nonoccurrence of a specific event is last; however, the order makes no difference to the evaluation when a complete set of probabilities is specified.

Branches are labeled with the names of the choices or events they represent. Terminal nodes may be labeled with a symbolic description of the outcome, as in Figure 1, or with an expression indicating the value or utility of the outcome, as in Figure 3. Branches of chance nodes may also be labeled with the probability of that branch as shown in Figure 4. Note that the probability of "disease present" is the same for both decision branches, but the probability of "cure" is higher

for the "empiric treatment" than for "observation." Similarly, utilities can be represented by numbers as shown in Figure 4. The lowest utility is for the worst outcome, which is having the disease, being treated, but not being cured. The highest utility is for the best outcome, which is being observed and not having the disease. Others are intermediate, and their exact values will depend on the specifics of the disease and the treatment. For example, the utility loss due to untreated disease may be worse than the utility loss due to the treatment.

Elements of the model that require assignment of quantitative values (probabilities, utilities, and others) are called model *parameters*.

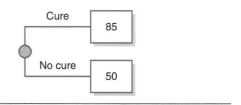

Figure 3   Numerical utilities

Navigation and Orientation

Upstream Versus Downstream

Nodes and branches closer to the root of the tree are said to be *proximal* or *upstream*. Those farther from the root are said to be *distal* or *downstream*. The designation of upstream versus downstream has additional meaning in terms of applying bindings and context-specific variables. A *path* through the tree is defined as the sequence of nodes and branches between any two points in the tree. In general, proximal events occur earlier in time than distal events, but this is not an absolute rule, and nodes at many levels of the tree may represent events that occur simultaneously.

Tree Context

The context of a branch or node in a decision tree is defined as the path from the root of the tree to that branch or node and incorporates all the decisions and consequences that precede them. So, for example, in Figure 1, the context of "cure" indicated by the dotted ellipse is (empiric therapy given, disease present, cured), whereas the context of "cure" indicated by the solid ellipse is (observation, disease present, cured). These often differ in their impact on the probabilities of any downstream events and in determinants of the utilities of the terminal nodes or economic costs.

Variables and Expressions

In the above discussion, probabilities and utilities were expressed either as descriptive labels (Figure 1) or as numerical quantities (Figure 4). It is convenient to represent these quantities symbolically using mathematical expressions composed of variables (Figure 5). There are several reasons for using symbolic variables:

1. To express the model in terms of the meanings of values, allowing alternate values to be specified as input.

2. To facilitate sensitivity analysis by allowing model parameters to vary systematically. For example, the value of pDIS represents the probability of disease and can be varied to determine how the model is affected by changes in disease prevalence.

3. To permit values in specific tree contexts to depend systematically on previous, upstream values. The value of pCure in contexts downstream from "Empiric Treatment" will differ from the value of pCure in contexts downstream from "Observation."

4. To permit the use of subtrees that permit reusing elements of tree structure while allowing values of parameters to change.

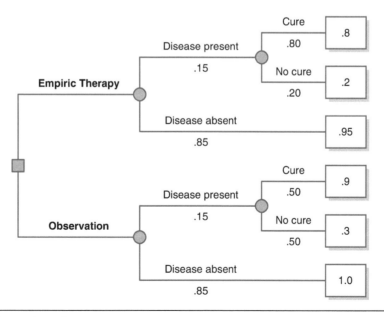

Figure 4   Probabilities on branches

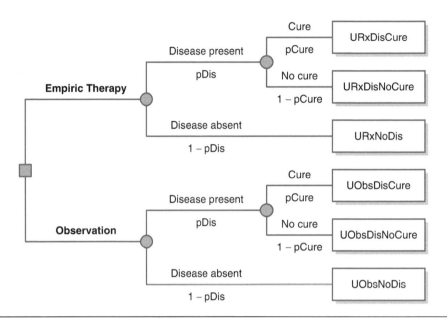

Figure 5   Symbolic probabilities and utilities

5. To express and maintain relationships (*linkage*) between variables during model evaluation using mathematical expressions, thus promoting greater consistency and clarity. This is especially important when parameters are defined functionally, rather than prespecified. For example, the posttest probability of disease may be calculated from the pretest probability in terms of the sensitivity and specificity of a diagnostic test. This not only ensures that the posttest probability is calculated correctly, but linkage of these variables avoids errors during sensitivity analysis. It would be incorrect to vary only the pretest probability of disease or the test sensitivity without also varying the posttest probability. Variables and expressions ensure that these relationships are maintained as models are constructed, modified, and evaluated.

6. To maintain internal statistics of the events that occur at various points in a model.

Expressions

The use of algebraic expressions to express probabilities and utilities permits building them up systematically from more elemental parameters.

More complicated expressions can be constructed in models using a variety of mathematical operators and functions. Application of Bayes's rule is one example. Other examples include the computation of disease prevalence and probabilities in terms of varying factors such as age, and calculating costs as a function of events in specific tree contexts, and employing counting and tracking variables to determine whether and how often specific events occur in a model. Modern decision analysis software implements a full complement of mathematical operators and functions, permitting a great deal of representational power in creating expressions.

The use of variables rather than fixed parameters also facilitates maintenance of the model by enabling the analyst to make lists of parameters. Entire sets of variables can be substituted in the model to represent distinct scenarios or decision contexts.

Utilities

The values of terminal nodes (leaves) of the tree are referred to generically as utilities. The underlying theory and method of assessing and assigning utilities is discussed elsewhere. In practical terms,

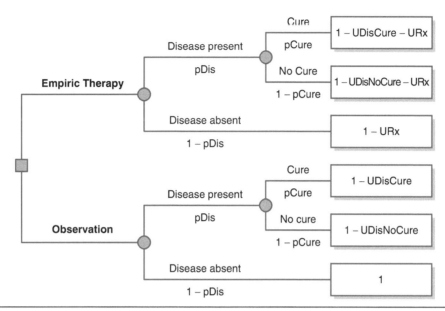

Figure 6   Tree with algebraic expressions

the values of terminal nodes are expressed in terms of health outcomes and financial costs.

The use of algebraic expressions to express utilities is illustrated by the terminal nodes in the tree in Figure 5. There are six unique utilities in this model. While it is feasible to assign each of them a unique variable name as is done in Figure 5, it can be easier to express these utilities in terms

of four parameters as in Figure 6. Each utility is calculated by subtracting all applicable disutilities from 1, the value of the "no disease, no treatment" state. When there is a much larger number of terminal nodes, this approach can greatly simplify the assignment of utilities and can greatly reduce the number of parameters the analyst needs to maintain.

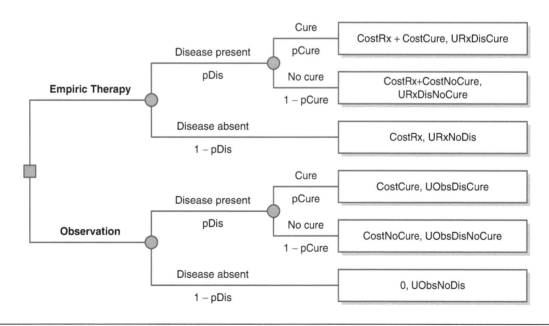

Figure 7   Costs at terminal nodes

Dual Utilities in Cost-Effectiveness Models

In cost-utility analysis, a financial cost must be applied to each path through the tree in addition to its quality measures. Most conveniently, these costs are assigned to the terminal nodes along with the utilities, as shown in Figure 7. Each cost can be calculated as the sum of component costs attributed to treatment, testing, and costs of any of the effects of the disease itself. For the outcome of "observation-disease absent," there are no costs.

Computer Applications for Tree Construction and Evaluation

Several software applications are available for constructing and evaluating decision trees. Using software has many advantages over constructing models manually. By integrating the graphical and mathematical components of the model, such tools greatly speed model construction and minimize errors, allowing much more complicated, clinically realistic models to be considered than would be possible by manual calculation. The ability to load complete sets of variables permits evaluating a model for different scenarios, without manually changing the variables one at a time. Furthermore, the ability to automate the evaluation of models encourages more complete exploration of a model through sensitivity analysis. Graphical representations of models and their results can then be generated, often automatically, for papers and presentations. Models can also be built incrementally and adapted in future applications or work sessions allowing components to be reused, thus providing a systematic means for sharing knowledge and models among analysts.

Frank A. Sonnenberg and C. Gregory Hagerty

See also Cost-Utility Analysis; Decision Trees, Evaluation; Decision Trees: Sensitivity Analysis, Deterministic; Disutility; Expected Utility Theory; Multi-Attribute Utility Theory; Tree Structure, Advanced Techniques

Further Readings

Howard, R. A., & Matheson, J. E. (Eds.). (1984). *The principles and applications of decision analysis, Volume I: Professional collection.* Menlo Park, CA: Strategic Decisions Group.

Information for Authors. (2008). *Medical Decision Making, 28*(1), 157–159.

Pauker, S. G., & Kassirer, J. P. (1981). Clinical decision analysis by personal computer. *Archives of Internal Medicine, 141*(13), 1831.

Sonnenberg, F. A., & Pauker, S. G. (1987). Decision maker: An advanced personal computer tool for clinical decision analysis. *Proceedings of the 11th annual symposium on Computer Applications in Medical Care.* Washington, DC: IEEE Computer Society Press.

DECISION TREES, EVALUATION

A decision tree is a branched structure used as a tool to support decision making by displaying key elements of the choices among alternatives and the consequences of each choice. This entry uses several examples to illustrate the evaluation of decision trees.

The following examples of surgery versus radiation therapy for Stage 1 (early stage) versus Stage 4 (late stage) disease demonstrate the visual benefits of a decision tree without needing to completely elaborate the tree or to perform any calculations. These examples also explore why the decision analyst in charge of the construction and elaboration of a decision tree needs to be in full control of the key aspects of the decisions that may influence (a) the patient's decision in each stage of this disease process, from Stage 1 (early in life) to Stage 4 (later in life), when the disease is identified early enough in a patient's care, or (b) the patient who presents at the time of diagnosis with Stage 1 disease versus the patient who presents at the time of diagnosis with Stage 2 disease. These examples also explore the difficulties in capturing alternative strategies open to patients in a simple decision tree structure.

Decision Tree for Early Stage 1 Disease

The following decision tree lays out the decision for early Stage 1 disease in a patient for whom physicians believe there are two options open: surgery for Stage 1 disease versus radiation for Stage 1 disease. The decision node (■) represents the decision for surgery for Stage 1 disease and radiation therapy for Stage 1 disease (Figure 1).

Even at this point in the elaboration of the decision tree in a patient with early Stage 1 disease, many patients would say that this tree is complete. Because both surgery and radiation therapy have outstanding chances for survival in this individual, complications become the focal point. Here, there would be a shift in discussion away from the decision tree representing short-term survival to discussions related to differences in quality of life after surgery and quality of life after radiation therapy. Here, after hearing about the 100% chance of surgical cure of the disease and the quality of life after surgery and the 97% cure rate for radiation therapy and the complications of radiation therapy, the patient may well decide to accept the surgery without any additional exposition of the decision tree or discussion of quality of life. Here, the demonstrated strength of the decision tree is to show the outcomes and features of the comparison between surgery versus radiation therapy for early Stage 1 disease and a simplification for the patient in understanding options.

Laying Out a Decision Tree

The expression "laying out a decision tree" refers to the structuring of a decision tree, with tree growth through the addition of alternatives, outcomes, and their related chances (probabilities) of occurring. We will now structure a set of decision trees to represent a patient's decision problem related to consideration of surgery versus radiation therapy for a progressive disease. Here, we will represent this progression of disease process and disease state in terms of early disease (labeled Stage 1) to the most severe form (labeled Stage 4). We will also consider an intermediate form of progression of this disease (labeled Stage 3). With consideration of these stages, we will examine two strengths of a decision tree: (1) using a decision tree to help visualize the patient's decision problem and (2) using a decision tree in a calculation to determine which of the two treatments would have a survival advantage in a patient with intermediate Stage 3 disease.

In a more complicated patient with Stage 4 disease, the decision tree might take the form as shown in Figure 2.

Here, the complexity of the decision in terms of the questions raised even at the point of the

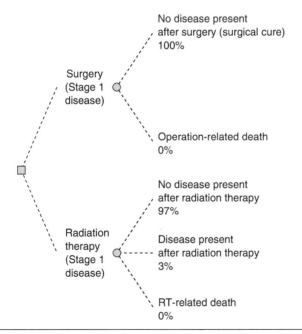

Figure 1   Decision tree for early Stage 1 disease

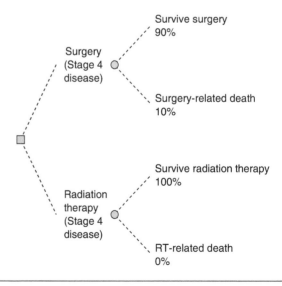

Figure 2   Decision tree for Stage 4 disease

elaboration of the decision tree can be seen. In Stage 4 disease, the patient notes that there is a 10% chance of dying with the surgery and no chance of dying with the radiation therapy and also the suggestion that there is disease still present (which will continue to progress after each therapy).

While one might take this opportunity to further elaborate this tree in terms of the amount of residual disease left after each therapy, another approach would be to see how the disease behaves over time and proceed with an elaboration of a graphical comparison of the 5-year survival curve for surgery and the 5-year survival curve for radiation therapy; the visual comparison of each curve may drive the patient's decision, seeing the difference in 5-year survival at Year 5 after surgery (e.g., 35% of patients sill alive after surgery) in contrast to 5-year survival at Year 5 after radiation therapy (e.g., 25% of patients still alive after radiation therapy).

Here, the patient's decision may be driven by the chance of 5-year survival. However, the 5-year survival curve comparison would also demonstrate the crossover point, which is the point where the shorter-term benefit of survival after radiation therapy is lost and the longer-term benefit of survival after surgery is realized and continues to 5 years, where there would be a 10% 5-year survival benefit at Year 5 with surgery as opposed to radiation therapy (35% − 25% = 10%). Here, a 5-year survival curve comparison between surgery and radiation therapy could be used along with the decision tree to provide the patient fuller information about the decision over time, from Year 0 to Year 5, a time 5 years after the initial treatment.

A decision tree for Stage 3 disease may be more complex because both therapies (a) may not have a clearly defined peer-reviewed medical literature, in contrast to Stage 1 and Stage 4 disease, and (b) there will be more questions about what is going on with survival and quality of life during the time period from Stage 3 to Stage 4 disease (Figure 3).

Given that phase 1 of this decision tree shows the same rates of cure (0%) and disease presence (100%) in this Stage 3 disease, one can simplify the construction by eliminating the first part of the decision tree and move on to Phase 2.

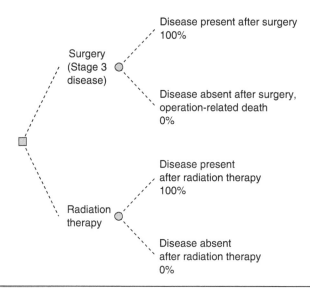

Figure 3   Decision tree for Stage 3 disease, Phase I

Calculating a Decision Tree

Once a decision tree is laid out, it can be evaluated or calculated. One needs to recognize that for many situations where a specific mathematical calculation is not needed, the process of laying out the decision tree (reviewing the peer-reviewed medical scientific literatures, acquiring expert opinion, eliciting an individual's preferences regarding outcomes, and allowing individuals an opportunity to see the risks and benefits associated with alternatives) is a powerful visual procedure in its own right, without the need for any specific mathematical calculation. This laying out of a decision tree may be very useful in areas of consent and informed consent in medicine and in information disclosure in economic and legal contexts. This said, this entry now discusses how a decision tree is evaluated.

Decision Tree Evaluation

The term *decision tree evaluation* usually refers to the calculation of a decision tree. A decision tree is calculated by *folding back* (averaging out or rolling back) the decision tree.

Referring to the above example, in Phase 2 of the decision tree, we go to the peer-reviewed medical literature and find that there are no studies on Stage 3 disease, so we go to local experts (the physicians who actually are doing the surgery and performing the radiotherapy). These local experts may rely on their own data collection on the patients that have been treated in both departments (surgery and radiation therapy), and we need to rely on these data.

From these data, derived from the database in both departments, we see that patients with Stage 3 disease who had surgery on average have 15 years of life expectancy, or 15 life years (LY), and that patients with Stage 3 disease who underwent radiation therapy have 10 years of life expectancy, or 10 LY (Figure 4).

Folding Back the Decision Tree

Once reliable baseline probabilities and outcome values are attained from the peer-reviewed medical scientific literature, expert opinion, and patient preferences (through the elicitation of patient preferences from a standard gamble), the tree is ready to be folded back or rolled back. Theoretically, the expression *folding back* (averaging out or rolling back) the decision tree is an overall calculation that is executed at a particular point in time, when all outcomes are enumerated and listed, all probabilities have been gathered,

and all preferences have been elicited. However, with any expressions where the term *all* is used, as in the above expressions, including *all outcomes*, *all probabilities*, and *all preferences*, caveats are in order and must be examined.

We will now perform the calculations based on the data set obtained from the hospital that is providing the patient's care (Figures 5, 6, and 7).

Based on this decision tree, surgery (13 years − 10 years = 3 years) would offer the patient a better survival than radiation therapy, and for the patient whose primary preference is survival, surgery would be the dominant choice given the above numbers.

Pruning

The above example of radiation therapy versus surgery for early Stage 1 disease did not consider chemotherapy as one of the alternative treatments. Here, the medical-scientific point may be that this early-stage disease does not respond well to existing chemotherapies. And even if chemotherapy did exist for Stage 1 disease, the patient may not want to consider any therapeutic options. In both cases, the chemotherapy alternative was pruned away from the decision structure in Tree 1 above.

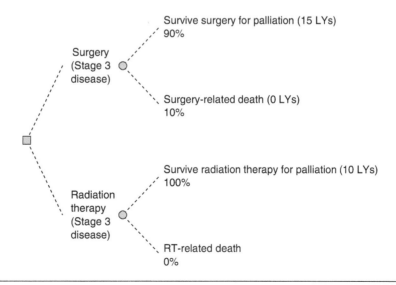

Figure 4   Decision tree for Stage 3 disease, Phase 2

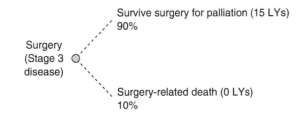

Figure 5   Calculation of the average life years for surgery

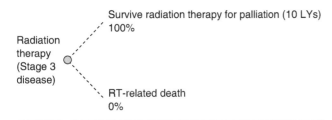

Figure 6   Calculation of the average life years for radiation therapy

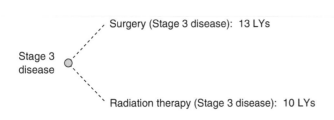

Figure 7   Calculations of the average life years for surgery and radiation therapy

Future Treatment Options

In later stages of the disease under consideration after either surgery or radiation therapy (or both surgery and radiation therapy) have been exhausted, there may be a role for palliative chemotherapy, that is, therapy intended to palliate, not cure, the disease. Early surgery, for example, may well have been intended to offer an option for cure for the patient, based on review of the peer-reviewed medical scientific literature. However, if a cure was not secured and the disease returned, radiation therapy could be offered. And when the disease recurs after both surgery and radiation therapy, there may be a role for palliative chemotherapy in a patient whose main goal is to survive as long as possible.

Certain patients may want to see how surgery followed by chemotherapy versus radiation therapy followed by chemotherapy look in a decision tree. In Figure 8, one can see that when chemotherapy for palliation is considered as an option after surgery and after radiation therapy as requested by the patient, the surgery alternative becomes stronger in terms of survival over radiation therapy because the palliative chemotherapy after surgery provides a longer survival than palliative chemotherapy after radiation therapy. Thus, the addition of a future treatment option (palliative chemotherapy) may change a patient's mind toward surgery as an initial therapy after seeing the tree in Figure 8.

Addition of a Wait-and-See Alternative

It is important to recognize that decision trees are not optimal for structuring all types of decisions. One of the key alternatives in patient care is the wait-and-see alternative (or watchful waiting). Here, no intervention is made in a disease state. Rather, the patient elects to wait and see how his or her disease acts over time and then decides to act at the time when there is an increase in tumor activity noted on the basis of a worsening of symptoms, a change in physical examination suggesting an increase in growth of tumor mass, a change in laboratory testing measurement, or a change in biopsy results suggesting a move from a lower-stage tumor to one that is more aggressive.

In this case, one can construct a decision tree that considers surgery for palliation versus radiation therapy for palliation versus watchful waiting (wait and see) and then palliative chemotherapy for survival for Stage 3–4 disease in a patient whose main goal is to live as long as possible regardless of quality of life. Given the added emphasis that is being placed by oncologists on the offering of palliative care options to patients with oncologic diseases, one can add a wait-and-see palliative care decision option with palliative chemotherapy to the tree in Figure 8, creating the tree shown in Figure 9.

Figure 9 illustrates the pruning of the tree in Figure 8 and the elimination of branches from the tree structure.

Figure 10 shows the pruning of the tree in Figure 9 and the LY expectancy with the three approaches that can be offered to the patient. Figure 11 shows the comparison of the LY expectancy of three

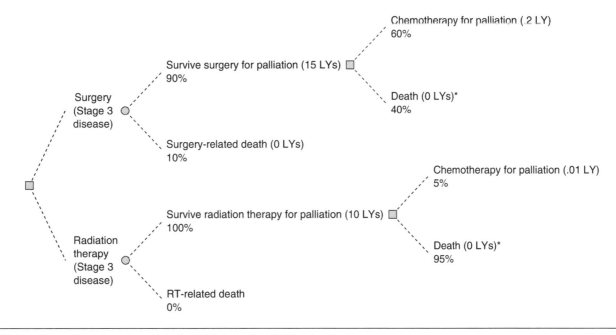

Figure 8   Decision tree with the addition of palliative chemotherapy

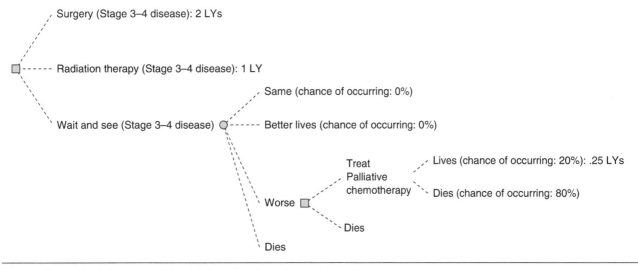

Figure 9   Decision tree with addition of wait-and-see alternative

treatments—palliative surgery versus palliative radiotherapy versus wait-and-see and then treat with palliative chemotherapy—for a patient who is focused on survival rather than quality of life in his or her decision making.

The problem with the trees in Figures 9 through 11 is that by displaying wait-and-see as simply

another alternative similar to surgery and radiation therapy, there is no reflection of the fact that there may be vast differences in time that is accorded to a wait-and-see state, such that a patient may spend various times (from days, weeks, months to years) in a wait-and-see state, and this time variability is not reflected in the basic decision tree structure.

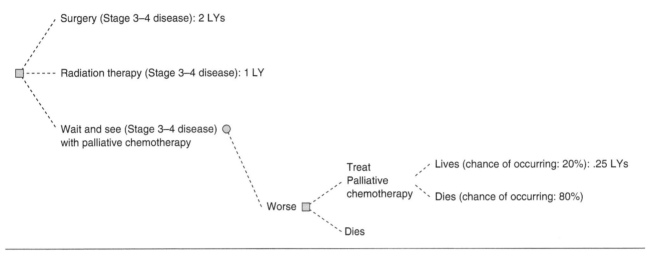

Figure 10   Decision tree showing life years expectancy of three treatments

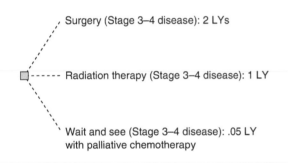

Figure 11   Decision tree showing the years of life expectancy for three treatments

Here, there is a call for procedures and analyses, such as Markov models, to portray wait-and-see states, to allow for a more real and dynamic interpretation of wait-and-see attitudes and alternatives in patient decision making.

Caveats

The fact of the matter is that in any decision analysis, all the outcomes, all the probabilities, and all the preferences will not have been derived and enumerated as extensively as required by physicians and providers. And there will be missing, problematic, or illusory numbers appearing in the tree as considered by physicians and other providers. Decision scientists may examine the same tree and find it to be acceptable. Viewed from another perspective, a physician may view a decision tree and see all the unanswered questions that exist

regarding outcomes, probabilities, and preferences and say that more work is needed before the tree can be folded back.

Decision to Stop Building a Decision Tree

Folding back a decision tree is a procedure that can begin only when one stops building a decision tree or pauses in the building of a decision tree. Some authors will say that one can stop building a decision tree at any point, with one provision: that one is able to describe the terminal outcome at each endpoint in such a way that the unmodeled future from that endpoint onward in time can be accounted for and approximated. Other authors will argue that one can elaborate the tree to the point where one feels comfortable with the approximations made and their analytical implications for the immediate choice of action that needs to be made.

Each attempt at approximation will be made by those who will agree with the approximation or those who will accept the approximation to see where it leads (how it performs), while others will reject the approximation as outlandish from its outset of construction to its conclusion. At some point, some will be happy with the probabilities as gathered; others will be insistent that the peer-reviewed medical literature, expert opinion, and patient preference must be more thoroughly searched for. The only limitation on continued folding back of a decision tree in the case of an individual's decision making is the estimated length of time a decision can be postponed or delayed without significant impact on the patient's survival and quality of life.

Dennis J. Mazur

See also Decision Trees, Evaluation With Monte Carlo; Expected Utility Theory; Markov Models

Further Readings

Audrey, S., Abel, J., Blazeby, J. M., Falk, S., & Campbell, R. (2008). What oncologists tell patients about survival benefits of palliative chemotherapy and implications for informed consent: Qualitative study. *British Medical Journal, 337,* a752.

Pratt, J. W., Raiffa, H., & Schaifer, R. (1995). *Introduction to statistical decision theory.* Cambridge: MIT Press.

Pratt, J. W., & Schlaifer, R. (1988). On the interpretation and observation of laws. *Journal of Econometrics, 39,* 23–52.

Raiffa, H. (1968). *Decision analysis: Introductory lectures on choices under uncertainty.* Reading, MA: Addison-Wesley.

Raiffa, H., & Schaifer, R. (2000). *Applied statistical decision theory.* New York: Wiley. (Original work published 1961)

Savage, L. J. (1972). *The foundations of statistics* (2nd rev. ed.). New York: Dover. (Original work published 1954)

Decision Trees, Evaluation With Monte Carlo

Monte Carlo simulations are based on Monte Carlo methods. *Monte Carlo method* refers to a method of solving sets of equations using an algorithm dependent on repeated random sampling. The Monte Carlo method is used in the process of simulating (approximating) a system. Monte Carlo methods are computational algorithms that rely on repeated random sampling to compute their results. *Monte Carlo simulation* involves repeated random sampling from input distributions and subsequent calculation of a set of sample values for the output distributions with the repeating of the process over several iterations.

The term *Monte Carlo method* was used in the 1940s in the more rapid solving of equations and algorithms possible on the first electronic digital computer, the ENIAC computer. The term was used by Nicholas Metropolis and Stanislaw Ulam in 1949. Metropolis attributed the initial insights on the use of the method to Enrico Fermi. The reference to the gaming tables of Monte Carlo, Monaco, shows the importance of randomness and chance events in the entities that are being simulated.

Today, the major uses of the Monte Carlo method involve examining real-life phenomena that need to be approximated or simulated rather than tested in the sense of real-world testing of scientific hypotheses. In testing, for example, in research on humans, there would be the tasks of developing scientific protocols, collecting data in trials, and conducting research on humans that in turn would need to be derived in conjunction with existing federal laws and approved by an institutional review board. If alternative strategies can be effectively modeled, sparing humans lives and costs, then real-world testing may not be needed as extensively as it is needed today.

Use of Monte Carlo simulation has expanded exponentially into many areas where random behavior, uncertainty, and chance events characterize the system being simulated in a diverse range of real-world endeavors: economics; finance (interest rates and stock prices); business (inventory, staffing needs, and office tasks); the sciences; and medical decision making with economic implications (e.g., impact of colonoscopic referral for small and diminutive polyps detected on CT colonography screening).

Monte Carlo Simulation

Monte Carlo simulation selects value variables at random in the attempt at simulating a real-life situation whose outcome needs to be estimated or predicted. The variables of interest will have a known range or at least a range that can be estimated.

A variable may be uncertain, but if that variable is known to have a range of values (or estimated to have a range of possible values), this range of possible values can define a probability distribution. A simulation calculates multiple scenarios by repeatedly sampling values from the probability distributions for the uncertain variables.

Monte Carlo simulations depend on the computational tools available at the time a simulation is run. Simulations run during the days of the Manhattan Project in the 1940s are dwarfed by computations performed on a laptop computer today.

Deterministic Models Versus Iterative Models

When a model is created with a spreadsheet, one has a certain number of input parameters and a few equations that use those inputs to give a set of outputs (or response variables). This type of model is usually termed *deterministic* in that one gets the same result no matter how many times one performs a recalculation.

A basic decision tree is an example of a deterministic model. Although inputs may differ in terms of the chance success of a surgery versus a radiotherapy intervention on a cancer at different medical centers based on the specific patient data found in one medical center versus another medical center, when one calculates the model based on the same data, everyone who performs the calculation should come up with the same result.

One sense of Monte Carlo simulation is as an *iterative model* for evaluating a deterministic model. Here, the Monte Carlo simulation uses a set of random numbers as the input numbers for the model.

The Monte Carlo method is one of many methods that can be used to understand how (a) random variation, (b) lack of knowledge, or (c) error rates affect the sensitivity, performance, or reliability of the system being modeled. Monte Carlo simulation is categorized as a sampling method because the inputs are randomly generated from probability distributions used to simulate the process of sampling from an actual population. Hence, there must be a choice of a distribution for the inputs that most closely matches the data that is available on the question about which an answer is sought. The data generated from the simulation can be represented as probability distributions and in turn converted to confidence intervals.

Input and Output Variables

A simulation begins with the development of a model of a system that one wishes to test. The model comprises mathematical equations describing relationships between one or more input (independent) variables and one or more output (dependent) variables. By selecting specific values for the input variables, corresponding output values may be calculated for the output variables. In this manner, one can determine how the system, to the extent that it is accurately represented by the model, will respond to various situations represented by the input values. Note that, as used herein, a "system" may comprise virtually anything that can be represented by an appropriately constructed mathematical model, for example, the impact of referral to a colonoscopist for direct visualization of small and diminutive polyps detected on indirect imaging, for example, visualization on a CT scan.

In Monte Carlo simulations, a range of plausible input values is designated for each input variable. Likewise, a distribution for each input variable (i.e., a probability distribution function) is also designated. Thereafter, the Monte Carlo simulation generates random inputs for each input variable based on the designated range of values and distributions for the corresponding variables. The random input values are then used to calculate corresponding output values. This process is repeated many times, typically numbering in the hundreds, thousands, ten thousands, or more, and is used to create statistically meaningful distributions of one or more of the output variables. In this manner, the analyst performing the Monte Carlo simulation can develop insight into how the model will perform under certain sets of assumed input conditions. The analyst needs to have intimate knowledge of the underlying system and its simulation model.

Incorporation of Monte Carlo Simulation Into a Decision Tree

The incorporation of Monte Carlo simulation into a decision tree allows examination of "probability distributions" rather than "single expected values" or "ranges of expected values." Some describe Monte Carlo simulation as replacing the analysis of point estimates with fuzzy values (or better, ranges of fuzzy values).

For example, monetary values can be replaced with normal distribution functions (e.g., a normal distribution with a specified mean and a standard deviation). One can present the distribution of results for the expected value after a Monte Carlo simulation with 10 trials, 100 trials, 1,000 trials, 10,000 trials, and so on.

Probability Distributions

The probability distributions selected must describe the range of likely values for each parameter. This is a selection problem for the analyst, who must be able to represent the best probability distribution for a particular setting.

Probability distributions may be of standard form (normal or lognormal distributions) or may have empirical forms (rectangular, triangular, among others). Here, an analyst can start with the historical data of the parameters being considered and attempt a "best-fit" approach of a distribution to the historical data.

The parameters of the distribution (mean and standard deviation in the case of normal distributions) may be based on data derived from (a) the peer-reviewed medical scientific literature (if present and available), (b) historical data as is contained in the databases of surgery departments or radiation therapy departments in medical centers (if accessible), or (c) the experience of experts.

In absence of specific knowledge about the form of a distribution, assumptions are made about what the distributions should look like, and certain distributions may be selected, for example, normal or lognormal distributions. Some properties may need to be bounded, as it may not be possible to have specific properties outside of specific ranges.

Statistics Obtained From a Monte Carlo Simulation

The statistics obtained from any simulation are estimates of the population parameters; the exact values of the population parameters will never be known. The assumption is that as the number of iterations increases, the probability that an estimate of a population parameter is within a specific amount of the actual population also increases.

The analyst himself or herself selects the number of iterations, the accuracy required from the procedure. The analyst's assumptions regarding number of iterations and accuracy required in a task are

issues that can be argued about and taken up with the analyst. Nonanalyst-related impacts on Monte Carlo simulation include the complexity of the initial problem being modeled and cost of the procedure (e.g., analyst's time, computing time).

Simulation Analysis

In simulation analysis, a decision tree is "rolled forward." A bank of data is generated by the simulation analysis that, if interpreted correctly, can give a probabilistic picture of the consequences of a decision strategy.

Example

Let us take a medical example using a Monte Carlo simulation. A patient with adult respiratory distress syndrome (ARDS) has a diffuse injury to lung tissue due to diffuse damage to the smallest air sacs of the lungs (alveoli) in the absence of congestive heart failure. (The fluid in the lung of the ARDS patient is not due to heart failure.) ARDS is a serious medical condition of acute onset with infiltrates found in both lungs on chest X-ray and has as its origin a diverse array of predisposing conditions causing fluid buildup in the lungs, including direct pulmonary injury (lung infection or aspiration of materials into the lung) and indirect injury (blood infection, pancreatitis, moderate to severe trauma). Here, a patient with ARDS may undergo care in the following states:

- Patient intubated in the intensive care unit
- Patient nonintubated on a hospital ward
- Patient in offsite long-term care
  - In an offsite long-term care facility that accepts respirators
  - In an offsite long-term care facility that does not accept respirators
- Patient in home care

The patient will not stay in any one state but will transition between states (home care, long-term care facility without respirator, long-term care facility with respirator, medical ward extubated, intensive care unit intubated until death) with time at home decreasing and time in all care states increasing until death.

In this setting, neuromuscular blocking (NMB) has potential benefits (NMB drugs may facilitate mechanical ventilation and improve oxygenation) and potential risks (NMB drugs may result in prolonged recovery of neuromuscular function and acute quadriplegic myopathy syndrome [AQMS]). The researchers attempted to answer the question whether a reduction in intubation time of 6 hours and/or a reduction in the incidence of AQMS from 25% to 21% provide enough benefit to justify an NMB drug with an additional expenditure of $267 (the difference in acquisition cost between a generic and brand name NMB drug, the neuromuscular blocker). They performed this task by (a) constructing a Markov computer simulation model of the economics of NMB in patients with ARDS (b) using Monte Carlo simulation to conduct a probabilistic sensitivity analysis considering uncertainties in all probabilities, utilities, and costs.

If one attempted to model ARDS in terms of decision trees (a deterministic approach), these trees and their analysis would be limited in their abilities to model the events of ARDS because of the need to model "multiple times" in the care of a patient who transitions from state to state, moving from one extreme, the most severe state with most intensive care (patient intubated), to the least severe state, the stable state of having resolved ARDS and being now with minimal care at home.

The researchers, Macario and colleagues, used probabilistic sensitivity analysis to consider uncertainties in all probabilities, utilities, and costs simultaneously. In their model, mean values of the net monetary benefit were calculated for results of N = 10,000 Monte Carlo simulations, where triangular distributions were used for parameter values, with the mode being the case and the 5th and 95th percentiles of the lower and upper limits of the ranges reported. They reported all costs in year 2004 U.S. dollars and discounted all future costs and quality-adjusted life years at 3% per annum.

This report of the results of a Monte Carlo simulation followed the recommendation of Doubilet and colleagues that the following results be recorded:

- The mean and standard deviation of the expected utility of each strategy
- The frequency with which each strategy is optimal

- The frequency with which each strategy "buys" or "costs" a specified amount of utility relative to the remaining strategies

Macario and colleagues reported the results of the simulation by noting that the net monetary benefit was positive for 50% of simulations with a ceiling ratio of $1,000 versus 51% if the ceiling ratio was increased to $100,000. They argued that lack of sensitivity was caused by the mean changes in quality-adjusted life year (QALY) and cost being small relative to their standard deviations.

Their Markov model noted that the following variables had the largest influence on their results: (a) probability from ICU intubated to death, (b) probability from ICU intubated to extubated, and (c) probability from ICU extubated to ward. The model showed that the better the patients do overall, the larger the net monetary benefit of a drug that reduces AQMS and/or intubation times.

First-Order and Second-Order Uncertainty

There are two categories of uncertainty related to the ARDS model above and similar models. *First-order uncertainty* refers to variability among individuals. *Second-order uncertainty* refers to parameter uncertainty. First-order uncertainty can be captured in the phrase *overall variability between patients* and is reflected in standard deviation associated with a mean value. Second-order uncertainty is *parameter uncertainty,* where uncertainty exists in mean parameter values and is reflected in standard error of the mean.

To understand the uncertainty within a model, Monte Carlo simulation techniques can be applied using both first-order and second-order simulations. A first-order simulation is also called a *run of a random trial,* a *microsimulation,* or a *random walk.* A first-order simulation is performed by running each patient in the hypothetical cohort through the model, one at a time. First-order simulation trials can be used to model the variability in individual outcomes. First-order simulation reflects what can be described as first-order uncertainty involving the variability among individuals.

Variability between individuals can be modeled using first-order Monte Carlo microsimulation. But what about questions of second-order uncertainty? In practice, the most commonly used measures are those that are based on formulating uncertainty in the model inputs by a joint probability distribution and then analyzing the induced uncertainty in outputs, an approach which is known as probabilistic sensitivity analysis. Probabilistic sensitivity analysis is more readily applied to an aggregate cohort of patients.

Probabilistic Sensitivity Analysis

Probabilistic sensitivity analysis uses a probabilistic approach where all the input parameters are considered random variables, endowed with known prior probability distributions. Why is probabilistic sensitivity analysis needed? First, there are numerous parameters in decision models. Second, each parameter has an estimated uncertainty. There is a need to "propagate" parameter uncertainty. The use of an analysis approach to estimate the effect of uncertainties on model prediction is referred to as *uncertainty propagation*. Second-order simulation as an analysis approach—relies on sampling parameter values to estimate the effect of uncertainties on model prediction.

Probabilistic sensitivity analysis requires one to identify sources of parameter uncertainty, to characterize uncertain parameters as probability distributions, and to propagate uncertainty through the model using Monte Carlo simulation.

When applied to groups of patients rather than individual patients, Halpern and colleagues note that implementing a probabilistic sensitivity analysis may lead to misleading or improper conclusions. The authors argue that the practice of combining first- and second-order simulations when modeling the outcome for a group of more than one patient can yield an error in marginal distribution, thus underrepresenting the second-order uncertainty in the simulation. It may also distort the shape (symmetry and extent of the tails) in any simulated distribution, resulting in premature or incorrect conclusions of superiority of one strategy over its alternatives being modeled.

The complexity of Monte Carlo simulations—how they are conducted and how they are interpreted—is still being unraveled in relation to first- and second-order effects.

Dennis J. Mazur

See also Decision Trees, Evaluation; Expected Utility Theory; Markov Models; Quality-Adjusted Life Years (QALYs)

Further Readings

Doubilet, P., Begg, C. B., Weinstein, M. C., Braun, P., & McNeil, B. J. (1985). Probabilistic sensitivity analysis using Monte Carlo simulation. A practical approach. *Medical Decision Making, 5,* 157–177.

Eckhardt, R. (1987). Stan Ulam, John von Neumann, and the Monte Carlo method. *Los Alamos Science* (Special issue), *15,* 131–137.

Halpern, E. F., Weinstein, M. C., Hunink, M. G., & Gazelle, G. S. (2000). Representing both first- and second-order uncertainties by Monte Carlo simulation for groups of patients. *Medical Decision Making, 20,* 314–322.

Macario, A., Chow, J. L., & Dexter, F. (2006). A Markov computer simulation model of the economics of neuromuscular blockade in patients with acute respiratory distress syndrome. *BMC Medical Informatics and Decision Making, 15*(6), 15.

Metropolis, N., & Ulam, S. (1949). The Monte Carlo method. *Journal of the American Statistical Association, 44*(247), 335–341.

Pickhardt, P. J., Hassan, C., Laghi, A., Zullo, A., Kim, D. H., Iafrate, F., et al. (2008). Small and diminutive polyps detected at screening CT colonography: A decision analysis for referral to colonoscopy. *American Journal of Roentgenology, 190,* 136–144.

Student. (1908). Probable error of a correlation coefficient. *Biometrika, 6,* 302–310.

Student. (1908). The probable error of a mean. *Biometrika, 6,* 1–25.

Sullivan, P. W., Arant, T. W., Ellis, S. L., & Ulrich, H. (2006). The cost effectiveness of anticoagulation management services for patients with atrial fibrillation and at high risk of stroke in the US. *PharmacoEconomics, 24,* 1021–1033.

DECISION TREES: SENSITIVITY ANALYSIS, BASIC AND PROBABILISTIC

Sensitivity analysis is defined as systematically varying one or more parameters in a decision model over a specified range and recalculating the expected utility of the model for each value. There are four reasons to employ sensitivity analysis:

1. to determine the effect of reasonable variations in the estimates of parameters on the results of the analysis;

2. to determine which variables are most critical to the analysis—and, therefore, may justify further efforts to estimate them more precisely;

3. to determine what the analysis would recommend for various *scenarios* (combinations of parameters); and

4. to explore the model for bugs or anomalies.

The best estimate of the value of each parameter in a model is called the *baseline* value. When all parameters are at their baseline values, the model is said to be the *base case* model. Without sensitivity analysis, one can say only that the results of the analysis apply to the base case model. When small changes in a parameter affect the recommended choice or cause significant changes in the results, the analysis is said to be *sensitive* to that parameter. Some changes in parameters affect the decision only if they are combined with specific changes in one or more other variables. Therefore, complete sensitivity analysis must examine more than one variable at a time. Sensitivity analyses may examine any number of variables at a time, although in practical terms, only one-, two-, or three-way sensitivity analyses can be illustrated graphically. Examination of more than three variables simultaneously requires probabilistic sensitivity analysis (PSA).

One-Way Sensitivity Analysis

The decision tree shown in Figure 1 models a simple decision between Observation and Treatment. The prior probability of disease (.3) and the utilities of each combination of treatment and disease state are indicated. The expected utilities are 21.98 for the Treatment strategy and 22.38 for the Observation strategy. Figure 2 shows a one-way sensitivity analysis on the probability of disease. When pDis = 0, the difference between the Observe and Treatment strategies represents the "cost" of treatment (in this case the morbidity cost). When pDis = 1, the difference in utility between the Observe and Treatment strategies represents the net benefit of treatment. It is intuitive that when pDis = 0, Observation must be the preferred strategy and when pDis = 1, Treatment must be the preferred strategy. If not, then the treatment is worse than the disease and the analysis makes no sense.

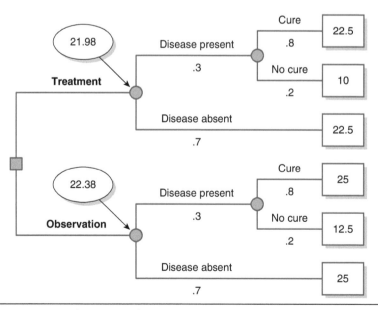

Figure 1   Empiric therapy versus observation decision tree

Threshold Approach

It is apparent from Figure 2 that the lines representing the two strategies cross at a point. This point is called a *threshold* because it represents the value of the independent variable above or below which the preferred strategy changes. In the case of the Observe/Treatment choice, the threshold is referred to as the *treatment threshold*. Figure 3 shows a simple geometric way of calculating the treatment threshold. Assuming that the expected utilities of both strategies are straight lines (i.e., they vary linearly with the independent variable), the combination of the expected utility lines forms a set of similar triangles. The "height" of the left-ward triangle is the threshold value. The width of the base of the left triangle is the cost of treatment. The width of the base of the right triangle is the benefit of treatment. For similar triangles, the ratios of the heights are equal to the ratios of the bases:

$$\frac{C}{B} = \frac{t}{1-t}.$$

Solving for t,

$$t = \frac{C}{C+B} \quad \text{or} \quad \frac{1}{1+\frac{B}{C}}.$$

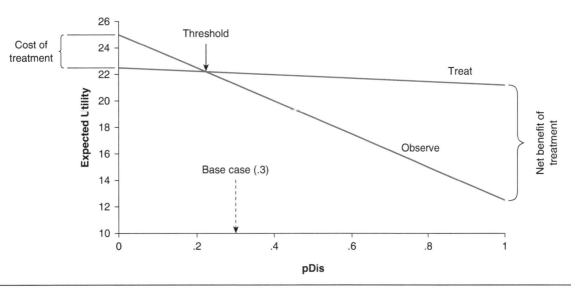

Figure 2   One-way sensitivity analysis on probability of disease

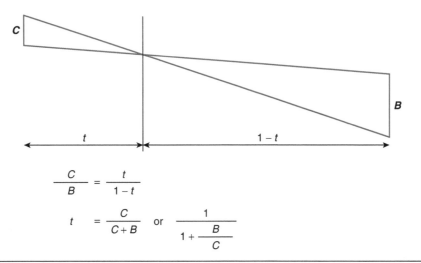

Figure 3   Geometric calculation of treatment threshold

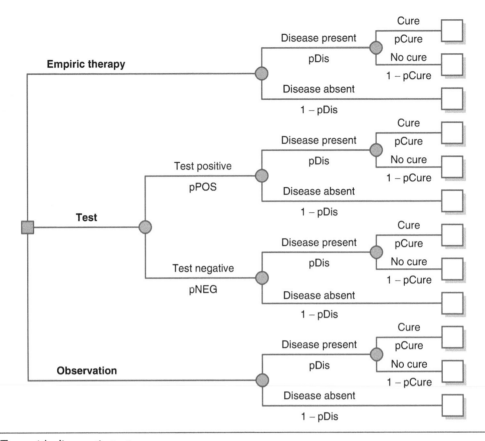

Figure 4   Tree with diagnostic test

C and B can be calculated by evaluating the model for pDis = 0 or pDis = 1, respectively.

Consider the more complicated tree shown in Figure 4, which adds a third Test strategy. Figure 5 shows a one-way sensitivity analysis on pDis, which now has three lines. There are now two new thresholds. The Testing threshold is the value of pDis above which Test is favored over Observe. The Test-Treatment threshold is the value of pDis above which Treat is favored over Test.

Two-Way Sensitivity Analysis

A two-way sensitivity analysis looks at variations in two independent variables simultaneously. Since a one-way sensitivity analysis requires a two-dimensional graph, as in Figure 2, a two-way analysis would require a three-dimensional graph, plotting one independent variable on each horizontal axis and the expected utilities on the vertical axis. However, a more convenient way

has been devised of representing a two-way analysis on a two-dimensional graph.

Figure 6 illustrates a two-way sensitivity analysis considering simultaneously pDis and SENS (test sensitivity). For each value of pDis, the Test-Treatment threshold is calculated and plotted on the vertical axis. The resulting points define a curve that divides the plane of the graph into two regions. Points above the curve represent combinations of pDis and SENS for which Test is favored. Points below the curve represent combinations of pDis and SENS for which Treat is favored. Figure 7 illustrates the same kind of two-way analysis in which all three strategies are considered. There is an additional curve representing the Testing threshold, thus dividing the plane of the graph into three areas, each favoring one strategy. Note that below the test sensitivity at which the Testing threshold equals the Test-Treatment threshold, testing is not favored regardless of the value of pDis.

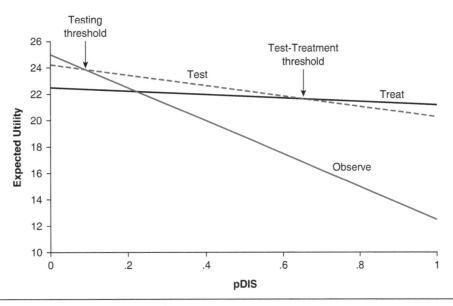

Figure 5   One-way sensitivity analysis with three strategies

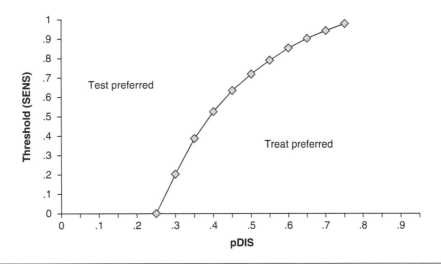

Figure 6   Two-way sensitivity analysis

Three-Way Sensitivity Analysis

As with the two-way analysis, a three-way sensitivity analysis can be represented on a two-dimensional graph by using threshold curves. Figure 8 shows a series of Test-Treatment threshold curves, one for each value of a third variable (test specificity, or Spec). Each curve divides the plane of the graph into a different pair of regions.

Probabilistic Sensitivity Analysis

Sensitivity analyses, as illustrated above, perform deterministic calculations on the model. While they explore variations in key parameters, they do not represent actual uncertainty in the parameters since nothing in the results indicates which scenario is more likely. In PSA, uncertainty in parameters is represented by using probability distributions to represent the values of parameters.

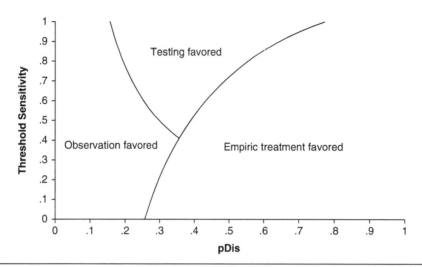

Figure 7   Two-way sensitivity analysis showing all three strategies

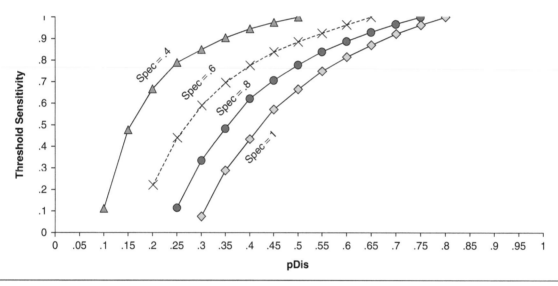

Figure 8   Three-way sensitivity analysis

Mathematical Distributions

A mathematical distribution describes the likelihood that the value of a parameter will be in a certain range. It is usually represented by a probability density function (PDF), as illustrated in Figure 9. The height of each bar (or point on the curve) represents the relative likelihood of the corresponding value (on the horizontal axis) occurring. Probability distributions are characterized by bounds (e.g., 0 to 1 or unbounded), mean value, and shape. A complete discussion of probability distributions is beyond the scope of this entry but may be found elsewhere.

Useful Distributions

The most important distributions in PSA are those representing probabilities. Thus, they must be bounded between 0 and 1. The *beta distribution* has many desirable characteristics for representing probabilities and is therefore commonly used. Parameters for determining the parameters of the distribution (mean and shape) may be determined by analyzing sets of data or by estimating the range of likely values.

In PSA, any number of variables may be represented by distributions. During evaluation, each value is drawn from its distribution according to

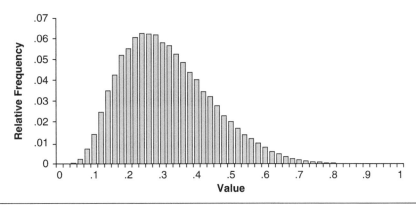

Figure 9   Probability density function for a distribution

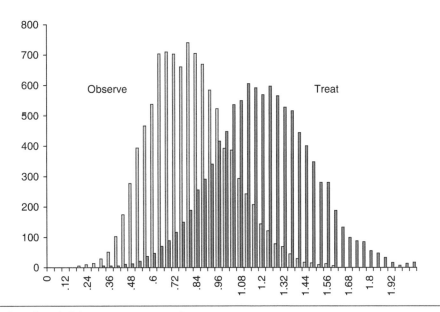

Figure 10   Results of probabilistic sensitivity analysis

its PDF, and the model is evaluated with the resulting set of parameters. This is repeated a large number of times, typically 1,000 to 10,000 times. Because each iteration has a different set of parameters and a different result, the process is said to be *stochastic* rather than *deterministic*. The resulting expected utilities of each of the model's strategies are themselves combined into a results distribution (Figure 10) and thus provide measures of the uncertainty of the results (e.g., variance). The results may be interpreted as the difference in the means of the distributions and also in terms of the percentage of

iterations for which one strategy is favored over the other.

Detecting Model Bugs and Errors With Sensitivity Analysis

Another important purpose of sensitivity analysis is detecting errors in the model. The sensitivity analysis illustrated in Figure 11 shows the expected utilities of medical management (MedRx) and cardiac catheterization (Cath) as a function of the probability of left main disease (pLeftMain). Because the

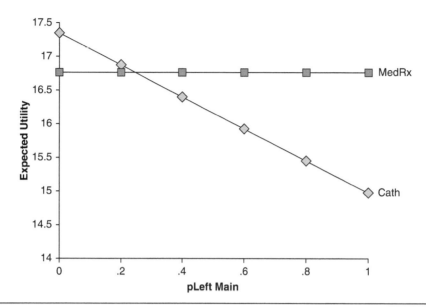

Figure 11   Model "bug" revealed by sensitivity analysis

analyst has neglected to include pLeftMain in the model for medical therapy, it appears that MedRx is favored more when pLeftMain is higher. The opposite is true. This is an example of *asymmetry* error, in which different strategies model the underlying disease or outcomes differently.

Frank A. Sonnenberg

See also Cost-Effectiveness Analysis; Decision Trees: Sensitivity Analysis, Basic and Probabilistic; Decision Trees: Sensitivity Analysis, Deterministic; Test-Treatment Threshold; Threshold Technique

Further Readings

Briggs, A. H. (2000). Handling uncertainty in cost-effectiveness models. *PharmacoEconomics, 17*(5), 479–500.

Doubilet, P., Begg, C. B., Weinstein, M. C., Braun, P., & McNeill, B. J. (1985). Probabilistic sensitivity analysis using Monte Carlo simulation. A practical approach. *Medical Decision Making, 5*(2), 157.

NIST/SEMATECH. (2003). Probability distributions. In *NIST/SEMATECH e-handbook of engineering statistics*. Retrieved January 27, 2009, from http://www.itl.nist.gov/div898/handbook/eda/section3/eda36.htm

Pauker, S. G., & Kassirer, J. P. (1980). The threshold approach to clinical decision making. *New England Journal of Medicine, 302*(20), 1109.

Decision Trees: Sensitivity Analysis, Deterministic

All decision analyses have to deal with various forms of uncertainty in a manner that informs the decisions being made. In particular, it is essential to establish the degree to which the results of an analysis are sensitive to a change in a parameter or an assumption and the extent to which the conclusions of the analysis are robust to such changes. The assessment of sensitivity or robustness is known as sensitivity analysis. Such an analysis would consider, for example, the fact that the mean length of inpatient hospital stay associated with a particular clinical event is estimated with uncertainty (reflected in its standard error) and would consider how the results of the study would change if a higher or lower value were used for this parameter. Two different forms of sensitivity analysis are used in this situation: (1) deterministic analysis, which varies the parameter (or assumption) in one or a small number of stages and assesses the implications for results, and (2) probabilistic analysis, which uses simulation methods to simultaneously vary a number of parameters in terms of a large number of possible alternative values they could take. This entry considers deterministic sensitivity analysis.

Different Types of Uncertainty in Decision Analysis

The uncertainties relevant to a decision model have been categorized in various ways in the literature. The main distinction is between parameter and model (or structural) uncertainty. The former refers to the uncertainty that exists in the parameter inputs that are incorporated into models—for example, the baseline risk of a clinical event in a particular patient group under current treatment, the risk reduction in the event associated with a new intervention relative to current practice, the mean cost of the event, or the mean decrement in health-related quality of life associated with the event. Model uncertainty relates to a range of possible assumptions that are made in developing a model. These could include the extent to which the baseline risk of an event changes over time, the duration of the risk reduction associated with a new intervention, or whether or not to include a particular study in a meta-analysis to estimate the relative treatment effect. The distinction between parameter and model uncertainty is blurred in that many forms of model uncertainty could be expressed in terms of an uncertain parameter.

Deterministic sensitivity analysis can also be used to address heterogeneity rather than uncertainty—that is, to assess the extent to which the results of an analysis change for different types of patients. For example, a treatment may be more effective in females than in males, so the results of the analysis could be separately reported for the two genders. This is probably more correctly labeled as a subgroup, rather than a sensitivity, analysis and is not further discussed here.

Different Forms of Deterministic Sensitivity Analysis

Deterministic sensitivity analysis can be characterized in a number of ways. One is whether a parameter is varied across a range or simply takes on discrete values. In the case of model assumptions that have not been formerly parameterized, the use of discrete values is usually required. Table 1 shows an example of this form of sensitivity analysis (which can also be described as a scenario analysis) in the context of a cost-effectiveness model of endovascular abdominal aortic aneurysm repair (EVAR) compared with open surgery for abdominal aortic aneurysm. It shows the impact of variation on the difference in costs, quality-adjusted life years (QALYs), and the incremental cost-effectiveness ratio relative to the "base-case" or primary analysis. It also shows the results of a probabilistic sensitivity analysis in terms of the probability that EVAR is more cost-effective conditional on a threshold cost-effectiveness ratio. The table mostly includes assessment of uncertainty in the parameter estimates used in the model. However, there are also examples of modeling assumptions that have been varied, for example, Scenario 6 (source of a parameter); and some subgroup analyses are reported (e.g., Scenarios 10 and 11).

An alternative form of deterministic sensitivity analysis is to vary a parameter along a continuous scale and to present this diagrammatically. An example of this is presented in Figure 1, which shows how the incremental cost per QALY gained of primary angioplasty, relative to the use of thrombolysis, in patients with ST-elevation myocardial infarction varies with the additional capital cost per patient required for the angioplasty service. The results are shown for two assumptions regarding the time delay to provide angioplasty compared with thrombolysis.

A second way in which deterministic sensitivity analysis can be characterized is in terms of the number of uncertain parameters/assumptions that are varied simultaneously. Table 1 generally shows analyses that vary one parameter/assumption at a time (one-way sensitivity analysis). There are, however, examples of analyses where two parameters are varied at a time (e.g., Scenarios 12 and 13) (two-way sensitivity analysis). Figure 1 also represents an example of two-way sensitivity analysis in that two uncertain parameters are being varied together: the additional capital cost of angioplasty per patient (as a continuous variable) and the time delay associated with angioplasty (as a categorical variable) compared with thrombolytics.

It becomes very difficult to present deterministic sensitivity analyses when more than two variables are being varied at a time—this is one of several reasons why probabilistic sensitivity analysis might be preferred. One way of looking at multiple

Table I   Example of deterministic sensitivity analysis

Scenario	Base-case assumption	Secondary analysis	Difference in cost (£)	Difference in QALYs	ICER for EVAR versus open*	Probability EVAR is cost-effective[†]	
						Λ = £20,000	Λ = £40,000
1	Base case		3758	−0.020	EVAR dominated	0.012	0.080
2	Hazard of cardiovascular death is twice that of the general population	Baseline hazard of cardiovascular death is the same as the general population	4105	0.017	239,000	0.028	0.161
3	Lower rate of cardiovascular death following open surgery	Same hazard of cardiovascular death following each treatment strategy	3687	0.087	42,000	0.098	0.481
4	1 CT and 1 outpatient visit per year after EVAR	Same cost of monitoring following each treatment strategy	2613	−0.020	EVAR dominated	0.045	0.145
5	Cost of EVAR device is £4800	Cost of EVAR device is £3700	2669	−0.020	EVAR dominated	0.048	0.147
6	Odds ratio of 30-day mortality from EVAR 1 only	Odds ratio from a meta-analysis of DREAM[2] and EVAR trials	3765	−0.015	EVAR dominated	0.012	0.084
7	Discount rate of 3.5%	No discounting of costs nor health benefits	4103	−0.041	EVAR dominated	0.016	0.084

8	Odds ratio of AAA-related death during follow-up from EVAR 1	No difference between EVAR and open repair of the long-term rate of AAA-related death	3859	0.080	48,000	0.076	0.419
9	5% die within 30 days of open repair	8% die within 30 days of open repair	3795	0.090	42,000	0.147	0.463
10	Age 74 years	Age 66 years	4513	−0.144	EVAR dominated	0.001	0.025
11	Age 74 years	Age 82 years	3072	−0.015	EVAR dominated	0.047	0.138
12	Age 74 years and lower long-term rate of cardiovascular death after open surgery	Age 66 years and no difference in rate of cardiovascular death after open repair or EVAR	4468	−0.075	EVAR dominated	0.006	0.068
13	Age 74 years and lower long-term rate of cardiovascular death after open surgery	Age 82 years and no difference in rate of cardiovascular death after open repair or EVAR	2960	0.110	27,000	0.262	0.670

Source: Modelling the long-term cost-effectiveness of endovascular or open repair for abdominal aortic aneurysm. Epstein, D. M., Sculpher, M. J., Manca, A., Michaels, J., Thompson, S. G., Brown, L. C., et al. *British Journal of Surgery, 95,* 183–190. Copyright © 2008 British Journal of Surgery Society Ltd., first published by John Wiley & Sons Ltd.

Note: AAA, abdominal aortic aneurysm; CT, computed tomography; EVAR, endovascular abdominal aortic aneurysm repair; ICER, incremental cost-effectiveness ratio (difference in mean cost divided by difference in mean health benefits); QALY, quality-adjusted life year.

*"EVAR dominated" means EVAR, on average, costs more and has fewer QALYs than open repair and is not expected to be cost-effective.

†The probability EVAR is cost-effective is evaluated at threshold ICERs (λ) of £20,000 and £40,000 per additional QALY20. The National Institute for Health and Clinical Excellence in the United Kingdom has not to date funded interventions with an ICER above £40,000. Given the uncertainty in the model parameters, this represents the probability that a decision to implement EVAR will be better than open repair.

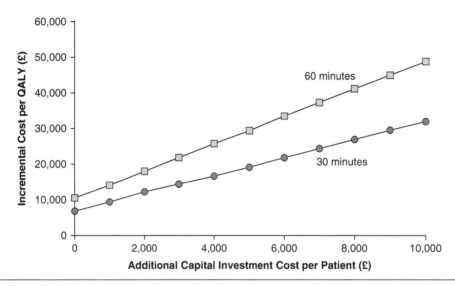

Figure 1   Example of a graphical deterministic sensitivity analysis

Source: Bravo Vergel, Y., Palmer, S., Asseburg, C., Fenwick, E., de Belder, M., Abrams, K., et al. (2007). Results of a comprehensive decision analysis. Is primary angioplasty cost effective in the UK? *Heart, 93,* 1238–1243. Reprinted with permission of BMJ Publishing Group Ltd.

sources of uncertainty is to undertake threshold analysis, a variant on sensitivity analysis. This involves identifying a particular threshold in the results of an analysis that is expected to trigger a policy shift—for example, a point where the incremental cost-effectiveness ratio is equal to a policy maker's cost-effectiveness threshold or when an intervention is expected to generate a net cost saving. The uncertain parameters/assumptions are then varied across a range until the threshold in results is reached, indicating the value(s) of the uncertain variable(s) that, if true, would potentially change a policy decision.

Figure 2 presents an example of a threshold analysis. The context is a cost-effectiveness study of alternative hip prostheses. The analysis provides a general framework for addressing the question of how effective a particular new prosthesis needs to be (in terms of a reduction in the rate of revision procedures) for a given additional cost (compared with a standard prosthesis) to be cost-effective. The example defines *cost-effectiveness* in terms of combinations of additional cost and effectiveness that result in the new prosthesis meeting three alternative thresholds: cost neutrality (including the cost of the prosthesis and other costs of care),

an incremental cost per QALY gained of £6,500, and an incremental cost per QALY gained of £10,000.

Mark Sculpher

See also Applied Decision Analysis; Decision Trees: Sensitivity Analysis, Basic and Probabilistic; Managing Variability and Uncertainty; Uncertainty in Medical Decisions

Further Readings

Bravo Vergel, Y., Palmer, S., Asseburg, C., Fenwick, E., de Belder, M., Abrams, K., et al. (2007). Results of a comprehensive decision analysis. Is primary angioplasty cost effective in the UK? *Heart, 93,* 1238–1243.

Briggs, A. H. (2000). Handling uncertainty in cost-effectiveness models. *PharmacoEconomics, 17*(5), 479–500.

Briggs, A., Sculpher, M., Britton, A., Murray, D., & Fitzpatrick, R. (1998). The costs and benefits of primary total hip replacement. How likely are new prostheses to be cost-effective? *International Journal of Technology Assessment in Health Care, 14*(4), 743–761.

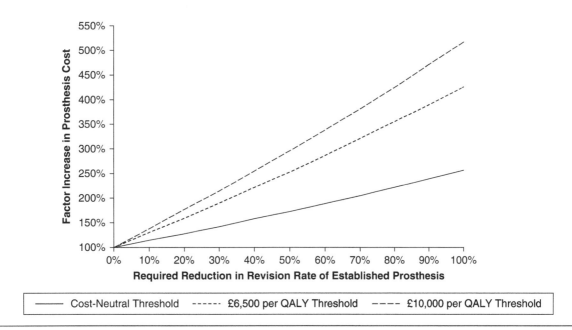

Figure 2   Example of a threshold analysis

Source: Briggs, A., Sculpher, M. J., Britton, A., Murray, D., & Fitzpatrick, R. (1998). The costs and benefits of primary total hip replacement: How likely are new prostheses to be cost-effective? *International Journal of Technology Assessment in Health Care, 14,* 743–761.

Claxton, K., Sculpher, M., McCabe, C., Briggs, A., Akehurst, R., Buxton, M., et al. (2005). Probabilistic sensitivity analysis for NICE technology assessment: Not an optional extra. *Health Economics, 14,* 339–347.

Epstein, D. M., Sculpher, M. J., Manca, A., Michaels, J., Thompson, S. G., Brown, L. C., et al. (2008). Modelling the long-term cost-effectiveness of endovascular or open repair for abdominal aortic aneurysm. *British Journal of Surgery, 95,* 183–190.

DECISION WEIGHTS

A decision weight reflects a person's subjective interpretation of an objective probability. Almost all medical decisions involve probabilistic outcomes. For example, there is some chance that a treatment will cure a disease and some chance that the treatment will have a side effect. Data are often available to help patients and providers know the probability that an outcome, such as a serious side effect, will occur. When people face decisions involving uncertain outcomes, how do they use these probabilities?

Theories of rational decision making recommend using the exact value of the probability in evaluating a decision. For example, in expected utility theory, a rational decision maker should evaluate the overall worth of an option by (a) multiplying the probability of each possible outcome by the utility of that outcome and (b) summing the products across all possible outcomes. However, people making actual decisions do not use the real, or "objective," probability when making decisions; the subjective sense of a given probability p is not necessarily the same as p. This phenomenon is analogous to the psychophysics of light perception, in which the brightness a person perceives does not have a 1:1 relationship with the actual luminous energy in the environment.

In the most well-known descriptive theory of decision making, prospect theory, the subjective sense of a probability is known as the *decision weight* corresponding to that probability, denoted by π. Understanding how a person uses objective probabilities in decision making requires knowledge of that person's *decision weight function*, which describes how probabilities are related to decision weights.

Figure 1 shows a typical decision weight function and illustrates some typical findings from research on decision weights.

First, people tend to overweight small probabilities. Because people have difficulty conceptualizing small probabilities, they translate them into decision weights that are greater than the actual probabilities. This finding might help explain why, for example, both patients and investigators overestimate the small chances of benefit and harm associated with participation in early-phase oncology trials.

Second, people tend to be less sensitive to the differences among probabilities near the middle of the probability scale. Theories of rational decision making state that changes in objective probabilities should make a difference to people. However, actual decision weight functions are relatively flat for intermediate objective probabilities. Thus, a patient might appear to disregard information about the probabilities of success or failure when those probabilities are in the intermediate range (e.g., $p = .25$ to $.75$). In fact, the patient might be attending to the probabilities presented but assigning them similar decision weights.

Third, the decision weight function is usually steepest as it approaches 0 and 1.00. People tend

to prefer changes in probabilities that will result in a state of certainty, something known as the *certainty effect*. Consider a patient deciding between medical and surgical therapies for a heart condition. If the probabilities of success are .80 and .90, respectively, there is a .10-point difference between the treatments. Now imagine that the .10-point difference arises from the probabilities of .90 and 1.00. In expected utility theory, these two scenarios should not be different, because the difference between the options is .10 in both. Yet people do not typically experience these scenarios as equivalent. The decision weight function shows that this is the case because people assign greater weight to the elimination of uncertainty.

Another feature of decision weights is that they are not necessarily additive. Consider a treatment in which only one of two outcomes can occur: (1) a .40 probability of cure and normal life expectancy and (2) a .60 probability of immediate death. Because these are the only possible outcomes, the probabilities sum to 1.00. However, a patient with the decision weight function shown in Figure 1 would convert the probabilities to decision weights that do not sum to 1.00. When people operate according to nonadditive decision weights, their behavior may be contrary to most tenets of rational decision making.

Decision weight functions make it possible to describe many types of situations. For example,

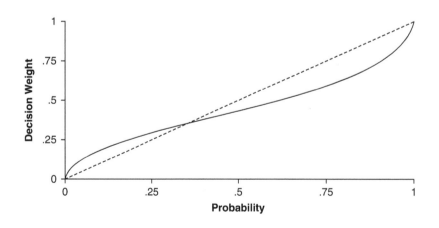

Figure 1   Decision weight function for a hypothetical person

Note: Dotted reference line denotes 1:1 relationship; solid line denotes actual decision function.

some people appear to use a decision weight function that has only three regions. They interpret a probability of 0 as a decision weight of 0 (i.e., there is no chance that the outcome will occur), probabilities between 0 and 1.00 as decision weights equal to .50 (i.e., there is some chance that the outcome will occur), and a probability of 1.00 as a decision weight of 1.00 (i.e., the outcome will occur). Alternatively, some people use a *threshold function*. For example, in deciding which potential side effects to discuss with a patient, a physician might regard all side effects with an objective probability less than .001 to be essentially 0. Because the physician's decision weights for the outcomes are 0, the physician might not mention the side effects to the patient.

Decision weights have implications for the *standard gamble method* of eliciting health utilities. In a simple standard gamble, a patient might be asked to choose between two treatments. Treatment 1 will produce Health state A with a probability of 1.00. Treatment 2 will produce either perfect health (utility = 1.00) with probability p or instant death (utility = 0) with a probability of $1 - p$. The value of p is the point at which the patient is indifferent between Treatments 1 and 2. Assume that $p = .60$. In expected utility theory, the utility of Health state A is calculated as .60. However, this conclusion is only correct if the patient's decision weight for the probability is .60; that is, there is no subjective distortion in the underlying probability. Because the patient's decision weight is generally not known, most researchers interpret standard gamble results as though there is a 1:1 relationship between probabilities and decision weights.

Approaches other than prospect theory extend the use of decision weights to more complex situations. For example, *rank-dependent* models can order multiple possible outcomes in terms of how good or bad they are for the person. In these approaches, it is desirable to understand how people interpret the *cumulative probabilities* of the outcomes. Imagine that a patient with advanced cancer is examining different treatment options. The possible outcomes of treatment are disease progression, stable disease, partial tumor response, and complete tumor response. Here, the patient is less likely to think about the probabilities of each outcome one at a time. Rather, the patient might think about the chance that a treatment will result in an outcome "at least as good as," say, stable disease. A model of such ranked outcomes posits a cumulative decision weight function to correspond to the cumulative probabilities of the outcomes. This promising approach has yet to take hold in studies of medical decision making.

Kevin Weinfurt

See also Expected Utility Theory; Probability; Prospect Theory

Further Readings

Birnbaum, M. H., & Chavez, A. (1997). Tests of theories of decision making: Violations of branch independence and distribution independence. *Organizational Behavior and Human Decision Processes, 71*, 161–194.

Kahneman, D., & Tversky, A. (1979). Prospect theory: An analysis of decision under risk. *Econometrica, 47*, 263–291.

Tversky, A., & Kahneman, D. (1992). Advances in prospect theory: Cumulative representation of uncertainty. *Journal of Risk and Uncertainty, 5*, 297–323.

Declining Exponential Approximation of Life Expectancy

The declining exponential approximation of life expectancy (DEALE) is a model that simplifies the problem of handling life expectancy calculations in clinical decision analyses. During the early years of clinical decision analysis, much of the focus was on tree construction and probability estimation. Utility or outcome measures were less of a focus; measures such as "percent chance of cure" or "5-year survival" were commonly used in lieu of life expectancy values. In large part, this was because the clinical literature reported results that way. Combining medical risks to estimate survival was rarely done. As decision modelers focused on chronic diseases over short-term problems, the need arose to model life expectancy for healthy persons and those battling disease.

The Mathematical Formulation

Life expectancy has been studied for 180 years. Benjamin Gompertz, a self-educated English mathematician, published a demographic model in 1825. The Gompertz function is a sigmoid curve, shallow at the beginning and at the end, that represents general-population survival with a fair degree of accuracy. The Gompertz survival function is

$$S(t) = e^{-be^{ct}},$$

where

b is the base rate (i.e., initial mortality) and is negative (decreasing survival),

c is the growth rate (i.e., accelerating mortality), and

e is Euler's constant (= 2.71828 ...).

Figure 1 shows the Gompertz survival curve for a healthy population near 70 years. The curve falls slowly at the beginning, with 90% of the population alive after 7 years. By 10 years, however, only 80% of the population is alive, and after 20 years, less than 15% of the cohort is surviving. Thereafter, the curve flattens out, as the still increasing force of mortality acts on the fewer people remaining alive.

Although the Gompertz curve reflects the survival of a healthy population rather well, it offers a basic mathematical challenge: Its integral does not have a closed-form solution. Therefore, the expected value of t in Figure 1 (expected survival time, or life expectancy) cannot be solved exactly. Of course, with modern computational assistance, the area under the survival curve can be calculated to any degree of precision, which would be fine if the only issue were to calculate life expectancy for the general population.

The problem faced in medical decision making adds complexity to this mathematical issue. In a clinical decision analysis, the mortality attached to a disease, or disease-specific mortality, needs to be considered. In many cases, however, the mortality attached to a disease can be estimated from the literature. For many chronic illnesses, a constant specific mortality force can be applied. Assuming that disease-specific mortality rate is independent and additive, the survival function for a person with a chronic disease with constant-mortality rate m would be

$$S(t) = e^{-(be^{ct} + m)}.$$

This additional mortality force would depress the Gompertz curve, more at the beginning than later, as the constant additive risk acts on a larger population early. Of course, this function also cannot be integrated directly, so an expected survival cannot be calculated exactly.

However, if the population mortality were a constant M, then the joint survival function would be

$$S(t) = e^{-(M + m)t},$$

which would be easy to calculate and simple to integrate. The expected value of a probability function is

$$\int_{-\infty}^{\infty} tf(t)dt.$$

For the joint mortality function, which is a probability, the expected value (i.e., life expectancy) is $\int_0^\infty te^{-(M + m)t}dt$. The value of this integral is $1/(M + m)$; that is, the life expectancy associated with a constant mortality μ is $1/\mu$.

Of course, the population mortality is not constant. The conceptual attractiveness of the mathematics led Beck, Kassirer, and Pauker to model Gompertz mortality with various clinically plausible constant excess mortality rates, to determine how this constant-mortality assumption would affect overall-survival calculations. They discovered that this DEALE tended to overestimate mortality, especially in later years, and underestimated survival. For diseases with overall life expectancy at or below 10 years, the DEALE model proved a good approximation to detailed calculations using the "correct" formulation.

The DEALE in Medical Decision Making

The first application of the constant-mortality model was in traditional clinical decision analyses, where life expectancy was the desired outcome

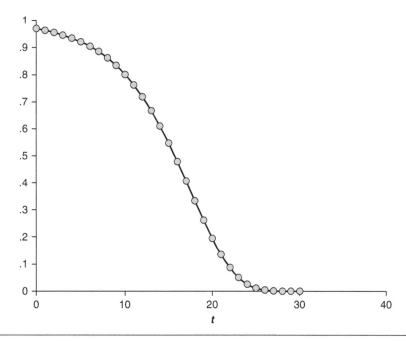

Figure 1   Gompertz survival function

measure. General-population mortality was sub-divided by many authors into age-, gender-, and race-specific rates, taken from *Vital Statistics of the United States.* One to three competing disease-specific mortalities, modified by surgical and medical therapies, were added to the population mortality, and reciprocals were taken to generate outcome measures. Until these models were super-seded by Markov cohort software, they were stan-dard practice for medical decision analyses where life expectancy was the clinically relevant out-come. Over 30 papers employed this strategy in the 5 years after the DEALE was first published, and the method diffused into many areas of clini-cal medicine over the ensuing 20 years. Somewhat surprisingly, articles continue to appear in the lit-erature that use the DEALE model as an outcome measure, although with the worldwide availability of personal computers that run decision analysis software, stochastic modeling approaches should be in routine use.

The DEALE as a Bedside Approximation of Mortality

The fact that mortality and life expectancy are reciprocals under the assumption of constant-mortality rate (the negative exponential function) led to another early use of the DEALE, one that has persisted. Suppose a male patient is 65 years of age. According to a life table, his life expec-tancy is 14.96, or approximately 15 years. The reciprocal of this is .067, or 6.7%. If this patient has a malignancy that has a 10% excess-mortal-ity rate, then his risk of death due to cancer is 1.5 times as great as his general-population mortal-ity. Thus, he has a 60% lifetime risk of death from cancer versus a 40% risk of death from other causes. This approach can be extended to multiple risk factors. Over the past several years, this comparison has been used in oncology to compare therapeutic regimens for patients of varying ages.

The DEALE as a Technique for Probability Estimation

As clinical decision models became more complex, and as trees were supplanted by Markov models for chronic diseases, the DEALE's role as an out-come estimator waned, to be replaced by its endur-ing value as an aid to probability calculation. The approach has several steps:

1. Obtain a life-expectancy-related value from a study or the literature.

2. Determine what form the value takes: overall-mortality rate, excess mortality, 5-year survival, median survival, and so on.

3. Transform the value into an excess-mortality rate.

4. Transform the excess-mortality rate into a probability.

Table 1 illustrates the first three of these steps (adapted from Beck et al., 1982). Four types of data are commonly found in the literature. Mortality rates are often presented as overall values, which include the underlying population mortality as well as disease-specific excess mortality. These rates are transformed into excess mortality (μ_D) by simply subtracting the population mortality (μ_{pop}) from the overall or compound mortality (μ_C). Life expectancy values are reported as time units, most often years. Taking a reciprocal gives the corresponding constant-mortality rate (an approximation given the Gompertz behavior of general-population mortality). From this, one proceeds as above to obtain μ_D.

Five-year survivals require a bit more calculation. From the survival function $S(t)$ above, some algebra transposes it to $\mu = -(1/t)\ln S$. Substituting 5 for t (5-year survival), the reported value for S (38% in Table 1) will yield μ_C. Similarly, median survival is transformed into mortality by substituting the survival time for t and .5 for S (median survival is the time at which half of the cohort, or 50%, has died).

The final step in using the DEALE to generate transition probabilities is to use the equation

$$p = 1-e^{-rt},$$

where r is the rate, in this case a mortality rate, t the time period (in most cases 1 year or one unit, but not necessarily so), and e the natural logarithm base. Of the nearly 150 articles from 2000 to 2008 that cite the original DEALE papers (and several hundred more that do not), most use probability transformation techniques.

Extensions to the DEALE

Although the DEALE was developed to simplify the problem of handling life expectancy calculations in clinical decision analyses, the "fun" mathematics of the model led to refinements and extensions. Stalpers, van Gasteren, and van Daal extended the model to handle multiple time periods, each with different partial DEALE calculations. Durand-Zaleski and Zaleski showed that the DEALE model could admit discounting of present values as a pseudomortality. Keeler and Bell, and van den Hout looked at other mortality functions and showed how some could admit direct or approximate closed-form solutions that would improve the fidelity of the model. These extensions have found uses in clinical decision analyses. Other refinements essentially put the cart before the horse: The math involved in some sophisticated remodeling was so complex that computer assistance was required to use it.

Gompertz functions and mortality modeling have helped increase the rigor of formal clinical

Table 1   Examples of excess mortality rates

Source	Study Population	Reported Data	Compound Rate (μ_C)	Baseline Rate (μ_{pop})	Excess Rate (μ_D)
Mortality rate	66-year-old men	.230 per year	.230	.070	.160
Life expectancy	55-year-old women	4.5 years	.222	.037	.185
5-year survival	60-year-olds	38%	.194	.045	.148
Median survival	44-year-old men	7.2 years	.096	.032	.065

decision analyses and risk analyses. Despite the limitations of the approximation, over the past 25 years the approach has meant a good "DEALE" for medical decision making.

J. Robert Beck

See also Decision Tree: Introduction; Life Expectancy; Markov Models

Further Readings

Beck, J. R., Kassirer, J. P., & Pauker, S. G. (1982). A convenient approximation of life expectancy (The "DEALE"). I. Validation of the method. *American Journal of Medicine, 73,* 883–888.

Beck, J. R., Pauker, S. G., Gottlieb, J. E., Klein, K., & Kassirer, J. P. (1982). A convenient approximation of life expectancy (The "DEALE"). II. Use in medical decision making. *American Journal of Medicine, 73,* 889–897.

Durand-Zaleski, I., & Zaleski, S. (1994). DEALE-ing and discounting: A simple way to compute the accrued costs of preventive strategies. *Medical Decision Making, 14,* 98–103.

Gompertz, B. (1825). On the nature of the function expressive of the law of human mortality. *Philosophical Transactions of the Royal Society of London, 115,* 513–585.

Keeler, E., & Bell, R. (1992). New DEALEs: Other approximations of life expectancy. *Medical Decision Making, 12,* 307–311.

Life expectancy tables. Retrieved February 10, 2009, from http://www.annuityadvantage.com/lifeexpectancy.htm

Stalpers, L. J. A., van Gasteren, H. J. M., & van Daal, W. A. L. (1989). DEALE-ing with life expectancy and mortality rates. *Medical Decision Making, 9,* 150–152.

van den Hout, W. B. (2004). The GAME estimate of reduced life expectancy. *Medical Decision Making, 24,* 80–88.

DECOMPOSED MEASUREMENT

The decomposed approach to the measurement of preferences for health states, services, or treatments expresses the overall preference as a decomposed function of the attributes of the health state, service, or treatment. It requires the systematic decomposition of the decision problem into smaller parts. It enables the investigator to obtain values for all health states, services, or treatments without requiring the judge to assign values to every one. Decomposition of complex decisions has been shown to aid the decision-making process and its outcomes.

Valuing Health States, Services, or Treatments

Basically, there are two different approaches to measuring preferences for health states, services, or treatments. The holistic approach requires the rater to assign values to each possible health state or treatment, where a state or treatment represents a combination of many attributes. The rater is thus required to simultaneously consider all the relevant attributes during the assessment. The decomposed approach expresses the overall value as a decomposed function of the attributes. The decomposed approach can also be used to simply obtain values for aspects (attributes) of health states or treatments.

As an example, preoperative adjuvant radiotherapy for rectal cancer may increase survival and local control over surgery alone, but at the expense of continence and sexual functioning. The relative value patients place on each of these attributes will determine whether they are prepared to undergo radiotherapy as an adjunct to surgery.

The decomposed models that reveal how a patient values different attributes can be based on statistical inference or explicit decomposition. They have several purposes. First, as in the case of multi-attribute utility theory (MAUT), discussed below, relative importance ratings for attributes can be used to identify global preferences for health states or treatments. Second, where there are individual differences in preferences, the values underlying those preferences can be identified. Such an analysis can highlight the key issues that carers should raise when discussing treatments with patients. For example, conjoint analysis may reveal that lack of energy is an important determinant of preferences for the management of non-metastatic prostate cancer. With this in mind, patient treatment could focus on increasing the energy levels. Such analysis may thus identify new treatment packages that, with minimum cost or effort, create a much preferred alternative. Third, knowledge of other patients' preference patterns may aid individuals in making choices about their own treatment.

Multi-Attribute Utility Theory

The best-known application of a decomposed method is that based on MAUT, which uses explicit decomposition. Each attribute of a health state (or similarly of a treatment) is given an importance weight. Next, respondents score how well each health state (or treatment) does on each attribute. These scores are weighted by the importance of the attributes and then summed over the attributes to give an overall multi-attribute score for each state (or treatment). For this summation, the theory specifies utility functions and the independence conditions under which they would be appropriate. Gretchen Chapman has used a MAUT model to assess prostate cancer patients' preferences for health states. She describes metastatic prostate cancer by the attributes pain, mood, sexual function, bladder and bowel function, and fatigue and energy, each at three levels of functioning. The attributes had been predefined, and the patients were asked to rate the relative importance of these by dividing 100 points among them. Next, the patients indicated their current level of health for each attribute. MAUT scores were computed by multiplying, for each attribute, the level by the attribute importance weight and summing across the attributes.

Analytical Hierarchy Process

The analytical hierarchy process (AHP) decomposes options into a hierarchy of criteria that include a person's ultimate goal for the decision. First, participants identify their ultimate goal (e.g., maximum possible health and well-being) and the subgoals (criteria) that contribute to it (e.g., avoiding side effects, decreasing the risk of cancer). The participants compare options in a pairwise fashion in terms of these criteria: They give them a rating to indicate which is better or whether they are similar. These pairwise ratings can be combined to give each option a score in terms of each criterion and to work out how the attributes describing an option contribute to achieving the criteria. The participants then prioritize these criteria, giving them a weight to indicate how much they contribute to achieving the ultimate goal. These can be combined to give each option a score in terms of the ultimate goal.

Health State Classification Systems

Both MAUT and statistically inferred regression methods have found well-known applications in the health state classification systems. The two most often used systems are the Health Utilities Index (HUI) and the EQ-5D. Health state classification systems, or health indexes, are customarily composed of two components: a descriptive system and a formula for assigning a utility to any unique set of responses to the descriptive system. The descriptive system consists of a set of attributes, and a health state is described by indicating the appropriate level of functioning on each attribute. For instance, in the EQ-5D, the attributes, or domains, are mobility, self-care, usual activities, pain/discomfort, and anxiety/depression. Each domain is divided into three levels of severity, corresponding to no problem, some problem, and extreme problem. By combining each of the three levels from each of the five domains, a total of 3^5—that is, 243—EQ-5D health states are defined. The formula is generally based on utilities that have been obtained in part from direct measurement and in part from application of MAUT (in the HUI) or statistical inference (in the EQ-5D) to fill in values not measured directly. In both instances, only a limited number of valuations have been obtained from the surveyed population, usually the general public. Of more recent date is a scoring formula based on the SF-36 descriptive quality-of-life instrument. Researchers in the United Kingdom have created from this instrument a six-dimensional health classification system called the SF-6D.

Valuing Aspects of Health States and Treatments

Whereas the ultimate aim of techniques such as MAUT is to assess preferences for health states, or treatments, via decomposition, other techniques aim to measure how treatment or health state attributes in themselves are valued. Judgment analysis, conjoint analysis, discrete choice experiments, and the repertory grid method each examine how aspects of a treatment or health state influence preferences. In these methods, a holistic valuation technique is used to derive the underlying value of the dimensions described in scenarios. In these cases, a rater holistically values a set of scenarios in which the dimensions appear together in various combinations. The full set of these holistic scores is then analyzed with multiple regression techniques to derive the underlying value each rater was assumed to have assigned to each dimension while making a holistic judgment.

Conjoint Analysis

Conjoint analysis has been widely used to examine consumer preferences, particularly in marketing, and its use in examining patient preferences is increasing with the availability of both generic and specialist software. The principle of conjoint analysis is that evaluations of options are compared to reveal the importance of differences between them. Similar to the statistically based decomposition techniques described above, participants judge hypothetical cases (health states or treatments) that are described in terms of combinations of attributes at particular levels. Statistical analysis reveals the relative importance weights of attributes and identifies sets of attribute-level utilities. Discrete choice experiments are variations on forced-choice conjoint analysis with their roots in economics. Analysis of the data is based on random-utility theory. Judgment analysis is technically similar to conjoint analysis but has its roots in a Brunswikian tradition of psychology, seeking to describe participants' natural judgment processes as they happen, rather than what they would prefer if they had a range of options.

Repertory Grid Technique

The use of repertory grid techniques has been proposed as a bottom-up approach to analyzing what is of more or less importance to patients choosing between treatments. While conjoint analysis and other statistical inference techniques have their roots in psychophysics, perception, and cognition, repertory grid techniques emerged from Kelly's construct theory in social psychology. It has been used to assess patients' quality-of-life measures in relation to their previous and desired states of health. In the statistical inference techniques discussed above, option attributes are defined or identified by the researcher prior to analyzing their relative importance. In the case of the analytical hierarchy process, this may happen after discussion with respondents. In repertory grid analysis, the defining attributes, and their hierarchical combinations, emerge from participants' contrasts between options.

Repertory grid analysis involves four steps. First, in a series of judgments, a participant indicates which of three options (such as treatments) differs from the other two and in what way. This is repeated for all possible triplets of options. Second, each option is rated to indicate to what degree it has this characteristic. Third, characteristics are rated to indicate how important they are. Fourth, a grid of options by characteristics (termed constructs) is analyzed, using simple frequency counts (the number of times a particular construct appears in the option set or the number of overlapping constructs that options have is counted) or using some sort of computer-based cluster analysis. Principal components analysis identifies the correlations between patterns of constructs for each option to reveal which are similar to each other and which constructs tend to co-occur and form a principal component. Generalized procrustes analysis (GPA) is similar to principal components analysis, but it can summarize results across participants even if they have not produced an identical set of constructs.

Anne M. Stiggelbout

See also Conjoint Analysis; Discrete Choice; EuroQoL (EQ-5D); Health Utilities Index Mark 2 and 3 (HUI2, HUI3); Holistic Measurement; Multi-Attribute Utility Theory; SF-6D; Social Judgment Theory

Further Readings

Chapman, G. B., Elstein, A. S., Kuzel, T. M., Nadler, R. B., Sharifi, R., & Bennett, C. L. (1999). A multi-attribute model of prostate cancer patients' preferences for health states. *Quality of Life Research, 8,* 171–180.

Dolan, J. G. (1995). Are patients capable of using the analytic hierarchy process and willing to use it to help make clinical decisions? *Medical Decision Making, 15,* 76–80.

Harries, C., & Stiggelbout, A. M. (2005). Approaches to measuring patients' decision-making. In A. Bowling & S. Ebrahim (Eds.), *Handbook of health research methods: Investigation, measurement and analysis* (pp. 362–393). Maidenhead, UK: Open University/ McGraw-Hill.

Kelly, G. A. (1955). *The psychology of personal constructs*. New York: Norton.

Morera, O. F., & Budescu, D. V. (1998). A psychometric analysis of the "divide and conquer" principle in multicriteria decision making. *Organizational Behavior and Human Decision Processes, 75,* 187–206.

Rowe, G., Lambert, N., Bowling, A., Ebrahim, S., Wakeling, I., & Thomson, R. (2005). Assessing patients' preferences for treatments for angina using a modified repertory grid method. *Social Science Medicine, 60,* 2585–2595.

Ryan, M., & Farrar, S. (2000). Using conjoint analysis to elicit preferences for health care. *British Medical Journal, 320,* 1530–1533.

Von Winterfeldt, D., & Edwards, W. (1986) *Decision analysis and behavioral research.* Cambridge, UK: Cambridge University Press.

DELIBERATION AND CHOICE PROCESSES

Deliberation is consideration of the reasons for and against an action, issue, or measure. Deliberation may be carried out with attention and without attention. The notion of deliberation without attention brings to realization the notion of dual (or multiple types of) processing of information underlying and affecting acts of deliberating.

Much attention is directed to the notion of how individuals can better focus mentally on their decision problems and structure (formulate) their decision problems to better optimize the decisions they make. These issues become even more of a concern for individuals with declining brain function. A population whose members have a susceptibility to developing neurodegenerative diseases focuses public attention on the loss of the affected individuals' contribution to society and their increased dependence on societal resources to care for them as they continue to age. Today, we have rough estimates of the levels of success in slowing cognitive deterioration from neurodegenerative disease through various modalities. A Dutch team of investigators used brighter daytime lighting to improve patients' sleep and mood and cut aggressive behavior. These researchers found that brighter daytime lighting can slow cognitive deterioration by 5%. This figure is judged at this time to compare well with the rate of slowing of cognitive deterioration in humans through the use of current prescription medicines.

Deliberations With Attention

Research on deliberations with attention may be carried out in nonmedical and medical contexts. In the research arena, investigators have studied nonmedical deliberations involving purchase decisions, which they describe as "simple" (a choice of which towels to buy among a set of towels available at a time) or "complex" (a choice of which car to buy among a set of cars available). One characteristic shared by such simple and complex product purchase decisions is that deliberations with attention regarding such purchases (barring extenuating circumstances) do not have to necessarily be made at that time but can be delayed until a future time, as long as the items are available and the price is right.

Medical Decision Making

While investigators may study simpler and more complex choices in medical deliberations, medical deliberations have a unique quality: the nondelay factor. Many decisions in medicine are a matter of life and death—act now or face the consequences later. Deliberations may not be delayed without adverse consequences for the patient.

The issue of nondelay of medical decisions arises because of the chance that a medical condition will advance if it is not acted on quickly or soon enough. A delay in medical intervention in an individual may cause consequences for that individual in the future. The delayed decision may no longer be about the initial medical condition or disease process but may evolve into a different decision wherein the medical condition or disease considered for intervention is more advanced than it was at that earlier time when first identified.

Consider the following example. The treatment decision in an oncologic disease, such as early-stage

Hodgkin's disease, when it is first diagnosed in a patient is much different from a delayed decision. In the latter case, Hodgkin's disease may have progressed because the intervention was not applied in the early stage. Here, because the competent adult (for whatever reason) chooses not to undergo treatment when the disease is first diagnosed (and is most responsive to therapy), the decision is delayed. Delaying this particular decision means that the disease will continue to grow and continue to progress in its development; the disease may evolve from being curable to being potentially curable and then to being incurable. At the incurable stage, the only treatment option available will be palliation.

Medical Care and Medical Research

Deliberation is at the very heart of some conceptions of decision making in two very different areas: medical care and medical research. The fact that medical care needs to be distinguished from medical research is a view traceable to *The Belmont Report* (1979), created by the National Commission for the Protection of Human Subjects of Biomedical and Behavioral Research.

Medical care and medical research are distinguished in the following ways. In medical care, (a) the care is being provided with one purpose only—that is, to best screen, diagnose, and treat the individual patient, and (b) the patient bears all risks of the screening, diagnostic, and treatment interventions that are undertaken with the patient's permission, but the interventions themselves for the most part have undergone study with the approval of regulatory bodies within government for their use in the population. This is particularly true of medical care with the use of medical products such as prescription medicines and medical devices. These medical products have gone through preapproval research studies, which have developed an evidentiary base for the medical product, and the medical product is approved based on the scientific evidence developed during its research and development phases. In medical care, it is recognized that a competent adult individual—except in the context of a medical emergency—chooses to come to the physician for medical care.

In medical research, the principal investigator (or designee) pursues the individual as part of an act of recruitment, where the individual in many cases is not aware at all of the study's existence prior to being pursued as a study volunteer. Here, the individual is made aware of the study's existence by the pursuit and recruitment processes that have been put into place for a particular research study. This individual is asked to consider study participation and asked to engage in an informed-consent session, where the principal investigator or designee presents the research study, its goals, its methods, its risks, and how liability for injury will be handled within the research study, among other points. Part of the information provided to the individual being recruited into a research study is a discussion of the nature of "research" itself as an activity with one focus only: to attempt to develop new scientific knowledge that might benefit future generations. This new scientific knowledge will then become the evidentiary base for the medical product or medical intervention that may result in approval for its use in the population.

Legal Concepts

Disclosure

The imparting of information for deliberation is termed *disclosure*. The notion of disclosure in the court-defined concepts of consent and informed consent refers to disclosure of information by the physician to the patient (or by the principal investigator to the study volunteer) for the purposes of the patient's deliberations about whether to accept a physician-recommended intervention for the patient's care (or the deliberations of an individual being recruited into a medical research study considering whether or not he or she will enroll in a research trial as a study volunteer). Yet the courts—for example, the landmark 1972 U.S. federal decision in *Canterbury v. Spence*—are also very clear that a competent adult patient in medical care can base his or her decision on whatever grounds the patient sees fit. Similarly, an individual can not enroll in a research study and, even after enrolling, can terminate his or her enrollment in the research study within the bounds of safety for any reason that the individual sees fit.

Autonomy, Trust, and Accountability

Autonomy and self-decision have been foundational concepts in court and medical decision making in the United States, Canada, and Australia. In England, Onora O'Neill has argued that there are foundational truths besides autonomy and self-decision on which legal structure can be based for the protection of patients and study volunteers. Here, O'Neill argues for "trust" in decision making and "accountability" of those responsible for medical care and medical research as the focus of attention in consent and informed consent. Accountability in this sense involves increased institutional efforts to check on the responsibilities of those overseeing decision making in medical care or medical research to ensure that the best decisions are being made and carried out on the patient's or study volunteer's behalf in medical care and in medical research on humans, respectively.

O'Neill argues that trust and accountability in issues of informed consent can provide a level of protection that is more durable in decision making in medical care and in medical research than considerations solely of individual autonomy. Neil C. Manson and O'Neill discuss the notion of informed consent in terms of waivers against receiving certain types of information. Ethicists continue to examine the conceptual developments related to consent, informed consent, choice, and decision making as conscious choices involving deliberation with attention.

Deliberation Without Attention

Ap Dijksterhuis and colleagues have described what they call the *deliberation-without-attention effect*. The authors argue that it is not always advantageous to engage in thorough conscious deliberation before choosing in the arena of product purchases. As noted earlier, the authors studied simple choices (choices between or among different towels or different sets of oven mitts) and complex choices (choices between different houses or different cars). The authors found that simple choices produce better results after conscious thought but that choices in complex matters should be left to unconscious thought (deliberation without attention).

Neuroeconomics

Alan G. Sanfey and Luke J. Chang define "neuroeconomics" as the science that seeks to gain a greater understanding of decision making by combining theoretical and methodological principles from the fields of psychology, economics, and neuroscience. Key among the early findings of neuroeconomics is evidence that the brain itself may be capable of employing dual-level (or even multiple level) processing of information when making decisions. Sanfey and Chang argue that while behavioral studies provide compelling support for the distinction between automatic and controlled processing in judgment and decision making, less is known about to what extent these components have a corresponding neural substrate. Yet there are other effects on judgment and decision making that need further clarification with neuroeconomics.

Deliberation Deficits

Disinhibition is a process whereby an individual with a measurable capacity to edit his or her immediate impulsive response to a stimulus or situation is rendered to have a deficit in this capacity. Such incapacities are found (a) after brain injuries to the orbitofrontal and basotemporal cortices of the right hemisphere of the brain (caused by closed-head traumatic brain injuries, brain tumors, stroke lesions, and focal epilepsy), which selectively inhibit or release motor, instinctive, affective, and intellectual behaviors elaborated in the dorsal cortex; (b) after the application of agents such as alcohol; and (c) after the use of prescription medicines such as the benzodiazepines alprazolam and flunitrazepam. Benzodiazepines have an effect on gamma-aminobutyric acid, the chief inhibitory neurotransmitter in the central nervous system and the retinas of humans.

Future Research

Future research in the area of deliberations and choice will continue to clarify three areas: deliberation with attention, deliberation without attention, and the impact of brain lesions, agents, and prescription medicines on choice and deliberation. Research is also needed on how best to define and measure nonrisky and risky options over which deliberations are carried out in research trials on medical decision making.

Dennis J. Mazur

See also Decisions Faced by Institutional Review Boards; Informed Consent

Further Readings

Bhugra, D. (2008). Decision making by patients: Who gains? *International Journal of Social Psychiatry, 54,* 5–6.

Griffin, R. J., Yang, Z., ter Huurne, E., Boerner, F., Ortiz, S., & Dunwoody, S. (2008). After the flood: Anger, attribution, and the seeking of information. *Science Communication, 29,* 285–315.

Lane, S. D., Cherek, D. R., & Nouvion, S. O. (2008). Modulation of human risky decision making by flunitrazepam. *Psychopharmacology (Berlin), 196,* 177–188.

Lau, H. C., & Passingham, R. E. (2007). Unconscious activation of the cognitive control system in the human prefrontal cortex. *Journal of Neuroscience, 27,* 5805–5811.

Manson, N. C., & O'Neill, O. (2007). *Rethinking informed consent.* New York: Cambridge University Press.

National Commission for the Protection of Human Subjects of Biomedical and Behavioral Research. (1979). *The Belmont report: Ethical principles and guidelines for the protection of human subjects of research.* Washington, DC: U.S. Department of Health, Education, and Welfare.

O'Neill, O. (2004). Accountability, trust and informed consent in medical practice and research. *Clinical Medicine, 4,* 269–276.

O'Neill, O. (2004). Informed consent and public health. *Philosophical Transactions of the Royal Society of London. Series B, Biological Sciences, 359,* 1133–1136.

Riemersma-van der Lek, R. F., Swaab, D. F., Twisk, J., Hol, E. M. Hoogendijk, W. J. G., & Van Someren, E. J. W. (2008). Effect of bright light and melatonin on cognitive and noncognitive function in elderly residents of group care facilities: A randomized controlled trial. *Journal of the American Medical Association, 299,* 2642–2655.

Sanfey, A. G., & Chang, L. J. (2008). Multiple systems in decision making. *Annals of the New York Academy of Sciences, 1128,* 53–62.

DETERMINISTIC ANALYSIS

Deterministic analysis and decision analysis are not interchangeable. Instead, deterministic analysis is one of the analytical approaches under decision analysis. Under the framework of decision analysis, deterministic analysis conducts mathematical calculations to compare the outcomes of interest.

In medical decision making, the outcome of medical interventions is usually measured by clinical efficacy, effectiveness, or cost-effectiveness. Deterministic analysis compares outcomes of alternative interventions by developing a mathematical model to calculate the value of the outcomes associated with each intervention. The model is often structured in the form of a decision analytical model and contains a number of parameters that affect the outcome of interventions. Deterministic analysis uses the best available estimate of each parameter as the model input and the report point estimate, such as means or median, of the outcome of interest as the model output. For example, deterministic analysis of a cost-effectiveness analysis comparing two interventions may include probabilities of the occurrence of certain clinical events, utilization patterns of healthcare resources, and unit cost associated with each type of healthcare resource as the model inputs and may report the results in terms of a point estimate of the incremental cost-effectiveness ratio (ICER), calculated as the difference in the mean cost between the two competing interventions divided by the difference in the mean effectiveness between these two interventions. Deterministic analysis is not only a terminology used in the field of medical decision making, it is also mentioned in the literature of operational research, civil engineering, and risk assessment, among others.

Sensitivity Analyses

Findings from deterministic analyses serve as the base case scenario of the model output, and researchers apply sensitivity analyses to evaluate whether the conclusions derived from the model are sensitive to the model parameters. Sensitivity analyses vary the model parameters within reasonable ranges to examine the effect of these parameters on the conclusion of the analyses. The number of parameters assessed in sensitivity analyses often ranges from one (known as the one-way sensitivity analyses) to three (three-way sensitivity analyses) because it becomes extremely difficult to interpret the findings of sensitivity analyses if the number of parameters exceeds three. For ease of illustration, one-way sensitivity analyses are most frequently used to address uncertainties in deterministic modeling. In these analyses, researchers will vary parameters of interest one at a time to determine which parameter(s) has the largest effect on the study findings.

When reporting findings from deterministic analyses, it is common to add a *tornado diagram* to summarize the results of one-way sensitivity analyses graphically. Tornado diagrams are charts that use horizontal bars to describe the magnitude of effect associated with each parameter. Decision makers can visually identify the most influential parameters based on the width of each bar in the diagram. Another analysis commonly added to sensitivity analyses, but not limited to one-way sensitivity analyses, is the *threshold analysis*, in which the deterministic model calculates the parameter value or values indicating that decision makers are indifferent between two interventions (i.e., the break-even point). The idea of threshold analysis is to inform decision makers of the minimum or maximum value (i.e., the threshold value) of a certain model parameter for an intervention to be considered effective or cost-effective. Readers who are looking for straightforward examples and clear graphical illustrations of various forms of sensitivity analyses should read the chapter "Sensitivity Analysis" in Petitti (2000).

Advantage

The advantage of deterministic analyses is that the output of the model is summarized in an exact number (e.g., life expectancy, quality-adjusted life years [QALY], and ICER), which makes it easier for decision makers to select the best intervention. For example, in a deterministic analysis comparing the life expectancy of various interventions, decision makers can simply identify the best intervention by picking the intervention that yields the highest mean life expectancy calculated from the model. Similarly, in a deterministic cost-effectiveness analysis comparing a new intervention with a standard-of-care intervention, decision makers can determine whether the new intervention is cost-effective by assessing whether the ICER calculated from the model is lower than the level of willingness to pay society sets forth for new medical interventions

(e.g., $50,000 or $100,000 per QALY). However, as the model becomes more complex, the number of parameters involved increases accordingly, and it becomes more difficult to understand the results of sensitivity analyses due to the excessive number of parameters (for one-way sensitivity analyses) or combinations of parameters (for two- or three-way sensitivity analyses) to be explored.

Relationship With Stochastic Analyses

Although deterministic analyses have the advantage of being exact, the information presented in these analyses is not sufficient to perform hypothesis testing. Therefore, in studies comparing two interventions, deterministic analyses are able to calculate the mean difference in effectiveness between these two interventions but cannot inform decision makers whether the calculated difference can be considered statistically significant. For the purpose of hypothesis testing and to obtain information on the uncertainties associated with model parameters or estimates, it is necessary to conduct another type of analysis known as *stochastic analysis* (or *probabilistic analysis*). The distinction between deterministic and stochastic analyses can be clearly understood in the context of assessing the effectiveness of health interventions, in which deterministic analyses are viewed as analyses that use information on *the average number of events per population*, whereas stochastic analyses use randomization to simulate *the probability distributions of events that may occur*.

There are a number of important differences between deterministic and stochastic analyses. First, deterministic analyses report results as exact numbers, while stochastic analyses present findings either in 95% confidence intervals or as the probability that one treatment is more effective (or more cost-effective) than the other(s). The former presentation is based on analyses taking a classical statistical approach (also known as the frequentist approach), and the latter uses the Bayesian approach. Second, deterministic analyses assume certainty about parameter values that are used as model inputs, whereas stochastic analyses explicitly acknowledge uncertainties in parameter values and describe them in probability distributions. For example, when incorporating hospitalization cost as one of the components in the estimation of total medical costs, deterministic analyses will include the average cost per hospitalization as the model input, but stochastic analyses will use either lognormal or gamma distribution to characterize this parameter. Last, the lack of knowledge about model parameters was addressed with sensitivity analyses in deterministic analyses and probabilistic sensitivity analyses in stochastic analyses. As discussed previously, sensitivity analyses vary the model parameters within a reasonable range to determine the impact of each parameter (or a combination of two or more parameters) on the study findings. In probabilistic sensitivity analysis, model parameters are described as random variables, each with its own designated probability distribution, and researchers can perform Monte Carlo simulations to estimate the mean and standard deviation of the expected outcome(s) or calculate the probability that one strategy performs better than the other(s). Doubilet and colleagues provided a clear illustration of probabilistic sensitivity analysis. In their article comparing the expected utility among three treatment strategies, (1) biopsy but no treatment, (2) treat but no biopsy, and (3) no biopsy and no treatment, deterministic analyses showed that the expected utilities associated with the above three strategies were .558, .566, and .494, respectively. That is, the strategy "treat but no biopsy" had the highest expected utility. However, such an analysis did not inform the decision maker whether this strategy was significantly better than the other two strategies. On the contrary, the results from the probabilistic sensitivity analyses indicated that the likelihood that "treat but no biopsy" was the best strategy was 80%, as compared with 18% and 2% for the "biopsy but no treatment" and "no biopsy and no treatment" strategies, respectively.

Deterministic and stochastic analyses should not be viewed as rival analytical approaches. Indeed, a comprehensive study is expected to present results from both deterministic and stochastic analyses. Perhaps the best way to describe the relationship between these two types of analysis was expressed in a review article by Corner and Corner in 1995. The authors envisioned a decision problem from a systems engineering perspective and characterized the decision-making process in four steps. In Step 1, a basic structure was developed to model the decision problem and identify the relevant parameters in the model. In Step 2, deterministic analysis was performed, along with sensitivity analysis, to remove those variables that would not affect the final results. Step 3 involved a complete analysis of uncertainty using stochastic analysis and concluded with a recommendation of the best (or most cost-effective) strategy. Step 4 related to model validation and the value of information analysis. Together these four steps complete a decision analysis cycle. The decision-making process can become iterative as information gained from Step 4 may lead to modification of the model structure, thus starting the decision cycle from Step 1 again.

Recent methodological development has made substantial improvements in the statistical and computational methods used in stochastic analysis. This does not mean that deterministic analysis has lost its role in medical decision making. Regardless of how sophisticated the analytical techniques have become, the exact value calculated from deterministic analyses is often what matters most to decision makers, or at least what is most remembered by them.

Ya-Chen Tina Shih

See also Bayesian Analysis; Confidence Intervals; Cost-Effectiveness Analysis; Cost-Utility Analysis; Expected Value of Perfect Information; Frequentist Approach; Hypothesis Testing; Life Expectancy; Managing Variability and Uncertainty; Marginal or Incremental Analysis, Cost-Effectiveness Ratio; Probability; Quality-Adjusted Life Years (QALYs); Statistical Testing: Overview; Threshold Technique; Tornado Diagram; Uncertainty in Medical Decisions; Variance and Covariance

Further Readings

Briggs, A. H. (1999). A Bayesian approach to stochastic cost-effectiveness analysis. *Health Economics, 8*(3), 257–261.

Briggs, A. H. (2000). Handling uncertainty in cost-effectiveness models. *PharmacoEconomics, 17*(5), 479–500.

Claxton, K., Sculpher, M., McCabe, C., Briggs, A., Akehurst, R., Buxton, M., et al. (2005). Probabilistic sensitivity analysis for NICE technology assessment: Not an optional extra. *Health Economics, 14*(4), 339–347.

Corner, J. L., & Corner, P. D. (1995). Characteristics of decisions in decision analysis practice. *Journal of the Operational Research Society, 46*(3), 304–314.

Doubilet, P., Begg, C. B., Weinstein, M. C., Brawn, P., & McNeil, B. J. (1985). Probabilistic sensitivity analysis using Monte Carlo simulation: A practical approach. *Medical Decision Making, 5*(2), 157–177.

Mandelblatt, J. S., Fryback, D. G., Weinstein, M. C., Russell, L. B., Gold, M. R., & Hadorn, D. C. (1996). Assessing the effectiveness of health interventions. In M. R. Gold, J. E. Siegel, L. B. Russell, & M. C. Weinstein (Eds.), *Cost-effectiveness in health and medicine* (Chap. 5). New York: Oxford University Press.

Petitti, D. B. (2000). *Meta-analysis, decision analysis, and cost-effectiveness analysis: Methods for quantitative synthesis in medicine* (2nd ed.). New York: Oxford University Press.

Shih, Y. C. T., & Halpern, M. T. (2008). Economic evaluation of medical interventions for cancer patients: How, why, and what does it mean? *CA: A Cancer Journal for Clinicians, 58*, 231–244.

DEVELOPMENTAL THEORIES

Developmental theories concern changes that occur over the lifespan as a result of maturation and experience. The nature of decision making shifts as children become adolescents and, as more recent research shows, as adolescents become adults and adults age. Two major theories of decision making are discussed that are also theories of development: the prototype/willingness model and fuzzy-trace theory. When discussing decision making in a medical context, it is important to keep in mind the key concepts of risk perception and informed consent (including issues of autonomy). How these theories address each of these issues and their implications for development and rationality are discussed.

In discussing what rationality in decision making is, it important to note two approaches offered as criteria: coherence and correspondence. The coherence criterion for rational decision making is that a decision is rational if the process used is internally consistent. For example, decision makers use a logical rule to combine their assessments of the costs and benefits of each option. Furthermore, the choice made must reflect the decision makers' goals. This coherence criterion is what is traditionally referred to when a process is described as rational. For the coherence criterion, the outcome of the decision is not involved in denoting a decision as rational. The correspondence criterion argues that outcomes do matter. To the extent that the decisions made correspond with good outcomes in reality (e.g., they cause no harm to the decision maker or to others), the decision can be considered rational. Researchers who focus on the health of children and youth often emphasize positive outcomes. However, coherent reasoning is also relevant for issues such as whether young people are capable of giving informed consent for medical treatments.

The two theories discussed here are dual-process theories of decision making. These theories argue that there are two ways in which a decision maker can arrive at a decision. One process is rational (in the traditional sense) and analytic. This process involves the decision maker combining relevant factors using a logically defensible decision rule; behavior resulting from this process is a planned and intentional action. The other process is described as intuitive. This process is quick and does not involve deliberation. Although both theories are similar in that they propose a dual-process distinction, they differ in what is proposed for developing and what is considered rational. Crucially, intuition in prototype/willingness theory is developmentally primitive, whereas intuition in fuzzy-trace theory characterizes advanced thinking.

Prototype/Willingness Model

A standard dual-process theory, the prototype/willingness model has been applied to many health decisions, such as the decision to smoke or drink, and to health-promoting behaviors, such as cancer screening and family planning. The prototype/willingness model argues that there are two paths to a decision, a reasoned path and a reactive path. For the reasoned path, intentions are the direct antecedent to behavior. In turn, intentions are a function of subjective norms and attitudes. Decisions using the reasoned path are deliberative and planned and characterize more mature decision makers. The reactive path was proposed to capture behavior that is not deliberative and is captured by the construct of willingness. Research has shown that willingness is able to explain unique variance when included in a model with behavioral intentions. For the reactive path, individuals are said to form images of the prototypical person who regularly performs the behavior. What dictates behavior from this process is the reaction that the individual has to this prototype. For instance, producing a prototype of a smoker, an individual can have a positive reaction to the prototype, increasing the probability that the individual will smoke, or a negative reaction to the prototype, decreasing the probability that the individual will smoke. (The theory also holds that a negative image can sometimes be viewed as a cost of engaging in the behavior.) Furthermore, individuals recognize that the more they do the behavior, the more they will come to be perceived as similar to the prototype.

For the prototype/willingness model, development progresses from greater use of the reactive path as children get older to greater reliance on the reasoned path as adults. Therefore, the reasoned path is considered the rational process. Because adolescents are said to be preoccupied with social images and identities, they are more likely to rely on the reactive path than adults. Studies have shown that a positive relationship between intentions and behavior increases with age. Risk perception for the reactive path is defined by the reaction the individual has to the prototype, yet for the reasoned path, it is dictated by the knowledge the individual has of the risk.

Fuzzy-Trace Theory

A more recent dual-process theory, fuzzy-trace theory is based on studies of memory, reasoning, social judgment, and decision making. The theory has been applied to children, adolescents, younger adults, and older adults as well as to groups varying in expertise, such as medical students and physicians. The phrase *fuzzy trace* refers to a distinction between gist memory representations that are fuzzy (i.e., they are vague and impressionistic) and verbatim memory representations that are vivid. Reasoning gravitates to using gist (or fuzzy) representations, which minimizes errors. Moreover, this adaptive tendency to use gist representations—the fuzzy-processing preference—increases with development as children and youth gain experience. Studies of children (comparing older with younger children) and of adults (comparing experts with novices in a domain of knowledge) have demon-

strated that reliance on gist representations increases with development. People make decisions using simple gist representations of information, often processing it unconsciously, and engage in parallel rather than serial processing of that information (leaping ahead based on vague gist impressions of the relations and patterns in information without fully encoding details). This kind of thinking is what is meant by "gist-based intuitive reasoning." What develops with age and experience, therefore, is a greater reliance on gist-based intuition in decision processes. Fuzzy-trace theory has been used to describe developmental trends in adolescent risky decision making, HIV prevention, cardiovascular disease, and cancer prevention.

Specifically, fuzzy-trace theory relies on four basic principles in explaining decision making: (1) parallel encoding, (2) the fuzzy-to-verbatim continua, (3) the fuzzy-processing preference, and (4) task calibration. Parallel encoding states that people extract patterns from the environment and encode them along with exact surface form information. These traces (verbatim and gist) are independent, as previously discussed. The second principle, the fuzzy-to-verbatim continua, states that people encode multiple representations at varying levels of precision. At one end are factual, detailed verbatim representations, and at the other end are simplified, abstracted gist representations. These representations are sensitive to environmental cues, meaning that either could be used in the decision process, depending on which representation is cued in context. Verbatim representations support a quantitative, analytic process, while gist representations support an intuitive/holistic process. Since problems are represented at multiple levels of specificity, the same problem can be approached analytically (verbatim) or intuitively (gist) depending on which representation is retrieved. The third principle, task calibration, states that the lowest level of gist required is used to perform the task. For instance, when deciding between Option A, gaining $5, or Option B, gaining $7, one need only remember the ordinal distinction between the two, B > A, to choose B. Finally, the fuzzy-processing preference states that individuals prefer to operate on the simplest representation (gist) needed to accomplish their goals. For development, studies have shown that young children are more likely to make decisions based on quantitative differences and that what develops with experience is a greater reliance on gist representations, a finding predicted by fuzzy-trace theory. Therefore, consistent with fuzzy-trace theory, gist-based intuitive reasoning has been shown to be the more advanced (and consequently more rational) mode of processing.

Risk perception can vary along the fuzzy-to-verbatim continua in that it can be precise, for example, remembering the exact risk that was conveyed if the surgery were done, or it can be fuzzy, for example, remembering that there is a risk with surgery but not the exact number. Fuzzy-trace theory explains and predicts the major findings in risk perception and risk taking—for example, that risk perceptions vary greatly depending on how they are elicited. The theory also predicts reversals in the relation between risk perception and risk taking depending on whether people use gist-based intuition or verbatim-based analysis. Paradoxically, adolescents often take risks that compromise health because they logically analyze the details of decisions. Adults avoid unhealthy risk taking by considering the gist, or bottom line, of the decision. Fuzzy-trace theory also explains most of the biases and fallacies exhibited in judgment and decision making (ratio bias, framing effects, hindsight bias, base-rate neglect, conjunction fallacy, disjunction fallacy, and others). Many of these biases and fallacies have been demonstrated in medical decision making by patients and healthcare professionals. Fuzzy-trace theory also predicts (and this prediction has been borne out by data) that many biases increase from childhood to adulthood because they are caused by gist-based intuition.

Informed Consent

Recently, there has been an emphasis on increasing the role the patient has in his or her medical decisions. The patient-practitioner relationship has been steadily growing from paternalism to egalitarianism. Evidence has shown that involving patients in their own medical decisions has a positive effect on their well-being. One of the central issues of this move centers on the concept of informed consent. Informed consent involves a decision, or authorization, given without coercion and involves the decision maker having a fundamental understanding of the risks and benefits.

Informed consent is given with volition and is usually assumed to involve an underlying rational process. Given that it is rational, it is assumed that to give fully informed consent, the decision maker must be intellectually competent and mature. In discussing the matter of young children, the issue is not one of consent, in that it is clear that children are not considered on par in maturity and cognitive capacity with adults. For young children, decisions are left up to the parent or guardian. However, the case of whether or not an adolescent is capable of providing informed consent is still an ongoing debate. Evidence supporting both sides of the issue has been found. For instance, older adolescents were found to perform on par with adults in a task involving hypothetical medical scenarios. These adolescents were able to select options based on logical reasoning and give valid evidence for their choices, and they had a clear understanding of the costs and benefits of the options. However, other studies have shown that real differences between adults and adolescents do exist. For example, adolescents' goals are more likely than adults' to maximize immediate pleasure, adolescents take more risks in the presence of peers than adults, and the brain is still not fully mature in adolescence. Therefore, the issue of autonomy in adolescence and of whether adolescents can make a rational decision is still unresolved. How each theory handles consent is important with respect to medical decision making.

Prototype/willingness does not specifically address the concept of consent. For the prototype/willingness model, however, using the reasoned path is considered the preferred process. Therefore, deliberating about details and precise knowledge of the options involved in the process matter greatly. For fuzzy-trace theory, making an informed decision requires a grasp of the bottom-line meaning of the situation (e.g., there is a fatal risk involved in the surgery), not simply regurgitating the minutia. For example, imagine that two patients are informed that the risk of death from surgery is 2% and each is later asked to recall what the risk they were informed is. One patient says 0% and the other 10%. Although the patient reporting 0% is objectively more correct (2% off is closer than 8% off), the patient reporting 10% is more informed because he or she understands that the surgery does have some risk. Research has shown that patients often cannot recall the details of surgical risks and that consent is driven instead by their understanding of the gist of the options. People low in numeracy, the ability to understand and use numbers, have difficulty getting the gist of health information, which impairs informed medical decision making. In sum, developmental differences related to age, experience, and knowledge determine informed consent and the quality of medical decisions.

Steven Estrada, Valerie F. Reyna, and Britain Mills

See also Dual-Process Theory; Fuzzy-Trace Theory; Intuition Versus Analysis; Risk Perception

Further Readings

Fischhoff, B. (2008). Assessing adolescent decision-making competence. *Developmental Review, 28*, 12–28.

Gerrard, M., Gibbons, F. X., Houlihan, A. E., Stock, M. L., & Pomery, E. A. (2008). A dual-process approach to health risk decision-making: The prototype–willingness model. *Developmental Review, 28*, 29–61.

Jacobs, J., & Klaczynski, P. A. (2005). *The development of judgment and decision making in children and adolescents*. Mahwah, NJ: Lawrence Erlbaum.

Kuther, T. L. (2003). Medical decision-making and minors: Issues of consent and assent. *Adolescence, 38*, 343–358.

Reyna, V. F. (2004). How people make decisions that involve risk. A dual-processes approach. *Current Directions in Psychological Science, 13*, 60–66.

Reyna, V. F., & Adam, M. B. (2003). Fuzzy-trace theory, risk communication, and product labeling in sexually transmitted diseases. *Risk Analysis, 23*, 325–342.

Reyna, V. F., & Farley, F. (2006). Risk and rationality in adolescent decision making: Implications for theory, practice, and public policy. *Psychological Science in the Public Interest, 7*, 1–44.

Reyna, V. F., & Lloyd, F. (2006). Physician decision making and cardiac risk: Effects of knowledge, risk perception, risk tolerance, and fuzzy processing. *Journal of Experimental Psychology: Applied, 12*, 179–195.

DIAGNOSTIC PROCESS, MAKING A DIAGNOSIS

The diagnostic process is central to clinical medicine. Patients come to a physician with complaints, and the physician attempts to identify the illnesses responsible for the complaints. The physician accomplishes this task by eliciting from patients their collection of signs (manifestations of the disease perceived by the physician, brought forth during the physical examination) and symptoms (manifestation of the disease perceived by the patient and brought forth during the history taking). Generally, physicians make treatment errors as the result of diagnostic errors. If the disease responsible for the complaints is correctly diagnosed, the correct treatment has a high probability of being prescribed. This makes good sense. Treatments can be looked up in reference materials; making the correct diagnosis is more complex.

Methods of Diagnosis

How physicians make a medical diagnosis has received considerable study and attention, although our understanding remains incomplete. Traditionally, physicians were thought to first systematically collect a complete clinical data set on the patient. This included the chief complaint, the history of present illness, the patient's complete past medical history, the patient's social history, a detailed family history, a comprehensive review of systems, and, finally, the complete physical exam. Only as a second and separate step were physicians thought to analyze the data and diagnose the responsible disease.

Despite the belief of some physicians that this method is central to diagnostic success, when psychologists study the process of diagnosis, they find that expert physicians do not blindly collect clinical information. In fact, expert physicians are often observed to collect less information than novice physicians when making diagnoses but are much more likely to make the correct diagnosis. While the novice physician collects a great deal of information, the novice can miss collecting the data needed to make the diagnosis. Expert physicians might be expert in knowing which data to collect as well as expert in knowing which data are irrelevant to the diagnostic task.

It appears that physicians use intuition, deliberate reasoning, or a combination of these two processes when engaged in making medical diagnoses. Many psychologists describe two different and complementary mental systems used by humans:

an automatic, experiential, recognition-based system and a rational, conscious, analytic system. The recognition-based system generates impressions of the attributes of objects of perception and thought. These impressions are not necessarily voluntary and often cannot be explained by the person. In contrast, the conscious, analytic system involves deliberate reasoning, which is much slower and effortful but more controlled. Although these two cognitive systems operate independently, there is reason to suspect that skilled diagnosticians learn to use their analytical brains to double-check their intuitive brains. In the discussion below, three distinct diagnostic methods are presented. These are presented as prototypes; physicians might use one of these three methods and a mixture of these methods when involved in medical diagnosis.

Pattern Recognition Method

In many studies, physicians appear to use pattern recognition when making diagnoses; that is, they make diagnoses based on sensory input and without deliberate or conscious analysis. This process is typically fast and accurate but difficult for the physician to explain. For example, when an experienced physician sees a psoriatic plaque on a patient's elbow, the physician will instantly diagnose the disease as psoriasis. Ask why it is psoriasis, one might observe a pause, and only after a few seconds will the physician come forth with the observation that the skin plaque is salmon-colored and covered with distinct, silvery scales. The explanation of the diagnosis takes considerably longer and more effort than does making the diagnosis itself!

Recognized patterns can be visual (the plaque of psoriasis), olfactory (the smell of an anaerobic infection), tactile (the hard, gritty feel of a cancer), or auditory (the confined speech of a patient with a peritonsillar abscess). Patterns can be learned through instruction or clinical experience, but novices frequently need a guiding mentor to point out clinically important patterns.

Pattern recognition has another interesting characteristic—the accuracy of a diagnosis is inversely correlated with the time it takes the physician to make the diagnosis. Thus, diagnoses that are made almost instantaneously are more likely to be correct than those made only after a more drawn-out review. This finding suggests that pattern recognition involves a cognitive process that is not based on deliberate reasoning.

Pattern recognition is a powerful and impressive tool when it works, but it also has weaknesses. The patient's signs and symptoms might resemble the patterns of two or more diseases. Again turning to the discussion of psoriasis, a physician might come across an isolated scalp lesion that is scaling, but it is not clear whether it is psoriasis or seborrheic dermatitis. In this situation, the physician needs to use more than pattern recognition. Physicians can also perceive specific patterns when they are not present, because visual pattern recognition appears to be influenced by nonvisual data. For example, researchers showed that they could manipulate the findings expert radiologists report on radiographs by manipulating the brief clinical histories that accompany each radiograph.

Prediction Rules Method

Another strategy used by physicians for arriving at a medical diagnosis is the prediction rule. When using a prediction rule, the clinician moves through a series of predetermined steps of an algorithm based on the presence or absence of clinical findings at branch points. Prediction rules can also be presented as mathematical functions that generate scores based on clinical findings. In contrast to pattern recognition, the use of prediction rules is slow, deliberate, effortful, and controlled.

Often, prediction rules are in the form of algorithms that are branching flow diagrams. Following a flow diagram does not require great domain knowledge. Therefore, this is a powerful method for physicians and other clinicians when they encounter a problem that they infrequently see and are unfamiliar with. As long as the algorithm is followed, the physician has a good chance of ending with the correct diagnosis.

Prediction rules can be stored mentally, on paper (now a prominent feature in review articles, textbooks, and practice protocols), or as Web pages. Some prediction rules used by physicians come from more expert physician colleagues and are transmitted via curbside consults. The systematic use of a prediction rule can improve physicians' diagnostic accuracy. For example, a short algorithm for diagnosing acute myocardial infarction in patients with chest pain was shown to perform at least as well as third-year internal medicine residents.

Despite this power, prediction rules also have a weakness: If a sign or symptom is not in the algorithm, it can not be used in the diagnostic process. For example, egophony is a specific finding for pneumonia, but its sensitivity is low. In the effort to keep a prediction rule manageably simple so that it can be easily presented and followed, egophony would not be included in the rule. Therefore, the examiner using the prediction rule would not be prompted to look for this finding. The lean and mean prediction rule might be efficient and helpful but not particularly nuanced.

A second problem with using prediction rules to make diagnoses is that they force a physician to lumber through a series of decision steps that an expert would bypass because of a more expert way of approaching a diagnostic problem. A final problem is that while prediction rules are readily available to physicians, many have never been validated.

Hypothetico-Deductive Method

The hypothetico-deductive approach to medical diagnosis can be placed between the sudden insight of pattern recognition and the slow, deliberate movement through a prediction rule. This is the method of medical diagnosis probably most frequently used by physicians. The method involves rapidly generating a differential diagnosis based on limited information about the chief complaint and then deliberately collecting additional clinical information to assess the likelihood of the different diseases in the differential.

Imagine that a physician is seeing a middle-aged patient in the office and has collected some initial information about chest pain. Instead of recognizing a single diagnosis, he or she might have several competing hypotheses (the differential diagnosis) and will usually set off to collect specific pieces of data (e.g., location, duration, provokers and relievers of the pain) that increase the probability of one diagnosis and decrease the probabilities of others. The additional data can come from further questioning, maneuvers on the physical exam, the laboratory, or the radiology suite or by using time to observe the change in signs and symptoms.

Central to the hypothetico-deductive method is the differential diagnosis. This list of competing diagnoses is typically short, usually three to five diseases, and is formulated by the physician early in the clinical encounter, usually within the first few minutes. Physicians spend much of their time during the patient visit collecting data to evaluate these different diagnostic possibilities. Data not pertinent to the differential are not collected by the expert clinician because it is not relevant to the task at hand.

Physicians use a number of approaches to judge the probabilities for the different diseases in a differential. One approach is to look up this information in a medical reference, although this information is often unavailable or difficult to find. A more commonly used approach is that of employing heuristics—simple, efficient rules, which are either hard-coded or learned. These work well under many circumstances but in certain situations are linked to systematic cognitive biases. These biases have gained a great deal of notoriety.

One frequently used heuristic is based on availability—diseases that come more easily to the physician's mind after learning the initial symptoms are taken to be more probable. This strategy is taught as part of the informal curriculum in most medical schools, transmitted through aphorisms such as "If you hear hoof beats, think horses, not zebras." However, attributes other than greater likelihood might make a disease come easily to mind. For example, when a physician has recently attended a talk about an uncommon disease, it might be more mentally available to him or her when he or she next goes to see patients. If a physician errs by missing an important diagnosis, the disease will often easily come to mind when encountering a future patient with similar symptoms. If the physician has recently been diagnosed with a disease, it may more readily come to mind when the physician is evaluating patients.

A second commonly used heuristic is basing the probability of a disease on the representativeness of the symptoms. Using this heuristic, a physician will estimate the probability that a person with symptom complex A, B, and C has disease X by judging the degree to which the complex of symptoms A, B, and C is representative or typical of disease X. This heuristic is often taught to medical students using the aphorism "If it walks like a duck and quacks like a duck, it probably is a duck." However, this heuristic ignores the underlying probably of a disease in a population. Because it ignores base rates, this heuristic can lead to errors in probability estimation. For example, a middle-aged woman who recently developed truncal obesity, excess sweating, telangiectasia, and hypertension might fit our image of Cushing's disease; but this is an uncommon disease. Despite the close match to our profile of Cushing's disease, simple obesity accompanied with hypertension is much more common and therefore a much more likely diagnosis.

The hypothetico-deductive method not only requires that physicians determine the correct prior probability for a disease, but physicians must also correctly revise this probability given the additional information uncovered during the clinical evaluation. Bayes's theorem is a normative standard by which intuitive probability revision can be assessed. Researchers have raised considerable doubt about physicians' abilities to intuitively revise this probability after gathering new information. Using Bayes's theorem as a comparison, physicians have been shown to badly err when asked about the effect of new information on the likelihood of a disease. More recently, other researchers have suggested that physicians are quite skilled at probability revision. They suggest, however, that the format in which physicians are provided with the information about probabilities is a major determination of whether they revise probabilities in a way consistent with Bayes's theorem. These researchers suggest that physicians do poorly with likelihood information in the format of probabilities but perform well when the information is in the format of natural frequencies.

George Bergus

See also Cognitive Psychology and Processes; Decision Psychology; Errors in Clinical Reasoning; Hypothesis Testing; Judgment; Learning and Memory in Medical Training; Pattern Recognition; Problem Solving; Teaching Diagnostic Clinical Reasoning

Further Readings

Ark, T. K., Brooks, L. R., & Eva, K. W. (2006). Giving learners the best of both worlds: Do clinical teachers need to guard against teaching pattern recognition to novices? *Academic Medicine, 81,* 405–409.

Brooks, L. R., LeBlanc, V. R., & Norman, G. R. (2000). On the difficulty of noticing obvious features in patient appearance. *Psychological Science, 11*(2), 112–117.

Elstein, A. S., & Schwartz, A. (2002). Clinical problem solving and diagnostic decision making: Selective review of the cognitive literature. *British Medical Journal, 324*(7339), 729–732.

Eva, K. W., Hatala, R. M., Leblanc, V. R., & Brooks, L. R. (2007). Teaching from the clinical reasoning literature: Combined reasoning strategies help novice diagnosticians overcome misleading information. *Medical Education, 41*(12), 1152–1158.

Gigerenzer, G. (1999). *Simple heuristics that make us smart.* Oxford, UK: Oxford University Press.

Gilovich, T., Griffin, D., & Kahneman, D. (Eds.). (2002). *Heuristics and biases: The psychology of intuitive judgment.* New York: Cambridge University Press.

Hogath, R. (2001). *Educating intuition.* Chicago: University of Chicago Press.

Kahneman, D. (2002). *Maps of bounded rationality* (The Sveriges Riksbank Prize Lecture in Economic Sciences in Memory of Alfred Nobel 2002). Retrieved February 10, 2009, from http://nobelprize.org/nobel_prizes/economics/laureates/2002/kahneman-lecture.html

Norman, G. (2005). Research in clinical reasoning: Past history and current trends. *Medical Education, 39,* 418–427.

Rikers, R. M., Schmidt, H. G., Boshuizen, H. P., Linssen, G. C., Wesseling, G., & Paas, F. G. (2002). The robustness of medical expertise: Clinical case processing by medical experts and subexperts. *The American Journal of Psychology, 115*(4), 609–629.

Diagnostic Tests

Numerous diagnostic tests exist that can provide information to guide medical decision making. In a broad sense, diagnostic tests include symptoms and signs (e.g., chest pain, fatigue, varicose veins, ankle edema); measurements on physical examination (e.g., height, weight, blood pressure); special measurements (e.g., ankle-brachial pressure index, electrocardiogram [ECG], electroencephalogram [EEG]); blood tests (e.g., cholesterol, lipid profile, glucose); cytology and histology (e.g., Papanicolaou smears, biopsy); and imaging tests (e.g., endoscopy, ultrasound, computerized tomography [CT], magnetic resonance imaging [MRI], single photon emission computed tomography [SPECT], positron-emission tomography [PET]).

Tests results can be dichotomous—that is, the result is either positive or negative, or the test may have multiple possible results on a categorical, ordinal, or continuous scale. Interpreting information obtained from diagnostic tests correctly is key in optimizing medical decision making.

Tests With Two Results, Positive Versus Negative

A test result is said to be "positive" if it shows a particular finding to be present and "negative" if the finding is absent. Note that a positive test result suggests that a patient has the disease in question—which is usually not a positive thing for the patient—and vice versa.

Most diagnostic information is not perfect but rather subject to some degree of error. A positive test result may be

- *true positive (TP)*—the test result indicates disease, and the patient has the disease, or
- *false positive (FP)*—the test result indicates disease, but the patient does not have the disease.

A negative test result may be

- *true negative (TN)*—the test result indicates no disease, and the patient has no disease, or
- *false negative (FN)*—the test result indicates no disease, but the patient has the disease.

Whether a patient has the disease or not is determined by the "truth" as established by a reference (gold) standard test, which is generally an invasive and/or expensive test and one that many patients would like to avoid. The occurrence of false-positive (FP) and false-negative (FN) test results implies that medical professionals need to be careful in interpreting diagnostic test information to minimize the impact of such errors.

Diagnostic performance (also referred to as accuracy or validity) of a test is its correspondence with the underlying truth and is expressed using the test's characteristics, sensitivity, and specificity. Alternatively, the diagnostic test performance may be characterized with true- and false-positive

ratios, which is particularly convenient when a test has more than two possible results. Sensitivity and specificity describe how often the test is correct in the diseased and nondiseased groups, respectively. True- and false-positive ratios describe how often the test yields a positive result in the diseased and nondiseased groups, respectively.

Sensitivity, or *true-positive ratio* (TPR), is the probability of a positive test result given that the disease is present, denoted by $p(T+|D+)$. *Specificity*, or *true-negative ratio* (TNR), is the probability of a negative test result given that the disease is absent, denoted by $p(T-|D-)$. The *false-negative ratio* (FNR) is the complement of sensitivity, that is, $1.0 - TPR$, and is the proportion of patients with disease who have a negative test result, denoted by $p(T-|D+)$. The *false-positive ratio* (FPR) is the complement of specificity, that is, $1.0 - TNR$, and is the proportion of patients without disease who have a positive test result, denoted by $p(T+|D-)$.

Algebraically, these can be summarized as follows:

- Sensitivity = $p(T+|D+)$ = TPR = TP/(TP+FN).
- Specificity = $p(T-|D-)$ = TNR = TN/(TN+FP).
- $1 - $ Sensitivity = $p(T-|D+)$ = FNR = FN/(TP+FN).
- $1 - $ Specificity = $p(T+|D-)$ = FPR = FP/(TN+FP).

There is an analogy between diagnostic tests and research studies. The FPR is the rate of Type I errors (α value) that are errors of commission: We are saying there is a finding that is in fact not there. The FNR is the rate of Type II errors ($1 - \beta$ value) that are errors of omission: We omit to identify the finding.

Although sensitivity and specificity are important characteristics of a test, they are not the conditional probabilities required to decide how to treat a patient. Sensitivity and specificity are the probabilities of test results conditional on the presence versus absence of disease. In practice, medical professionals do not know whether or not someone has the disease, but rather, they find a test result is positive or negative, and from this information, they infer the probability of disease. Thus, medical professionals usually need to know the probabilities of disease given positive or negative test results, which are very different. Posttest revised (or posterior) probabilities are defined as follows:

- The *post-positive-test probability of disease*, or *positive predictive value (PPV)*, is the conditional probability of disease given a positive test result, $p(D+|T+)$—that is, the probability that a patient with a positive test result has the disease.
- The *post-negative-test probability of disease* is the conditional probability of having the disease given a negative test result, $p(D+|T-)$—that is, the probability that in spite of a negative test result, the patient does have the disease.
- The *post-positive-test probability of absence of disease* is the conditional probability of absence of the disease given a positive test result, $p(D-|T+)$—that is, the probability that in spite of a positive test result, the patient does not have the disease.
- The *post-negative-test probability of absence of disease*, or *negative predictive value (NPV)*, is the conditional probability of not having the disease given a negative test result, $p(D-|T-)$—that is, the probability that a patient with a negative test result does not have the disease.

If the number of TP, FN, FP, and TNs in the population is known, then these probabilities can be calculated as follows:

- Post-positive-test probability of disease = $p(D+|T+) = TP/(TP + FP) = PPV$.
- Post-negative-test probability of disease = $p(D+|T-) = FN/(TN + FN)$.
- Post-positive-test probability of absence of disease = $p(D-|T+) = FP/(TP + FP)$.
- Post-negative-test probability of absence of disease = $p(D-|T-) = TN/(TN + FN) = NPV$.

Estimates of probabilities of disease conditional on test results are not readily available, and if they are available, they are highly influenced by the pretest (prior) probability of the disease in the patient population studied. Sensitivity and specificity values are, however, generally available and under certain conditions can be transferred from one population to another in spite of a different prior probability because they are conditional on disease status. Converting the probabilities of test results given the disease to probabilities of disease given the test results is done with Bayes's theorem.

Tests With Multiple Results

Many tests have multiple possible test results, which may be on a categorical, ordinal, or continuous scale. In the setting of multiple test results, diagnostic test performance is best characterized with true- and false-positive ratios of each of the test results and the corresponding likelihood ratio. The likelihood ratio (*LR*) for test result *R* is the ratio of the conditional probability of *R* given the disease under consideration to the probability of *R* given absence of the disease under consideration. The *LR* summarizes all the information medical professionals need to know about the test result *R*. A high *LR* indicates that the test result argues in support of the diagnosis. A low *LR* indicates that the test result argues against the diagnosis.

In the setting of multiple test results, medical professionals frequently need to choose a cut-off value that defines a positive test result that requires treatment or further workup versus a negative result that does not require further action. Shifting the chosen cut-off value will yield pairs of FPR and TPR rates that together give the receiver operating characteristic (ROC) curve of the test.

M. G. Myriam Hunink

See also Bayes's Theorem; Conditional Probability; Likelihood Ratio; Receiver Operating Characteristic (ROC) Curve

Further Readings

Hunink, M. G. M., Glasziou, P. P., Siegel, J. E., Weeks, J. C., Pliskin, J. S., Elstein, A. S., et al. (2001). *Decision making in health and medicine: Integrating evidence and values.* Cambridge, UK: Cambridge University Press.

DIFFERENTIAL DIAGNOSIS

The term *differential diagnosis* is generally thought of as both a noun and verb by clinicians. The noun form of differential diagnosis is the list of all possible conditions that could explain the collection of signs, symptoms, and test results observed in a particular patient at a particular point in time. This list of conditions is organized from most likely (high on the list) to least likely (low on the list). The verb form of differential diagnosis is the medical decision-making process whereby this list is continually updated by eliminating conditions that are considered to be ruled out and adding conditions that may not have been previously considered based on the acquisition of new information. Conditions that remain on the list are also moved up and down in priority based on a continual reanalysis of their likelihood. The goal of diagnostic investigation and problem solving is the elimination of all conditions from the differential diagnosis until a single unifying diagnosis remains.

Casting a Broad Net

The number of conditions contained in a differential diagnosis is referred to as its breadth. Generally, the smaller the number of signs, symptoms, and test results available for consideration, the broader the differential diagnosis. A clinician always has the least amount of information available at the time of the patient's initial presentation, and so it behooves him or her to "cast a broad net" by adding many conditions to the list even if they are only remote possibilities. An initial broad differential can be winnowed down later using additional information obtained during the course of further diagnostic investigation. The choice of which conditions to add occurs by pattern recognition, whereby clinicians recognize patterns of signs and symptoms present in disease states that they have seen before. The process of recognizing these patterns, identifying the condition, and adding it to the differential diagnosis is referred to as hypothesis generation.

Accurate pattern recognition and hypothesis generation are the foundation of accurate differential diagnosis, because if a condition does not make it onto the list of differential diagnoses, it can never be confirmed or refuted via further investigation. Research has shown that the source of the improved accuracy of expert diagnosticians is not better acquisition of the signs and symptoms that provide the data set for hypothesis generation, nor is it the number of hypotheses generated from a given data set, but instead, it is the generation of more accurate hypotheses compared with novice diagnosticians. The source of this improved accuracy has

been the topic of much debate. However, a rule of thumb that is used frequently by clinicians to describe hypothesis generation is "common things are common." This seemingly obvious adage means that a given sign or symptom is more likely to be an uncommon manifestation of a common disease than a common manifestation of an uncommon disease. In other words, one should focus on generating hypotheses that are epidemiologically most likely even if they do not seem to fit the pattern perfectly. Recall or availability bias is a type of cognitive error in this process wherein the clinician has a distorted sense of the prevalence of a particular condition based on his or her own personal experience rather than that reported in the scientific literature.

While the amount of data available to the diagnostician is the principal determinant of the breadth of an initial differential diagnosis, the particular characteristics and the quality of the data being considered can also have a profound effect. Certain findings are considered pathognomonic for particular diseases, meaning that the finding is so specific and sensitive that a patient should be considered to have the condition until proven otherwise. An example would be the presence of Kaiser-Fleischer rings in the eyes of patients with Wilson's disease. This single observation on the physical exam would eliminate nearly all other conditions from consideration. Similarly, the quality of the data also has dramatic effects on the breadth of the differential. Demented, mentally ill, or malingering patients may supply a wealth of historical details; however, the reliability of this information would remain suspect, and it might add little value despite its abundance. In these situations, the differential would remain broad despite obtaining a relatively large amount of data.

Narrowing the Differential Diagnosis

Once a broad differential has been established based on initial data gathering and hypothesis generation, the list is narrowed by either confirming (ruling in) a single diagnosis or eliminating (ruling out) conditions one by one until a single diagnosis remains. Usually, both approaches are used simultaneously. The order in which conditions in the differential are investigated depends on (a) the urgent or emergent nature of diagnoses on the list,

(b) the logistical expediency of obtaining a definitive answer for a particular diagnosis, and (c) the particular cognitive preferences of the diagnostician. Diagnoses that threaten loss of life or function are always investigated first even if they are low on the differential. Dissecting thoracic aortic aneurysm is a relatively rare cause of chest pain and is often near the bottom of the differential. However, it is investigated rapidly, as the consequences of a delayed diagnosis would be devastating. Once all the life-threatening diagnoses have been eliminated from the differential, diagnostic investigation can proceed at a more leisurely pace. If a condition can be excluded simply and easily, it is often pursued next. These are the so-called low-hanging fruit of the diagnostic process, and an example would be excluding a diagnosis of anemia with a simple complete blood count. In general, ruling in is a quicker way to narrow the differential than ruling out because one need only be correct once in the former approach and one needs to be correct $N - 1$ times (N being the number of conditions in the differential) in the latter.

Once a diagnosis has been ruled in, the remainder of the diagnoses are assumed to be ruled out based on the principle of parsimony, or Ockham's razor. The principle is attributed to the 14th-century logician William of Ockham and states that "the explanation of any phenomenon should make as few assumptions as possible, eliminating those that make no difference in the observable predictions of the explanatory hypothesis." Practically, this means that all of the observable signs, symptoms, and test results should be explained by a single diagnosis. If a single condition has crossed the threshold of evidence to be accepted as the unifying diagnosis, then all other diagnoses must be rejected. Even if a diagnosis has been confirmed, the particular cognitive preferences of a diagnostician will still factor into the ongoing investigation. Some diagnosticians may continue to rule out conditions as they prefer to "leave no stone unturned."

Cognitive Bias

All diagnosticians are subject to bias in the medical decision making involved in narrowing the differential diagnosis. Two common types of cognitive bias are confirmation bias and anchoring bias. Confirmation bias arises when a clinician only performs further testing in an effort to confirm a diagnosis that he or she already believes to be true and does not test other hypotheses that might refute the favored diagnosis. Anchoring bias is similar but distinct in that it results from a failure to add new diagnoses to the differential or adjust the position of old diagnoses based on new information. The clinician becomes anchored to the original differential and is blinded to new possibilities.

Negative Diagnostic Workups

"No evidence of disease is not evidence of no disease" is a phrase often used to describe the fact that a clinician's inability to detect a condition at a particular point in time does not mean that it is not present currently or was not present in the recent past. This is especially true for conditions that have waxing-and-waning courses, such as occult gastrointestinal bleeding. Commonly, 80% of upper gastrointestinal bleeding has stopped by the time of presentation to medical attention. Nonbleeding ulcers or varices are often found on esophagogastroduodenoscopy and presumed to be the source, but in a significant number of cases, the source of the bleeding cannot be found because active bleeding is no longer visible at the time of the diagnostic investigation. Failure to find a source of bleeding despite thorough investigation does not mean that gastrointestinal bleeding has been ruled out as a cause of the patient's presenting signs and symptoms, and consequently, it cannot be eliminated from the differential diagnosis.

When a workup is entirely negative and the differential diagnosis still contains more than a single diagnosis, watchful waiting is sometimes employed as a passive diagnostic strategy if the patient's condition is stable. The hope is that the condition causing the presenting symptoms will reactivate and new observations can be made at that time, which will allow the differential diagnosis to be narrowed.

When a workup is negative but the differential is relatively small and/or the patient's condition is deteriorating, a strategy of diagnostic and therapeutic intervention can be employed to confirm a diagnosis. If the therapy is narrowly directed at a particular diagnosis and the patient responds to treatment, the individual diagnosis in question is considered to be ruled in, and further diagnostic workup is unnecessary. When this strategy is employed, it is important that a diagnostic response to treatment be defined clearly and prospectively and that only a single, narrowly directed therapy be used at any one time. If multiple therapies are employed simultaneously, a causal relationship between treatment and disease cannot reliably be inferred, and therefore, a diagnosis cannot be reliably confirmed based on response to treatment. This type of obfuscation of the differential diagnosis often occurs when broad-spectrum antibiotics are used to treat an infection of unclear etiology. The patient may have improvement in fever, white blood cell count, and bacteremia, but the signs and symptoms that would have helped localize the infection have not been allowed to develop.

The process of differential diagnosis is critical to medical decision making, because without an accurate diagnosis, decisions about treatment become extremely difficult. The medical decision making involved in differential diagnosis is complex and subject to the underlying cognitive biases of clinicians. Diagnostic testing is not without the potential to harm patients. Consequently, risk/benefit decisions must be made to determine whether the additional diagnostic information provided by a test or procedure is warranted. Skilled differential diagnosticians balance these risks with their degree of confidence that the correct single unifying diagnosis has been selected from the list of possibilities generated during the process of differential diagnosis.

Robert Patrick

See also Diagnostic Process, Making a Diagnosis; Errors in Clinical Reasoning; Heuristics

Further Readings

Adler, S. N., Adler-Klein, D., & Gasbarra, D. B. (2008). *A pocket manual of differential diagnosis* (4th ed.). Philadelphia: Lippincott Williams & Wilkins.

Barrows, H. S., & Feltovich, P. J. (1987). The clinical reasoning process. *Medical Education, 21*(2), 86–91.

Bordage, G. (1999). Why did I miss the diagnosis? Some cognitive explanations and educational implications. *Academic Medicine, 74*(Suppl. 10), S138–S143.

Elstein, A., Shulman, L., & Sprafka, S. (1978). *Medical problem solving: An analysis of clinical reasoning.* Cambridge, MA: Harvard University Press.

Eva, K. W. (2005). What every teacher needs to know about clinical reasoning. *Medical Education, 39*(1), 98–106.

Groves, M., O'Rourke, P., & Alexander, H. (2003). The clinical reasoning characteristics of diagnostic experts. *Medical Teacher, 25*(3), 308–313.

Norman, G., Young, M., & Brooks, L. (2007). Non-analytical models of clinical reasoning: The role of experience. *Medical Education, 41*(12), 1140–1145.

Disability-Adjusted Life Years (DALYs)

The disability-adjusted life year (DALY) measure combines nonfatal outcomes and mortality in a single summary measure of population health. One DALY represents 1 lost year of healthy life. The basic philosophy associated with the estimation of DALYs is (a) use the best available data, (b) make corrections for major known biases in available measurements to improve cross-population comparability, and (c) use internal consistency as a tool to improve the validity of epidemiological assessments. For the latter purpose, a software application, DISMOD II, is available from the World Health Organization (WHO) Web site.

Uses

DALYs were first employed in the 1993 *World Development Report* to quantify the burden of ill health in different regions of the world. The Global Burden of Disease (GBD) study, edited by Murray and Lopez and published in 1996, used a revised DALY measure. The DALY was developed to facilitate the inclusion of nonfatal health outcomes in debates on international health policy, which had often focused on child mortality, and to quantify the burden of disease using a measure that could also be used for cost-effectiveness analysis. DALYs have been widely used in global- and national-burden-of-disease studies and to assess disease control priorities. They have also been used to make the case for primary prevention programs for disorders such as stroke prevention in Australia and in assessing funding allocations in medical research programs in Australia, Canada, and the United States in relation to the burden associated with different diseases.

DALYs are also frequently used in economic evaluations of public health interventions, particularly in low- and middle-income countries. The DALY is the health effect measure that is recommended by the WHO's Choosing Interventions that are Cost Effective (WHO-CHOICE) program for generalized cost-effectiveness analysis (GCEA) and is also used in the World Bank's Disease Control Priorities in Developing Countries program. In GCEA, the costs and effectiveness of all possible interventions are compared with the null set for a group of related interventions to select the mix that maximizes health for the given resource constraints. DALYs and quality-adjusted life years (QALYs) are both health-adjusted life year (HALY) measures that use time as a common metric. QALYs were developed for the economic evaluation of clinical interventions and remain the dominant outcome measure used in cost-utility analyses that compare the costs and health effects of specific interventions using a preference-based measure of health. It is standard for cost-utility analyses using QALYs to subtract averted direct costs of care (cost offsets) from intervention costs to calculate the net cost of interventions used to calculate cost-effectiveness ratios, which can be negative. In contrast, most analyses that use DALYs do not calculate cost offsets, primarily because reliable information on such costs is extremely scarce in low- and middle-income countries.

Components

DALYs are composed of two components, years of life lost (YLL) due to premature death and years lived with disability (YLD) associated with nonfatal injuries and disease. YLL represents the stream of lost healthy life due to premature death at a particular age. It is calculated as the product of the number of deaths due to a specific cause and the years lost per death. YLD is calculated as the product of incidence of a specific cause and its average duration, multiplied by a disability or severity weight for that condition. Disability weights are assigned on a scale from 0 (representing *perfect health*) to 1 (representing *death*), in addition to an optional age-weighting parameter. The scale of DALY weights is inverted from that used to calculate QALYs. Consequently, when DALYs are used as the denominator in cost-effectiveness ratios, one

refers to the cost per DALY averted as opposed to cost per QALY gained. Equivalently, the DALY is a health gap measure, whereas the QALY is a health gain measure. When different interventions are evaluated by some studies using DALYs and by others using QALYs, ranking interventions according to cost-effectiveness ratios may be possible even though there is no systematic formula for converting between the two measures, as long as the same approach is used in each study to calculate costs.

Weights

The GBD study derived DALY weights for 22 indicator conditions through a person trade-off (PTO) process, in which panels of health experts from various countries were asked to assess the expected relative burden of conditions in two trade-off exercises. In one exercise (PTO1), participants were asked to trade off extending the lives of different numbers of "healthy" people and people with a condition such as blindness. In the second exercise (PTO2), participants were asked to choose between prolonging life for 1 year for people with perfect health and restoring to perfect health a different number of people with the same condition used in PTO1. If the results of the PTO1 and PTO2 exercises differed, participants were required to individually reconcile their estimates in order to reach internal consistency using PTO1-PTO2 equivalence tables. Afterward, participants shared their PTO1 and PTO2 assessments through a deliberative group process in which participants were confronted with the implications of their choices and allowed to discuss the basis for their viewpoints, to reflect on the implications of their preferences, and to revise their assessments. Subsequently, DALY weights were derived for several hundred other conditions by comparison with the indicator conditions. The PTO exercises have been repeated in many countries and have generally yielded comparable weights, which supports the use of the same weights in different populations. Potential facilitator biases in the PTO valuation process can be reduced through the training of facilitators, and potential participant biases are minimized by the deliberative process and by replication across multiple groups of participants.

The standard DALY used in the GBD study is calculated using a 3% discount rate to calculate present values and an age-weighting parameter (which is optional). Discounting of future benefits is standard practice in economic analysis, but the use of age weighting is more controversial. The age-weighting parameter gives greater weight to young-adult years, peaking at around age 20 years, than to years lived in childhood or older adulthood. It is also possible to calculate DALYs with discounting but without age weighting or with neither discounting nor age weighting (see Figure 1), as has been done, for example, in the Australian burden-of-disease study.

One distinctive feature of DALYs as estimated in the GBD study is the use of Standard Expected Years of Life Lost (SEYLL). To define the standard, the highest national life expectancy observed was used, 82.5 years for Japanese females and 80.0 years for Japanese males. The use of a standard life expectancy, regardless of local life expectancy, is to express the social value of people being equal regardless of country or location. For the calculation of DALYs in cost-effectiveness analyses, as opposed to burden-of-disease studies, national life expectancies are typically used.

"Disability," as used in DALYs, encompasses all nonfatal outcomes and aggregates various aspects of an individual's health such as mobility, anxiety, and pain. The calculation of YLD does not entail an empirical assessment of functional or activity limitations experienced by individuals with impairments, which is how disability is conventionally defined and measured. The DALY weights reflect the preferences regarding different disease/health states or impairments in relation to the societal "ideal" of good health. The health state valuations used to estimate the burden of disease in terms of DALYs lost do not represent the lived experience of any disability or health state or imply societal value of the person in a disability or health state. A relatively high DALY weight for a condition means that 1 year lived in that condition is less preferable than 1 year lived in health states with lower disability weights. For example, the disability weight of .43 for blindness implies that 1 year spent with blindness is preferable to 1 year with paraplegia (weight .57) and 1 year with paraplegia is preferable to 1 year with unremitting unipolar major depression (weight .76). Equivalently, these weights imply that 1 year of living in good health

followed by death (1 year × [1.0 − 0.0 disability weight] = 1.0 healthy life year) is less preferable than 3 years of living with paraplegia followed by death (3 years × [1.0 − .57 disability weight] = 1.3 healthy years). Based on these weights, other things being equal, it is preferable to prevent or cure a case of paraplegia (weight .57) rather than a case of low back pain (weight .06) if the prevention or cure for each case would cost the same and there were not enough resources to do both.

In the GBD study, disability weights for selected conditions and sequelae were adjusted according to whether a person was assumed to have received medical treatment and whether the treatment was believed to decrease the severity of the condition. For example, the disability weight was .583 for patients with untreated bipolar disorder and .383 for bipolar patients whose condition improved due to the treatment but was not in remission. For most disabling conditions (e.g., spina bifida, limb loss, spinal cord injuries), disability weights reflected the assumption that no improvement in functioning occurred as the result of rehabilitation. Disability weights could also be modified to incorporate data on the effectiveness of rehabilitation therapies.

A major attraction for the use of DALYs in comparison with QALYs is that they provide a means of comparing the health impact of a wide range of medical conditions through the use of a standardized set of disability weights. However, additional sources of disability weight estimates are appearing. The Dutch Disability Weights study has provided additional estimates for disorders or sequelae that were not fully included in the GBD study, and these have been used in national burden-of-disease studies conducted in the Netherlands, Australia, and the United States. In particular, the Dutch Disability Weights study estimated disability weights stratified on the basis of disease stages and complications. For example, that study estimated a weight of .07 for Type 2 diabetes, with weights of increasing severity for complications, such as a weight of .17 for moderate vision loss and .43 for severe vision loss. To take one more example, the GBD study assigned a weight of .73 for adults with dementia, whereas the Australian and Dutch studies calculated weights of .27 for mild dementia (with impairments in daily activities of living),

Formulas for DALY calculations without discounting or age weighting

$DALY_i = YLL_i + YLD_i$

YLL_i = Number of deaths due to cause i * Years lost per death

YLD_i = Number of incident cases of cause i * Average duration$_i$ * DW_i

$DALY_i$ = Disability-adjusted life years due to cause i

YLL_i = Years of life lost due to cause i

YLD_i = Years lived with disability due to cause i

DW_i = Disability weight for cause i

Example using individual-level data (for population data, incidence would be used):

Motor vehicle collision results in two fatalities and two injuries

A 55-year-old woman dies, resulting in 29.37 standard expected years of life lost (SEYLLs)

A 60-year-old man dies, resulting in 21.81 SEYLLs

Total YLL = 51.18 (without discounting or age weighting)

A 35-year-old woman gets a fractured skull, for which she is treated, but the effects are lifelong. The duration is equal to 48.38 SEYLLs, with a disability weight of .35. YLD for this injury is 48.38 * .35 = 16.933

A 40-year-old man treated for fractured sternum. The average duration is .115 years, with a disability weight of .199. YLD for this condition is .115 * .199 = .022885

Total YLD = 16.95589 (without discounting or age weighting)

Total DALY loss = 68.13589 (without discounting or age weighting)

Figure I   How disability-adjusted life years (DALYs) are calculated

Source: The SEYLL and DW estimates were taken from Murray and Lopez (1996), in which discounting and age weighting were used in the estimation of DALYs.

.63 for moderate dementia (unable to live independently), and .94 for severe dementia (requiring permanent supervision). Future empirical studies may provide still more detail and better reflect the heterogeneity among health conditions. Currently, efforts are being undertaken to update disability weights for DALYs both globally and in the United States, to address the relevance of the social values that have been incorporated in the calculation of DALYs, and to assess changes in weights due to new developments in treatments for various diseases and conditions.

Cost-Effectiveness Ratios

The use of fixed thresholds for cost-effectiveness ratios to conclude that a particular intervention is or is not cost-effective is widespread but still controversial. Because of the interaction between cost-effectiveness, disease burden, and available resources, a single threshold for maximum cost per health gain cannot be specified. Nonetheless, a consensus has emerged that an intervention with a cost-effectiveness ratio less than three times the per capita gross domestic product (GDP) in a given country can be considered cost-effective, and one with a cost-effectiveness ratio less than one time the GDP per capita is "very cost-effective." This does not mean that clinical interventions with higher cost-effectiveness ratios do not provide good value but that more health gains could be achieved by prioritizing funding to interventions with lower cost-effectiveness ratios, which is the rationale for the Disease Control Priorities in Developing Countries program. However, even cost-effective interventions may not be feasible to implement if the costs are monetary and come from a public budget and the benefits are nonmonetary and diffused over the population.

Scott D. Grosse and Armineh Zohrabian

Authors' Note: Authors have contributed equally and are listed alphabetically. The findings and conclusions in this article are those of the author and do not necessarily represent the official position of the Centers for Disease Control and Prevention.

See also Cost-Effectiveness Analysis; Cost-Utility Analysis; Person Trade-Off; Quality-Adjusted Life Years (QALYs)

Further Readings

Gold, M. R., Stevenson, D., & Fryback, D. G. (2002). HALYs and QALYs and DALYs, oh my: Similarities and differences in summary measures of population health. *Annual Review of Public Health, 23,* 115–134.

Grosse, S. D., Lollar, D. J., Campbell, V. A., & Chamie, M. (in press). Disability and DALYs: Not the same. *Public Health Reports.*

Jamison, D. T., Breman, J. G., Measham, A. R., Alleyne, G., Claeson, M., Evans, D. B., et al. (Eds.). (2006). *Disease control priorities in developing countries* (2nd ed.). New York: Oxford University Press (published for the World Bank).

Mathers, C. D., Vos, T., Lopez, A. D., Salomon, J., & Ezzati, M. (Eds.). *National burden of disease studies: A practical guide* (2nd ed.). Geneva: World Health Organization. Retrieved February 10, 2009, from http://www.who.int/healthinfo/nationalburdenof diseasemanual.pdf

Mathers, C., Vos, T., & Stevenson, C. (1999). *The burden of disease and injury in Australia.* Canberra, Australian Capital Territory, Australia: Australian Institute of Health and Welfare. Retrieved February 10, 2009, from http://www.aihw.gov.au/publications/ phe/bdia/bdia.pdf

McKenna, M. T., Michaud, C. M., Murray, C. J. L., & Marks, J. S. (2005). Assessing the burden of disease in the United States using disability-adjusted life years. *American Journal of Preventive Medicine, 28,* 415–423.

Murray, C. J. L., & Lopez, A. D. (Eds.). (1996). *The global burden of disease: A comprehensive assessment of mortality and disability from diseases, injuries, and risk factors in 1990 and projected to 2020.* Cambridge, MA: Harvard University Press.

Stouthard, M. E. A., Essink-Bot, M. L., Bonsel, G. J., & Dutch Disability Weights Group. (2000). Disability weights for diseases: A modified protocol and results for a Western European region. *European Journal of Public Health, 10,* 24–30.

World Health Organization. (2003). *Making choices in health: WHO guide to cost-effectiveness analysis* (T. Tan-Torres Edejer, R. Baltusse, T. Adam, A. Hutubessy, D. B. Acharya, D. B. Evans, et al., Eds.). Geneva: Author. Retrieved February 10, 2009, from http://www.who.int/choice/publications/p_2003_ generalised_cea.pdf

World Health Organization—software tools: http://www .who.int/healthinfo/global_burden_disease/tools_ software/en/index.html

DISCOUNTING

Why does a person engage in behaviors, such as eating high-calorie foods or keeping a sedentary lifestyle, that provide an immediate reward over behaviors that offer health benefits in the long run? Understanding the time dimension of health preferences, or intertemporal health preferences, has been an important area of inquiry for medical decision making. The concept of discounting over time has been central to this understanding. Time discounting of preferences refers to the common situation where money, goods, services, and other outcomes are more highly valued when obtained in the present than those occurring in the future. When all things are equal, a given reward is more desirable when obtained sooner than later. The section below provides an introduction to discounting in intertemporal choices and discusses the importance of these concepts in medical decision making.

Preferences for Early Versus Late Rewards

The question as to why money, goods, services, and health are more desirable in the present than in the future has been answered in several ways. Money and some goods can increase in value with time, so that it is better to obtain them in the present to obtain future growth. Having $100 now allows one to invest it and accrue interest over time. Waiting a year to receive $100 means that a year of interest is lost. Also, waiting for a reward may increase the risk of losing it in the future, so it is better to have it in the present. For example, a person may choose to spend money on a vacation this year over investing in a retirement fund that would allow a vacation in the future. Waiting introduces the risk that one may not be healthy enough to enjoy a vacation during retirement. In medical decision making, the concept of discounting provides a way to understand why people engage in behaviors, such as smoking, that provide immediate gratification but that may contribute to risks to health in the future.

Discounting in Health and Medicine

Consideration of the value of health outcomes over time is critical to decision analysis and in analyses of the costs and benefits of preventive health regimens, diagnostic tests, and medical treatments. The results of decision analyses and cost-and-benefit analyses are important considerations in the development of policy on healthcare. In these types of analyses, discounting rates are used to provide an adjustment of the present value of an outcome for the costs and benefits occurring at different time points. While a variety of discounting rates have been used in these studies to estimate the value of future outcomes, the U.S. Preventive Service Task Force suggests the use of a 3% discount rate for cost-and-benefit analyses with a rate of 5% used for sensitivity analyses. However, discount rates have been shown to vary in studies of time preferences, and higher rates of 40% and 50% have been observed. The selection of discount rates for decision and economic analyses should depend on whether the interest is in group preferences or individual preferences. The lower rates may be reasonable to use for group analyses, but the higher rates may be appropriate to examine individual preferences.

Discounted Utility Theory

Discounted utility theory (DUT) has been used as a framework to understand preferences over time. Similar to expected utility theory (EUT), DUT is a normative decision model. Both models are based on the assumption that choices among alternatives depend on a weighted sum of utilities where decision makers seek to maximize the utility of their choices. While EUT describes preferences in situations of uncertainty, DUT describes preferences in the domain of time. DUT assumes a single discounting rate over time; the discounting rate serves as the utility weights in DUT. DUT also posits a single discount function that is exponential.

The axioms of DUT specify that preferences for outcomes over time are monotonic, complete, transitive, continuous, independent, and stationary. Monotonicity of preferences over time means that if an outcome is preferred at Time A over Time B, then Time A occurs before Time B. Thus, outcomes are more desirable if they occur earlier in time. Based on the propositions of DUT, the same discounting rate should be observed for all choices in time and should be positive in most cases. The axiom of completeness of preferences posits that there are preferences across different points in time. Transitivity of preferences over time means that if Outcome 1 is preferred to Outcome 2 at a later time and if Outcome 2 is preferred to Outcome 3 at a time that is still later, then Outcome 1 will be preferred over Outcome 3. Continuity of preferences assumes that there are points of indifference in preferences for outcomes between an earlier time and a later time, where outcomes are equally preferred. This axiom ensures that there exists a continuous utility function over time. The axiom of independence over time means that the order of preferences for outcomes should not reverse at different points in time. If one outcome is preferred to another at one time, this order of preferences should be preserved over time. Stationarity requires that when preferences are ranked across time, this ranking should not change even if the time interval changes.

Sign Effect

While DUT has proved to be useful in describing intertemporal preferences in a range of situations, violations in the axioms have been observed. For example, based on the assumption of a single discounting rate, DUT would suggest that preferences should be equal over time whether the health outcome is a gain or a loss. However, a number of studies provide evidence that the discount rate for losses is lower than that for gains. In other words, preference for a desirable outcome is discounted more over time than preference to avoid a loss. This has been termed the *sign effect*.

The Value of Health Versus Money

The idea that a single discounting rate can be used to describe preferences in all decisions also has been challenged. These arguments are especially important to medical decision making, where health is the desired outcome rather than money. Both money and health have been found to have relatively large discount rates, especially as compared with what is recommended for use in economic analyses. In contrast to what is predicted by DUT, decision makers appear to use different rates for health as compared with money. This observation has been used to understand why it can be difficult to encourage people to adopt preventive health behaviors to improve future health. A large discounting rate would mean that future health does not seem attractive enough in the present to overcome the desire to engage in behavior that is highly rewarding in the short term, such as smoking.

Choice Sequences

Another violation of DUT has been described with respect to a series of decisions made over time. For example, many health decisions occur in a sequence rather than as single choices. A person diagnosed with cancer may make a series of decisions about surgery, radiation therapy, and adjuvant chemotherapy. A person who is diagnosed with diabetes may face a series of choices about diet, exercise, medication, and self-monitoring. The sequence effect refers to the tendency to observe a negative discount rate when choices occur in a sequence. In other words, people prefer to defer desirable outcomes, to savor the rewards, and to want to hasten undesirable outcomes in order to get them out of the way sooner and reduce dread of an adverse event.

Hyperbolic Discounting

Alternative theories to DUT have been suggested to explain these anomalies. For example, it has been suggested that, as compared with the constant discounting posited by DUT, a hyperbolic model may better describe the preferences reversals over time. A hyperbolic discounting model describes preferences where delayed outcomes are discounted in a way that is inversely related to the time delay between the early review and the late review. Thus, short-term outcomes are discounted more than long-term outcomes. This could happen if the decision maker is more impatient in making judgments about reviews in the short run than in the long run. This might describe the case where a smoker has greater difficulty deferring a cigarette in the short run than in deferring the purchase of cigarettes in the long run.

The Neurobiology of Intertemporal Preferences

Recent work on discounting has been directed toward understanding the neurobiology of intertemporal preferences. These studies often employ functional magnetic resonance imaging to examine the brain activity of research participants who are engaged in a choice experiment. Results of these studies have described two systems relevant to making choices over time. In making intertemporal decisions, humans show several cognitive processes: ones that focus on the present and others that consider the future. These findings—that there may be several cognitive processes that distinguish between events in time—provide some support for the hyperbolic discounting models. These studies, while not conclusive, have offered innovative methods to more fully understand the processes underlying intertemporal choice.

Sara J. Knight

See also Cost-Effectiveness Analysis; Cost-Effectiveness Ratio; Cost-Utility Analysis; Marginal or Incremental Analysis

Further Readings

Cairns, J. A., & Van Der Pol, M. M. (1997). Saving future lives: A comparison of three discounting models. *Health Economics, 6,* 341–350.

Chapman, G., & Elstein, A. E. (1995). Valuing the future: Temporal discounting of health and money. *Medical Decision Making, 15,* 373–386.

Kalenscher, T., & Pennartz, C. M. A. (2008). Is a bird in the hand worth two in the future? The neuroeconomics of intertemporal decision-making. *Progress in Neurobiology, 84,* 284–315.

Kamlet, M. S. (1992). *The comparative benefits modeling project: A framework for cost-utility analysis of government health care programs.* Washington, DC: Office of Disease Prevention and Health Promotion, Public Health Service.

Khwaja, A., Silverman, D., & Sloan, F. (2007). Time preference, time discounting, and smoking decisions. *Health Economics, 26,* 927–949.

Loewenstein, G., & Prelec, D. (1991). Negative time preference. *American Economic Review, 81,* 347–352.

Loewenstein, G., & Prelec, D. (1992). Anomalies in intertemporal choice: Evidence and interpretation. *Quarterly Journal of Economics, 107,* 573–597.

Loewenstein, G., & Prelec, D. (1993). Preferences for sequences of outcomes. *Psychological Review, 100,* 91–108.

McClure, S. M., Laibson, D. I., Loewenstein, G., & Cohen, J. D. (2004). Separate neural systems value immediate and delayed monetary rewards. *Science, 306,* 503–507.

Redelmeier, D. A., & Heller, D. N. (1993). Time preferences in medical decision making and cost-effectiveness analysis. *Medical Decision Making, 13,* 212–217.

Discrete Choice

A discrete choice experiment (DCE) is a type of stated preference method used to elicit values for goods and services. DCEs rely on the premise that any good or service can be described by its characteristics and the extent to which an individual values a good or service depends on the levels of these characteristics. DCEs have long been used by consumer products companies to design new products to meet customer preferences by measuring the relative importance of different product attributes, but they have only more recently been applied in the context of health and environmental goods. This approach typically provides more detailed, yet substantively different, information compared with traditional stated preference methods, such as contingent valuation or health state utility assessment.

Comparison With Other Stated Preference Methods

Stated preference methods, in which respondents value hypothetical descriptions of products or choices, are useful in valuing nonmarket goods, such as health. They are useful in situations in which the market for a good, or for the full range of attributes of a good, does not exist and "revealed preference" studies cannot be conducted. In a revealed preference study, preferences are estimated by observing the actual choices that have been made in a real-world setting. For example, the relative value of individual attributes of automobiles, such as size, color, make, and model, could be measured by analyzing retrospective data on automobile sales prices along with the specific characteristics of the automobiles sold. For a new model, a revealed preference approach would not be possible since data are not yet available for the new model; instead, a stated preference approach could be used. Other stated preference methods typically used to value health outcomes are health state utility assessment or contingent valuation. Elicitation techniques for these stated preference methods include standard gamble, time trade-off, or willingness to pay. Compared with these methods, DCEs can be used to value health, nonhealth, and process attributes and provide information about the trade-offs between these attributes. DCEs can also be used to value willingness to pay for an attribute, whereas traditional methods provide a single numerical rating for the whole service.

All stated preference methods have the limitation that the valuation task asks about hypothetical choices and, therefore, may not fully predict future choices. Using stated preference methods can often provide a valuable starting point for further research given the difficulty of obtaining preference data on nonmarket goods. All stated preference methods allow data to be collected on programs and interventions while they are still under development, similar to how studies might be conducted to develop new consumer products. Once a program or intervention has been introduced, additional research could combine revealed and stated preference data to provide even more detailed information about user preferences.

Understanding preferences for different aspects of health and health interventions and incorporating these values into clinical and policy decisions can result in clinical and policy decisions that better reflect individuals' preferences and potentially improve adherence to clinical treatments or public health programs.

Terminology

The terms *discrete choice experiments* or *conjoint analysis* are typically used to describe a type of stated preference method in which preferences are inferred according to responses to hypothetical scenarios. These terms are often used interchangeably. Conjoint analysis comes from marketing applications and DCEs from transportation and engineering applications. The common element of DCEs and conjoint analysis is that they both allow the researcher to examine the trade-offs that people make for each attribute, attribute level, and combinations of attributes. They differ in that the term *conjoint analysis* is more generally used to refer to a method whereby the respondent rates or ranks a scenario and DCEs involve a discrete choice between alternative scenarios. DCEs, and the related approach of conjoint analysis, have been successfully applied to measuring preferences for a diverse range of health applications, and the use of these approaches is growing rapidly.

Example of a Discrete Choice Experiment

An example of the attributes used in a DCE designed to identify preferences for a pharmacogenetic testing service is shown in Table 1. The service offers a test to identify a person's risk of developing a side effect (neutropenia) from azathioprine. This example has five attributes, and the attributes have different numbers of levels. Both health and nonhealth outcomes are included in the evaluation of the service.

Table 2 shows an example of one choice question. It is also possible to design discrete choices with more than two options.

Conducting a Discrete Choice Experiment

Conducting a DCE includes proper design, fielding, and analysis. Elements of design include designing the experiment and overall survey development, as the survey should include survey questions in addition to the discrete choice questions.

Designing and Administering a Discrete Choice Experiment

The first step in a DCE is to identify and define the attributes of the health intervention or program. Once the attributes or characteristics have been identified, the levels of each attribute must also be defined, which must be realistic options for the service being valued. Attributes and levels should be developed through an iterative process including literature review, experts in the field, focus groups, and one-on-one interviews.

The second step is to identify the choice task. Discrete choice task options include forced choice, in which the respondent chooses between one or more options. Alternatively, the respondent can be offered an opt-out option, which must then be addressed in the analysis step. The selection of the choice task will have implications about the type of analytic approach that is appropriate.

The third step is to set the experimental design for the DCE. Depending on the numbers of attributes and levels, it may be possible to use a full-factorial design in which all possible combinations of attributes and attribute levels are used to create scenarios. If the number of possible combinations exceeds the likely sample size, then efficient combinations of a subset of choices can be identified through the use of design libraries or other methods. This is called a fractional-factorial design, which uses mathematical properties to ensure non-association between the variables in the design (orthogonality). Choice sets must then be created from these scenarios, and again different methods exist, including pairing the scenarios or using fold-over techniques. It is important that key design principles are followed when creating the choice sets from the scenarios to ensure that the main effects—and, if necessary, two-way interactions—can be estimated.

The fourth step is to construct the survey that includes the DCE. A successful DCE survey will include an introductory section to provide the respondents with enough information to understand the choices they are about to be presented in the survey. This will involve a section that describes the attributes and levels and introduces the valuation task. This section should also include a practice question. Key questions for survey design will include mode of administration and sample selection. Mode of administration may determine the number of choices that can be included for each respondent. Depending on the numbers of attributes and attribute levels, choices may need to be divided into *choice sets*. A choice

Table 1   Possible attributes and levels

Attribute	Level
Process attributes	
The level of information given to the patient about the test	None Low Moderate High
How the sample is collected	Blood test Mouthwash Finger prick Mouth swab
Who explains the result to the patient	Primary-care physician Pharmacist Hospital physician Nurse
Cost	£0 £50 £100 £250
Health outcome	
The ability of the test to predict the risk of the side effect (neutropenia)	50% 60% 85% 90%
Nonhealth outcomes	
How long it takes before the patient receives a result	2 days 7 days 14 days 28 days

Table 2   Example of a pairwise choice

	Test A	Test B
The level of information given to the patient about the test	Moderate	High
The ability of the test to predict the risk of the side effect (neutropenia)	50% accurate	60% accurate
How the sample is collected	Finger prick	Mouth swab
How long it takes before the patient receives the result	28 days	2 days
Who explains the result to the patient	Pharmacist	Hospital doctor
Cost	$50	$250
Tick (✓) one option only	❑	❑

set is a fixed set of choices presented to a single respondent. For example, if the DCE has a total of 64 choices, then the choices may be split into 8 choice sets of 8 choices each to reduce respondent burden. An essential part of survey development is to pretest the questionnaire with respondents one-on-one until the survey instrument is stable. The survey should also include a section on respondent demographics and other characteristics that may relate to choices, such as experience with the health condition or intervention being valued.

Survey administration should follow the recommended approaches for the mode of administration involved. Most DCEs are administered via computer (online) or on paper via a mail survey.

Additional Design Considerations

Additional design considerations include the definition of the value attribute, inclusion of an opt-out option, and internal validity tests. The value attribute is the attribute used to infer value for the program or intervention; in health, it is typically represented by money or time. Other metrics can also be considered, such as risk, but to date there has been little research that explores how respondents value risk estimates in a DCE. The important characteristic of this attribute is that it is a continuous variable and can be analyzed as such. The inclusion of an opt-out option will be appropriate in any situation in which it would be a realistic option for the respondent in a real-world choice situation. In the survey design process, the development of attributes, levels, and choices should aim at keeping the hypothetical situations presented as close to reality as possible while still maintaining the objectives of the study.

Analysis of Discrete Choice Experiments

Analyzing data from a DCE requires the use of discrete choice analysis. The survey should have been designed to have an appropriate number of levels and attributes to produce robust estimates of the value for each attribute/level. For example, using the sample discrete choice question in Table 2, a utility function U is specified for each of the two alternatives of Test A or Test B:

$$U_i = \beta_1 X_{1i} + \beta_2 X_{2i} + \beta_3 X_{3i} + \ldots + \beta_k X_{ki} + \varepsilon_i$$
$$= \beta X_i + \varepsilon_i, \quad (i = A, B).$$

X_{ki} ($k - 1, \ldots, K$) are the causal variables for alternative i and consist of both the attributes of the alternatives (e.g., effectiveness of the test). Further analyses can explore preferences in subgroups of the population (e.g., race/ethnicity, income). ε_i is the random error.

Assuming utility-maximizing behavior and ε_i iid (independent and identically distributed), extreme value distributed leads to the logit probability of choosing alternative i:

$$P(i) = \frac{exp(\beta X_i)}{\sum_{j=A,B,C} exp(\beta X_i)}.$$

The survey responses are used to make inferences on the coefficients β. This is performed by maximizing the log-likelihood of the sample over the unknown coefficients. Variables that should be statistically tested for inclusion in the model will include all attributes and all levels of each attribute; respondent characteristics such as race/ethnicity, age, sex, and income; appropriate interaction variables if these were included in the design. Other variables that could affect patient choices should also be considered as covariates in the analysis, such as a patient's familiarity with the service in question.

The sign of a statistically significant coefficient provides a decision maker with information about the effect of an attribute. A positive coefficient suggests that improved effectiveness as an attribute of the recommendation would make the program more attractive. Furthermore, the ratio between two coefficients can provide information about the trade-off, or marginal rate of substitution, between the two corresponding variables. For example, the ratio of the coefficient for benefit to the coefficient for cost represents the willingness to pay for a particular level of benefit. Results from a DCE survey can also quantify how an individual's value of effectiveness of an intervention compares with, for example, having a fast turnaround time. The results can provide additional information on which programs are likely to provide the most value to patients and clues on how to improve participation by aligning program characteristics with patient preferences.

In the past, the results of DCEs have been used to place the attributes in relative order of importance according to the size of the coefficient. Analysts have also attempted to compare the results from DCEs conducted in two populations by directly comparing the size of the coefficients. Both these approaches are problematic because they do not make allowances for the scale parameter.

The analytic approach described above uses standard discrete choice methods. Advanced discrete choice methods can be used to both (a) improve the statistical efficiency of the coefficient estimates (by capturing serial correlations over multiple responses from the same individual) and (b) capture unobserved heterogeneity through estimation of random coefficients.

Future Research

Future research opportunities, some of which are under way, include methodological issues such as identifying optimal design sets, including risk as an attribute, understanding potential bias in using the cost attribute to estimate willingness to pay, estimating individual preferences, accounting for heterogeneity in preferences, and measuring the external validity of DCEs.

Lisa Prosser and Katherine Payne

See also Utility Assessment Techniques; Willingness to Pay

Further Readings

Bridges, J. F. P. (2003). Stated preference methods in health care evaluation: An emerging methodological paradigm in health economics. *Applied Health Economics and Health Policy, 2*(4), 213–224.

Elliott, R., & Payne, K. (2005). Valuing preferences. In *Essentials of Economic Evaluation in Healthcare* (Chap. 11). London: Pharmaceutical Press.

Hensher, D. A., Rose, J. M., & Greene, W. H. (2005). *Applied choice analysis: A primer.* Cambridge, UK: Cambridge University Press.

Lancsar, E., & Louviere, J. (2008). Conducting discrete choice experiments to inform healthcare decision making: A user's guide. *PharmacoEconomics, 26*(8), 661–677.

Ryan, M., & Gerard, K. (2003). Using discrete choice experiments to value health care programmes: Current practice and future research reflections. *Applied Health Economics and Health Policy, 2*(1), 55–64.

Street, D. J., & Burgess, L. (2007). *The construction of optimal stated choice experiments.* London: Wiley.

Discrete-Event Simulation

Discrete-event simulation (DES) is a very flexible modeling method that can be used when the research question involves competition for resources, distribution of resources, complex interactions between entities, or complex timing of events. The main advantage and disadvantage of DES is its large but constrained modeling vocabulary. That is, though there is more to learn initially, there is more freedom regarding the kinds of systems one can model.

DES was originally developed in the 1960s to model industrial and business processes, finding its first home in industrial engineering and operations research. Since then, DES has been used to gain insight into a wide range of research and business questions. Because of its unique strengths, DES began to be applied to healthcare problems in the mid-1980s.

Since its introduction, DES has been used to examine a broad array of healthcare and healthcare-related problems. Areas in which it has been applied have been mental health; disease management; infectious disease; disaster planning and bioterrorism; biology model and physiology; cancer; process redesign and optimization in laboratories, clinics, operating rooms, emergency services, healthcare systems, and pathways of care; geographic allocation of resources; trial design; policy evaluation; and survival modeling. DES is often the preferred simulation method in healthcare when (a) there is competition for resources, (b) systems are tightly coupled, (c) the geographic distribution of resources is important, (d) information or entity flow cannot be completely described a priori, (e) the timing of events may be asynchronous or cannot be modeled on a fixed clock, and (f) entities in the system require memory.

Simulation Modeling

In general, models allow researchers to explicitly explore the elements of a decision/problem and mediate understanding of the real world by rendering it comprehensible. Simulation modeling is any activity where the actual or proposed system is replaced by a functioning representation that approximates the same cause-and-effect relationship of the "real" system. Simulation allows researchers to generate evidence for decision making or to develop understanding of underlying processes in the real world when direct experimentation (due to cost, time, or ethics) is not possible. Experimentation with simulation models is performed through sensitivity analyses, where the parameters of the system are varied, or through what-if experiments, where the number or types of resources of the system are varied.

Decision trees and Markov models have, to date, been the most common types of computer simulation models used in healthcare. These methods are used to create highly structured representations of decision processes and alternative strategies. This is done by constraining the formulation of these models to a limited vocabulary, essentially three building blocks—decision nodes, chance nodes, and outcome nodes. The main advantage of this type of formulation is that the highly structured format is relatively transparent and easy to interpret. The disadvantage is that the highly structured framework restricts the types or problems that can be articulated, often forcing significant compromises on the model and the modeler. With over 100 building blocks, DES has a much broader vocabulary (than tree models), allowing a broader array of problems to be modeled, with fewer compromises. This means that though there is more to learn initially there, is a greater range of problems one can model.

DES models differ from decision trees and Markov models in several ways. First, unlike tree models, DES allows entities within a system (e.g., patients) to interact and compete with each other. For example, two or more end-stage liver patients may be competing for a newly available donor liver. Second, DES allows for more flexible management of time than in tree models. Unlike simple trees, which handle time in the aggregate, or Markov models, which restrict changes in the system to fixed time intervals (Markov cycles), in DES, the time interval between events can be either fixed or treated as completely stochastic. In DES, each interaction provokes a change in the state of the system. Every interaction of entities with each other or with the resources in the system is an event. Every interaction changes the state of the entity involved and of the system as a whole. The time between events may be handled probabilistically, using fixed time increments, or both depending on the nature of the system being modeled.

There are generally four approaches for managing events in DES platforms: the *process interaction, event-scheduling, activity-scanning*, and *three-phase methods*. The differences are in how the software reacts to or anticipates interactions in the system. Third, every entity in the system can have memory. This means that the modeler can not only have entities interact but also can have the entities carry the memory of the interaction and have this information influence future interactions.

Key Features

The key features of a DES model are entities, attributes, queues, and resources. *Entities* are objects. They can move or be static within the system. They have the ability to interact with other entities. They represent persons, places, or things and so, metaphorically, act like nouns. The types of objects represented are not constrained to physical objects. For example, entities may also represent packages of information, such as phone calls, e-mails, or chemical signals. DES packages have been primarily written in object-oriented computer programming (OOP) languages, and entities may be considered to represent a class of objects.

Attributes are variables local to the entity object. This means that entities may carry information with them describing, for example, their age, sex, race, and health state, acting metaphorically as both the memory of the entity and as an adjective describing the entity. This information may be modified during any interaction within the system and may be used to determine how an entity will respond to a given set of circumstances. In DES, much of the information driving changes in the state of the model are embedded in the entities themselves in the form of attributes. This is in contrast to other modeling methods (e.g., trees, Markovs), where the information and knowledge are embedded in the nodal structure of the model. As a result, entities in DES have potentially many more degrees of freedom in how they transit the system being modeled.

A *resource* is an entity or object that provides a service to a dynamic entity. A service can be described as any activity requiring the simultaneous presence of the active entity. Providing a service requires time. The number of entities a resource can serve simultaneously is the resource's capacity. For example, a bank with a single cashier can serve one person at a time. A bank with three tellers can serve up to three customers simultaneously. A mobile resource, such as a motorcycle, can transport 2 persons, whereas a school bus can transport 40 people. If a resource is occupied when a new entity seeks its use, the new entity must wait until the resource is free.

A *queue* is any place or list in which an entity waits for access to a resource. If an entity arrives seeking service and the resource is already occupied, it must wait somewhere. Queues have logic. For example, the line at a cashier may follow first-in/first-out (FIFO) logic, getting on or off an airplane may follow last-in/first-out (LIFO) logic, and the waiting room in an emergency department or the waiting list for a transplant may follow highest-value-first (HVF) logic. Queue theory is the mathematical study of queues or waiting lists.

Queue Theory

DES explicitly embeds queue theory. The simplest queuing model is the M/M/1 (Kendall's nomenclature), which translates as Markovian interarrival time/Markovian process time and one server, or M/G/1, which is Markovian interarrival time/ general or arbitrary and one server. Simple systems such as these may be solved analytically and give insight into the behavior of more complex systems that cannot be analytically solved. This is important because every system from sufficient distance may be modeled as an M/M/1 system.

Interarrival rate is the rate of entity arrival (λ) ($1/\lambda$ = mean interarrival time). For example, the time between patient arrivals at a clinic may average 1 patient every 10 minutes. This may be stationary or nonstationary; for example, patients may arrive every 5 minutes around lunchtime. The service rate (μ) ($1/\mu$ = mean service time) is the rate at which the resource/server can process entities. The utilization rate (β) is λ/μ. If the average interarrival time = 10 minutes and the average service time = 7.5 minutes, the average utilization = .75. Another way to conceive of utilization is busy time/ total time resource available. For example, if a nurse is busy 4 hours out of an 8-hour shift, then the utilization rate is .5. If the interarrival rate is

less than the service rate (e.g., patients are arriving at longer intervals than the time required to process them), then the system is stable. If entities arrive faster than the system can process them, then waiting list length rises rapidly. Bottlenecks are temporary or permanent disequilibria between processing capacity and arrival rate at some point in the system—for example, a person calling in sick or an out-of-order elevator serving an apartment complex. Congestion occurs when a stable system has a utilization rate that is very close but slightly less than 1; that is, mean process time is very close to mean arrival rate (e.g., a tunnel or bridge into a major city). These are interesting systems because, first, they are very common and, second, they often experience large variations in behavior over time. Unexpected bottlenecks may occur randomly. These systems generally require longer run times to estimate expected system behavior. The breaks from normal behavior may be more interesting than the typical system behavior.

Flow time is the time from the moment an entity enters a system to the time the entity exits. The average flow time for a simple system may be described as $((\sigma^2_{server}\lambda + \beta^2\lambda)/2(1-\beta)) + \mu$, where σ = standard deviation of process time, μ = mean process time, and λ = arrival rate. The average wait time is the flow time number minus μ. The average number in queue is $\beta^2(1+\mu^2\sigma^2_{server})/2(1-\beta)$.

Measures of Performance

In addition to the standard outputs, such as quality-adjusted life years and cost, DES also provides operational outcome measures, such as throughput, utilization, flow time, and wait time. *Flow time* is usually defined as time from entry into the system to time of exit. *Wait time* is usually defined as time from entry into the system to time of receipt of service. *Throughput* is usually defined as total system production over measurement period. *Utilization* is usually defined as total busy time of a resource over total time resource available. Queue theory allows researchers to predict or approximate these measures.

Software

There are many software packages available for conducting DES. However, most of these are custom built for specific purposes. The Institute for Operations Research and the Management Sciences provides an extensive list of vendors on its Web site. Currently, some of the most commonly used general-purpose DES packages are GPSS, Arena/SIMAN, AutoMod, Extend, ProModel, Simu18, and Witness. There is also freeware available on the Internet, although these tools generally require a higher degree of computing skill to use.

James Stahl

See also Decision Trees, Construction; Markov Models

Further Readings

Banks, J. (1998). *Handbook of simulation.* New York: Wiley.

Davies, H., & Davies, R. (1987). A simulation model for planning services for renal patients in Europe. *Journal of the Operational Research Society, 38*(8), 693–700.

Institute for Operations Research and the Management Sciences: http://www.informs.org

Nance, R., & Sargent, R. (2002). Perspectives on the evolution of simulation. *Operations Research, 50*(1), 161–172.

DISCRIMINATION

In statistics, discrimination is the ability of a prediction (judgment scheme, statistical model, etc.) to distinguish between events and nonevents (or cases from controls, successes from failures, disease from nondisease, etc.). In the simplest form, a prediction scheme focuses on a single event with two possible states and assigns some estimate of the chance that one state will occur. This prediction comes from the set of cues and other factors, both measurable and immeasurable, available to the researcher.

Whether it is meteorologists forecasting the weather, business analysts predicting the rise and fall of the stock market, bookmakers predicting the big game, or physicians diagnosing disease, predictions have some degree of "correctness" relative to the actual occurrence of some unknown or future event. In medicine, we commonly predict the presence or absence of disease (diagnosis) or the likelihood of development of disease progression (prognosis). Measures have arisen to gauge the quality of a given set of predictions and to quantify prediction accuracy.

Multiple methods for forming these predictions exist, and each has associated strengths and weaknesses. One aspect is the "difficulty" that is set by nature. Outcome index variance is a measure of this difficulty. In addition, calibration addresses the relationship of the subgroup-specific predictions to the subgroup-specific observed event rate. The part of prediction accuracy that is often of highest interest is discrimination. The task of discrimination is to determine with some degree of certainty when the event will or will not occur. It measures the degree to which the prediction scheme separates events from nonevents. Discrimination is therefore influenced by variation in the predictions within the event/nonevent groups. Discrimination strength is related to the degree to which a prediction scheme assigns events and nonevents different probabilities—in other words, how well a scheme separates events into distinct "bins" (e.g., alive vs. dead or first vs. second vs. third). The sole focus of discrimination is this ability to place different events into different categories. The labels placed on those categories are somewhat arbitrary.

"Perfect" discrimination will occur when each appropriate category contains 100% or 0% of events. Perfect nondiscrimination, or nil discrimination, occurs when the group-specific event rate is the same as the overall percentage of events (also called the prevalence or mean base rate). In this case, the prediction scheme is no better than chance, and the groups are essentially assigned at random. One can, however, do worse than this by predicting groups in the wrong direction. However, this is, in a sense, still better than nil discrimination, but it is classifying groups incorrectly. Any discrimination that is better than the overall event prevalence improves the discrimination. In this case, simply reversing the labels of event and non-event associated with the predictions can improve the discrimination.

Discrimination Types

Discrimination can be thought of in three distinct ways, each of use in different situations. These three types of discrimination arise from thinking of discrimination like types of data. Data can be *nominal*, having no order but simply labels (e.g., color or gender). *Ordinal* data have associated order (e.g., mild/moderate/severe) but no measurable distance between groups. *Continuous* data have a distance between two groups that can be measured. Discrimination can be thought of along a similar continuum: nominal, ordinal, and continuous.

The simplest conceptualization is to partition items into similar event groups—that is, strictly labels without an associated order. Separation occurs through labeling similar predicted event groups with the same name or probability. These labels have no rank or relative position. The labels have no intrinsic meaning and serve no purpose other than to form bins to place the groups into. Discrimination is measured by the degree to which these bins are used for distinct event types. This level of discrimination can be measured when no probability measurement is assigned to the groups. Observations need only be assigned to differing groups with a similar likelihood of event occurrence (e.g., Group A vs. Group B, red vs. blue, or common vs. rare).

The Normalized Discrimination Index (NDI) is typically used to measure this type of discrimination and is most often found in the meteorological literature. A hypothetical example of looking at the NDI would be a study comparing the ability of two new screening exams to separate cancerous lesions from noncancer lesions. All other things being equal, it would be favorable to choose the new test that has the higher NDI.

Next, one can conceive a measure of rank order discrimination—for example, when only rank order predictions are available. In this case, the available information separates groups into situations where "A will have a higher event rate than B." With rank order discrimination, a group of events can be placed in terms of least to most likely. Rank order discrimination occurs when the events have predictions consistently higher (or lower) than the nonevents. Rank order discrimination measures the ability of a judge to correctly assign the higher likelihood of occurrence when the outcome of interest actually occurs. This is similar to nominal discrimination, but bins now have an associated rank, thus requiring at least ordinal predictions.

The area under the receiver operating characteristic (ROC) curve, or C statistic, best measures this sort of discrimination and is the most used method in medicinal research. The C statistic ranges from 0 (*perfect discrimination, wrong labels*) to 1.0 (*perfect discrimination*), with *nil discrimination* at .50. Returning to the hypothetical example, we would look to the C statistic if instead of the lesion being declared cancerous versus noncancerous, the screening tests returned a four-level scale (e.g., high, medium, low, or no risk of being cancerous).

Finally, actual probability estimates used can be compared among the groups. By comparing actual probabilities, the focus is on a continuous discrimination, drawing an arbitrary cut-point where separation is most distinct. Continuous discrimination determines how far apart groups are on a probability scale, and it requires continuous predictions to be calculated. The difference between the mean probabilities assigned to events and nonevents defines the slope index (SI), the primary measure of this type of discrimination. If we had two screening models that returned the exact probability of the lesion being cancerous, we could use the SI to compare the models' discrimination ability.

Discrimination Measurements

Except for the C statistic, these measures are on a −1 to +1 scale, where 1 is *perfect discrimination*, 0 is *nil discrimination*, and −1 indicates *perfect discrimination with the wrong labels*. The C statistic can be transformed into Somer's D by subtracting 0.5 and doubling the result. Somer's D is on the same −1 to +1 scale as NDI and SI. Unfortunately, no rule of thumb exists to define "weak" or "strong" discrimination. Since what might be "strong" discrimination in one area might be "weak" in another, discrimination strength is relative to the scientific area of interest; thus, this entry is reluctant to provide a rule of thumb for good versus poor discrimination. Whether a .7 score (70% of the total scale) is a strong discrimination really depends on the situation under study. In areas where little is known and any relationship is of value, a smaller amount of discrimination might be more important than in an area where much is understood and the research is trying to distinguish between degrees of perfection.

Any given prediction scheme will have degrees of the three types of discrimination. So long as predictions are given in terms of probabilities, for example, the results of a logistic regression, all three of these measures can be calculated. By creating ordered bins of probability of some fixed width, the SI, Somer's D, and NDI can all be calculated. This can be especially useful when discrimination ability of one type is capped and the goal is to determine tests that are "more perfect," or stronger but on a differing scale. For example, when taking a drug from the ideal conditions of a randomized clinical trial and using it in day-to-day practice, "ROC shrinkage" or a slightly less effective test is often observed. Examinations of continuous discrimination can help gauge the degree of ROC shrinkage, that is, the reduction in rank order discrimination expected to be observed, when variation in predictions increases.

Matthew Karafa

See also Calibration; Diagnostic Tests; Logistic Regression

Further Readings

Dawson, N. V. (2003). Physician judgments of uncertainty. In G. B. Chapman & F. A. Sonnenberg (Eds.), *Decision making in health care: Theory, psychology, and applications* (p. 211). Cambridge, UK: Cambridge University Press.

Yaniv, I., Yates, J. F., & Smith, J. E. K. (1991). Measures of discrimination skill in probabilistic judgment. *Psychological Bulletin, 110*(3), 611–617.

Yates, J. F. (1990). *Judgment and decision making* (p. 56). Englewood Cliffs, NJ: Prentice Hall.

Yates, J. F. (1994). Subjective probability accuracy analysis. In G. Wright & P. Ayton (Eds.), *Subjective probability* (pp. 381–410). New York: Wiley.

Zhou, X.-H., Obuchowski, N. A., & McClish, D. K. (2002). *Statistical methods in diagnostic medicine.* New York: Wiley.

DISEASE MANAGEMENT SIMULATION MODELING

Simulation is a general term describing a method that imitates or mimics a real system using a *model* of that system. Models vary widely and may be a physical object, such as a mannequin used in training healthcare providers, or a conceptual object, such as a supply-demand curve in medical economics. This entry is confined to computer models that are based on a logical or mathematical/statistical structure and use the computer to examine a model's behavior. Models can represent various types of healthcare systems that are engaged in disease management of patients, allowing, for example, examination and comparisons of alternative clinical decisions for patient care, insurance coverage policies, or the processes for delivering safe, effective, and efficient preventive or therapeutic care.

The best practices for disease management use evidence-based medicine, such as the outcomes from observational and experimental human studies, including clinical trials. However, such studies are not always possible and may be impractical. Consider, for example, studies that seek to determine the most effective (balancing risks and benefits) and cost-effective (balancing costs and effectiveness) strategies for colon cancer screening. An effective strategy might include ignoring small polyps in low-risk people, but a prospective human study that includes such a component might never be approved. Determining the best age to initially screen for colon cancer would require an experiment that tested perhaps 25 different ages. Determining the frequency and type of follow-up testing based on a person's family history, biological and social profile, and past test results, including the size and type of past polyps, would require such a large study over such a long period of time as to be essentially impossible. In engineering and in the physical sciences, computational models have been frequently used to complement and to substitute for direct experimentation.

Key Components of Simulation Models

Simulation models can be used to integrate evidence from observational and experimental human studies and extend insights into the consequences of different disease management strategies. The fundamental concept involves constructing a model of the natural history of the disease in an individual patient from a specific patient group. The model can be simulated on the computer to produce the experience of many patients with this disease over their lifetimes. Then the model is altered to represent a medical strategy of care that includes an intervention, such as a screening test, a diagnostic test, medical therapy, or a surgical procedure. The population of patients with the intervention is simulated using the new model, and the results for the new model are compared with the results from the baseline model. Statistical comparisons can readily be made across myriad clinical strategies.

Validating the Simulation Model

A model is a representation of reality, not reality itself. As a representation, it attempts to replicate the input and the essential logical structure of the real system. A valid model can be exercised and the results inferred to the real world being studied. Consider Figure 1.

Here, the real world is the experience of real patients. The modeled world is the simulated experience of those patients. In addition to the proper representation of the logical and temporal relationships among the patients and their disease and the accurate description (including higher-order moments beyond the mean) of the probabilities of events and the importance of the outcomes of the various events, a third important key to any successful modeling activity is its validation. For purposes of assessing strategies for disease management, *construct validity* is supported by including model elements, relationships, and data derived from the published literature and assessed as appropriate by clinical experts. *Criterion-based validity*, comparing a model's output with real-world data when input conditions are held similar, provides significant assurance of the overall validity of the model for the purposes for which it is intended.

Notably, all models have limitations in their ability to represent the totality (complete detail) of actual patients or systems of care. Nonetheless, the simulation model should ideally represent patient- and/or system-level experiences that are indistinct from real patients or systems of care. For example, when computer-generated (simulated) histories are compared with a set of real patient histories (at the same level of detail), physicians (or other medical personnel) should not be able to tell them apart. Ultimately, the level of detail should depend on the questions being asked of the model, and sufficient detail should be included to allow model validation and provide for useful results.

Performance Measures From the Simulation

The amount of detail in a disease management simulation model is a direct reflection of the purpose for doing the simulation, such as comparing health outcomes or healthcare system performance. For example, the model can record the

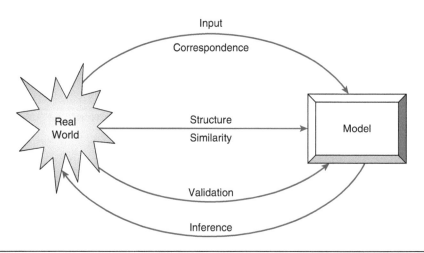

Figure 1   Relationship of model to real world

time a simulated patient spends in various health states (precancerous, healthy, cancerous, etc.), with each health state representing a different level of quality of life. A summary estimate from many simulated patients of the overall *quality-adjusted life years* (QALYs) can then be computed. Costs could be collected as a patient moves through the care system and summarized for many simulated patients to assist in the assessment of cost-effectiveness. Various healthcare resource utilization metrics may also be collected, such as the number of screening or diagnostic tests, laboratory procedures, or days of hospitalization. Performance measures need to be delineated during the construction of the simulation model so that appropriate data are being collected during execution of the model and summarized for analysis.

Data collections relative to performance measures are implemented in the simulation as patients traverse the care system. These performance measures are generally statistically presented at the end of the simulation. By sampling a statistically sufficient number of people, adequate statistical confidence intervals for the averages can be constructed. Fortunately, since individual patients are being individually simulated, the performance measures for the patients provide independent and identically distributed observations, which make traditional statistical analysis applicable. Advanced statistical methods related to statistical design of experiments can also be applied to simulation models.

Modeling the Care Cycle

A disease management simulation model should be a model of the care cycle for that disease, namely, from onset of the disease to eventual resolution or death. For example, a woman who died from colon cancer may have experienced the medical timeline shown in Figure 2.

In this case, two undetected adenomas occur (A1 and A2), each of which would eventually result in invasive cancer (C1 and C2). Surgery is performed to remove the invasive cancer from C1 at time CO. But because of late detection, she dies from this colon cancer at CD, which occurs before the second adenoma develops into invasive cancer (C2). Had A1 been detected and removed with a screening strategy, she would have survived to natural death (i.e., from some cause other than colon cancer). Each of these occurrences is considered an "event" since each changes the health status of the individual.

A valid model of this "natural history" must recognize that almost all the causes for these events that affect the timeline need be described by *random variables*. A random variable is a variable whose exact value is unknown but is described by a probability distribution or probabilistic process. The time for an undetected adenoma to become invasive cancer is an example of a "time until" random variable, whereas the incidence of undetected adenomas is a random process. Also, note that there is an "order" or pathway to the events in that an invasive cancer cannot occur without first being an undetected adenoma.

So a comprehensive model of the natural history for this case would include the following: (a) incidence of the disease based on an overall risk modified by the individual risk, (b) the disease pathways, (c) the rate and trajectory of

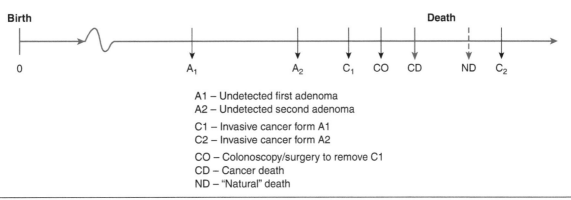

Figure 2   Medical timeline for a colon cancer death

progression, (d) the state and progress of the end disease, and (e) the time until natural death. Corresponding to the intervention (e.g., a screening strategy), the model changes would potentially alter any of the processes to produce longer life or more quality-adjusted life years or different costs in relation to quality-adjusted life years.

Modeling Details

There are several possible approaches to modeling these kinds of disease processes. One approach would be a state-based model, such as a Markov process. The modeling approach would identify patient states and the potential transitions between states. Figure 3 is an example of a Markov model.

Here, the "ovals" represent states relative to cancer, and the "arrows" represent the possible transitions between states at fixed points in time. Transitions are usually probabilities and may be a function of patient characteristics, such as age, gender, and genetic profile. The arrows that are directed back to the same state indicate that one possible transition is to remain in the same state. An alternative is to model "time in state" as a random variable. If the arrows represent transition probabilities, then the total probability "out" for each state must sum to 1.

Markov models are usually used to compute change in the state of a particular population. Time is incremented, and the transitions are applied, yielding populations in different states.

For example, if 100 people start with no cancer, then after one time step, some people may move to the "Death" state, while others may move to the "Local cancer" state. Yet, depending on the probabilities, most will remain in the "No cancer" state. When a Markov model is used to model individual experiences, the simulation must be manipulated to employ tracker variables to report the events that a patient has suffered over time. In general, when the model employs random variables to describe state transitions and time-in-state variables, the simulation is called a Monte Carlo simulation. One of the popular uses of Monte Carlo simulations is in *probabilistic sensitivity analysis*, in which the parameters of a decision model are represented by random variables and the decision model is examined by sampling from these uncertain parameters.

A generalization of the Monte Carlo simulation model is the *discrete-event simulation*. Discrete-event simulations typically focus on the experiences of individuals throughout a process (such as healthcare delivery) and statistically aggregate the individual experiences to a population at risk. The description of a discrete-event simulation begins with the identification of *events*. Events are points in time when the individual changes health state—namely, when a patient experiences something that moves him or her from one state to another. The simulation operates by maintaining a calendar of future events, removing one event at a time, updating time to the time of that event, and executing all the processes associated with that event. Execution

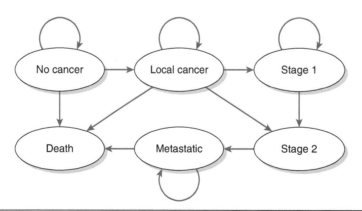

Figure 3   A Markov model

of these processes may add new events to the calendar of future events. What makes a discrete-event simulation most flexible is that it deals with only the immediate event. The immediate event may change other potential future events, so that, for example, more than one adenoma can be represented in the colon and each has its own characteristics. Diseases with multiple precursors and multiple consequences are readily included in the model. A discrete model can be visualized as an event diagram, as shown in Figure 4.

In this diagram, the "boxes" represent events, while the arrows represent the event-scheduling requirements. For example, suppose a "Nonvisible adenoma" event occurs. From this event, three possible new events are scheduled: (1) possibly another nonvisible adenoma event, (2) an advanced adenoma event if the progression type is progressive, and (3) a cancer event when the progression type is progressive or if the cancer is immediate. Note that an event graph is not a flowchart, since it only schedules future events. Furthermore, the time when a future event is scheduled may be described by a random variable. Thus, time to the next event is also part of the "arrow." It is the scheduling of future events that distinguishes the discrete-event simulation from its Monte Carlo counterpart.

Choosing to Do a Simulation

Simulation modeling provides a very flexible and powerful method to represent the evolution of disease and the management of its treatment. However, part of the power of the technique is derived from the detailed data input requirements, which is also a challenge when using the method. While a simulation of the natural history of a disease may employ local and national databases, it is often the case that critical information related to the stochastic nature of the disease and treatment process must be estimated or inferred from experience and nominal group or survey techniques.

Disease management simulation models provide a viable method to synthesize the complex natural history of a disease replete with the stochastic and statistical elements that describe real experiences. Interventions in the process make it possible to consider alternative management choices quantitatively.

Stephen D. Roberts and Robert S. Dittus

See also Discrete-Event Simulation; Markov Models

Further Readings

Caro, J. J. (2005). Pharmacoeconomic analyses using discrete event simulation. *PharmacoEconomics, 23*(4), 323–332.

Banks, J., Carson, J. S., Nelson, B. L., & Nicol, D. M. (2005). *Discrete-event simulation* (4th ed.). Upper Saddle River, NJ: Prentice Hall.

Doubilet, P., Begg, C. B., Weinstein, M. C., Braun, P., & McNeil, B. J. (1985). Probabilistic sensitivity analysis using Monte Carlo simulation: A practical approach. *Medical Decision Making, 5*(2), 157–177.

Freund, D. A., & Dittus, R. S. (1992). Principles of pharmacoeconomic analysis of drug therapy. *PharmacoEconomics, 1*(1), 20–31.

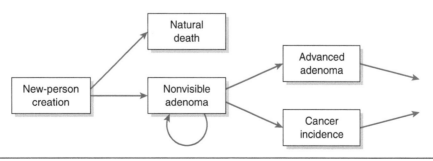

Figure 4   An event diagram for discrete-event simulation

Gold, M. R., Siegel, J. E., Russell, L. B., & Weinstein, M. C. (Eds.). (1996). *Cost-effectiveness in health and medicine.* New York: Oxford University Press.

Puterman, M. (1994). *Markov decision processes.* New York: Wiley.

Roberts, S., Wang, L., Klein, R., Ness, R., & Dittus, R. (2007). Development of a simulation model of colorectal cancer. *ACM Transactions on Modeling and Computer Simulation, 18*(4), 1–30.

Sonnenberg, F. A., & Beck, J. A. (1993). Markov models in medical decision making: A practical guide. *Medical Decision Making, 13*(4), 322–339.

DISTRIBUTIONS: OVERVIEW

In medical decision making, distribution functions are used for two main purposes. The first is to model variability in data at the individual observation level (often subjects or patients). The second is to model uncertainty in the parameter estimates of decision models.

Distributions for Modeling Variability

Distributions that are used to model variability can be either discrete or continuous. Examples of discrete distributions include the binomial distribution, commonly used to model the occurrence or not of an event of interest from a total sample size, and the Poisson distribution, commonly used to model counts of events. Examples of continuous distributions that are used to model data variability are the normal distribution and gamma distribution. The modeling of variability is particularly important for discrete-event simulation (DES) models, which are often employed to look at service delivery methods that involve queuing problems. For example, patients might be assumed to arrive at an emergency room and queue up to see the receptionist before waiting to see a physician. Arrival times could be modeled as random while following an underlying exponential distribution, and different methods of organizing the procedures for receiving and attending to patients could be modeled to maximize throughput and minimize waiting time. More generally, individual patient simulation models describe medical decision models that model an individual's pathway through disease and treatment. Monte Carlo simulation is typically used to represent the stochastic nature of this process and is termed "first-order" simulation when the focus is on variability in the patient experience rather than uncertainty in the parameters.

Distributions for Modeling Parameter Uncertainty

The use of probability distributions to represent parameter uncertainty in decision models is known as probabilistic sensitivity analysis. Distributions are chosen on the basis of the type of parameter and the method of estimation. Monte Carlo simulation is then used to select parameter values at random from each distribution, and the model is evaluated at this set of parameter values. By repeating this process a large number of times, the consequences of uncertainty over the input parameters of the model on the estimated output parameters is established. In contrast to modeling variability, only continuous distributions are used to model parameter uncertainty. Monte Carlo simulation used in this way is termed "second order" to reflect the modeling of uncertainty of parameters. Probability parameters are commonly modeled using a beta distribution, since a beta distribution is constrained on the interval 0 to 1. Parameters such as cost of quality-of-life disutility, which are constrained to be 0 or positive, are often modeled using the lognormal or gamma distributions since these distributions are positively skewed and can only take positive values. Relative-risk parameters are often used as treatment effects in decision models and can be modeled using a lognormal distribution, reflecting the standard approach to the statistical estimation of uncertainty and confidence limits for these measures.

Central Limit Theorem

The normal distribution is of particular note for two reasons. First, it turns out that many naturally occurring phenomena (such as height) naturally follow a normal distribution, and therefore, normal distributions have an important role in modeling data variability. Second, the *central limit theorem* is an important statistical theorem that states that whatever the underlying distribution of the data, the sampling distribution of the arithmetic mean will be normally distributed with sufficient sample size. Therefore, the normal distribution is always a candidate distribution for modeling parameter uncertainty, even if the parameters are constrained (in technical terms, if there is sufficient sample size to estimate a parameter, the uncertainty represented as a normal distribution will result in negligible probability that a parameter will take a value outside its logical range).

Statistical Models

Decision models in the medical arena often include statistical models as part of their structure. For example, a multivariate logistic regression may be used to estimate the probability of an event, or an ordinary least squares regression model may be used to explain how quality-of-life disutility is related to a particular clinical measure. Statistical regression models are of interest in that they simultaneously assume a distribution for the data and for the parameters of interest. For example, suppose that a transition probability in a Markov model is to be estimated from a survival analysis of time to event. A common parametric distribution for the time-to-event data themselves might be a Weibull distribution, which is capable of modeling time dependency of the underlying hazard function of the event of interest. However, the parameter uncertainty relates to the estimated coefficients from the regression of how the (log) hazard depends on patient characteristics. Since the scale of estimation in survival analysis is the log hazard scale and since a multivariate normal distribution of regression coefficients is assumed, this means that the underlying distribution of any particular parameter (coefficient) of the model is lognormal.

Bayesian Interpretation

As a brief aside, it is perhaps worth noting that the use of parametric distributions to represent uncertainty in decision models underlies the fundamentally Bayesian nature of medical decision making. The classical approach to probability does not allow uncertainty in the parameters themselves; rather, uncertainty relates to the estimation process and the likelihood that the true (but unobserved) parameter takes a particular value given the data. The Bayesian paradigm more naturally allows distributions to be chosen to reflect not only the data (equivalent to the frequentist data likelihood) but also the parameter itself.

Effective Modeling

Many distributions exist and have potential applications in medical decision making. Nevertheless, the appropriate distribution typically depends on the purpose of the model, on the constraints on the data or parameter, and on the method of estimation. Careful consideration of the appropriate distribution is required for effective modeling. Typically, such careful consideration will reduce a wide set of all possible distributions to a small set of candidate distributions for a particular application within the model.

Andrew H. Briggs

See also Bayesian Analysis; Decision Trees: Evaluation With Monte Carlo; Decision Trees: Sensitivity Analysis, Basic and Probabilistic; Decision Trees: Sensitivity Analysis, Deterministic; Discrete-Event Simulation; Managing Variability and Uncertainty; Parametric Survival Analysis

Further Readings

Briggs, A., Claxton, K., & Sculpher, M. (2006). *Decision modelling for health economic evaluation*. Oxford, UK: Oxford University Press.

Gelman, A., Carlin, J. B., Stern, H. S., & Rubin, D. B. (1995). *Bayesian data analysis*. London: Chapman & Hall.

Johnson, N. L., Kemp, A. W., & Kotz, S. (2005). *Univariate discrete distributions* (3rd ed.; Wiley Series in Probability and Statistics). Hoboken, NJ: Wiley.

Johnson, N. L., Kotz, S., & Balakrishnan, N. (1995). *Continuous univariate distributions* (Vol. 2; Wiley Series in Probability and Statistics). New York: Wiley.

Kotz, S., Balakrishnan, N., & Johnson, N. L. (1994). *Continuous univariate distributions* (Vol. 1; Wiley Series in Probability and Statistics). New York: Wiley.

Parmigiani, G. (2002). *Modeling in medical decision making*. Chichester, UK: Wiley.

DISTRIBUTIVE JUSTICE

Distributive justice is the branch of theories of justice that is concerned with the distribution of available resources among claimants. Theories of distributive justice all accept the central claim of formal justice that "equal claims should be handled equally" but differ in terms of what features they accept as relevant to the judgment of equality in claims and in outcomes. Considerations of distributive justice in health and healthcare are important because being healthy is a prerequisite for full or equal participation in a whole range of social activities, from employment to politics.

Within healthcare, considerations of distributive justice are especially important in the context of priority setting or rationing of healthcare services. This raises specific problems because one of the main outcomes of interest, namely, health, cannot be distributed directly. Health is not fungible and not detachable from the person who is healthy. Many discussions about justice in health therefore focus on access to healthcare, on the social determinants of health, or on justice in aggregate outcomes for groups of claimants. A further issue of current debate is whether justice in health or healthcare can be detached from much more general questions of social justice.

The main approaches to distributive justice that are of relevance to medical decision making are egalitarianism, maximization, equal opportunity, and procedural.

Egalitarianism

The most stringent theory of distributive justice is egalitarianism, which simply states that the resource in question should be distributed equally among claimants. Egalitarianism also implies that if complete equality cannot be obtained, then the distribution must at least reduce any preexisting inequalities.

In the healthcare context, most egalitarians hold that what determines the strength of a healthcare claim is exclusively the size of the healthcare need. The further from complete health a person is, the stronger is his or her claim to healthcare. However, the concept of health need probably also contains elements related to urgency and to the possibility of intervention.

Most people hold egalitarian views of varying strengths, and such views probably underlie the common idea that healthcare resources should be allocated primarily to those who have the greatest need, that is, those who are most ill.

Egalitarianism is open to two significant counterarguments: (1) the leveling-down objection and (2) a potential conflict between equality and making people better off. The leveling-down objection is simply that one of the ways of making people (more) equal is to take something away from those who have the most without redistributing it. In the medical context, health equality could be increased by taking health away from those who are completely healthy. A strict egalitarian would have to claim that that is an improvement, but that judgment seems highly counterintuitive. A world where some people have been harmed and no one benefited cannot be ethically better than the one before the change.

The potential conflict between equality and making people better off arises in its starkest form when one is contemplating a change that will improve the situation of everyone while also widening inequalities. A strict egalitarian would have to say that the position after the intervention is worse than before, and this is again strongly counterintuitive, at least in cases where the improvement for the least well-off is significant.

Maximization

Another prevalent theory of justice is the theory held by consequentialists. For consequentialists, what matters is the maximization of good outcomes from a distributive decision, not whether the distribution increases or decreases equality. The strength of a claim is thus not based on need but on how much good can be generated if the claim is met. In the healthcare context, this view underlies or is at least compatible with many health economic approaches to resource allocation—for instance, the quality-adjusted life year (QALY) approach. This compatibility with health economics is partly a result of an isomorphism between consequentialism and economic theory in their approach to maximization.

Most people hold maximizing views of some strength, and this underlies the general belief that a healthcare system has a strong, but perhaps not overriding, obligation to allocate resources in order to get the largest benefit possible.

The most significant counterarguments to understanding distributive justice as the maximization of good outcomes are (a) that it is completely need independent, unless need is redefined as "possibility of benefiting," and (b) that maximization may in some cases be achieved by distributive decisions that take away resources from those who are a priori worst off and thus increase inequalities.

Prioritarianism

Prioritarianism is a recent revision of the consequentialist maximizing approach, aimed at dealing with some of the counterintuitive distributive effects of maximization. Prioritarians argue that when good consequences are assessed and added up, benefits to the worse off should count for more than comparable benefits to the better off. This will have the effect of strengthening the claims of those who are worse off and make it less likely that resources are taken away from them to benefit others. In the healthcare context, a prioritarian approach will thus lead to more resources being directed to those who are most ill than nonprioritarian maximization.

Equal Opportunity

A third approach to distributive justice argues that what is important is not equality in or maximization of outcomes but equality in initial opportunities or capabilities. If we distribute so that everyone has an equal starting point in relation to whatever resources are important for success in a given area, then we have distributed justly. This implies that the claims of those who are worst off in terms of opportunities or capabilities should be given priority. In the healthcare context, this would, for instance, imply that public health interventions aimed at socioeconomically deprived groups should be given priority; and this view also has significant implications for the distribution of resources for healthcare research.

The main counterargument against the equal opportunity approach is that it is often difficult to define who is worst off in a given situation because a person may be worst off on one parameter and not worst off on another. For instance, should priority be given to the claim of the poor person with a minor illness or the rich person with a major illness?

A further problem arises in the healthcare area because there are good reasons to believe that this is an area where it is impossible to create equality of opportunity. There are people with such severe disabilities or illnesses that there is no intervention that can improve their health to such a degree that they have equal opportunities with respect to health status.

The equal opportunities approach is very similar to an approach toward compensation for bad outcomes, including bad health outcomes that depend on a distinction between "brute luck" and "option luck." Brute luck refers to those outcomes that are not dependent on the choices of the person; it is, for instance, a matter of brute luck whether a person is born with a disability. Option luck refers to those outcomes that are dependent on a person's prior choices; it is, for instance, a matter of option luck if a smoker develops chronic obstructive lung disease. On the basis of this distinction, an argument can be made that persons should be compensated for large differences in brute luck, but that differences in option luck do not justify compensation or redistribution.

Procedural Approaches

It has long been recognized that there are situations where we know what the just outcome is but do not have any easy way of achieving it except by devising a procedure leading as close to the just outcome as possible. If X children are to share a birthday cake they should each get 1/X of the cake, but given the practical difficulties in cutting cakes, this is difficult to achieve. The procedural solution is to let one child cut the cake, knowing that he or she will be the last to pick a piece.

In healthcare it has recently been argued that the situation is even more complex. Not only do we not know how to bring about the just outcome (e.g., equal access to tertiary services if we believed that that was what justice required), there are many cases where we cannot fix the just outcome with any degree of precision. We may be able to identify clearly unjust distributions of resources but find it difficult to identify which of the remaining distributions is the most just. This argument has led many to shift focus from further elaboration of the details of the theories of distributive justice to procedural approaches that can ensure that our distributive decisions are (a) not clearly unjust and (b) legitimate to those who are affected. These developments have been linked with the more general developments of ideas concerning deliberative democracy.

A number of different procedural approaches have been developed, but all aim at ensuring that (a) all stakeholders have a voice, (b) all reasonable arguments are put on the table, and (c) the decision processes are transparent.

The currently most popular and well-researched procedural approach is the so-called accountability for reasonableness (or A4R) approach. It has four distinct components: publicity, relevance, appeals, and enforcement. In conjunction, these four components emphasize reason giving and create a process with successive opportunities for all interested parties to challenge priority decisions.

Publicity is a call for explicitness. *Relevance* entails a requirement for reasonableness in priority setting. That is, priority decisions must be made in accordance with reasons that stakeholders will agree are relevant and adequate. The *appeals* component is an institutional mechanism that provides patients with an opportunity to dispute and challenge decisions that have gone against them. Finally, *enforcement* entails public or voluntary regulation of the decision process to ensure that the three other components are maintained. Proper enforcement of the decisions that are made through agreement on fairness will ensure that reasoning is decisive in priority setting and not merely a theoretical exercise.

Søren Holm

See also Bioethics; Rationing

Further Readings

Daniels, N. (1985). *Just health care.* Cambridge, UK: Cambridge University Press.

Daniels, N. (2000). Accountability for reasonableness: Establishing fair process for priority setting is easier than agreeing on principles. *British Medical Journal, 321,* 1300–1301.

Nozick, R. (1977). *Anarchy, state and Utopia.* New York: Basic Books.

Rabinowicz, W. (2001). *Prioritarianism and uncertainty: On the interpersonal addition theorem and the priority view.* Retrieved August 14, 2008, from http://mora.rente.nhh.no/projects/EqualityExchange/ressurser/articles/rabinowicz2.pdf

Rawls, J. (1999). *A theory of justice* (Rev. ed.). Harvard, MA: Belknap Press.

Sen, A. (1992). *Inequality reexamined.* Oxford, UK: Clarendon Press.

Temkin, L. S. (1993). *Inequality.* Oxford, UK: Oxford University Press.

DISUTILITY

Where utility reflects the positive value of a health state to an individual (its desirability) and is expressed as the fraction of perfect health it entails, disutility reflects the complement of this fraction (its undesirability), 1 minus the utility. Thus, if a disability state is assigned a utility of .85, its disutility, relative to good health, is .15. Disutility is mostly used in comparative contexts, where states are compared relative to one another. In these cases, disutility is the difference in the average utility reported by persons with a given problem compared with those without the problem. An example is that of a treatment for menopausal symptoms that is 80% effective. If the utility for the health state "living with menopausal symptoms" is .6, a way to calculate utility with treatment is the following: The disutility of the remaining symptoms will be (1 − Effectiveness of treatment) × Disutility from symptoms = .20 × .40 = .08, and thus, the utility for "living with the remaining menopausal symptoms" will be 1 − .08 = .92.

Expected Utility Theory

The utility of a health state is a cardinal measure of the strength of an individual's preference for particular outcomes when faced with uncertainty, on a scale from 0 to 1, where 0 generally reflects *death* and 1 reflects *perfect health*. A distinction is usually made in the decision-making literature between utilities, or strengths of preferences under uncertainty, and values, strengths of preferences under certainty. This concept of utilities dates back to 1944, when John von Neumann and Oskar

Morgenstern developed a normative model for decision making under uncertainty—expected utility theory. This model calculates the utility that can be expected from each option in terms of the desirability of its outcomes and the probability with which they will occur. For most decisions in healthcare, outcomes may occur with a certain probability, and the decision problem is thus a problem of choice under uncertainty. Decision analysis is indeed firmly grounded in expected utility theory, and the most common use of utilities is in decision analyses. In decision analyses, the strategy of preference is calculated by combining the utilities of the outcomes with the probabilities that the outcomes will occur.

Anne M. Stiggelbout

See also Utility Assessment Techniques; Values

Further Readings

Franks, P., Hanmer, J., & Fryback, D. G. (2006). Relative disutilities of 47 risk factors and conditions assessed with seven preference-based health status measures in a national U.S. sample: Toward consistency in cost-effectiveness analyses. *Medical Care, 44,* 478–485.

Hunink, M., Glasziou, P., Siegel, J., Weeks, J., Pliskin, J., Elstein, A., et al. (2001). *Decision making in health and medicine. Integrating evidence and values.* Cambridge, UK: Cambridge University Press.

Morgenstern, O., & von Neumann, J. (2004). *Theory of games and economic behavior.* Princeton, NJ: Princeton University Press. (Original work published 1944)

DOMINANCE

In cost-effectiveness analyses, costs and effectiveness of different decision alternatives are estimated. They can then be presented in the two-dimensional cost-effectiveness plane (Figure 1).

A decision alternative A is called strongly dominated (or dominated) by a different alternative B if the costs and effectiveness of Alternative B are at least as favorable as those of Alternative A:

$$\text{Effect}_A \leq \text{Effect}_B \text{ and } \text{Cost}_A \geq \text{Cost}_B,$$

with strict inequality for either effectiveness or costs. In Figure 1, all alternatives in the light gray top-left area are strongly dominated by Alternative B.

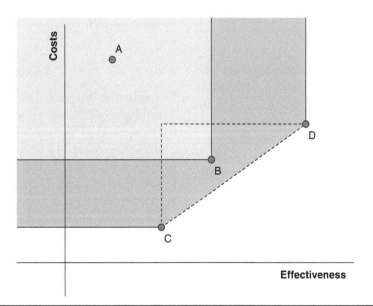

Figure 1   Cost-effectiveness plane

Note: The light gray area is (strongly) dominated by Alternative B. The dark gray area is weakly dominated by Alternatives C and D together.

Decision alternative A is called weakly dominated by two different alternatives C and D if Alternative A is strongly dominated by a mixture of those alternatives C and D:

$$Effect_A \leq \alpha \times Effect_C + (1 - \alpha) \times Effect_D$$

and

$$Cost_A \geq \alpha \times Cost_C + (1 - \alpha) \times Cost_D,$$
$$\text{for some } 0 \leq \alpha \leq 1,$$

with strict inequality for either effectiveness or costs. Mixtures can be thought of as if one alternative is applied to a fraction α of the patients and the other to a fraction $(1 - \alpha)$ of the patients. All such mixtures together form a straight line segment between alternatives C and D. In Figure 1, all alternatives in the dark gray area are weakly dominated by Alternatives C and D.

The main difference between strong dominance and weak dominance is illustrated by the dashed triangle in Figure 1. Decision alternatives in this triangle (like Alternative B) are not strongly dominated by Alternative C or by Alternative D, but they are weakly dominated by Alternatives C and D together. Strong and weak dominance are also referred to as strict and extended dominance.

Preference

Dominance is closely related to preference. Which alternative is preferred, in general, depends on the properties of the utility function on effectiveness and costs. In Figure 1, Alternative A has lower effectiveness and higher costs than Alternative B. Nevertheless, an individual is free to prefer A over B. However, it is more reasonable to assume that higher effectiveness and lower costs are preferred. The utility function $U(\cdot)$ is then strictly increasing in effectiveness and strictly decreasing in costs:

$$Effect_A < Effect_B \Rightarrow U(Effect_A) < U(Effect_B),$$

$$Cost_A > Cost_B \Rightarrow U(Cost_A) < U(Cost_B).$$

If Alternative A is strongly dominated by Alternative B, then this strict monotonicity of the utility function is sufficient for B to be preferred over A:

$$U(Effect_A, Cost_A) \leq U(Effect_B, Cost_A)$$
$$\leq U(Effect_B, Cost_B),$$

with strict inequality for either of the inequalities.

For weak dominance, strict monotonicity of the utility function is not sufficient to determine preference. For example, in Figure 1, Alternative B may be preferred over Alternatives C and D. A common stronger assumption is that the utility function is linear in costs and effectiveness—that is, the utility function equals the net benefit:

$$U(Effect, Cost) = WTP \times Effect - Cost,$$

where the positive WTP stands for the willingness to pay in monetary terms for one unit of effectiveness. For this linear utility function, a weakly dominated alternative cannot be preferred; if A is weakly dominated by Alternatives C and D, then A is less preferred than the hypothetical mixture (due to strong dominance) and the hypothetical mixture is not more preferred than the better of alternatives C and D (due to the linearity of the line segment and the utility function). This reasoning holds regardless of whether the decision alternatives C and D are actually divisible into mixtures. Therefore, weakly dominated alternatives are not the most preferred in standard cost-effectiveness analyses (i.e., with linear utility functions and positive WTP).

Example

Consider the numerical example presented in Table 1 and Figure 2. Alternative A is strongly dominated by B, C, and D because A has lower effectiveness and higher costs. Therefore, Alternative A is not preferred if the utility function is strictly increasing in effectiveness and decreasing in costs.

Alternative B is not strongly dominated by any of the alternatives. If the utility function were nonmonotone, then Alternative B could be the most preferred alternative. However, Alternative B is weakly dominated by Alternatives C and D, since it is above the line segment through C and D. The cost-effectiveness ratio of Alternative D compared with Alternative C is ($20,000 − $5,000)/ (.8 − .3) = $30,000 per QALY. For WTP below $30,000 per QALY, B may be preferred over D but B is not preferred over C. For WTP above

Table I   Example of cost-effectiveness analysis results, presented numerically

Decision alternative	A	B	C	D	E
Effectiveness (in QALYs)	.2	.4	.3	.8	.9
Costs	$25,000	$15,000	$5,000	$20,000	$35,000

Note: QALYs, quality-adjusted life years.

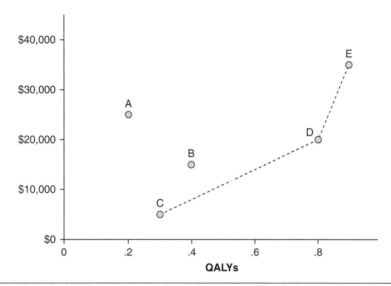

Figure 2   Example of cost-effectiveness analysis results, presented graphically

$30,000 per QALY, B may be preferred over C but B is not preferred over D. Regardless of the WTP, B is not preferred over both C and D. Therefore, Alternative B is not the most preferred alternative if the utility function is linear (with positive WTP per QALY).

Alternatives C, D, and E are neither strongly nor weakly dominated by any of the alternatives. Even if the utility function is linear, depending on the WTP, C, D, or E can be preferred. The cost-effectiveness ratios for Alternative C compared with D and for Alternative D compared with E are $30,000 and $150,000 per QALY, respectively. Alternative C is preferred for low WTP (up to $30,000 per QALY), Alternative B is preferred for intermediate WTP (between $30,000 and $150,000 per QALY), and Alternative C is preferred for high WTP (above $150,000 per QALY).

Wilbert van den Hout

See also Cost-Effectiveness Analysis; Economics, Health Economics; Net Monetary Benefit

Further Readings

Cantor, S. B. (1994). Cost-effectiveness analysis, extended dominance, and ethics: A quantitative assessment. *Medical Decision Making, 14,* 259–265.

Drummond, M. F., O'Brien, B. J., Stoddart, G. L., & Torrance, G. W. (1997). *Methods for the economic evaluation of health care programmes* (2nd ed.). New York: Oxford University Press.

Gold, M. R., Siegel, J. E., Russell, L. B., & Weinstein, M. C. (1996). *Cost-effectiveness in health and medicine.* New York: Oxford University Press.

Postma, M. J., de Vries, R., Welte, R., & Edmunds, W. J. (2008). Health economic methodology illustrated with recent work on chlamydia screening: The concept of extended dominance. *Sexually Transmitted Infections, 84,* 152–154.

DUAL-PROCESS THEORY

Dual-process theories of cognition (also referred to as "two-system" theories) posit two distinct systems of judgment operating in parallel. Dual-process theories have been described since 1975, with a variety of different names for the two processes. Since 2000, however, the two processes have been conventionally referred to as System 1 and System 2.

System 1 is an intuitive judgement system that shares many features with the perceptual system. It operates by tacitly encoding and retrieving associations between perceived cues in the environment. System 1 is fast, holistic, and automatic and underlies pattern recognition, prototypicality judgments, and heuristic processing. Because it is driven by associations acquired through experience, it is sensitive to the features of learning context and environmental exposure. It is also influenced by the emotional state of the judge and the emotional content of the judgment.

In contrast, System 2 is a rule-based system for forming judgments. It is slow, effortful, and analytic and applies rules in an emotionally neutral manner. When appropriate data are available, System 2 yields the most normatively rational reasoning, but because it is relatively difficult and demanding, it is easily disrupted by high cognitive load or time pressure. The figure, reproduced from the psychologist Daniel Kahneman's Nobel Prize lecture on dual-process theories, compares the attributes of the two judgmental systems and the perceptual system.

A key feature of dual-process theories is that System 1 and System 2 operate simultaneously and in parallel. Because System 1 is considerably faster, System 1 judgments typically emerge first and serve as additional inputs to System 2. If a System 1 judgment does not emerge, the judge must resort to System 2 alone; similarly, if a lack of time or cognitive resources curtails System 2, the judge must resort to System 1 alone.

The two systems can interact in several ways. When a System 1 judgment has been made, System 2 may endorse the judgment, may use the System 1 judgment as an anchor and adjust the judgment on the basis of other situational features, or may identify the System 1 judgment as incompatible with a subjectively valid rule and block it from overt expression. Because System 1 processing itself (as distinct from the judge's response) cannot be suppressed, judges often feel drawn to the System 1 judgment even when they recognize that it is incorrect.

Kahneman has illustrated this effect with the bat-and-ball problem: "A baseball bat and a ball together cost one dollar and 10 cents. The bat costs one dollar more than the ball. How much does the ball cost?" Most people who hear this problem initially conclude that the ball costs 10 cents, but

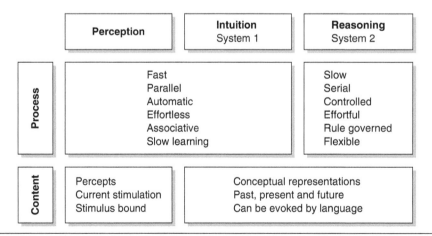

Figure 1   A comparison of the features of the human perceptual system with human judgment Systems 1 and 2

Source: Kahneman, D. (2003). Maps of bounded rationality: A perspective on intuitive judgment and choice. In T. Frangsmyr (Ed.), *Les Prix Nobel 2002* [The Nobel Prizes 2002]. Stockholm: Almqvist & Wiksell International. © The Nobel Foundation 2002. Reprinted with permission.

they realize, after a moment of reflection, that this (System 1) answer is incorrect and, in many cases, suppress the response in favor of the System 2 answer (5 cents), which emerges later.

Paul Slovic provides a more distressing example of the power of System 1 and the need for System 2 regulation. He reviews extensive research on willingness to provide life-saving interventions and argues that because the perceptual basis of System 1 is attuned to small changes at the margins, it can lead to increasing disregard for absolute numbers of lives saved. Saving a small number of lives is highly valued; saving 10,000 times as many lives (as in the case of preventing genocide), while more valuable, is intuitively treated as much less valuable than a factor of 10,000.

Dual-process theories posit System 1 as the source of heuristics in judgment; when the results of such heuristics produce normatively incorrect judgments, they are referred to as biases. However, Gerd Gigerenzer and colleagues have argued extensively for the adaptive nature of "fast and frugal" System 1 heuristics. Fuzzy-trace theory specifically argues that gist processing (a System 1 function) represents the apex of the development of reasoning.

Alan Schwartz

See also Bias; Fuzzy-Trace Theory; Heuristics; Intuition Versus Analysis; Judgment

Further Readings

Gigerenzer, G., Todd, P. M., & ABC Research Group. (2000). *Simple heuristics that make us smart.* Oxford, UK: Oxford University Press.

Hogarth, R. M. (2005). Deciding analytically or trusting your intuition? The advantages and disadvantages of analytic and intuitive thought. In T. Betsch & S. Haberstroh (Eds.), *The routines of decision making* (pp. 67–82). Mahwah, NJ: Lawrence Erlbaum.

Kahneman, D. (2003). Maps of bounded rationality: A perspective on intuitive judgment and choice. In T. Frangsmyr (Ed.), *Les Prix Nobel 2002* [The Nobel Prizes 2002] (pp. 449–489). Stockholm: Almqvist & Wiksell International.]

Slovic, P. (2007). "If I look at the mass I will never act": Psychic numbing and genocide. *Judgment and Decision Making, 2*(2), 79–95.

Stanovich, K. E., & West, R. F. (2000). Individual differences in reasoning: Implications for the rationality debate? *The Behavioral and Brain Sciences, 23*(5), 645–726.

DYNAMIC DECISION MAKING

Most real-life decisions occur in multiple stages—individuals experience a series of actions and their consequences over time. Medical decision making, in particular, often involves anticipating uncertain future consequences where subsequent decisions are contingent on (or constrained by) the outcomes of patients' earlier choices. There has been a great deal of research on the basic principles underlying single-stage decision making but very little work on multistage decisions. Decision field theory has begun to examine many of the principles underlying multistage decision making and could be used to inform real-life choices involving both uncertainty and multiple stages.

Decision Field Theory

Most psychological research focuses on static decisions in isolation—a single decision followed by a single outcome. Dynamic decisions involve a sequence of decisions in which the choices and outcomes available at a later stage depend on the choices and outcomes that occurred earlier. Decision field theory tries to quantify such multistage decisions. A typical study asks subjects to take an initial gamble, and then they are given the option of taking a second gamble; this process is repeated.

Subjects are instructed to make three kinds of decisions:

1. A *planned decision:* Before subjects begin, they are asked to predict what they will decide at the end of the decision-making task, contingent on both winning and losing the initial gambles.

2. A *final decision:* This is what the subjects actually decide once they have gone through to the end of the task.

3. An *isolated decision:* All the initial gambles are eliminated so that only the final gamble remains.

Subjects are then asked to make the same final decision as above but without the experience of going through the previous decision-making tasks.

The normative procedure for selecting a strategy for these three decisions involves three consistency principles: dynamic, consequential, and strategic. The first requires the decision maker to follow through with his or her plans to the end, the second requires the decision maker to focus solely on future events and final outcomes given the current information available, and the third is the conjunction of the first two.

Decision field theory predicts (and has found that) there will be

1. a difference between planned and final decisions—a violation of dynamic consistency, that is, the plan for action differs from the final choice taken;

2. *no* difference between isolated and final decisions—*no* violation of consequential consistency; and

3. a difference between planned and isolated decisions—a violation of strategic consistency.

Dynamic Inconsistency

Two types of dynamic inconsistencies can be found: (1) Subjects who planned to take the second gamble but then won the second gamble (i.e., experienced a gain) become risk-averse and reverse their original plan; that is, they now want to play it safe and keep their winnings, so they choose not to take the gamble. (2) Subjects who planned *not* to take the second gamble but then lost the second gamble (i.e., experienced a loss) become risk seeking and reverse their original plan; that is, they now want to recoup their losses, so they are willing to take the risk and gamble.

The explanation for this reversal of preference was a change in the reference point. The planned decision was made against a reference point of zero (i.e., nothing gained or lost yet), but the final decision was made by incorporating the outcome of the first gamble. Consequently, the reference point was shifted such that the gamble seemed more or less risky, as shown above.

An alternative explanation is that the planned decision was made in a "cold" or rational state, whereas the final decision was made during the actual decision-making task, when subjects were in a "hot" or emotional state. Therefore, the final decision may be based more on immediate hedonic and affective processes, leading subjects to make a different choice in the "heat of the moment" from what they had planned to do.

Consequential Consistency

The consequential consistency finding is supported by the goal-gradient hypothesis. This hypothesis comes from approach-avoidance theories, which state that a decision anticipated from a distance feels very different from the decision one experiences as one gets closer to actually having to make a choice. Therefore, the hypothesis argues that the decision maker faces identical consequences from the same distance in both the final- and the isolated-decision conditions and, therefore, the two choices should also be identical.

Multistage Medical Decision

An important multistage medical decision individuals commonly face today involves cancer screening tests. Prostate and breast cancer are the most commonly occurring cancers in U.S. men and women and the second leading cause of cancer deaths. However, both tests are surrounded by controversy.

Prostate-specific antigen (PSA) testing has led to both overdiagnosis of and unnecessary treatment for prostate cancer. It is estimated that 75% of early-stage prostate cancers detected through PSA testing would never have become clinically significant. Therefore, men may be exposed to unnecessary prostate cancer treatment and suffer from the side effects of impotence and incontinence needlessly. Even professional organizations disagree about whether PSA screening is more beneficial than harmful.

Increased mammography screening has quadrupled the diagnosis of ductal carcinoma in situ (DCIS). Neither the prognosis nor the treatment for DCIS is known, and it is not necessarily a precursor to invasive breast cancer. However, this diagnosis has led some young women to undergo prophylactic mastectomies that are potentially unnecessary in order to avoid developing cancer.

Therefore, the multistage decision individuals face for these screening tests is (a) whether to have prostate or breast cancer screening tests and, if so, when to have them done; (b) whether to undergo an invasive diagnostic procedure after a potentially false-positive test result; and (c) how to proceed if something is detected that may not lend itself to standard treatment options. A dynamic decision theory could be used to guide patients through this process.

Strategies for Success

According to dynamic decision theories, two tasks are crucial for success: goal setting and information collection. The most accomplished dynamic decision makers are able to integrate the goals of the decision-making task with the current state of the environment in order to identify tactics that have worked in analogous situations from their past. If no such situations exist, they are able to generate strategies using problem-solving techniques. Second, they systematically gather information relevant to achieving their goals. Third, they continually evaluate their advancement toward their goals.

Those who are less successful tend to shift from one goal to another or focus too narrowly on a single goal. To improve performance, dynamic decision theories suggest three strategies. First, constrain information processing. This may be accomplished by asking patients to focus on the next two or, at most, three goals rather than thinking about everything at once, which is the tendency of many newly diagnosed patients. Second, encourage a more focused information-gathering strategy, perhaps by pointing patients toward specific educational materials or online resources, as the nearly endless amount of medical information available both in print and online can quickly become overwhelming.

Finally, if patients do not have relevant past experiences to inform their decision making, introduce them to more experienced others from whom they can learn, such as former patients who have successfully completed their treatment. This may help patients envision what it is like to face the decisions they are contemplating and to experience the outcomes. By doing so, they may be better able to anticipate the "hot" or more emotional state of mind they are likely to be in as they get closer to making their treatment choice.

Julie Goldberg

See also Biases in Human Prediction; Decision Psychology; Decisions Faced by Patients: Primary Care; Gain/Loss Framing Effects; Gambles; Hedonic Prediction and Relativism; Managing Variability and Uncertainty; Preference Reversals; Prospect Theory; Risk Attitude; Value Functions in Domains of Gains and Losses

Further Readings

Barkan, R., & Busemeyer, J. R. (2003). Modeling dynamic inconsistency with a changing reference point. In "Time and decision" [Special issue]. *Journal of Behavioral Decision Making, 16*(4), 235–255.

Busemeyer, J. R., & Townsend, J. T. (1993). Decision field theory: A dynamic-cognitive approach to decision making in an uncertain environment. *Psychological Review, 100*(3), 432–459.

Busemeyer, J. R., Weg, E., Barkan, R., Li, X., & Ma, Z. (2000). Dynamic and consequential consistency of choices between paths of decision trees. *Journal of Experimental Psychology: General, 129*(4), 530–545.

Johnson, J., & Busemeyer, J. R. (2001). Multiple-stage decision-making: The effect of planning horizon length on dynamic consistency. *Theory and Decision, 51*(2–4), 217–246.

Roe, R. M., Busemeyer, J. R., & Townsend, J. T. (2001). Multialternative decision field theory: A dynamic connectionist model of decision making. *Psychological Review, 108*(2), 370–392.

DYNAMIC TREATMENT REGIMENS

A dynamic treatment regimen (DTR) is a sequence of individually tailored decision rules that specify whether, how, and when to alter the intensity, type, or delivery of treatment at critical decision points in the medical care process. DTRs operationalize sequential decision making with the aim of improving clinical practice. Ideally, DTRs realize this goal by flexibly tailoring treatments to patients when they need it most, thereby improving the efficacy and effectiveness of treatment and reducing inappropriate variance in treatment delivery. DTRs can be used to develop clinical guidelines, including clinical decision support systems. All the following are types of DTRs: (a) structured treatment interruptions in the HIV/AIDS literature; (b) clinical strategies, treatment strategies, or treatment algorithms in the psychiatric disorders literature; (c) adaptive therapy or multiple-treatment courses in the cancer literature; and (d) adaptive treatment strategies, stepped-care models, or continuing-care models in the alcohol and other substance abuse treatment literature. A variety of statistical methods exist to inform the development of DTRs.

Structure

A DTR consists of four key ingredients. The first ingredient is a *sequence of critical decision points* in the medical care process. These decision points may represent time in the form of patient visits to the clinic (first visit, second visit, and so on); or if critical decisions are to be made on a monthly basis, the decision points may represent calendar time in months since disease diagnosis. More generally, though, the sequence of critical decision points is not required to be aligned with a pre-specified set of discrete time points. For example, critical decision points may, instead, be defined by patient events, such as the point at which a patient fails to respond to prior treatment.

The second ingredient is a set of one or more *treatment options* at each critical decision point. Possible treatment options may be switch medication, augment medication, or continue medication; or there may be more complex options, such as any of the three-way combinations of treatment type (medication, physical therapy), treatment intensity (high, medium, low), and treatment delivery (specialty clinic, general clinic). The set of potential treatment options may differ at different decision points. For example, initially, the emphasis may be on treatment suitable for an acute episode of the illness, whereas subsequent decisions may involve options for intensifying or augmenting treatment for nonresponding patients or transitioning to lower-intensity treatments or monitoring for responding patients.

The third ingredient is a set of one or more *tailoring variables* at each critical decision point. The tailoring variables form the set of key measures that will determine subsequent treatment. For example, tailoring variables may include patient severity, number and type of comorbidities, side effects resulting from prior treatment, treatment preference, adherence to prior treatment, and, perhaps most important, response to prior treatment. Tailoring variables can also be summary measures over the full course of prior treatment; for example, subsequent treatment could depend on the rate of improvement in symptoms during prior treatment or the pattern of nonadherence to prior treatment. The set of tailoring variables may differ at different time points; for instance, history of comorbidities or genetic background may be used to choose from the options for initial treatment, while the choice of subsequent treatment might be based on response to the present treatment and the type of present treatment.

The final ingredient in a DTR is the specification of a *decision rule* at each of the critical decision points. For every patient and at each time point, the decision rule inputs values of the tailoring variables and outputs one or more recommended treatments from the set of treatment options. Importantly, the decision rules specify recommended treatment(s) for every feasible level of the tailoring variables. In the context of treatment for alcohol abuse, for example, a decision rule may state that as soon as the patient incurs 2 or more heavy drinking days following initiation of the medication, augment the medication with one of a set of cognitive behavioral therapies; otherwise, if the patient incurs less than 2 heavy drinking days during the 8 weeks following initiation of the medication, then keep the patient on medication and provide telephone disease monitoring.

The full set of decision rules over all of the critical decision points, taken together, constitutes one DTR. From the patient's point of view, a DTR is a sequence of treatments over time. This sequence of treatments is dynamic and patient specific because it is tailored in response to the patient's variable and evolving clinical status.

Clinical Settings

DTRs can be used to enhance clinical practice in any clinical setting in which sequential medical decision making is essential for the welfare of the patient. In settings in which treatment response is widely heterogeneous and/or patients are insufficiently responsive to any one treatment, clinicians must often consider a series of treatments to achieve a desired response. Furthermore, in settings in which relapse rates are high, treatment decisions during the acute phase of the disease are often followed by decisions concerning the best suitable treatment to prevent subsequent relapse. The treatment of many chronic disorders such as cardiovascular disease, HIV/AIDS, cancer, diabetes, epilepsy, obesity, substance abuse disorders, mental disorders, and behavioral disorders require these types of sequential decisions. Furthermore, since chronic disorders are often characterized by a waxing-and-waning course, it is important to reduce treatment burden by reducing treatment intensity whenever possible. DTRs are ideally suited for these settings because they can be designed to respond over time to the changing course of a patient's illness.

Development

Currently, DTRs are formulated using a combination of expert opinion, clinical experience, and biological/behavioral theory. Either by scientific consensus or by relying on more quantitative methods (e.g., meta-analyses), scientists using this approach rely on summarizing the results of separate randomized trials to inform their view about DTRs. This strategy does not involve research designs or data-analytic methods designed explicitly for the purpose of developing DTRs.

A variety of statistical methods currently exist that can be used to inform the development of DTRs. These methods can be used either with longitudinal data arising from specialized trials designed to inform their development or with existing longitudinal data sets. These tools are used in conjunction with clinical experience and biological/behavioral theory to arrive at recommended DTRs for implementation in clinical practice.

Basic Structure and Sources of Data

Data Structure

To be useful for developing a DTR, a data set must have both treatment measures and potential tailoring measures (or time-varying covariates)

observed at each of the critical decision points. In addition, the data set should have (possibly time varying) measures that define a clinically meaningful primary outcome measure. The choice of the primary outcome is crucial because the DTR will be developed explicitly to improve (or optimize) this outcome variable. In most cases, the primary outcome is a summary measure of response to treatment over time. For example, the outcome variable may be the percentage of time in remission over the full (dynamic) treatment course, or the outcome may involve a measure of functionality or may even be a composite measure involving cost and patient burden.

Existing Longitudinal Data

Longitudinal data sets having the characteristics described above are commonly collected as part of observational studies or can be extracted from large medical databases. In addition, longitudinal data sets of this type may arise from experimental studies. These include intervention studies that randomize patients to one of two (or more) single-shot treatments at baseline and follow them repeatedly over time, measuring the actual receipt of the assigned treatment and other treatments as well as a variety of other outcomes and time-varying covariates.

One of the primary challenges with using existing longitudinal data sets is the likely existence of unknown or unobserved, fixed or time-varying variables that affect both actual treatment receipt and the primary outcome. These variables confound (bias) the comparisons of different treatment regimens and present an important obstacle in data analyses aimed at informing the development of DTRs.

Sequential Multiple-Assignment Randomized Trials

Sequential multiple-assignment randomized trials (SMARTs) have been proposed explicitly for the purpose of developing new DTRs or refining already established ones. The key feature of a SMART is that patients are randomized multiple times over the course of the trial; that is, they are randomized at each critical decision point among feasible treatment options. Randomizing patients multiple times in this fashion ensures comparability among patients assigned to different treatment options at each time point, thereby resolving the problem of confounding described earlier.

Statistical Methods

A variety of statistical models and methods are currently available that allow researchers to compare the effectiveness of different decision rules, examine the effect of different timing and sequences of treatments, and discover the important tailoring measures for use in a DTR. These methods can be used with data arising from a SMART or with existing longitudinal data sets. They include the marginal mean model and the structural nested mean model, and adaptations of them; Bayesian methods; methods to discover DTRs connected with time-to-event outcomes; and methods designed explicitly for discovering optimal DTRs. Recently, as well, methods and models from computer science, called *reinforcement learning algorithms*, are emerging as viable options for informing the development of DTRs.

Susan A. Murphy and Daniel Almirall

See also Decision Rules; Dynamic Decision Making; Evaluating and Integrating Research Into Clinical Practice; Evidence-Based Medicine; Expert Systems

Further Readings

Gaweda, A. E., Muezzinoglu, M. K., Aronoff, G. R., Jacobs, A. A., Zurada, J. M., & Brier, M. E. (2005). Individualization of pharmacological anemia management using reinforcement learning. *Neural Networks, 18*, 826–834.

Lavori, P. W., & Dawson, R. (2004). Dynamic treatment regimens: Practical design considerations. *Clinical Trials, 1*, 9–20.

Lunceford, J., Davidian, M., & Tsiatis, A. A. (2002). Estimation of the survival distribution of treatment regimens in two-stage randomization designs in clinical trials. *Biometrics, 58*, 48–57.

Murphy, S. A. (2003). Optimal dynamic treatment regimens. *Journal of the Royal Statistical Society, Series B, 65*(2), 331–366.

Murphy, S. A. (2005). An experimental design for the development of adaptive treatment strategies. *Statistics in Medicine, 24*, 1455–1481.

Pineau, J., Bellemare, M. G., Rush, A. J., Ghizaru, A., & Murphy, S. A. (2006). Constructing evidence-based treatment strategies using methods from computer science. *Drug and Alcohol Dependence, 88*, S2, S52–S60.

Robins, J. M. (2004). Optimal structural nested models for optimal sequential decisions. In D. Y. Lin & P. Haegerty (Eds.), *Proceedings of the 2nd Seattle symposium on biostatistics* (pp. 189–326). New York: Springer-Verlag.

Thall, P. F., Logothetis, C., Pagliaro, L. C., Wen, S., Brown, M. A., Williams, D., et al. (2007). Adaptive therapy for androgen-independent prostate cancer: A randomized selection trial of four regimens. *Journal of the National Cancer Institute, 99*, 1613–1622.

Thall, P. F., Millikan, R. E., & Sung, H. G. (2000). Evaluating multiple treatment courses in clinical trials. *Statistics in Medicine, 19*, 1011–1028.

Wahed, A. S., & Tsiatis, A. A. (2004). Optimal estimator for the survival distribution and related quantities for treatment policies in two-stage randomization designs in clinical trials. *Biometrics, 60*, 124–133.

E

ECONOMICS, HEALTH ECONOMICS

Health economics investigates how scarce resources are used, or should be used, to satisfy health wants. Although in high-income countries 10% or more of wealth is spent on healthcare, resources are still scarce compared with the potentially unlimited want for physical, psychological, and social health.

The health market is not a competitive market in which price setting resolves differences between demand and supply, among others because insurance interferes with the relation between price and demand; new healthcare providers are often not free to enter the market and patients do not have perfect information about their needs. As a result, active decision making may be necessary to prevent supply of inefficient healthcare. Health economics intends to provide information on the economic aspect of such decision making.

Health economics includes several fields such as organization, management, finance, and insurance. Most relevant for medical decision making is the field of economic evaluation, which investigates whether costs of different medical decisions are justified by the value of associated effectiveness. Economic evaluation is a component of the wider research field of health technology assessment, which also includes evaluation of ethical, social, and legal aspects. It has its roots in evidence-based medicine, in trying to derive conclusions from explicit and judicious use of the best available evidence.

Types of Analysis

Economic evaluation in healthcare requires that costs and effectiveness of interventions are somehow measured and analyzed. Different types of analysis can be distinguished, depending on how costs are related to effectiveness. Two types of cost analysis that do not compare decision alternatives are cost price analysis and cost of illness analysis. Cost price analyses estimate the costs of a particular intervention. They are an essential starting point for economic evaluations, but by themselves they are often only part of the picture. Cost of illness analyses estimate the costs associated with a particular illness or condition, without comparing decision alternatives. As a result, they are largely irrelevant to decision making: How high costs are is not necessarily linked to whether these costs are justified.

For medical decision making, analyses that explicitly compare decision alternatives are more relevant: cost-minimization analysis (CMA), cost-consequence analysis (CCA), cost-benefit analysis (CBA), cost-effectiveness analysis (CEA), and cost-utility analysis (CUA). These types of analyses differ in how costs are compared with effectiveness. CMA only looks at which alternative is the least expensive, without considering the effectiveness. It is therefore only applicable when effectiveness is known to be equal for all alternatives, for example, when different ways to provide the same care are compared. CCA provides a list of both cost and effectiveness outcomes, but without explicitly combining these outcomes: The overall judgment is left to the decision maker. CBA, CEA, and CUA do explicitly combine costs and effectiveness, to suggest which decision alternative provides best value for the money. They differ in how effectiveness is quantified. CBA measures effectiveness by its monetary value, for example, by asking patients how much they would be willing to pay for effectiveness. Converting effectiveness to money is problematic, but does facilitate a direct assessment of whether the value of effectiveness exceeds the costs. CEA measures effectiveness in physical units, rendering cost-effectiveness ratios such as the costs per identified cancer patient, costs per prevented death, or costs per gained life year. CEAs can be used to compare the relative efficiency of interventions with the same goal, but are not useful for a more general framework for economic assessment across the wide field of healthcare. For that purpose, CUAs are advocated. CUAs are a special case of CEAs, measuring effectiveness in terms of quality-adjusted life years (QALYs). QALYs measure the two general goals of healthcare: to prolong life and to improve life.

Measuring Value of Effectiveness

Effectiveness of medical interventions can be measured in many ways. Intermediary outcome measures, such as cholesterol levels, bone density, and cancer recurrence, are relatively easy to measure and are essential to understanding how interventions work. However, to assess whether an intervention actually helps improve patients' health requires measures for disease burden, which includes both survival and quality of life. In addition, economic evaluation requires measuring the *value* of improving survival and quality of life.

Key to measuring value in economic evaluations is the concept of utility, which is the value of quality of life at a particular moment in time. Utility is measured on a scale anchored at 0 (*as bad as death*) and 1 (*perfect health*). It may even be less than 0 (for quality of life worse than being dead). Since utility tries to aggregate the multifaceted concept of health into a single index, measuring utility is not without problems. The simplest approach is to ask respondents to indicate the overall value of their quality of life on a visual analog scale (Figure 1). Other, more complicated, utility assessment techniques (such as the time trade-off and the standard gamble) are considered

more valid ways to directly assess utility, because they value quality of life compared with some other commodity (lifetime and mortality risk, respectively). These direct methods can be used to assess utility from the patients' perspective. Indirect utility measures, such as the EQ5D, HUI, and SF6D, ask the respondents not to value their health but to describe their health on a classification system. An existing formula is then used to assign a utility value to that description. Such formulae reflect the general public's valuation of the health described by the patient, which is preferred for economic evaluations from a societal perspective.

Life expectancy has long been an accepted measure of health. QALYs combine life expectancy with utility, to obtain a single generic value measure for both survival and quality of life. QALYs measure the value of a patient's health over a period of time by the product of the length of that period and the average utility during that period. This is equivalent to measuring the area under the utility curve. This way, both prolonged life and improved quality of life lead to higher QALYs. Conceptually, QALYs are very similar to DALYs (disability-adjusted life years) and Q-TWiST (quality-adjusted time without symptoms or toxicity).

As a schematic example of QALYs, consider the course of life shown in Figure 2. This person had depression from age 20 to age 40, contracted cancer at age 74, and died at age 80. The depression led to an average 25% utility loss over a 20-year period, which corresponds to a loss of 5 QALYs. The cancer period of 6 years has an associated QALY loss of 3 QALYs. Therefore, adjusted for quality of life, the 80 life years correspond to 72 QALYs. Measured in terms of QALYs, postponing cancer and death by 2 years would gain 2 QALYs. Reducing the severity of depression by 50% would gain 2.5 QALYs.

Measuring Costs

In economic evaluation, costs represent the monetary value of the investments that are associated with a particular medical decision. An important first step is to determine the relevant perspective of the cost evaluation, which can be the healthcare perspective, the societal perspective (including productivity and patient costs), or a particular institution (such as a hospital or insurer). The perspective determines not only which cost categories should

Perfect health is a state of complete physical, mental, and social well-being. Please indicate on the line below how good or bad your health was in the past week. Mark the appropriate point on the line with a cross, somewhere between 0 (as bad as dead) and 100 (perfect health).

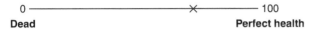

0 ————————————✕——————— 100
Dead   **Perfect health**

Figure I   Visual analog scale (indicating a 70% utility)

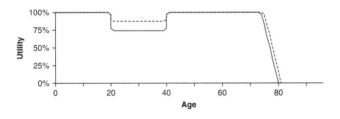

Figure 2   A schematic example of utility throughout life

be included but also how they should be valued. In the end, it is the differences in costs between the decision alternatives that need to be estimated, so all cost categories that can be expected to show an appreciable cost difference should be measured.

An essential part of a cost evaluation is usually the costs of a primary intervention. For this intervention, a detailed cost price analyses should be performed, including costs of personnel, equipment, materials, housing, and overhead. For other cost categories, standard prices or cost estimates from the literature can be used. For evaluations from an institutional perspective, charges may be relevant, but it should be realized that charges are not necessarily good approximations of costs. For example, costs of radiotherapy are partly proportional to the number of sessions and partly fixed per treatment, whereas charges for radiotherapy are often either fixed per session or fixed per treatment. When the number of sessions per treatment is changed, then estimating costs from charges per session or from charges per treatment will, respectively, overestimate and underestimate the impact on costs.

For many types of costs, costs can be distinguished as the product of volumes and prices. Volumes, such as the number of GP (general practitioner) visits or days absent from work, are more generalizable to other settings than costs. Patients can be asked to report volumes, using diaries, questionnaires, or interviews. They are aware of all the care they receive

but may have difficulty in accurately remembering less salient types of care. Providers of care can rely on the accuracy of information systems but can only report on care that they themselves are involved in.

Study Designs

Typically, two types of study designs are used for economic evaluations. On the one hand, there is research measuring costs and effectiveness in one single patient population. On the other hand, there are modeling studies, aggregating data from different sources.

In patient research, data should ideally originate from research in which patients are first selected and then randomly allocated to the different decision alternatives. This procedure ensures that the decision alternatives are all applied to the relevant patient population, without selection bias. Measuring costs and effectiveness in a single patient population is important to provide internal validity of the research. For external validity, it is important to use a pragmatic design with conditions that are close to those in practice, in how treatments are provided and to which patients. Typical for pragmatic trials is that it is more relevant to study whether and how much a treatment helps than why.

For many reasons, performing patient research to compare decision alternatives may not be feasible. The number of alternatives may be too large (e.g., when evaluating follow-up strategies), the differences between alternatives may be too small (to be demonstrated with the number of patients available), one of the decision alternatives may be generally considered unethical (obstructing new research), or the time to make a decision may be too limited (more limited than the duration of patient follow-up). In such situations, mathematical models may help evaluate decision alternatives and to aggregate effectiveness and cost data, obtained from different sources. Models can have varying degrees of detail, ranging from aggregate epidemiological models to patient-level models for day-to-day disease progression, and can be evaluated with techniques ranging from spreadsheet calculations and regression models to microsimulation. The use of models allows for sensitivity analysis to see how model parameters influence the conclusions, in order to validate the model's reliability for supporting decision making.

Cost-Effectiveness Analysis

Once costs and effects of different decision alternatives have been determined, CEA is used to decide which decision is optimal. CEA is intrinsically two-dimensional. When comparing two decision alternatives, one option is clearly preferred over the other alternative if it has lower costs and better effectiveness. The decision becomes difficult when one option is preferred based on better effectiveness and the other is preferred based on lower costs. In that case, a trade-off needs to be made between costs and effectiveness, to decide whether the more expensive decision alternative is justified by its better effectiveness.

Because of their two-dimensional nature, cost-effectiveness results are best presented graphically. Figure 3 shows costs and effectiveness for five different decision alternatives. Alternative A is said to be (strongly) dominated by Alternatives B, C, and D, because A has higher costs and lower effectiveness. As a result, Alternative A will not be the optimal decision, at least with respect to the economic aspect.

Alternative B is not dominated by any of the other alternatives, but it is dominated by a mixture of Alternatives C and D. This type of dominance is called weak, or extended, dominance. If Alternatives C and D were both applied to half of the patient population, then overall effectiveness and costs would be $(.3 + .8)/2 = .55$ and

($5,000 + $20,000)/2 = $12,500. Alternative B is (strongly) dominated by this 50:50 mixture of Alternatives C and D. The straight line CD between Alternatives C and D depicts the results that would be obtained by all possible mixtures of Alternatives C and D. The lines CD and DE together form the so-called efficient frontier. All alternatives above or to the left of this frontier are strongly or weakly dominated. All possible optimal alternatives are on the efficient frontier.

Which alternative on the efficient frontier is optimal depends on how much one is willing to pay to improve effectiveness. Cost-effectiveness should always be considered incrementally, that is, compared with the next best alternative. Compared with Alternative C, Alternative D provides .5 additional units of effectiveness and $15,000 additional costs, with a cost-effectiveness ratio of $15,000/.5 = $30,000 per unit. Similarly, the cost-effectiveness ratio comparing Alternatives D and E is $30,000/.1 = $300,000 per unit. The improvement by Alternative E is 10 times more expensive than the improvement by Alternative D, but without specifying the effectiveness measure, it is impossible to say which alternative is optimal. If effectiveness measures prevented mortality, then $300,000 per prevented death is likely to be acceptable and Alternative E would be optimal. If effectiveness measures prevented days with the flu, then $30,000 per day is unlikely to be acceptable and Alternative C would be optimal.

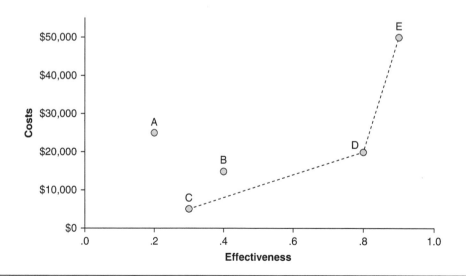

Figure 3   Cost-effectiveness plane

The economic aspect of a decision is rarely the only relevant aspect for decision making. Therefore, no strict thresholds exist for how much improved effectiveness is allowed to cost. Nevertheless, for effectiveness measured in terms of QALYs, there is some consensus on the rule of thumb that costs are definitely acceptable below $20,000 per QALY, are acceptable up to $50,000 per QALY, and are possibly acceptable up to $100,000 per QALY. According to this rule, Alternative D would be optimal: It provides good value for the money compared with Alternative C, and the costs of Alternative E would be too high.

Wilbert van den Hout

See also Cost-Effectiveness Analysis; Disability-Adjusted Life Years (DALYs); Evidence-Based Medicine; Marginal or Incremental Analysis, Cost-Effectiveness Ratio; Quality-Adjusted Life Years (QALYs); Quality-Adjusted Time Without Symptoms or Toxicity (Q-TWiST); Randomized Clinical Trials; Utility Assessment Techniques

Further Readings

Briggs, A., Sculpher, M., & Claxton, K. (2006). *Decision modelling for health economic evaluation*. New York: Oxford University Press.

Drummond, M. F., O'Brien, B. J., Stoddart, G. L., & Torrance, G. W. (1997). *Methods for the economic evaluation of health care programmes* (2nd ed.). New York: Oxford University Press.

Gold, M. R., Siegel, J. E., Russell, L. B., & Weinstein, M. C. (1996). *Cost-effectiveness in health and medicine*. New York: Oxford University Press.

EDITING, SEGREGATION OF PROSPECTS

In medical decision making, a prospect can be a medical treatment that will yield different outcomes with different probabilities. When patients are offered multiple treatment options, they will have to make a decision and follow one treatment that they think is the best. This selection process includes editing and segregation of the different prospects. A prospect $(x_1, p_1; \ldots; x_n p_n)$ is a contract

that yields outcome x_i with probability p_i, where $p_1 + p_2 + \ldots + p_n = 1$. To simplify this notation, we omit null outcomes and use (x, p) to denote the prospect $(x, p; 0, 1 - p)$, which yields x with probability p and 0 with probability $1 - p$. The riskless prospect that yields x with certainty is denoted by (x).

Within prospect theory, there are two distinct phases in the decision-making process: an early phase of editing and a subsequent phase of evaluation. The editing phase consists of a preliminary analysis and process of the offered prospects, which often yields a simpler representation of these prospects. In the second phase, the edited prospects are evaluated, and the prospect of highest value is chosen.

The objective of the editing phase is to organize and reformulate the options so as to simplify subsequent evaluation and choice. Editing is a mental process that transforms the probabilities of the various prospects. In medical decision making, the patient will edit the prospect of every treatment and then segregate the obvious undesirable treatments from the others according to the preliminary results from the editing phase.

Editing can be divided into six separate phases: (1) coding, (2) combination, (3) segregation, (4) cancellation, (5) simplification, and (6) detection of dominance.

Coding

Patients normally perceive the treatment outcomes as gains and losses, rather than as final states of health or life quality. This coding process will primarily rely on the choice of reference point. The reference point usually corresponds to the patients' current health level, in which case gains and losses can be interpreted as improvement or deterioration of their current health level. For example, consider a percentage as an indicator of people's health level, with 100% as *healthy* and 0% as *dead*. Also, consider the case of two patients, with health levels of 20% and 70%, respectively. Both patients are offered a treatment that provides an 80% chance of achieving an 80% health level and a 20% chance of decreasing to a 10% health level (.8, .8; .1, .2). Although the treatment is the same, the two patients would code this prospect differently. The first patient (current health level of 20%) will regard this as a good, acceptable gain choice, as his reference level is low and this treatment will increase his health level remarkably with a high probability. However, the second patient (current health level of 70%) would code this as a losing choice because she has a relatively high reference point. Therefore, she can increase her health level only trivially, while facing a 20% probability of losing most of her health.

In real medical decision-making cases, patients' reference points are usually influenced and shifted because of their expectation of the treatment, which comes from the prediagnosis, and their adaptation to the prognosis, which will also change their coding results over time.

Combination

Prospects can sometimes be simplified by combining the probabilities associated with identical outcomes. For example, a single treatment will result in four health outcomes with probabilities .1, .2, .3, and .4. The four health outcomes result in a life expectancy of 5, 10, 5, and 10 years, respectively. The patients will then combine the prospect into simply 5 years of life expectancy with probability .4 and 10 years of life expectancy with probability .6 (5, .4; 10, .6).

Segregation

Some prospects contain a riskless component along with an uncertain component. Patients can mentally segregate the risky part and simplify the decision making by addressing only the risky part. For example, a treatment has only two outcomes: (1) increase in life expectancy to 20 years with a probability of .3 and (2) increase in life expectancy to 30 years with a probability of .7. This can be naturally decomposed into a sure gain of 20 years of life expectancy and a risky prospect of 10 years of life expectancy with probability of .7 (10, .7).

Cancellation

Most patients tend to discard or exclude some components that are shared by the offered prospects. They rely on the cancellation of the common parts of the two prospects to help them make decisions. For example, consider two treatments. Both of them have a probability of success of .25. After the treatment is successful, Treatment A has an 80% chance of increasing life expectancy by 30 years (30, .8) while Treatment B has a 100% chance of increasing life expectancy by 20 years (20, 1.0). When facing this choice, most patients will ignore the precondition that both treatments have a 25% success rate, which is shared by both prospects. After they edit the two prospects, most of the patients will choose Treatment B. Interestingly, however, if we edit the prospects differently and apply the precondition, it will be a choice between (30, .20) and (20, .25), in which case most patients will choose Treatment A.

Simplification

This refers to the simplification of prospects by rounding probabilities or outcomes. For example, the prospect (101, .49) is likely to be recoded as an even chance to achieve 100.

Detection of Dominance

Many prospects may be dominated by the others. This can be mentally detected so that the dominated prospects will be segregated from the potential choices of patients. For example, Treatment A will achieve 10 years of life expectancy with a probability of .3 and 20 years of life expectancy with a probability of .7 (10, .3; 20, .7). Treatment B will achieve 8 years of life expectancy with a probability of .5 and 15 years of life expectancy with a probability of .5 (8, .5; 15, .5). It is obvious to the decision maker that Treatment A dominates Treatment B. Therefore, B is discarded without any further consideration.

One thing that needs to be stressed is that the editing process will vary between people, as well as within a single decision maker. The process is dynamic and highly dependent on the context of the problem, thus producing different results.

After editing the prospects, people will form a mental representation of all the existing prospects, which will segregate the prospects that they think are undesirable from the prospects that they would like to further evaluate. This editing and segregation phase simplifies the process of decision making and preclude some prospects so that the decision makers will reach their decision much more easily.

Lesley Strawderman and Yunchen Huang

See also Expected Utility Theory; Probability; Prospect
Theory

Further Readings

Emma, B. R., Kevin, P. W., & Kevin, A. S. (2005). Can
prospect theory explain risk-seeking behavior by
terminally ill patients? *Medical Decision Making, 25,*
609–613.

Jonathan, R. T., & Leslie, A. L. (1999). Health value and
prospect theory. *Medical Decision Making, 19,*
344–352.

Kahneman, D., & Tversky, A. (1979). Prospect theory:
An analysis of decision under risk. *Econometrica, 47,*
263–291.

EFFECT SIZE

In statistics, an effect size is a measure of the magnitude of a treatment effect. It is an indicator of how important an obtained effect is. Unlike statistical significance tests, effect size does not depend on the sample size of an underlying study. It is helpful to report the effect size, not just the statistical significance, when assessing the effectiveness of a specific intervention in medical studies as well as studies in other sciences. It has been also widely used in meta-analysis, which combines and compares estimates from different but relevant studies.

In medical studies, such as comparison of a new treatment with other traditional ones, the following question is often asked: How well does the new treatment work? In answering this question, the researchers are actually trying to quantify the difference between the effect of the new treatment and those of the traditional ones. Similar things happen in social studies and studies in educational and behavioral sciences. Effect size is a simple way of answering the question, and it has many advantages over the use of tests of statistical significance alone. Effect size measures directly the size of the difference rather than confounding this with the sample size of the study. It is easy to calculate and to interpret, and it can be applied to any measured outcome of medical, social, and educational sciences to quantify the effectiveness of a particular intervention in comparison with others.

Effect Size for Two Independent Groups With Continuous Outcomes

Let us consider comparing the outcome of two groups, the experimental group (the one for which a new treatment is going to be applied) and the control group (the one for which a traditional treatment is going to be applied). The outcome of the study is a kind of continuous measurement. The effect size in such a case is defined as the standardized difference in means between the two groups. In other words,

$$\text{Effect size} = \frac{[\text{Mean of experimental group}] - [\text{Mean of control group}]}{\text{Standard deviation}}.$$

It is very natural to take the difference of two group means when comparing the two groups of measurements. The standard deviation in the denominator, which is a measure of the spread of a set of values, is to standardize this difference. The same value of difference may represent totally different meanings when the standard deviations are different. It could be explained as a huge difference if the standard deviation is small, such that the two groups of values are completely separated; whereas if the corresponding standard deviation is large, the two sets of values might be well overlapped and the same value of difference might mean just nothing. The difference in means is standardized when it is divided by the standard deviation. In practice, however, the standard deviation is not known. It can be estimated either from the control group or from a pooled value of both groups.

The above-defined effect size is exactly equivalent to the z score of a standard normal distribution. For example, an effect size of 1 means that the average of the experimental group is 1 standard deviation higher than that of the control group. With the assistance of a graph of standard normal distribution curve, one can observe that the average of the experimental group, which is 1 standard deviation higher than that of the control group, is indeed the 84th percentile of the control group. In other words, 84% of the measurements of the control group are below the average of the experimental group. The value of 84% is calculated from the standard normal distribution as the probability that the standard normal random variable is less than or equal to 1. In case the effect size takes different values, the underlying effect size will replace the value 1 in the calculation. Another percentage rather than 84% will be obtained correspondingly. This provides an idea of how the two groups overlap with each other.

Effect Size for Experiments With Dichotomous Outcomes

Effect size can be defined differently within different settings of the studies. Another commonly used effect size in medical studies is the odds ratio. When the experimental outcome is dichotomous—for instance, success versus failure, or survival versus death, the comparison of a new treatment with a control experiment can be conducted based on the odds ratio. If success and failure are the only two possible outcomes, the odds of success is defined as the ratio of the probability of a success to that of a failure. For each group, an odds can be calculated that equals the ratio of the number of successes to the number of failures in the group. The odds ratio is then defined as the ratio of the two odds. Let $n_{S,exp}$ denote the number of successes in the experimental group, $n_{F,exp}$ the number of failures. Let $n_{S,con}$ and $n_{F,con}$ denote the numbers of successes and failures in the control group, separately, then the odds ratio can be calculated as

$$OR = \frac{ODDS_{experimental}}{ODDS_{control}} = \frac{n_{S,exp}/n_{F,exp}}{n_{S,con}/n_{F,con}}.$$

If the treatment effect is remarkable, the odds ratio should be much greater than 1. Otherwise, it should be very close to 1.

Examples

Example 1

Suppose that there was a study conducted to investigate the weekly weight gain of 3-month-old infants fed with different formulae. There were 20 infants randomly assigned to Group A and 30 infants assigned to Group B. The infants in Groups A and B were fed with Formulae A and B, separately. Formula B is newly developed. The infants were followed up for 4 weeks, and their individual average weekly weight gains (oz.) were recorded as

Group A:

10.41 10.38 9.16 10.01 11.07 10.47 10.18 9.59 8.77 9.75 8.37 8.95 10.27 9.70 11.61 9.43 8.36 10.23 10.23 9.69

Group B:

13.13 13.88 14.04 10.48 13.06 10.13 11.49 11.03 10.17 10.71 11.05 12.42 13.03 11.67 11.50 11.06 10.86 12.26 11.95 13.49 11.18 13.43 11.91 13.43 13.53 12.58 12.02 11.43 11.65 12.62

The mean of Group A is $\mu_A = 9.83$ oz. The mean of Group B is $\mu_B = 12.04$ oz. Group A has standard deviation $\sigma_A = .84$. Group B has standard deviation $\sigma_B = 1.13$. The pooled standard deviation of both groups is

$$\sigma_{pooled} = \sqrt{\frac{(n_A - 1)\sigma_A^2 + (n_B - 1)\sigma_B^2}{(n_A + n_B - 2)}}$$

$$= \sqrt{\frac{(20 - 1)(.84)^2 + (30 - 1)(1.13)^2}{20 + 30 - 2}} = 1.03.$$

The effect size is then

$$ES = \frac{\mu_B - \mu_A}{\sigma_{pooled}} = \frac{12.04 - 9.83}{1.03} = 2.15.$$

If we treat Group B as the experimental group and Group A as the control group, the effect size of this treatment (Formula B) is 2.15. Looking at the standard normal distribution table, the value 2.15 corresponds to a probability of .9842. This tells us that about 98% or 19 of the 20 values observed from Group A are below the mean of Group B. This is a big effect size.

Example 2

Suppose that there was a medical study investigating the effect of a newly developed medicine. There were 100 patients assigned to a group where the new treatment (medicine) was applied, and 80 were assigned to the control group, where the placebo was applied. Within 2 weeks of this experiment, 80 patients from the experimental group and 45 patients from the control (placebo) group had been cured.

$$OR = \frac{ODDS_{experimental}}{ODDS_{control}} = \frac{80/20}{45/35} = 3.11.$$

This effect size is much greater than 1. It tells us that the patients assigned to the experimental group have a much better chance to be cured, or that the new medicine is very effective.

Alternative Measures of Effect Size

A number of statistics were proposed as alternative measures of effect size, other than the standardized mean difference and odds ratio. In studies that employ linear statistical models to analyze the experimental outcome, the effect size can be defined as the square of the correlation coefficient of the two involved variables, denoted by R^2. This measure is the proportion of variance in one variable accounted for by the other. It can extend automatically to the case of multiple regression models.

It can be shown that the effect size measured by standardized mean difference is sensitive to the assumption of normality of data. For this reason, many robust alternatives were suggested. Peter Tymms and colleagues proposed a method for calculating effect sizes within multilevel models. José Cortina and Hossein Nouri discussed the effect sizes in analysis of covariance designs and repeated measures designs. To understand different effect size measures under different models, the monograph of Robert Grissom and John Kim gives a comprehensive discussion on effect sizes.

Xiao-Feng Wang and Zhaozhi Fan

See also Meta-Analysis and Literature Review; Odds and Odds Ratio, Risk Ratio; Sample Size and Power; Statistical Testing: Overview

Further Readings

Bausell, R. B., & Li, Y. F. (2002). *Power analysis for experimental research: A practical guide for the biological, medical and social sciences*. New York: Cambridge University Press.

Cliff, N. (1993). Dominance statistics: Ordinal analyses to answer ordinal questions. *Psychological Bulletin, 114*(3), 494–509.

Cortina, J. M., & Nouri, H. (2000). *Effect size for ANOVA designs*. Thousand Oaks, CA: Sage.

Grissom, R. J., & Kim, J. J. (2005). *Effect sizes for research: A broad practical approach*. New York: Lawrence Erlbaum.

Murphy, K. R., & Myors, B. (2004). *Statistical power analysis*. Mahwah, NJ: Lawrence Erlbaum.

Rubin, D. B. (1992). Meta-analysis: Literature synthesis or effect-size surface estimation. *Journal of Educational Statistics, 17*(4), 363–374.

Tymms, P., Merrell, C., & Henderson, B. (1997). The first year at school: A quantitative investigation of the attainment and progress of pupils. *Educational Research and Evaluation, 3*(2), 101–118.

EFFICACY VERSUS EFFECTIVENESS

The terms *efficacy* and *effectiveness* refer to different concepts and are not interchangeable. In general, efficacy refers to whether an intervention works under ideal conditions for a specific outcome. Effectiveness refers to a broader view of the usefulness of an intervention in the routine care of patients in the day-to-day practice of medicine. Efficacy is measured using controlled clinical trials, using specific outcome measures, such as prespecified changes in rating scales or laboratory parameters. Examples of efficacy studies are medication registration trials testing drug versus placebo. Effectiveness is measured by a variety of methods, including synthesis of efficacy and tolerability clinical trial data, clinical trials that incorporate broad outcomes such as quality of life, longitudinal prospective naturalistic studies, and retrospective studies using large-scale clinical, pharmacy, and administrative databases. Examples of effectiveness studies are studies examining all-cause discontinuation in the use of antipsychotics for the treatment of schizophrenia.

Efficacy

Efficacy refers to whether an intervention works under ideal conditions for a specific outcome. Regulatory agencies such as the U.S. Food and Drug Administration require that medications demonstrate efficacy prior to their approval for commercialization. These premarketing studies are referred to as drug registration trials and generally aim to show superiority of the proposed agent versus placebo. This superiority is measured using a very specific outcome, such as reduction of symptoms using a rating scale designed and validated for that purpose, or a reduction in a laboratory measure, such as decrease in blood cholesterol levels. These clinical trials can be very large, enrolling multiple hundreds of patients across many study centers in several countries. Attempts are usually made to ensure a homogeneous test population. Intervention choice is randomized and subjects are followed double-blind. These clinical trials also monitor for adverse events, usually relying on spontaneous reporting but also including safety scales when certain tolerability problems are anticipated, such as extrapyramidal symptoms encountered with the use of antipsychotics. Clinical registration trial reports include information on both efficacy and tolerability under these artificial study conditions, but the aim of these reports is not to provide a synthesis for clinical guidance but to prove that the intervention is efficacious. Whether or not the intervention is efficacious and effective in a routine clinical practice is not certain. This is especially problematic when the patients who receive the intervention in clinical practice are unlike the subjects who received the intervention under controlled conditions. A good example of this are the registration trials of intramuscular antipsychotics for the treatment of agitation associated with schizophrenia or bipolar mania. Patients in these trials were required to provide informed consent and may represent a population that is very different from the agitated patient involuntarily brought to an emergency department by the police in terms of level of cooperation, degree of agitation, comorbid medical conditions, and presence of active alcohol or drug use. Perhaps the biggest objection to the use of registration trial data is that the comparator of placebo is not appropriate for the clinician whose main interest is to know how the new intervention compares with the old established one.

Effectiveness

Effectiveness is a term that refers to the broad utility of an intervention under the usual conditions of care. This utility includes efficacy (whether or not the intervention reduces the symptoms and signs of the disease), tolerability (whether or not the adverse events intrude on the well-being of the patient), and adherence (whether the patient complies with the treatment as prescribed). These three components are necessary for the intervention to be effective in the "real world." Efficacy is a necessary but not sufficient condition for an intervention to be useful.

Effectiveness can be estimated by the pooling together of clinical trial data that include information on both efficacy and tolerability. However, the predicted adherence or acceptability of the intervention in general clinical populations cannot be directly ascertained from this synthesis of efficacy studies. To accurately identify drug effects under the conditions of routine clinical care, different methods are needed. These methods include clinical trials that incorporate broad outcomes, longitudinal prospective naturalistic studies, and retrospective studies using large-scale clinical, pharmacy, and administrative databases. The subjects in effectiveness studies are usually more heterogeneous than those in a medication registration study, and this can facilitate the comparison of different active treatments.

An example of a controlled double-blind effectiveness trial is the Clinical Antipsychotic Trials of Intervention Effectiveness (CATIE) study for schizophrenia, where patients were initially randomized to one of five antipsychotics for up to 18 months. This is in direct contrast to the usual efficacy trial of an antipsychotic whose design is to compare a drug with a placebo over a relatively brief period ranging from 3 to 8 weeks. CATIE's primary outcome measure was time to all-cause treatment failure marked by discontinuation of the medication. The assumption was that if a medication was continued to be prescribed, then it was thought to be of acceptable value by both the patient and the clinician. The three principal reasons for discontinuation were patient decision, lack of adequate efficacy, or poor tolerability. The study included three main phases that allowed for switching from one antipsychotic to another. When enrolled, patients were made aware that these switches were possible. This mirrors clinical practice in that switching of antipsychotics is not uncommon. Moreover, unlike registration trials, subjects were not excluded if they had psychiatric comorbidities such as substance use disorders.

Effectiveness studies such as CATIE can answer questions that registration trials cannot, but there are several practical limitations to conducting large-scale effectiveness trials, including their length, size, and expense. Informed consent is also required, limiting generalizability. This patient selection bias can be extreme when studying chronic mental disorders such as schizophrenia, where impaired decisional capacity is not unusual. The use of naturalistic data from large-scale clinical and administrative databases produced by the ordinary, day-to-day operations of healthcare delivery systems is another option. Data for very large numbers of patients (thousands and tens of thousands) are available. Advantages include generalizability (the whole population across multiple diagnoses can be studied as they receive routine care). Multiple interventions or sequences of interventions can be assessed. The major limitation is the lack of randomization and the presence of substantial treatment selection biases (e.g., more chronically ill patients may receive different and/or multiple medications). Another criticism is that the retrospective analysis of databases is prone to data mining, where many outcomes are evaluated but only a select few are ever reported.

Evidence-Based Medicine

Clinicians often struggle to find interventions that make a difference in the well-being of their patients. It is not always easy to discern whether or not a study result should actually change clinical practice. Evidence-based medicine (EBM) is a philosophy that can help answer a clinical question that a practitioner may have about two different interventions for an individual patient. Clinical judgment and clinical expertise are still required to make the best decision possible, but the ability to formulate the question, seek out clinical trial evidence, appraise this evidence, and then to apply it and assess the outcome forms the nucleus of EBM. The evidence base can vary in quality, from anecdotal reports that are subject to bias, and hence of lower value, to the gold standard of randomized clinical trials and systematic reviews of randomized clinical trials. Both efficacy and effectiveness studies can help answer the clinical questions, but the limitations of each approach need to be understood. The clinician will need to identify

evidence that can quantify the differences between treatments, ensuring that there are clinically significant differences. A discussion of effect sizes, such as the number needed to treat (NNT), is beyond the scope of this discussion but is integral to the clinical interpretation of efficacy and effectiveness studies.

Leslie Citrome

See also Confounding and Effect Modulation; Hypothesis Testing; Randomized Clinical Trials

Further Readings

Guyatt, G. H., & Rennie, D. (2001). *Users' guides to the medical literature: A manual for evidence-based clinical practice.* Chicago: AMA Press.

Jaffe, A. B., & Levine, J. (2003). Efficacy and effectiveness of first- and second-generation antipsychotics in schizophrenia. *Journal of Clinical Psychiatry, 64*(Suppl. 17), 3–6.

Lieberman, J. A., Stroup, T. S., McEvoy, J. P., Swartz, M. S., Rosenheck, R. A., Perkins, D. O., et al. (2005). Effectiveness of antipsychotic drugs in patients with chronic schizophrenia. *New England Journal of Medicine, 353,* 1209–1223.

EFFICIENT FRONTIER

Efficient frontier is an economics term commonly used in performance measurement, although it has more recently also been applied to decision analysis. Another term for it is *production possibilities curve.* It shows the maximum output attainable from various combinations of inputs: the boundary between what is possible with the given resources and technologies and what is not.

Performance of Firms

Economists speak of *firms* or decision-making units, which convert a variety of inputs (materials, capital, and labor) into outputs. These outputs can be goods and/or services, and the firms may be public, for-profit, or not-for-profit. A variety of methods have been used to measure the performance of firms. One common measurement is the productivity ratio, which is related to concepts of efficiency.

Defining Productivity and Efficiency

Productivity is defined as the ratio of outputs to inputs, both weighted by their prices. If it is possible to define the maximum output attainable from each input level, analysts can use this information to draw a production frontier. If a firm is operating on that frontier, they are classified as *technically efficient*; conversely, if they are beneath the frontier, they are technically inefficient. However, it may still be possible to move along the production frontier. One common way is to take advantage of economies of scale (or avoid diseconomies of scale). Technological changes may also shift the entire production frontier, allowing greater productivity for a given level of input.

Since most firms use multiple inputs, and produce multiple outputs, these must often be aggregated. Analysts may examine the productivity of particular inputs (e.g., labor productivity), but this can be misleading, particularly if substitution is possible. Total factor productivity refers to the productivity of all inputs used to produce the given outputs, each weighted by its price.

Productivity does not incorporate the costs of production but considers only the volume of outputs producible. *Allocative efficiency* for a given quantity of output is the term used to select the mix of inputs that will produce those outputs at minimum cost; this procedure assumes that the prices for the inputs are known and requires incorporating information about all firms that might produce the desired outputs. Depending on how broadly the outputs are defined, this may require assessment of the mix to produce a particular service (e.g., renal dialysis treatment), services within a particular sector (e.g., hospital care), or services across sectors within a society (e.g., trade-offs between education and healthcare). Data requirements increase with scope, such that determining allocative efficiency for an economy is extremely challenging. Total economic efficiency (also referred to as productive efficiency) must consider both technical and allocative efficiency. Economists will usually incorporate considerations of Pareto efficiency, defined as requiring that no alternative allocation

of goods is possible without causing a net loss to one or more consumers.

These concepts are similar, but not identical, to cost-effectiveness. Unlike allocative efficiency, cost-effectiveness does not fix the desired output levels and mix; instead, it looks at the marginal cost to produce an additional marginal unit of benefit.

Measuring Productivity and Efficiency

Although some authors use the terms *productivity* and *efficiency* interchangeably, others stress that they have slightly different meanings and different operational definitions.

Economists have devised a number of methods for measuring efficiency and productivity. Many require computing index numbers, to allow analysts to compute productivity compared with a reference case. These relative measures of performance may look at how much more output could be produced for a given level of inputs (the output-oriented measures) or, conversely, at how little input would be required to produce a given level of outputs (input-oriented measures), as compared with the reference case.

One problem with using these efficiency measures is the high data requirements. They assume that the production functions of maximally efficient firms are known; this is rarely the case. Various approaches for estimating these functions using various techniques have been suggested; good reviews can be found in Coelli et al. and Worthington.

One approach is to use statistical techniques to construct a deterministic frontier, which is taken to represent the most efficient approach. Accordingly, any deviation from this frontier is assumed to represent inefficiency. This approach assumes that there is no noise and no measurement error. It also requires a large sample size (often not available) and sufficient spread of the observations throughout the distribution. Accordingly, it is used less commonly than the alternatives noted below.

Another family of approaches, stochastic frontiers, uses econometric models to estimate the frontier. These resemble the deterministic models in that they use parametric models that require assumptions as to the functional form but differ in introducing a disturbance term to allow for measurement error and noise. A third family, Data

Envelopment Analysis (DEA), uses linear programming techniques and is classified as nonparametric. Because this approach does not include stochastic (i.e., random) components, it assumes that all deviations from the frontier represent inefficiency. DEA, however, is more flexible than the alternatives in its data requirements and in how models are specified. Note that all these modeling approaches differ in the underlying assumptions made (e.g., whether it is assumed that firms are fully efficient), the ability to deal with noise and outliers, the assumptions about functional forms, and the data requirements. All are also subject to omitted variable bias.

Applications to Healthcare

Frontier efficiency has been applied to a wide range of firms, typically within public or quasi-public sectors. More recently, some efforts have been made to use these techniques to study the productivity of various healthcare organizations, including hospitals, nursing homes, and physician practices. An ongoing issue has been whether efficiency measures should be incorporated into reimbursement schedules and, if so, whether these approaches might be helpful in determining them.

One set of issues is defining what is meant by outputs. Technical efficiency may be used to refer to intermediate outputs such as the number of patients treated or their waiting time. It may also be defined in terms of health outcomes, such as mortality or life expectancy. Because health outcomes are related to many factors, often outside the healthcare system, analysts may have difficulty in defining the production function linking particular interventions to overall outcomes. This dilemma becomes even more pronounced if efforts are made to aggregate outputs (e.g., to look at the performance of a healthcare system, as opposed to the results of a particular drug or surgical procedure).

In 2004, Worthington identified 38 studies that applied frontier efficiency approaches to the study of healthcare organizations. Over half referred to organizations in the United States, although examples were found for Spain, Sweden, the Netherlands, Finland, Taiwan, and the United Kingdom. Most studies (68%) analyzed the performance of hospitals, with other examples examining nursing homes,

health maintenance organizations, local area health authorities, and other settings.

More recently, these approaches have been applied to decision analysis through the construction of a cost-effectiveness frontier. This analysis equates cost efficiency with the production of technically efficient combinations of inputs and outputs at the least cost. If it is possible to create a cost function, one can construct a production frontier that represents the best currently known production techniques. Accordingly, Eckermann and colleagues have recommended shifting the two-dimensional representation of cost-effectiveness from the commonly accepted incremental cost-effectiveness (which plots difference in effectiveness against difference in cost) to a production function approach. This application shares advantages, and disadvantages, with the previously noted efforts to use these methods.

Cautions

As Worthington cautions, this approach may not always be appropriate. One problem is how to ensure that studies do not compare apples with oranges. One way to ensure homogeneous outcomes is to aggregate; studies have accordingly categorized outputs in terms of age or type of treatment. As Newhouse noted, such aggregation can be problematic. Frontier techniques appear to be designed for homogeneous outputs, which is rarely true in healthcare. It is particularly difficult to capture variations in quality unless these lead to unambiguous impacts on the chosen measure (e.g., mortality). In general, many important outputs will not be included, and their omission is likely to distort the findings. Similarly, many inputs may be omitted (e.g., capital, physicians), and case-mix controls are likely to be inadequate. Hospitals treating sicker patients may thus be seen as being inefficient rather than as delivering a different mix of services.

Despite these caveats, frontier analysis is being more widely used by policy makers seeking to increase accountability in the use of public funds. This has been particularly evident in the United Kingdom. These techniques are being used as an alternative to the "performance indicator" movement; they seek to aggregate multiple indicators into a single measure of efficiency, based on the difference between observed performance and that which would be predicted from the best case. A 2005 review by Jacobs and Street concludes that the approach is still not ready to be used to inform policy but recommends further research.

One key limitation to all these approaches is that they are not intended to deal with whether particular outputs are worth producing. Efficient markets assume that anything demanded should be produced as long as there are willing buyers and sellers. In contrast, appropriateness is a major concern for many healthcare services, and there is a widespread agreement that services that are not needed should probably not be provided, regardless of how efficiently they can be produced.

Raisa Deber and Audrey Laporte

See also Cost-Effectiveness Analysis; Cost-Identification Analysis; Cost-Minimization Analysis; Economics, Health Economics; Value Functions in Domains of Gains and Losses

Further Readings

Coelli, T., Rao, P. D. S., & Battese, G. E. (2002). *An introduction to efficiency and productivity analysis.* Boston: Kluwer Academic.

Eckermann, S., Briggs, A., & Willan, A. R. (2008). Health technology assessment in the cost-disutility plane. *Medical Decision Making, 28*(2), 172–181.

Jacobs, R., & Street, A. (2005). Efficiency measurement in health care: Recent developments, current practice and future research. In P. C. Smith, L. Ginnelly, & M. Sculpher (Eds.), *Health policy and economics* (pp. 148–172). Berkshire, UK: Open University Press.

Newhouse, J. P. (1994). Frontier estimation: How useful a tool for health economics? *Journal of Health Economics, 13*(3), 317–322.

Worthington, A. C. (2004). Frontier efficiency measurement in health care: A review of empirical techniques and selected applications. *Medical Care Research and Review, 61*(2), 135–170.

EMOTION AND CHOICE

It is increasingly recognized that emotions can have an important impact on judgment and decision making. However, in many respects, it remains an undeveloped area of judgment and decision making, particularly in medicine. First, emotions are difficult to characterize or define. Second, the causal mechanisms by which emotions influence decisions—independent of purely cognitive interactions—are poorly understood. Third, the circumstances in which emotions are most important in changing decisions are only partially understood. Finally, most of the well-controlled empirical data on emotions and decision making are outside the field of medicine, rarely involving physicians and patients. Each of these limitations is important when describing the role emotions play in medical decision making, so the sections that follow address each of these points in turn.

Defining Emotions

Clear definitions are crucial for outlining the role of emotions in judgment and decision making. Definitions or characterizations of emotion range across multiple disciplines. The philosopher Paul Griffiths proposes dividing what we commonly call emotions into two categories of mental phenomenon: lower-level "affect programs" and higher-level "irruptive emotional states." The first category of emotions consists of automated, stereotypical reactions that provide rapid responses to stimuli, seem rooted in evolutionarily justified patterns, are cross-cultural, and are correlated with survival needs in all higher animals. They are represented by the "lower" emotions of fear, anger, happiness, sadness, surprise, and disgust. The second category of emotions consists of those with complex mixtures of cognitive and emotional elements that occur more passively and interrupt other cognitive processes and tie together our mental lives in the long run. They are characterized by emotions such as love, guilt, envy, jealousy, and pride. They remain separate from other, more diffuse dispositional or visceral states referred to most accurately as "moods," such as anxiety, depression, and elation.

The political scientist Jon Elster presents a cluster of "features" that are robustly associated with human emotions, but none of which are essential to them. These features include being unbidden in occurrence, possessing cognitive antecedents, having intentional objects, being arousing, leading to action tendencies, and having specific valence. He specifically distinguishes human emotions from emotions that have a sudden onset, brief duration, and characteristic expressions. These correspond to the affect programs Griffiths describes, which we largely share with other animals and across human societies and cultures.

The psychologists Reid Hastie and Robin Dawes define emotions as reactions to motivationally significant stimuli and situations that usually include three components: (1) a cognitive appraisal, (2) a signature physiological response, and (3) an accompanying phenomenal experience. This captures, at least operationally, the features of emotions that are most relevant for decision making.

Overall, there seems to be agreement that there are two groups of emotions. The first group consists of those that are more basic and stereotypical, are rooted most obviously in evolutionary survival, and suddenly interrupt ongoing cognition to cause different behavior. The second group consists of more complex cognitive states, with cognitive antecedents, less obviously tied to our evolutionary roots and less obviously interrupting other cognitive states. A third category, which is left aside here, consists of moods, which are more diffuse mental states that seem to be predispositions or precursors to other states and less obviously tied to specific actions.

Impact of Emotions on Decisions

There are two methodological approaches to decision making: the economic approach and the psychological approach. The economic approach emphasizes rationality, response to incentives, and maximization of utility (i.e., benefits) subject to constraints (i.e., costs). Such an approach minimizes the role emotions play in decision making, treating them as inputs to valuation or utility. Choice is fundamentally cognitive and rational, with a dispassionate consideration of costs and benefits. The psychological approach focuses on two mental operations, judgments and decisions, both of which can be, and often are, influenced by emotions. Psychologists identify persistent exceptions to rational behavior, showing how systematic biases shape human behavior. The maturing field of behavioral economics brings psychological realism and attention to human biases, including the impact of emotions, to the rational utility-maximization

approach of economics. It is the approach taken here.

A causal framework for understanding the role of emotions in decision making from a behavioral economics perspective has been advanced by Loewenstein and Lerner. The framework highlights how emotions can influence decisions through two pathways: (1) immediate emotions and (2) expected emotions. Immediate emotions are experienced at the time a decision is made. These emotions can influence decision making in two ways: directly or indirectly. They can *directly* affect a decision as it is being made. For example, a patient might feel fearful at the time of choosing a treatment and therefore decline a riskier option, even if it has a better possible outcome. Immediate emotions can also *indirectly* influence a decision by altering expectations of the probability or desirability of an anticipated future outcome. In this case, a patient who is feeling happy may optimistically expect a good outcome from risky therapy and "go for it," even if it is it riskier. The second pathway of influence, expected emotions, are cognitive appraisals about the emotional consequences of decisions rather than the emotions currently being experienced. These are possible emotions that one considers when making a current decision. An example of an expected emotion's impact on decision making is a patient with prostate cancer projecting how he might feel if he developed impotence as a result of surgery, then choosing watchful waiting to avoid the undesired emotional consequences of that surgical outcome.

This general framework can be understood in specific circumstances based on the particular emotions involved and the context of the decision. Affect-program emotions—those that are most immediate, universal, and disruptive to current actions—can strongly influence immediate emotions. Consider, for example, a physician heading to the office after an unresolved spousal argument. Anger is a negative emotion, an activating one, and one that leaves one feeling less in control. The source of the anger is not relevant to the medical decisions that will be made that day; yet it is probable that those decisions will be more negative, aggressive, and definite, independent of the relevance of these features to the calculation of what is best for the patients. The important feature about affect-program emotions is that they can have big impacts on decisions with relatively little input from cognition.

When considering the other type of more complex emotions, the framework for application becomes more complicated. Other higher-level emotions seem to have longer-standing cognitive underpinnings that accompany them, making it more difficult to see their specific causal role. For example, emotions such as love, envy, vengeance, and empathy, to name a few, are quite different in character from those of the affect programs. Because they are accompanied by underlying, preceding thought processes that influence the emotions, it is more difficult to assign specific influences regarding decisions to these more complex emotional states. In the medical context, empathic physicians are thought to provide better care for their patients, all other considerations being equal, through more thoughtful decision making. However, characterizing the influence of empathy on decision making is very difficult.

Another reason emotions can be difficult to study with regard to choices is that many of the precursors of emotional responses are unconscious. Therefore, people are unaware that their decision processes are affected by these emotions, making them difficult to assess accurately. This is particularly true of the affect-program types of emotions. Evolutionarily, they are believed to protect the organism by causing certain actions to avoid specific situations. These more basic, universal emotions use neural pathways such as the amygdala that bypass other, more cognitive pathways such as the frontal cortex. Using animal models and functional magnetic resonance imaging (fMRI), neuroscientists have done an impressive job outlining the relevant neural pathways and showing how they bypass higher centers. For example, if one "sees" a snake in one's path and immediately reacts to get away, that might be important for survival from an evolutionary perspective. However, if that snake turns out to be a harmless stick, one has responded to a false judgment. These responses to fear, anger, and happiness still exist, but they can lead to false judgments and decisions in the modern world. A patient's fear about a disease such as cancer or Alzheimer's disease may derail his or her ability to consider rationally the probabilities involving a treatment decision.

In a similar vein, it has also been shown that damage to specific brain areas that disconnects our emotional responses from cognitive assessment can profoundly affect decision making. Damage to prefrontal cortex areas seems to disconnect our emotional centers from our more cognitive ones, leading those with such damage to become excessively risk taking and unable to conduct straightforward cost-benefit calculations. The mechanism seems to be a loss of the normal emotional response to losses, which makes undamaged individuals loss-averse. Patients with dementia are also prone to such behavior, and they may be unable to make decisions regarding their own care.

Typical Circumstances

The role of emotions in decision making is best understood in decisions that involve risky and/or uncertain choices over time. In the economic, utility-based conception of choice, risk and uncertainty are modeled with the assumption of expected utility represented by a "risk preference." Choices over time are modeled by discounted utility models in which future values are assumed to be worth less than the current values. However, a number of examples have been found showing that both of these models have important, persistent exceptions.

Under expected utility models of risky choice, risk is conceived as an outcome's expected value, the product of its likelihood of occurring and the subjective value of that outcome. People are said to have risk preferences if, when the expected values of competing outcomes are equal, they prefer one based on the distribution of it occurring. This explanation has been invoked to explain people's general willingness to purchase health insurance because they are risk-averse. However, there are a number of empirical situations in which people prefer riskier options in some situations and safer options in other situations, something that is inconsistent with expected utility. This is the result of the hedonics of valuing—people generally dislike a loss much more than they like the same-sized gain. As a result, people tend to avoid risks in a gain situation but to accept the same risks in a loss frame, an effect called loss aversion. One of the explanations of such findings is that emotions regarding risk change valuation.

Considering time-based decision making, the standard economic model is the discounted utility model. This model assumes that future values are worth less than current values at a constantly decreasing discount rate. Once again, a number of exceptions to this model have been found. For example, when asked to give the preferred time for a kiss from a chosen movie star, people choose 3 days from now rather than immediately, to "savor" the anticipation of the event. Once again, emotions are likely explanations for the failure of the economic models and the need for alternative explanations.

Emotions are thought to have important effects on decisions. However, characterizing the exact role emotions play in choices is very difficult. The best characterized emotions are the affect-program emotions, such as anger, fear, disgust, and happiness. These basic, evolutionarily preserved, and universal emotions appear to bypass the usual neural pathways and influence choices by disrupting other cognitive inputs. This is most important when the emotions are immediate but unrelated to the decisions being made, thereby deviating most strongly from balanced cost-benefit assessments. Other, more complex emotions have more cognitive underpinnings, and their effects on behavior are more indirect. Choices that involve risk, uncertainty, and "distance" are most likely to be influenced by emotions. There remains much work to be done to characterize how these emotions affect medical decisions.

William Dale

See also Decision Making and Affect; Decision Psychology; Fear; Mood Effects; Risk Perception

Further Readings

Elster, J. (1999). *Strong feelings: Emotion, addiction, and human behavior.* Cambridge: MIT Press.

Griffiths, P. E. (1997). *What emotions really are.* Chicago: University of Chicago Press.

Hastie, R., & Dawes, R. M. (2001). *Rational choice in an uncertain world: The psychology of judgment and decision making.* Thousand Oaks, CA: Sage.

LeDoux, J. (1996). *The emotional brain: The mysterious underpinnings of emotional life.* New York: Touchstone.

Loewenstein, G., & Lerner, J. (2003). The role of affect in decision making. In R. J. Davidson, K. R. Scherer, & H. H. Goldsmith (Eds.), *Handbook of affective sciences.* New York: Oxford University Press.

EQUITY

Equity in medical decision making is an area that has received little attention. One strategy to reduce disparities in care that often arise during the medical encounter, and thus increase equity, is shared decision making between providers and patients. The shared decision-making model includes a number of critical factors that can improve care: better communication; patient-centered, culturally competent care; and patient involvement in deliberations and decisions. Each of these elements can mitigate the sociopolitical factors that have been institutionalized in medicine through the unbalanced relationship between physician and patient. This model appears to be a powerful tool that could reduce disparate care and improve overall health outcomes for minority patients.

Background on Disparities in Healthcare

Disparities in healthcare in the United States are widespread and well documented. Multiple studies show that minorities are less likely to receive important healthcare services, including preventive services and regular physicals, as well as clinically appropriate interventions. They are also more likely to receive care from providers with fewer resources, lower qualifications, and less experience than whites. This disparate care results in less satisfaction with care, lower compliance with prescribed treatments, and poorer health outcomes for many minority Americans.

The poor quality of care provided to minority groups can be explained in part by failures in the healthcare system. Insurance status is a powerful predictor of healthcare use and type of provider seen, and minority groups are more likely to be uninsured than whites. Access problems, including geographic proximity to care and linguistic and cultural barriers, also hinder minority patients' ability to seek out high-quality care.

Disparities are not, however, solely a consequence of these system-level factors. Differences in care persist even when controlling for insurance status and access issues. Some researchers suggest that lower-quality care for minorities may be explained in part by patient preference, but the evidence is inconsistent, and the effect has been found to be small.

Given that patient preference cannot adequately explain disparities in care, researchers have begun to examine whether disparities emerge from the medical encounter and the process that physicians and patients go through to make important decisions about patients' health and healthcare. Provider bias in decision making, for example, can lead to disparate care for minorities. While providers resist believing that they provide disparate care, studies suggest that intentional and unintentional stereotyping and bias by race, ethnicity, and gender influence clinical decisions and lead to inferior care for minorities.

Poor communication, lack of information, and mistrust between patient and provider can influence patients' understanding of their health and the decisions they make regarding their care. Care for minority patients is often less patient centered than care for white patients, particularly when the patient-physician relationship is not racially or ethnically concordant. Minorities are less likely than whites to report that their physicians engage in participatory care and patient-centered communication and more likely to report that their physicians treat them with disrespect. Misunderstandings and a lack of culturally competent care on the part of the provider also contribute to disparate care.

A physician-patient interaction in which there is poor communication, bias, and mistrust is likely to result in uninformed decision making. Understanding and improving the decision-making process may mitigate some of these effects and substantially improve care for minority patients.

The Decision-Making Process and Disparities in Care

In their seminal research on shared decision making in the medical encounter, Cathy Charles et al. identify different theoretical approaches to medical decision making and espouse the benefits of shared decision making over the more traditional paternalistic model. In the paternalistic model, patients defer all decisions to the physician, who has the professional authority, training, and experience to make the "right" decisions for the patient. In each of the three stages of decision making—exchanging information, deliberating options, and deciding on

a treatment—the physician controls the process, with little to no input from the patient.

In this model, information exchange is restricted, flowing largely in one direction from the provider to the patient. During the deliberation stage, the physician alone or in consultation with other physicians considers the risks and benefits of alternative treatment options. Finally, the decision of the most appropriate treatment is made solely by the physician.

Within the context of social, economic, and political inequities experienced by minorities, the power asymmetry of the medical encounter is fraught with tension; the paternalistic model of decision making perpetuates this imbalance when the relationship is not racially or ethnically concordant. The one-way direction of information exchange (Phase 1) from physician to patient controls not only the amount but also the content of information shared with the patient. Minority patients might experience this information imbalance as a form of coercive authority and a way of dismissing patients' desire to be involved in their own care decisions. In fact, studies suggest that physicians' communication style is more verbally dominant with black patients than with white patients and that black patients have significantly less participatory visits with their physicians than white patients, particularly when the physician is white.

Without information provided by the patient, the physician may be unaware of important clinical concerns that could inform his or her treatment decisions and recommendations for certain interventions. For example, minority patients may experience illness differently than white patients; they may also have different expectations of the role of healthcare in their lives. In a paternalistic model, however, these issues are unlikely to emerge or be considered during the care process.

The deliberation and decision phases of the paternalistic model (Phases 2 and 3) also exclude the patient. For minorities, this is an especially important issue when their physician relationships are not concordant, and the physician is unlikely to be familiar with or knowledgeable about the unique racial and cultural contexts of their minority patients. Physicians who infer patients' needs and preferences rarely get them right, which can result in misunderstandings, confusion regarding care, lower patient compliance with treatments, distrust of the system, and overall dissatisfaction with care.

In the paternalistic model, the physician will provide the patient with a recommendation based on what he or she believes to be the "best" course of treatment despite imperfect information. Physicians' personal biases and stereotypes are reinforced as assumptions regarding what the patient wants and needs go largely unchallenged. Preconceived notions can very likely influence physicians' treatment recommendations and convey messages regarding minority patients' competence, self-efficacy, and deservingness.

The paternalistic model of decision making may still be the prevalent mode in which most physicians practice. Given its potential for inequitable practices and outcomes, however, a more patient-centered model of decision making should be considered. A model of shared decision making could be used to mitigate many of the negative factors inherent in the paternalistic model.

In the shared decision making model, the patient (sometimes including the patient's family) and the physician work together through all three stages of the decision-making process. At the core of this model is the concept of patient-centered care. Through communication, information exchange, and partnership in the deliberation and final decision processes, the physician and the patient together identify the patient's needs and preferences and incorporate them into their decision.

In a patient-physician relationship that is not racially or ethnically concordant, this model of decision making is critical to developing mutual trust and understanding of how the patient's social and cultural context influences his or her presentation of illness and compliance with care. Providers must approach minority patients in a manner that is appropriate and respectful of their cultural mores. This requires that the physician and patient participate in open communication, exchange information, and develop a relationship where both parties are partners in the decision-making process.

In this model, providers must also try to recognize their own limitations. For example, physicians must use interpreters and seek help in understanding racial and ethnic groups' styles of communication. They must learn about their patients' backgrounds and value systems to understand better the most appropriate course of action

for their minority patients—one that will be accepted and followed. Finally, physicians must be frank with themselves about their assumptions and beliefs regarding racial and ethnic groups and understand that they may be intentionally or unintentionally reinforcing disparate behavior based on stereotypes.

The exchange of information is critical to this process (Phase 1). In the shared decision-making model, the responsibility of exchanging information falls on both participants in the medical encounter. The provider is expected not only to provide information but also to elicit information from the patient regarding his or her needs, preferences, and values. The patient is also expected to share his or her experiences and expectations. If both participants are clear about their expectations and share their knowledge and values, then the decision-making process can be used to eliminate many of the inequities that may emerge from the patient-physician encounter.

As part of this process, the physician and patient should clearly establish the preferences of the patient regarding the roles each will play in decision making. It may be that not all patients want to take a participatory role in their own care process. For example, recent studies have suggested that black patients want information and full disclosure regarding medical tests and procedures but are hesitant to have autonomous decision-making power and prefer to follow the recommendations of their providers. For some ethnic groups, decision making is a family-centered process, including multiple family members. Understanding that some patients may prefer to delegate final responsibility of the treatment decision to others, including the physician, is part of the shared decision-making process.

Information exchange and patient involvement in this model of medical decision making may be able to reduce provider assumptions, improve communication, and achieve congruence in perspectives of health and approaches to treatment. It also sets the stage for the deliberation and final treatment decision phases of the care process. When engaged in shared decision making, the physician helps the patient weigh different treatment options with a better understanding of that patient's unique cultural context. When a decision regarding the best course of action is agreed on, the physician can probe the patient to ensure that he or she fully understands the implications of their (the physician and the patient's) choice. Understanding the patient's perspective is critical for the provider to fully comprehend the patient's experience of illness, how he or she perceives risks and benefits of treatment, and how he or she might accept and comply with medical intervention.

Katherine Mead and Bruce Siegel

See also Cultural Issues; Discrimination; Shared Decision Making

Further Readings

Aberegg, K., & Terry, P. B. (2004). Medical decision-making and healthcare disparities. *Journal of Laboratory and Clinical Medicine, 144*(1), 11–17.

Brian, D., Smedley, A. Y., & Nelson, A. R. (Eds.). (2002). *Unequal treatment: Confronting racial and ethnic disparities in health care.* Washington, DC: Institute of Medicine.

Burgess, D. J., Van Ryn, M., & Fu, S. S. (2004). Making sense of the provider role in promoting disparities. *Journal of General Internal Medicine, 19,* 1154–1159.

Charles, C., Whelan, T., & Gafni, A. (1999). What do we mean by partnership in making decisions about treatment? *British Medical Journal, 319,* 780–782.

Cooper-Patrick, L., Gallo, J. J., Gonzales, J. J., Vu, H. T., Powe, N. R., Nelson, C., et al. (1999). Race, gender, and partnership in the patient-physician relationship. *Journal of the American Medical Association, 282,* 583–589.

Johnson, R. L., Roter, D., Powe, N. R., & Cooper, L. A. (2004). Patient race/ethnicity and quality of patient-physician communication during medical visits. *American Journal of Public Health, 94*(12), 2084–2090.

Kaplan, S. H., Gandek, B., Greenfield, S., Rogers, W., & Ware, J. E. (1995). Patient and visit characteristics related to physicians' participatory decision-making style. *Medical Care, 33*(12), 1176–1187.

Murray, E., Pollack, L., White, M., & Lo, B. (2007). Clinical decision-making: Patients' preferences and experiences. *Patient Education and Counseling, 65*(2), 189–196.

Stewart, M., Brown, J. B., Weston, W. W., McWhinney, I. R., McWilliam, C. L., & Freeman, T. R. (1995). *Patient-centered medicine: Transforming the clinical method.* Thousand Oaks, CA: Sage.

Suurmond, J., & Seeleman, C. (2006). Shared decision-making in an intercultural context: Barriers in the interaction between physicians and immigrant patients. *Patient Education and Counseling, 60*(2), 253–259.

Torke, A. M., Corbie-Smith, G. M., & Branch, W. T. (2004). African American patients' perspectives on medical decision-making. *Archives of Internal Medicine, 164*(5), 525–530.

EQUIVALENCE TESTING

Frequently, the objective of an investigation is not to determine if a drug or treatment is superior to another but just equivalent. For instance, it is often of interest to investigate if a new drug, with say fewer side effects or lower price, is as efficacious as the one currently used. This situation occurs when new or generic drugs are evaluated for approval by the Food and Drug Administration (FDA).

In standard hypotheses testing, equivalence (i.e., equality) is the null hypothesis, and the alternative is the nonequivalence hypothesis. One problem with using this procedure, and determining equivalence when the null is not rejected, is that the test is designed to reject the null hypothesis only if the evidence against it is strong (e.g., $p < .05$). In other words, the burden of proof is in nonequivalence. The correct procedure to establish equivalence reverses the roles of null and alternative hypotheses so that the burden of proof lies in the hypothesis of equivalence. Consequently, the Type I error is tantamount to favoring equivalency when the drugs are not equivalent. This is the error that the FDA wants to minimize, and its probability is controlled at a low level (e.g., .05 or lower).

Some issues arise when testing for equivalence. A critical one is that perfect equivalence is impossible to establish. This problem is solved by introducing limits of equivalence that establish a range within which equivalence is accepted. Frequently, these limits are symmetric around a reference value. An example should help clarify the situation.

Suppose that a new drug for eliminating (or reducing to a prespecified level) a toxin in the blood is being evaluated. It has fewer side effects and the manufacturer is interested in proving that it is as efficacious as the currently used drug. Let p_C and p_N be the true (population) proportion of patients who respond to the current and the new drug, respectively. The problem consists of testing

H_0: $| P_C - P_N | \geq \delta$ (nonequivalency)
H_1: $| P_C - P_N | < \delta$ (equivalency).

A more informative way to write the alternative is H_1: $p_C - \delta < p_N < p_C + \delta$, which states that the efficacy of the new drug is within δ units from that of the current drug. The role of δ is crucial, and its value should be chosen with great care. Clearly, the probability of favoring equivalency increases as δ increases, so its value should be based on acceptable levels of deviation from perfect equivalence. The value of δ should be determined based on sound medical and biological considerations, independently of statistical issues. For example, if the potential benefits (fewer side effects) of the new drug are high, a larger value of δ could be justified. When the effect of the current drug is well established, the value of p_C is fixed and the test becomes a one-sample equivalence test.

Using data from the National Immunization Survey (NIS), in 2002, Lawrence Barker and colleagues investigated whether vaccination coverage was equivalent between children of three minority groups and white children. Since the NIS data for 2000 were supposed to detect coverages at the 5 percentage point level, δ was chosen to be 5. Thus, the alternative hypothesis was H_1: $-5 < p_M - p_W < 5$, where p_W and p_M are the coverage for white and minority children, respectively. The equivalence of the coverage was to be established if the data provided enough evidence to support H_1.

Procedure

An intuitive method to test equivalency is known as the two-one-sided test (TOST) procedure. At an α level, the TOST procedure will accept the hypothesis of equivalence if a $(1 - 2\alpha) \times 100\%$ confidence interval (CI) for the difference in proportions is contained in the interval $(-\delta, \delta)$. If either limit is outside the interval, nonequivalency cannot be rejected (i.e., equivalency cannot be established). The TOST procedure can be used in situations that involve other parameters (i.e., means, medians, odds ratios, etc.). It is

important to note that, even though the TOST procedure is two sided, it achieves an $\alpha = .05$, using a 90% CI.

Barker and colleagues found that the vaccination coverage for the 3-DTP vaccine was 95.0% for whites and 92.1% for blacks, with a 90% CI for the difference of (1.5, 4.3). Since this interval is included in the interval (−5, 5), equivalence was established at a .05 level. It is important to note that this interval does not include 0, so the standard procedure would have found a significant difference between the coverages (i.e., a lower coverage for black children). A contradiction also occurs when the CI includes 0, but is not within $(-\delta, \delta)$. In fact, Barker and colleagues found that contradictions occurred in 9 out of 21 comparisons (three minority groups and seven vaccines). In 7 of the 9 cases, the TOST procedure favored equivalence in contradiction with the standard procedure; in 2 cases the results were reversed.

In some cases, symmetric limits of equivalency are not appropriate. That would be the case when the "costs" of erring in either direction are not the same. In such a case, the procedure would be based on whether the CI is contained in an interval (δ_1, δ_2).

Sample-Size Considerations

The main problem in equivalence testing is that the samples needed to achieve acceptable levels of power are, frequently, fairly large. Using the TOST procedure with $\alpha = .05$, samples of $n = 2,122$ per group are needed to achieve a power of .95 to establish equivalence when $p_N = .4$, $p_C = .3$, and $\delta = .15$. Under the same circumstances, a standard procedure requires $n = 589$ per group to reject the null hypothesis of equivalence and conclude (incorrectly) nonequivalence. As mentioned earlier, larger values of δ increase the power to detect equivalence and thus reduce the required sample size. For example, if $\delta = .2$, the sample size needed to establish equivalence in the previous situation is $n = 531$.

Testing equivalence is particularly applicable in public health, where the sample sizes are usually large. The NIS contains millions of records of children nationwide, yielding a high power for any test. However, in clinical studies, large samples are hard to obtain, thus limiting the application of equivalence testing. In this respect, Stefan Wellek states,

> In equivalence testing power values exceeding 50% can only be obtained if either the equivalence range specified [δ] by the alternative hypothesis is chosen extremely wide or the sample size requirements are beyond the scope of feasibility for most if not all applications. (p. 63)

Noninferiority Testing

Noninferiority, or one-sided equivalence, testing is appropriate when the objective is to establish that one arm is not inferior to another (and possibly superior). Actually, the example of the toxin-reducing drug might be better suited for a noninferiority test. That is, the objective is to establish that the new drug is not inferior in efficacy to the drug in current use. As before, let p_C and p_N be the true efficacy of the current and the new drug, respectively. The test of interest is

$$H_0: P_C - P_N \geq \delta \text{ (inferiority)}$$
$$H_1: P_C - P_N < \delta \text{ (noninferiority)}.$$

It is informative to write the noninferiority hypothesis as $H_1: p_N > p_C - \delta$, which states that the efficacy of the new drug is not more than δ units lower than the efficacy of the current drug. In cases where higher values imply inferiority, the alternative hypothesis becomes $H_1: p_N - p_C < \delta$.

Noninferiority testing differs from a standard one-sided test only by the use of the "offset" term δ. Thus, noninferiority is established at an α level if the upper limit of a $(1 - 2\alpha) \times 100\%$ CI for the difference $p_C - p_N$ is less than δ. Significant confusion in the medical literature is caused by the fact that the upper limit of a $(1 - 2\alpha) \times 100\%$ CI is also the upper limit of a $(1 - \alpha) \times 100\%$ one-sided CI. That is, the upper limit of a 90% CI is also the upper limit of a 95% one-sided CI.

Warfarin prevents ischemic stroke in patients with nonvalvular atrial fibrillation, but dose adjustment, coagulation monitoring, and bleeding limit its use. In 2005, SPORTIF (Stroke Prevention Using an Oral Thrombin Inhibitor in Atrial Fibrillation) was created to conduct a study to compare ximelagatran with warfarin for stroke prevention. Ximelagatran has a fixed oral dosing, does not require coagulation monitoring, and has few drug interactions. The objective was to establish noninferiority of ximelagatran with respect to stroke prevention. An absolute margin of $\delta = 2\%$ per year was specified. Therefore, if p_X and p_W are the yearly stroke rates for ximelagatran and warfarin, respectively, the noninferiority hypothesis was $H_1: p_X < p_W + 2$. The observed yearly event rates were 1.62% and 1.17% for ximelagatran and warfarin, respectively. The difference was .45%, and the 95% upper limit of the CI for the difference was 1.03%. Since it was less than 2%, noninferiority was established. Note that for $\delta = 1\%$, the data do not support noninferiority.

Other Situations

Equivalence testing, just as standard testing, can be applied to a variety of problems. This includes differences or ratios of measures of location (e.g., means, proportions, medians) and dispersion (e.g., standard deviations). Wellek describes parametric and nonparametric tests of equivalence for dependent observations, multiple samples, linear models, survival times, hazard rates, and bioequivalence.

A natural application of the equivalence concept is in lack of fit where the objective is to determine if an observed distribution is equivalent to another. In the standard chi-square test for lack of fit, the null hypothesis is of equivalence, and thus, it is not designed to establish equivalence to the reference distribution and tends to favor equivalence too frequently. Wellek presents an equivalence test for this situation that has the desired properties.

p Values

Reporting p values in testing equivalence is not done routinely. This is unfortunate because p values are not difficult to calculate. In the noninferiority case, the p value is obtained from a standard test with an offset value of δ. This procedure can be carried out with any standard statistical program. To calculate the p value in the case of equivalence, one uses the fact that establishing equivalence is tantamount to establishing non-superiority and noninferiority, simultaneously. Thus, the p value for equivalence is the larger of the two p values.

Final Thoughts

Testing equivalence or noninferiority is the appropriate procedure for many biological and medical situations in which the objective is to compare a new therapy with a standard. The procedures to perform these tests are simple modifications of those used in standard testing but in many cases result in completely different conclusions. The margin of equivalence is critical and sometimes is the most critical issue. In spite of their apparent simplicity, there is still considerable confusion in the medical literature on how to perform and interpret equivalence and noninferiority tests. In a recent study, Le Henanff and colleagues found that out of 162 published reports of equivalence and noninferiority trials, about 80% did not justify the choice of the equivalence margin. They also observed that only about 50% of the articles reported a p value, and only 25% interpreted it.

The main obstacle in the application of these methods is the large samples needed to achieve acceptable levels of power. In the study by Le Henanff and colleagues, the median number of patients per trial was 333. However, 28% of the studies reviewed did not take into account the equivalence margin, so it is likely that many were underpowered to detect equivalency. Finally, the decision between testing equivalence or noninferiority involves similar issues as in choosing between a two-sided or a one-sided alternative in standard testing. This decision should be based on the objectives of the study and not on the observed data.

Esteban Walker

See also Efficacy Versus Effectiveness; Hypothesis Testing

Further Readings

Barker, L. E., Luman, E. T., McCauley, M. M., & Chu, S. Y. (2002). Assessing equivalence: An alternative to the use of difference tests for measuring disparities in vaccination coverage. *American Journal of Epidemiology, 156,* 1056–1061.

Barker, L., Rolka, H., Rolka, D., & Brown, C. (2001). Equivalence testing for binomial random variables: Which test to use? *The American Statistician, 55,* 279–287.

Le Henanff, A., Giraudeau, B., Baron, G., & Ravaud, P. (2006). Quality of reporting of noninferiority and equivalence randomized trials. *Journal of the American Medical Association, 295,* 1147–1151.

SPORTIF Executive Steering Committee. (2005). Ximelagatran vs. Warfarin for stroke prevention in patients with nonvalvular atrial fibrillation. *Journal of the American Medical Association, 293,* 690–698.

Wellek, S. (2003). *Testing statistical hypotheses of equivalence.* Boca Raton, FL: Chapman & Hall.

ERROR AND HUMAN FACTORS ANALYSES

The study of human error in diverse sociotechnical systems may be conducted by examining the human factors that contribute to error. A human error may be broadly defined as failure to take required action, failure to meet a performance standard for that action, or performing the wrong action. In the medical domain, human error may or may not adversely affect the patient. Patient safety is a medical providers' principal concern; thus, much attention has been placed on uncovering errors that have the potential to cause patient injury. Any patient injury (i.e., adverse medical event) that is attributable to human error is described as a preventable adverse event. Two prolific studies conducted in New York, Colorado, and Utah suggested that between 2.9% and 3.7% of hospitalizations produce adverse events. The proportion of these adverse events that was attributable to error (i.e., preventable adverse event) was between 53% and 58%. The New York study estimated that preventable adverse events in hospitals causes approximately 44,000 to 98,000 deaths annually when extrapolated to the 33.6 billion hospital admissions the United States experienced in 1997. Even if these statistics underestimate the magnitude of the problem, as some have argued, they would still place preventable adverse events among the leading causes of death in the United States, ranking higher than motor vehicle accidents, breast cancer, and AIDS. Results of these studies prompted the Institute of Medicine to produce the report *To Err Is Human: Building a Safer Health System,* which strongly recommended that the healthcare community look to other high-risk industries, such as nuclear power and aviation, for ways to improve their own record on the quality and safety of healthcare delivery. The authors of that report endorsed the study and application of human factors analyses to measure and improve human-system performance.

Human factors analyses are used to study how humans interact psychologically and physically with their particular environment (i.e., system). This includes the study of both human-human and human-system interactions. The objective of human factors analyses is to understand the nature of these interactions in order to improve system performance and human well-being. The field of human factors originated in aviation, but its current scope is as broad as it is deep, with specialization ranging from safety and human error to aging and virtual reality. The results of many years of research from the human factors community have yielded valuable insights into crucial aspects of human performance that can be affected by the design of work in light of human capabilities and limitations and the specialized nature of work involved in different aspects of healthcare.

Human factors analyses can be used to create assessments of the requirements of work involving demands on human performance in the physical, cognitive, and social domains. This includes the ways in which task demands, workload, and situational awareness are likely to interact to influence the performance of individuals. This knowledge can be translated to work process and system design such that human performance is optimized and system safeguards prevent human error from translating to patient injury. Formal human factors methods and measurement techniques are available, and many demonstrations of their uses exist to guide their application to healthcare. Each provides potentially useful information about factors that can limit or improve human performance. Measuring and accounting for human factors associated with healthcare delivery is likely to lead to safer and more reliable patient care.

The human factors analyses methods described in this entry are a subset of the methods most relevant to the study of error in medicine. This entry focuses on error in medicine and how human factors analyses may be applied to study and improve the quality and safety of healthcare delivery.

Human Error

Human error is often classified into one of two groups. The first group describes errors of *omission*—failing to perform a task or failing to act within a time period required by the situation. In this case, something that should have been done was not done because it was either skipped or not performed in time. The second group encompasses errors of *commission*—performing the wrong action or performing the right action incorrectly. Regardless of whether an action was performed or not, if it fails to meet an established performance standard, then it may be said to result in a state of error. Both errors of omission and commission describe a failure to achieve prescribed results in such a way that action was not performed or not performed to an acceptable standard. This includes both actions that are intentionally undertaken and those that are unintentionally committed.

Exposure to Human Error in Medicine

Medical systems function either directly or indirectly under the control of humans. This ranges from frontline medical care to the management and administrative work needed to support frontline care. For the patient, this encompasses a range of activities that begins at admission, continues through diagnosis and treatment, and ends with discharge or death. Patients may be exposed to errors through a variety of clinical and administrative activities over the course of their care. Lucian Leape and others categorized the most prevalent types of errors that patients are exposed to in an article titled "Preventing Medical Injury." *Diagnostic errors* were described as delays in diagnosis, failure to order appropriate tests, and failure to act on monitoring or test results. *Treatment errors* included, but are not limited to, errors in performance of a procedure, errors in administering a treatment, and errors in drug dose or administration. *Preventive errors* included failure to provide prophylactic treatment and inadequate monitoring or follow-up treatment. *Other errors* included communication failures, equipment failures, and other system failures. As the healthcare system has evolved to be more disaggregated and complex, it is helpful to study the causes of human error and preventable adverse events within the context of complex systems.

Human-System Error in Complex Systems

Medical specialization and advancements in medical knowledge and technology have created a complex healthcare delivery system. This complexity and disaggregation have greatly increased the opportunity for adverse events attributable to human error (i.e., preventable adverse events). Charles Perrow has discussed the propensity of human error in complex systems in other industries and attributes them in part to the nature of the systems themselves. Healthcare has been categorized as a complex and tightly coupled system. System complexity arises from the system's numerous specialized interdependent components (e.g., departments, providers, equipment). From a patient's perspective, complexity is reflected in the number of processes that must be accounted for and the dynamic nature of their relationships and response to medical treatment. Coupling refers to the degree of dependency between the system components and processes. Complex, tightly coupled systems are at greater risk for adverse events due to their inability to foresee the consequences of component interactions and the unique situations that are prone to error.

James Reason illustrates the human contribution to error in complex systems as either active or latent. Active errors occur only at the point of patient-provider interaction. The consequences of these errors are usually evident and experienced immediately. Latent errors are more suppressed, unknown, and await the appropriate initiating event or signal to trigger their effects on the system. In some cases, latent errors represent known or accepted conditions that either await correction or are not appreciated for the types of effects they may eventually unleash. Examples of latent errors include poor design, incorrect installation, poor management decisions, and poor communication processes. Latent errors are most dangerous in complex systems because of their ability to cause numerous active errors.

The study of human factors that contribute to error and preventable adverse events focuses on minimizing the risk of active and latent errors. Human factors methodologies assume that humans are imperfect and that errors are to be expected. However, there are specific factors within the work environment (i.e., system) that provoke the occurrence of errors. Just as the systems should be designed to minimize error-provoking circumstances, defense barriers and safeguards should be put in place to eliminate the ability of human error to create adverse medical events. Human factors analyses are meant to bridge the gap between system influences and human error and are especially relevant to complex systems such as healthcare. Human factors analyses may be used to study and understand human error within an environmental context and facilitate improvements, leading to better system performance and reliability.

Human Factors Analyses

Human factors analyses methods are concerned with the interaction of humans with the tools, systems, and other humans that make up their work environment. The design for these tools, systems, work, and communication processes are meant to strongly consider the characteristics, capabilities, and limitations of humans. Human factors analyses grew from work in aviation during World War II to improve cockpit design and aircrew performance. Cognitive psychology, engineering, computer science, sociology, anthropology, and artificial intelligence represent the roots of human factors methods. To date, human factors methods have been used extensively by other high-risk industries to improve human performance and organizational reliability. The application of human factors analyses in medicine has been less prevalent but is not necessarily new. Human factor analyses were first documented in medicine in the 1970s, and their application has steadily increased since then. Human factors analyses have been applied to a number of healthcare topics, including the following:

- Error reduction
- Hospital design
- Anesthesia delivery
- Patient safety
- Time and motion studies
- Workload management
- Communications and distractions
- Pharmacy operations and accuracy
- Team performance in operating rooms
- Curriculum development for medical schools
- The impact of information technologies on healthcare management and delivery

As is evident from this list, the field of human factors has always emphasized research and its application in work settings. As a result, a number of methods and tools are now available to analyze human performance. Although unique in purpose, these methods produce data that can be used within a workplace or system setting to assess requirements for safe, efficient, and economical operation in light of human capabilities and limitations. Three human factors methods that are among the most highly relevant to individuals and organizations involved in healthcare (i.e., task analyses, workload analyses, and situational awareness analyses) are described.

Task Analyses

The most common human factors method for studying human behavior in the work environment is task analysis. Task analysis involves the observation of people as they perform their work, structured interview techniques to elicit information from workers, and analysis of the resulting observations and data to describe an integrated set of activities that represent human performance in a work domain of interest. These methods employ a structured description or "decomposition" of work activities or decisions and classification of these activities as a series of tasks, processes, or classes. Each task is systematically described in terms of the mental and physical activities needed to perform the task successfully. The product of a task analysis is a description of tasks, the sequence and duration of their execution, conditions for task initiation and completion, the physical and mental dimensions of task performance, communications between work teams and between team members, and the tools and systems used to perform work. The results of task analysis are used to estimate the characteristics of predefined tasks, such as the frequency, complexity, time needed, equipment and tools needed, and communication performed.

Task analysis is an important analytical method for describing the way work is intended to be carried out. It works particularly well for sets of activities that occur in well-prescribed sequences. Results of task analysis are often ultimately used to develop or validate operational procedures, develop qualification requirements, develop training programs, and support the design of assistive tools employed in the workplace. The results may also be used to verify that the expectations for human activity are compatible with the capabilities and limitations of those expected to perform the work. This includes requirements for precision and accuracy, speed, strength, endurance, and other psychophysiological factors such as anthropometry (e.g., physical ability) and ergonomics.

Workload Analyses

Workload is a multidimensional, multifaceted concept that is difficult to define concisely. The elusiveness of a single satisfactory definition has challenged human factors researchers on many fronts and has fueled a lively and active debate among them. Even without consensus on a definition, human factors professionals agree that workload is a very valuable concept to understand and to measure in sociotechnical systems. Presently, the onset of technology and automation has greatly shifted the workload paradigm from the physical domain to the mental domain. Mental workload relates to the demands placed on a human's limited mental resources by a set of tasks being performed by an individual. The assumption behind this theory is that humans have a fixed amount of processing capacity. Tasks inherently demand processing resources, and the more difficult the task or tasks, the higher the processing capacity required for acceptable performance. If at any time the processing demands exceed the available processing capacity, performance quality may decrease. Thus, high levels of mental workload can lead to errors and poor system performance. Conversely, excessively low levels of mental workload can lead to complacency and errors, albeit for different reasons. As this implies, workload consists of an external, objective, observable referent as well as a subjective and mostly perceived referent. Both are important in understanding and predicting workload.

There are three primary methods for measuring workload: procedural, subjective, and physiological. Each of these methods can be applied in isolation, but generally, they are measured concurrently to obtain an integrated assessment of workload. *Procedural* measurement involves directly monitoring human behavior in the working environment. Task analysis, discussed above, is the most common method of procedural workload measurement.

Task analysis is used by observing a worker in an actual or simulated work setting and discerning changes in behavior as task loads vary. *Subjective* workload measures require a worker to rate or distinguish a level of workload required to perform a task. There are two major classes of subjective workload assessment techniques—unidimensional and multidimensional. Unidimensional techniques involve asking the subject for a scaled rating of overall workload for a given task condition. More comprehensive, multidimensional methods include various characteristics of perceived workload and are able to determine the nature of workload for a specific task or set of tasks. Validated workload measurement instruments include the NASA Task Load Index (NASA-TLX) and the Subjective Workload Assessment Technique (SWAT). *Physiological* techniques measure changes in subject physiology that correspond to different task demands. Most techniques emphasize cognitive task demands as opposed to actual physical demands. Studies have used physiological parameters such as heart rate, eye blink rate, perspiration, and brain activity to assess the state of workload of a human subject.

Situational Awareness Analyses

Mica Endsley defines situational awareness (SA) as a human's ability to perceive components within his or her environment (i.e., system), comprehend their meaning, and forecast their status in the future. This encompasses three distinct levels of SA. Level I SA refers to the perception of components within the environment. Level II SA involves comprehension of the current situation. Level III SA involves projecting the status of components and the situation picture in the near future. Progression through the levels of SA depends on the cognitive abilities and experience of an individual (and other team members) in performing mental operations on information from a dynamic process. SA is the product of cognitive activities and synthesis across the three levels of SA.

SA measurement can be used to evaluate system design and facilitate system improvements. Like workload measurement, SA measurement can be done using several methodologies. These methods include performance measures, subjective measures, questionnaires, and physiological measures. Again, these measurement techniques can be

administered separately, but usually, they are used simultaneously to obtain a more global assessment of SA.

Performance measures are the most objective way to measure SA. These measures are divided into two major types—external task measures and embedded task measures. External task measures involve removing information from a subject's environment and then measuring the amount of time it takes the subject to notice this difference and react. Imbedded task measures involve studying subtasks of subjects and noting subtle deviations in expected performance versus actual performance. *Subjective* measures of SA continue to be popular because of their ease of use, low cost, and applicability to real-world environments. One of the most well-known and validated ways to subjectively measure SA is by the Situational Awareness Rating Technique (SART), developed by R. Taylor in 1990. SART is a measure based on subjects' opinions that is broken up into 14 component subscales. All these subscales are integrated to create an overall SART score for a system. SART measures have shown high correlation with SA performances measures. *Questionnaires* allow for an objective assessment of SA, eliminating the disadvantages of subjective measures. They evaluate SA on a component basis and compare a subject's assessment of a situation with actual reality. The most popular questionnaire method is Endsley's Situational Awareness Global Assessment Technique (SAGAT). SAGAT executes randomized time freezes in simulation scenarios. At the time of the freeze, questions are asked of the subject about the situation to accurately evaluate the subject's knowledge of the situation. *Physiological* measures of SA are similar to physiological workload measures, but they have been proven thus far to be much more difficult to interpret. Electroencephalograms (EEG) and eye-tracking devices have been used to measure SA.

Bruce P. Hallbert, Scott R. Levin,
and Daniel J. France

See also Cognitive Psychology and Processes; Complications or Adverse Effects of Treatment; Human Cognitive Systems; Medical Errors and Errors in Healthcare Delivery; Unreliability of Memory

Further Readings

Bogner, S. (2003). *Misadventures in health care: Inside stories*. Hillsdale, NJ: Lawrence Erlbaum.

Brennan, A., Leape, L., Laird, M., Heber, L., Localio, A., Lawthers, A., et al. (1991). Incidence of adverse events and negligence in hospitalized patients: Results of the Harvard Medical Practice Study I. *New England Journal of Medicine, 324*, 370–376.

Cook, R., Woods, D., & Miller, C. (1998). *A tale of two stories: Contrasting views of patient safety*. Chicago: National Patient Safety Foundation.

Endsley, M. (1995). Toward a theory of situation awareness in dynamic systems. *Human Factors, 37*(1), 32–64.

Hart, S., & Staveland, L. (1988). Development of NASA-TLX (Task Load Index): Results of experimental and theoretical research. In P. Hancock & N. Meshkati (Eds.), *Human mental workload* (pp. 139–183). Amsterdam: North Holland.

Human Factors and Ergonomics Society: http://www.hfes.org

Institute of Medicine. (1999). *To err is human: Building a safer health system*. Washington, DC: National Academy Press.

Leape, L., Lawthers, A., Brennan, T., & Johnson, W. (1993). Preventing medical injury. *Quality Review Bulletin, 19*(5), 144–149.

Perrow, C. (1999). Organizing to reduce the vulnerabilities of complexity. *Journal of Contingencies and Crisis Management, 7*(3), 1450–1459.

Reason, J. (1990). *Human error*. Cambridge, UK: Cambridge University Press.

Salvendy, G. (1997). *Handbook of human factors and ergonomics* (2nd ed.). New York: Wiley.

Wickens, C. D. (2008). Multiple resources and mental workload. *Human Factors, 50*(3), 449–456.

ERRORS IN CLINICAL REASONING

Physicians make diagnostic and therapeutic decisions at every moment in their daily lives. Quality of care and patient outcomes, including sometimes distinction between life and death, come out of such decisions. In most cases, physicians' judgments are correct, but of course, they also fail. Errors, in fact, occur in medicine, and the Institute of Medicine's well-known report *To Err Is Human* recently called the public's and professionals' attention to this reality. Since then, the frequency and impact of adverse patient effects provoked by medical errors have been increasingly recognized. In the United States, it is estimated that medical errors result in 44,000 to 98,000 unnecessary deaths and around 1 million injuries each year. Even considering the lower estimate, deaths due to adverse events resulting from medical errors exceed the deaths attributable to motor vehicle accidents, breast cancer, or AIDS. Similar phenomena have been reported by studies in other countries. In Australia, for instance, medical errors are estimated to result in as many as 18,000 deaths, and more than 50,000 patients become disabled each year.

Medical errors occur in a variety of healthcare settings and in different stages of care. They may arise due to drug misuse or failures during the therapeutic phase, for instance, but due to their frequency and impact, diagnostic errors have received growing attention. Diagnostic error may be defined as a diagnosis that was unintentionally delayed (sufficient information for establishing the diagnosis was available earlier), incorrect (another diagnosis was made before the correct one), or missed (no diagnosis was ever made), as judged from the analysis of more definitive information. When a diagnosis is incorrect or does not entirely address the patient's problem, treatment can be delayed and/or wrong, sometimes with devastating consequences for patients and healthcare providers. Diagnostic mistakes represent a substantial and costly proportion of all medical errors. In the Harvard Medical Practice Study, the benchmark for estimating the amount of injuries occurring in hospitals, diagnostic errors represented the second largest cause of adverse events. In a recent study of autopsy, diagnostic discrepancies were found in 20% of the cases, and in half of them, knowing the correct diagnosis would have changed the case management. Indeed, postmortem studies indicate that the rates of diagnostic errors with negative impact on patient outcomes hover around 10%; this rate is stable across hospitals and countries and has not been affected by the introduction of new diagnostic technologies.

Undoubtedly, not all diagnostic errors can be attributed to faults in physicians' clinical reasoning. In a typology of medical errors that has been frequently used by Mark Graber and other authors, the so-called system-related errors come out from latent flaws in the health system that affect physicians' performance. This type of error derives from external interference and inadequate policies that affect patient care; poor coordination between care providers; inadequate communication and supervision; and factors that deteriorate working conditions, such as sleep deprivation and excessive workload. In a second category of errors, referred to as *no-fault errors*, the correct diagnosis could hardly be expected due to, for example, a silent illness or a disease with atypical presentation. However, a third category of errors, namely, *cognitive errors*, occur when a diagnosis is missed due to incomplete knowledge, faulty data gathering or interpretation, flawed reasoning, or faulty verification. As arriving at a diagnosis depends largely on a physician's reasoning, cognitive faults play an important role, particularly in diagnostic errors. Indeed, a recent study in large academic hospitals in the United States found that cognitive factors contributed to 74% of the diagnostic errors in internal medicine.

This entry addresses this latter category of errors: diagnostic failures generated by errors in clinical reasoning. First, the mental processes underlying diagnostic decisions are briefly reviewed, and subsequently, origins of medical errors are discussed. Finally, the nature of reflective reasoning in clinical problem solving and its role in minimizing diagnostic errors are discussed.

The Nature of Clinical Reasoning

Throughout the past decades, research on clinical reasoning has generated substantial empirical evidence on how physicians make diagnoses. Two main modes of processing clinical cases—nonanalytical and analytical—have been shown to underlie diagnostic decisions. Experienced doctors diagnose common problems largely by recognizing similarities between the case at hand and examples of previously seen patients. As experience grows, this so-called pattern-recognition, nonanalytical mode of clinical reasoning tends to become largely automatic and unconscious. Complex or uncommon problems, however, may trigger an analytical mode of reasoning, in which clinicians arrive at a diagnosis by analyzing signs and symptoms, relying on biomedical knowledge when necessary.

Cognitive psychology research indicates that these two different types of reasoning result from diverse kinds of knowledge used for diagnosing cases. According to Henk Schmidt and Henny Boshuizen, medical expertise development entails a process of knowledge restructuring, and therefore, knowledge structures available to medical students and physicians change throughout training and practice. In the first years of their training, medical students develop rich networks of biomedical knowledge explaining causal mechanisms of diseases. This biomedical knowledge is gradually "encapsulated" under clinical knowledge, and with clinical experience, illness scripts (i.e., cognitive structures containing little biomedical knowledge but a wealth of clinically relevant information about a disease) and examples of patients encountered are stored in memory. Experienced physicians' diagnostic reasoning is characterized largely by nonanalytical processing that relies extensively on illness scripts, examples of patients, and encapsulated knowledge. In fact, not only have illness scripts been shown to play a crucial role in hypotheses generation, but they also organize a search for additional data and interpretation of evidence, thereby acting on hypotheses refinement and diagnosis verification. However, the diverse knowledge structures developed throughout training apparently do not decay but remain as layers in memory, and earlier acquired structures may be used to deal with problems when necessary. Physicians have been shown to make use of knowledge of pathophysiological processes, for example, to understand signs and symptoms in a patient when cases are unusual or complex and when immediate explanations do not come to mind. Indeed, expert clinicians' reasoning seems to be characterized by complexity and flexibility, and apparently, different mental strategies are adopted in response to different problems' demands.

Origins of Medical Errors

Studies of medical errors point to possible failures in the generation of hypotheses, in hypotheses refinement through data gathering and interpretation, and in diagnosis verification. These failures may come from multiple sources. First, it is to be acknowledged that uncertainty is inherent to clinical decision making. Despite the high value attributed to the rational use of objective, well-established scientific knowledge within the medical domain and the growth of the medical knowledge base, this knowledge will always be insufficient to tell physicians what is to be done in a particular situation. Clinical judgment is a complex process that always involves perception and interpretation of findings within the context of a particular patient. The way diseases present themselves ranges from typical to very atypical manifestations, sometimes hardly recognizable. Physicians always have to interpret the scientific literature for making decisions in light of each patient's unique configuration of signs and symptoms, context, and needs. Second, traditional views of the physician as a neutral observer who objectively identifies and interprets a patient's signs and symptoms to make decisions have been increasingly questioned. Every physician always brings to a clinical encounter a body of medical knowledge that includes both theoretical knowledge from several disciplines and knowledge acquired through his or her own professional experience. From the interaction between this idiosyncratic body of knowledge and each unique patient, clinical knowledge required to solve the patient's problem is generated. Empirical studies have shown that physicians' experience, beliefs, and perspectives influence their perception and interpretation of features in a patient. Signs that corroborate a certain perspective may be recognized and emphasized, whereas another line of reasoning may not receive appropriate attention. Studies have shown that a suggested diagnosis influences identification and interpretation of clinical features in a patient. Misperceptions and misinterpretation of evidence, therefore, are not unusual in clinical problem solving and may compel physicians to make incorrect judgments.

Particular attention has been recently directed to the role of heuristics in medical errors. Heuristics are mental shortcuts or maxims that are used, largely unconsciously, by clinicians to expedite clinical decision making. Heuristics come out from professional experience or tradition, without being necessarily based on scientific evidence. They can be a very powerful instrument in the hands of experienced physicians, allowing them to take appropriate decisions, particularly within situations of time constraints. Nevertheless, heuristics can insert biases and distort reasoning throughout the diagnostic process, thereby generating cognitive errors.

A set of biases have been frequently pointed as underlying diagnostic errors and exemplify the potential negative effects of the use of heuristics. *Availability bias*, for instance, occurs when the judgment of the probability of a disease is influenced by readily recalled similar events. Recent or frequent experiences with a disease may, therefore, unduly increase the likelihood that it is considered as a diagnostic hypothesis. *Confirmation bias*, another frequent distortion, compels physicians to gather and value evidence that confirms a hypothesis initially considered for the case rather than searching for and considering evidence that refutes it. Confirmation bias is frequently associated with another bias, namely, *anchoring*, which occurs when the clinician remains fixed on the initial impression of the case instead of adjusting hypotheses in light of new data. As a last example, *premature closure*, accounting for a high proportion of missed diagnoses, occurs when an initial diagnosis considered for the case is accepted before all data are considered and other alternatives are verified. These are only examples of a large set of biases, of different types, that may distort diagnostic reasoning. Some of them tend to affect the generation of hypotheses, whereas others influence processing of information or hypotheses verification.

A diversity of mechanisms may act, therefore, as underlying causes of diagnostic errors. These mechanisms may be favored by an excessive reliance on nonanalytical reasoning. Nonanalytical, pattern-recognition reasoning allows physicians to efficiently diagnose most of the routine problems but may introduce distortions in clinical reasoning, thereby leading to errors. This tends to happen particularly when physicians are faced with complex, unusual, or ambiguous problems, which would require them to adopt a more analytical reasoning mode. Studies have indicated that expert doctors may in fact shift from the usual automatic way of reasoning to an analytical, effortful diagnostic approach in some situations. This happened, for instance, when doctors diagnosed cases out of their own domain of expertise and adopted an elaborate biomedical processing approach for understanding signs and symptoms. More recent empirical studies have confirmed that doctors may engage in effortful reflection for diagnosing cases, which affects the quality of their diagnoses. These studies reflect a recent interest in the analytical mode of diagnosing clinical cases. Research on clinical reasoning has traditionally focused on how physicians diagnose clinical problems through nonanalytical reasoning, and therefore, a substantial amount of empirical data about this mode of case processing are available. Not so much is known, however, about physicians' reasoning when they engage in reflection for solving clinical problems. Only recently, stimulated by concerns with avoidable medical errors, attention has been directed to the analytical diagnostic reasoning, and research conducted within the framework of reflective practice in medicine has contributed to shed some light on the nature and effects of reflection while solving clinical cases.

Reflective Reasoning and Diagnostic Errors

Reflective practice has been conceptualized as doctors' ability to critically reflect on their own reasoning and decisions while in professional activities. Critically reflecting on one's own practice has long been valued as a requirement for good clinical performance. Ronald Epstein suggested that by inserting "mindfulness" in their practice, physicians would become aware of their own reasoning processes during clinical problem solving. *Mindful practice*, as he called it, would compel physicians to observe themselves while observing the patient. It would then enable physicians to realize how their own body of knowledge, beliefs, values, and experiences influences their perception and interpretation of features encountered in a patient, thereby leading them to questioning and improving their own judgments.

Other authors, such as Pat Croskerry, have emphasized the potential role of metacognition, which means critically reflecting on one's own thinking processes as a crucial condition for good diagnostic performance. Metacognition consists of the ability to explore a broader range of possibilities than those initially considered for a case, the capacity to examine and critique one's own decisions, and the ability to select strategies to deal with decision-making demands.

Although they are easily encountered in the literature on medical errors, only recently did conceptualizations such as mindful practice, reflection, or reflective practice start to be investigated by empirical research. Recent studies provided empirical

evidence of the nature of reflective practice in medicine. Reflective practice comprises at least five sets of behaviors, attitudes, and reasoning processes in response to complex problems encountered in professional practice: (1) an inclination to deliberately search for alternative hypotheses in addition to the ones initially generated when seeking explanations for a complex, unfamiliar problem; (2) an inclination to explore the consequences of these alternative explanations, resulting in predictions that might be tested against new data; (3) a willingness to test these predictions against new data gathered from the case and synthesize new understandings about the problem; (4) an attitude of openness toward reflection that leads reflective doctors to engage in thoughtful, effortful reasoning in response to a challenging problem; and (5) a willingness and ability to reflect about one's own thinking processes and to critically examine conclusions and assumptions about a particular problem, that is, metareasoning.

A physician who is open to reflection tends to recognize difficulties in solving a problem and to accept uncertainty while further exploring the problem instead of searching for a quick solution. By engaging in reflective practice, physicians would bring to consciousness and critically examine their own reasoning processes. Patients' problems would, therefore, be explored more thoroughly; alternative hypotheses would be more easily considered and more extensively verified. Clinical judgments would improve, and errors would be reduced. Although theoretically justified, these statements have only recently been supported by empirical studies. Experimental studies with internal medicine residents have explored the effects of the two main modes of reasoning—nonanalytical and reflective—on the quality of diagnoses. Residents were asked to diagnose simple and complex cases by following, in each experimental condition, instructions that led to either a nonanalytical or a reflective approach. Reflective reasoning was shown to improve the accuracy of diagnoses in complex clinical cases, whereas it made no difference in diagnoses of simple, routine cases. In a subsequent study with internal medical residents, this positive effect of reflective reasoning on the diagnosis of difficult, ambiguous clinical cases was reaffirmed.

These recent studies indicate that diagnostic decisions would improve by adjusting reasoning approaches to situational demands. While nonanalytical reasoning seems to be highly effective for solving routine cases, complex, unusual, or unique clinical problems would require physicians to shift to a more analytical, reflective reasoning. This statement, however, is not so simple and obvious as it seems at first sight. As nonanalytical reasoning is inherently associated with expertise development, how would experienced physicians, who tend to reason highly automatically, recognize when a problem requires further reflection? It has been demonstrated that physicians in fact shift to analytical reasoning approaches, but conditions that break down automaticity are still under investigation. An experimental study with medical residents indicated that, as could be expected, the complexity of the case to be diagnosed seems to be one of these conditions. However, not only may the characteristics of the case itself trigger reflection, but apparently, contextual information may also play a role. In another study with residents, only information that other physicians had previously incorrectly diagnosed the case led participants to adopt a reflective approach. It is likely that factors related to the environment where the case is solved or to physicians' characteristics restrict or favor reflection. As an example, a study exploring correlates of reflective practice suggested that physicians with more years of practice and those working in primary-care settings in which high standards of performance are not so much valued tend to engage less frequently in reflection for diagnosing patients' problems.

These first studies shed some light on the conditions that trigger reflective reasoning and its effect on the quality of diagnoses, but much more remains to be explored. What seems clear now is that minimization of avoidable diagnostic errors depends on physicians' ability to adjust reasoning strategies to the problem at hand and appropriately, flexibly combine nonanalytical and reflective reasoning. While the usual pattern-recognition, nonanalytical approach allows physicians to efficiently solve familiar problems, diagnoses of complex or unusual problems would benefit from reflection. Much more, however, needs to be known about the knowledge structures and mental processes that constitute reflective reasoning, the conditions that lead physicians to effortful reflection while diagnosing cases, and the relative effectiveness of the different reasoning modes in various situations. By further investigating these issues, it would be possible to open perspectives for designing and testing educational interventions aimed at refining medical students' and practicing physicians' clinical reasoning.

Sílvia Mamede, Henk G. Schmidt,
and Remy Rikers

See also Automatic Thinking; Bias; Cognitive Psychology and Processes; Heuristics; Medical Errors and Errors in Healthcare Delivery

Further Readings

Corrigan, J., Kohn, L. T., & Donaldson, M. S. (Eds.). (2000). *To err is human: Building a safer health system.* Washington, DC: Institute of Medicine/ National Academy Press.

Croskerry, P. (2003). The importance of cognitive errors in diagnosis and strategies to minimize them. *Academic Medicine, 78,* 775–780.

Epstein, R. M. (1999). Mindful practice. *Journal of the American Medical Association, 282,* 833–839.

Graber, M. L., Franklin, N., & Gordon, R. (2005). Diagnostic error in internal medicine. *Archives of Internal Medicine, 165,* 1493–1499.

Kassirer, J. P., & Kopelman, R. I. (1991). *Learning clinical reasoning.* Baltimore: Williams & Wilkins.

Kempainen, R. R., Migeon, M. B., & Wolf, F. M. (2003). Understanding our mistakes: A primer on errors in clinical reasoning. *Medical Teacher, 25*(2), 177–181.

Kuhn, G. J. (2002). Diagnostic errors. *Academic Emergency Medicine, 9,* 740–750.

Mamede, S., & Schmidt, H. G. (2004). The structure of reflective practice in medicine. *Medical Education, 38,* 1302–1308.

Mamede, S., Schmidt, H. G., & Penaforte, J. C. (2008). Effect of reflective practice on accuracy of medical diagnoses. *Medical Education, 42,* 468–475.

Rikers, R. M. J. P., Schmidt, H. G., & Boshuizen, H. P. A. (2002). On the constraints of encapsulated knowledge: Clinical case representations by medical experts and subexperts. *Cognition and Instruction, 20*(1), 27–45.

Schmidt, H. G., & Boshuizen, H. P. A. (1993). On acquiring expertise in medicine. *Educational Psychology Review, 5,* 1–17.

Schmidt, H. G., & Rikers, R. M. J. P. (2007). How expertise develops in medicine: Knowledge encapsulation and illness script formation. *Medical Education, 41,* 1133–1139.

Weingart, S. N., Wilson, R. M., Gibberd, R. W., & Harrison, B. (2000). Epidemiology of medical error. *British Medical Journal, 320,* 774–777.

ETHNOGRAPHIC METHODS

The term *ethnography* describes both a literary genre (writings that attempt to capture people's cultural beliefs/practices) and a qualitative research methodology (a way of collecting social scientific data based on long-term, face-to-face interactions). In the current era, ethnographic analysis seems to have lost some of its authority, especially since human genomics and the statistical analysis of massive data sets are privileged in the search for contemporary solutions to social problems. Even still, ethnography is alive and well and can be used to inform medical decision making.

Data Collection

Anthropology and sociology are the two academic disciplines that traditionally cornered the market on ethnographic methods, but other social sciences have become more interested in the kinds of nuanced information that is gathered during intimate and ongoing interactions between qualitative researchers and their research subjects, interactions euphemized as "deep hanging out." Ethnographers spend time drinking beers with the folks they study, eating meals at their dinner tables, and shadowing them on the job—all in an effort to figure out what people's everyday lives actually look like and to determine how people make sense of those lives.

When they first start conducting research in a particular community, ethnographers may stand out like sore thumbs, drawing attention to themselves and making their research subjects self-conscious, which means that they run the risk of witnessing things that probably wouldn't have taken place at all without the conspicuous seductions of an outside audience. But as ethnographers spend more and more time observing and participating in the same community, among the same community members, they eventually begin to lose some of their distracting influence on people's behaviors. They transform into proverbial flies on the wall. The ethnographer is still there, asking questions and watching people's daily reactions, but is hardly noticed any more, not in ways that might compromise the reliability of what the ethnographer sees or hears.

Ethnography's value is based on the kinds of intimate and unguarded data that researchers gain from extended contact with one particular social group. When the discipline first emerged, this meant relatively small-scale and remote societies. Bronislaw Malinowski's early-20th-century work with Trobrianders is taken as a powerful marker for the birth of full-fledged ethnographic research within anthropology. He crossed the seas, pitched his tent, and found a way to live among people whose cultural world seemed radically different from his own. Part of the point, of course, was about making it clear to the European audience back home that those foreign practices could be understood only with the fullest knowledge of how people's entire belief systems fit together—even and especially when those cultural systems seemed spectacularly exotic to the Western eye.

Ethnography in Anthropology and Sociology

Anthropology was traditionally about studying societies unsullied by the advances of modernity. From the attempts at *salvage ethnography* among Native American tribes in the early 19th century (archiving cultural practices before they disappeared forever) to the constructions of primitive societies as examples of the modern Western world's hypothetical pasts, anthropologists used ethnographic methods to study those populations most removed from the taint of modern living.

Sociologists also embraced ethnographic methods in the early 20th century, and people like Robert Park at the University of Chicago helped institutionalize the *ethnographic imagination* as a method for studying not just faraway villages but also modern urban life in a teeming American city. That dividing line (between the anthropological ethnographer who studies some distant community and the sociological ethnographer who focuses her eyes on the modern Western metropolis) still defines most people's assumptions about how those two fields carve up the social landscape for qualitative examination (even though there are certainly sociologists who study small-scale societies and anthropologists who have been working in urban America for a very long time).

Both fields sometimes seem to place a premium on something close to the scientific equivalent of roughing it. They each have the highest regard for the "gonzo" ethnographer, the kind of heroic or mythical figure willing to put his or her very life at risk for the sake of ethnographic access. The more remote, removed, and potentially dangerous the location of the fieldwork experience, the more explicit and awestruck are the kudos offered up to any ethnographer bold enough to go where few have gone before. This search for dangerous exoticism can lead one halfway around the world or just to the other side of the tracks, the other end of town. But in either case, an added value is placed on access to the everyday lives of human beings and cultural perspectives that most middle-class Western readers know little about.

During the 1960s, anthropologists and sociologists in the United States wrote classic ethnographic offerings on the urban poor—specifically, the black poor, who were struggling to make ends meet in America's ghettos. Ethnographers were trying to explain the hidden realities of urban poverty, a tradition that continues today. Anthropologists and sociologists working in American cities still disproportionately study poor minority communities. That's because it may be harder to entice wealthier Americans to accept such scholarly intrusions. A $20 bill might suffice as an incentive for unemployed urbanites to answer some open-ended questions about their life history (and to allow an ethnographer to shadow them on an average afternoon), but it may not be enough to persuade middle-class citizens to expose their raw lives to an ethnographic gaze. Middle-class and wealthier Americans also sometimes live in gated communities or attend restricted social clubs, to which anthropologists may not have access. These same kinds of biases also tend to predetermine the kinds of communities ethnographers have access to abroad.

Traditionally, ethnographers have been taught that they must master the culture of the groups they study so completely that they should almost be able to see the world from that group's point of view, almost as if they were born into the community. Anthropologists call this an "emic" perspective, something that can only be acquired with long-term participant observation—many months, even years, of deep hanging out with the people being studied.

Medical Anthropology

The growing subfield of medical anthropology interrogates the often masked cultural assumptions that subtly inform medical decision making on the part of both doctors and their patients. Medical anthropologists deploy ethnographic methods (a) to uncover the hidden ethnocentricisms that might sometimes allow doctors trained in the West to underestimate the value of folk medicinal practices; (b) to describe how the roles of "doctor" and "patient" are constructed from social and cultural templates that usually go unexamined or unspoken; and (c) to emphasize how broader cultural expectations and interpretations configure the way medical practitioners conceptualize/ operationalize diseases and translate medical theories for a lay audience. Ethnographers such as Rayna Rapp and Paul Farmer mobilize ethnographic methods (studying medicine as an inescapably cultural—not just biological or genetic— domain) to mount critiques of presuppositions that sometimes obstruct professional attempts to negotiate the political, moral, and biological dilemmas of medical treatment.

Future Directions

Ethnographers have started to retool this methodological intervention for the newness of the empirical present, calling for (a) multisitedness, (b) a specific focus on the culture of medical research, and (c) particular emphasis on the challenges that come with studying a media-saturated world. Even still, there remains something inescapably troubling to some ethnographers about ethnographic attempts to study several places at once, to engage phenomena spread out over large expanses of space in ways that outstrip any ethnographer's ability to experience them directly and holistically. Does it mean sacrificing depth for breadth, and how much does that compromise ethnography's specific contribution to the constellation of methodological options open to social scientific researchers?

John L. Jackson Jr.

See also Cultural Issues; Qualitative Methods

Further Readings

Cerwonka, A., & Malkki, L. H. (2007). *Improvising theory: Process and temporality in ethnographic fieldwork.* Chicago: University of Chicago Press.

Clifford, J., & Marcus, G. E. (Eds.). (1986). *Writing culture: The poetics and politics of ethnography.* Berkeley: University of California Press.

Farmer, P. (1993). *AIDS and accusation: Haiti and the geography of blame.* Berkeley: University of California Press.

Madison, D. S. (2005). *Critical ethnography: Method, ethics, and performance.* Thousand Oaks, CA: Sage.

Marcus, G. E. (1998). *Ethnography through thick and thin.* Princeton, NJ: Princeton University Press.

Rabinow, P. (2003). *Anthropos today: Reflections on modern equipment.* Princeton, NJ: Princeton University Press.

Rapp, R. (1999). *Testing women, testing the fetus: The social impact of amniocentesis in America.* New York: Routledge.

Willis, P. (2000). *The ethnographic imagination.* Cambridge, UK: Polity Press.

EuroQoL (EQ-5D)

EuroQol, also referred to as EQ-5D, is one of the multi-attribute health status classification systems. It is a generic instrument for measuring the health-related quality of life. Along with other multi-attribute health status classification systems, such as Health Utilities Index (HUI) and Quality of Well-Being (QWB), EuroQol is used as an alternative to measure the utility or health preference. Measuring utilities or preferences can be a complex and time-consuming task. EuroQol is attractive due to its simplicity. Thus, it has been widely used throughout the world in both clinical investigations and health policy determinations.

The EuroQol questionnaire was developed by the EuroQol group, original members of which came from various research teams in Europe. The name EuroQol comes from European Quality of Life. There are three components within the EuroQol questionnaire. The first component, the most important one, comprises five dimensions (5D): mobility, self-care, usual activities, pain/discomfort, and anxiety/depression.

EuroQol Questionnaire

The EuroQol group was established in 1987, with investigators coming from various countries in western Europe. The group has expanded into an organization with members from all over the world in 1994. The EuroQol questionnaire is designed for self-completion by the respondents, and it was initially developed to complement other health-related quality-of-life measures. The primary component of the EuroQol questionnaire originally had six dimensions: mobility, self-care, main activity, social relationships, pain, and mood. EuroQol has become a stand-alone questionnaire subsequently, and the primary component was revised to five dimensions, including mobility, self-care, usual activities, pain/discomfort, and anxiety/depression. It has been publicly available since 1990.

The EuroQol questionnaire has three components. The first component is the primary one that includes five dimensions. Each dimension is measured by a question that has three possible responses: no problem, some problem, or severe problem. A preference-based index score can be created based on the answers to these five dimensions. The second component of the EuroQol questionnaire is a visual analog scale, where respondents can indicate their current health status on a "thermometer" scaled from 0, *the worst imaginable health state*, to 100, *the best imaginable health state*. The third component of the EuroQol questionnaire is for respondents to answer their background information, including disease experience, age, gender, smoking status, education, and others. The first two components are the instruments to be used if the researchers are only interested in knowing the health-related quality of life from the respondents.

Preference-Based Scoring Algorithm

Since the first component of the EuroQol questionnaire has five dimensions, with each having three levels of answers, the combination of responses results in 243 (3^5) possible health states. Methods were developed to assign preference scores to each of the 243 health states that represent an average preference for one state versus another. By adding two additional health states, "unconscious" and "dead" for a total of 245 health states, this method was initially developed based on a random sample of about 3,000 adults in the United Kingdom. The scoring function was developed using econometric modeling based on the time trade-off technique. The final preference-based index scores were assessed on a scale where 0 represents *a health state of being dead* and 1 represents *perfect health.*

The first component of the EuroQol has also been weighted according to the social preferences of the U.S. population. Similarly, the U.S.-based EuroQol preference-based scoring algorithm was developed using econometric modeling through the time trade-off technique. A representative sample of the U.S. general adult population with approximately 4,000 participants completed the interview. The interview was carried out in the United Kingdom and the United States in 1993 and 2002, respectively.

Application

As a quick and well-validated instrument, the EuroQol has been widely used in clinical and economic evaluations of healthcare as well as in population health surveys. The EuroQol is available in many languages. Most researchers use the first two components of the EuroQol questionnaire for respondents to rate their current health states. Both the preference-based index and the visual analog scale have been used in various ways, including establishing national and local population health status, comparing patients' health status at different times, and evaluating the seriousness of disease at different times. The EuroQol has also been used in a number of clinical areas to provide effectiveness outcomes during the drug approval process. Recent work has furnished a national catalog of the EuroQol preference-based index for all chronic conditions in the United States.

The score provided by the EuroQol is important in cost-effectiveness analysis, where quality-adjusted

life year (QALY) has become increasingly used to assess the treatment outcomes in clinical trials and health economic evaluations. However, EuroQol is designed to measure generic and global health-related quality of life. It is not sensitive or comprehensive enough to measure disease-specific quality of life.

Analyzing the EuroQol Preference-Based Index in Regressions

Previous research has noted that the EuroQol preference-based index score is, similar to other utility scores, far from being normally distributed. Methods designed for continuous data, such as the ordinary least squares (OLS) regression, are often inappropriate for such data. The OLS models the conditional mean as a linear function of the covariates. The idiosyncrasies of the EuroQol index distribution demand that the residuals should not be assumed to be normal or have constant variance. Although versions of OLS exist that are valid without any distributional assumptions on the residuals, the special features of the EuroQol index are neglected by only modeling the conditional mean.

Several other methods have been proposed, including the Tobit model and the censored least absolute deviations estimator (CLAD). One important feature of the EuroQol index score distribution is that many individuals reported perfect health with their EuroQol index at 1.0, thus forming a spike. The Tobit model and the CLAD model are extensions of the OLS that treat the health status of these patients as being *censored* at 1.0; that is, their health status, if it can be mapped onto the scale of EuroQol index, would be larger than 1.0. In other words, these methods assume that there is an underlying latent health status variable. When it is less than 1.0, it is observed as the EuroQol index; when it is larger than 1.0, we only observe EuroQol = 1 as an indicator of censoring. These methods then model the conditional mean of the latent variable, instead of EuroQol itself, as a linear function of the covariates. The difference between the Tobit model and the CLAD model is that Tobit model assumes that the latent variable has a normal distribution, while in the CLAD model, the latent variable can have any continuous distribution. Therefore, the Tobit model can be viewed as a special case of the CLAD model.

A two-part model approach has also been proposed to model the special features of the EuroQol index, particularly a large proportion of subjects having the score at 1.0. The first part is a logistic model for the probability of reaching the maximum score. The second part is a model for the rest of the scores that are less than 1.0, which can be either a least squares regression with robust standard errors for the conditional mean or a quantile regression for conditional quantiles such as the median. It has been shown that the two-part model has some desirable features that are not available in the aforementioned regression methods for the EuroQol preference-based index score.

Alex Z. Fu

See also Expected Utility Theory; Health Utilities Index Mark 2 and 3 (HUI2, HUI3); Quality of Well-Being Scale; Utility Assessment Techniques

Further Readings

Dolan, P. (1997). Modeling variations for EuroQol health states. *Medical Care, 35,* 1095–1108.

Drummond, M. F., Sculpher, M. J., Torrance, G. W., O'Brien, B. J., & Stoddart, G. L. (2005). Cost-utility analysis. In *Methods for the economic evaluation of health care programmes* (3rd ed., pp. 137–209). Oxford, UK: Oxford University Press.

Fu, A. Z., & Kattan, M. W. (2006). Racial and ethnic differences in preference-based health status measure. *Current Medical Research and Opinion, 22,* 2439–2448.

Li, L., & Fu, A. Z. (2008). Methodological issues with the analysis of preference-based EQ-5D index score. *Value in Health, 11,* A181.

Shaw, J. W., Johnson, J. A., & Coons, J. S. (2005). US valuation of the EQ-5D health states: Development and testing of the D1 valuation model. *Medical Care, 43,* 203–220.

Sullivan, P. W., & Ghushchyan, V. (2006). Preference-based EQ-5D index scores for chronic conditions in the United States. *Medical Decision Making, 26,* 410–420.

Sullivan, P. W., Lawrence, W. F., & Ghushchyan, V. (2005). A national catalog of preference-based scores for chronic conditions in the United States. *Medical Care, 43,* 736–749.

Evaluating and Integrating Research Into Clinical Practice

The impetus for evidence-based medicine (EBM), or its younger brother, evidence-based practice, has been that it takes too long for efficacious and effective treatments to be brought to bear in routine clinical practice. The usual time given is a 17-year delay between demonstration of efficacy and routine practice, although the evidence for this specific time frame is sparse. However, as a social value in medicine, most believe that it is better for patients to receive effective care than none, so regardless of the true time delay, researchers, healthcare administrators, policy makers, clinicians, and patients all now recognize as crucial the systemic issues that delay the integration of research into practice. Like medical care, addressing this issue requires diagnosis of the systemic issues that prevent the translation of research into practice (TRIP) and requires treatment based on those diagnoses.

Diagnosis

A number of different approaches have been used to diagnose the systemic barriers. One is the diffusion of innovation formalism. Rogers identified five components of diffusion: (1) relative advantage, (2) compatibility, (3) complexity, (4) trialability, and (5) observability. Berwick and Greenhalgh provide a general framework for applying these to medical care. Early studies documented the slow uptake of basic innovations and documented, for instance, from the physician's point of view, the need for observability—the need for a local champion. Later studies showed that apparently not much had changed; from the patient's perspective, only about 55% received recommendation-based care for preventive, acute, or chronic care. Cabana showed the application of a barrier-based framework to the (non)use of clinical practice guidelines (CPGs), touted as one solution to the TRIP problem. He discerned that barriers ranged from issues of physician self-efficacy to systemic difficulties in getting access to the guidelines as well as traditional concerns such as disagreement over applicability.

Treatment

There are two basic approaches to the incorporation of research-based evidence into practice: active and passive. *Active* means that the clinical practitioner must make the explicit effort of finding the evidence and evaluating it. *Passive* means that the environment has been architected to bring the evidence to bear automatically.

Active Approaches

The primary active approach has been to teach clinicians the process of EBM in the hope that they would use those methods at the bedside. Supporting this agenda has required several components. First, EBM resources have been needed. The primary one has been PubMed, which references several thousand journals and several million articles. Almost all EBM searches end up at PubMed (in English-speaking countries), because the latest, authoritative results are available there. Searches there depend on skillful use of the PubMed-controlled vocabulary—MeSH (Medical Subject Headings)—as well as free text and other specifics of the indexing system. The Cochrane Database of Systematic Reviews houses systematic reviews of studies (primarily randomized controlled trials) that, themselves, are often indexed on PubMed. However, these reviews are extensive, reproducible, and go beyond PubMed, to include unpublished articles or novel data provided by published authors. Perforce, these reviews are not as current as PubMed. CPGs go beyond Cochrane reviews in authority, because they include the definition of standard of practice, as defined by professional societies. Because of this added layer of vetting, CPGs are the least up-to-date but the most authoritative. Thus, a reasonable search strategy is to start with CPGs (as indexed or contained at the National Guideline Clearinghouse), then move on to Cochrane to see if there is anything newer, and then move on to PubMed to look for anything newer still.

Evidence searching goes beyond the searching of reference or full-text databases to include evaluation or appraisal of the report found. Tools that support this process include the *JAMA* reading guides and worksheets; both are available via the University of Alberta.

There are many sites on the Web that cater to clinicians. Each of them requires clinicians to go on their own through the cycle of searching and evaluating the retrieved evidence. Some sites such as the TRIP site in the United Kingdom search many sites for the user and bring them together. Choosing, appraising, and using any specific source is left to the user.

There are also a number of commercial tools that supply resources and levels of evidence, are kept up-to-date, and are available on handheld devices.

Finally, there is a small industry in teaching EBM methods to clinicians, whether in medical school, through journals, on the Web, or in continuing medical education (CME) classes.

Evidence shows that medical students can learn the methods, that physicians do not have time to use them, and that CME lecturing is the least effective way of learning a skill.

Passive Approaches

In passive approaches, barriers are broached by others. Pharmaceutical companies invest more than any others in educating clinicians about available evidence, but they are generally not thought to have the clinician's EBM process as their primary goal. On the other hand, pharmaceutical methods have been tried through *academic detailing*, where trained staff attempt to teach clinicians about the best evidence and most effective therapies with one-on-one encounters. While there have been successes, they have been frustratingly Pyrrhic and not clearly worth the investment required.

Decision support systems, embedded in clinicians' workflow, have been thought to offer the best possibility of getting the best evidence and practice before a clinician's eyes, with the system's blessing. There are several degrees of decision support relevant to TRIP.

The first type is generic access to relevant material. This access is usually to the CPG and leaves the user to read the text (if guided to it) and apply it as seen fit. The next level of access is more tailored, using an "Infobutton," where the computer system uses generic patient information to find generic information about that patient. So a patient's diagnosis of sickle-cell disease will be used by the system to provide the user with instant access to definitions, normal values, textbook entries, and CPGs on sickle-cell disease. The next level of access is customized, where the system takes several pieces of information about the patient and provides access to yet more specialized information, say, a relevant PubMed reference. Systems providing such access are rare and, because of the difficulty of automating the EBM process, end up leaving it to the user to judge the applicability or evidential quality of the linked article, since there can be no ante vetting by the system builders.

The next class of decision support is guided choice, where evidence can be put into the workflow by making it difficult to act on the basis of bad evidence. Thus, the generic guided choice may be a calculator for total parenteral solution ordering that would prevent generic conditions such as high osmolarity or simultaneous inclusion of calcium and bicarbonate in the solution. The next level of decision support is tailored guided choice, such as order sets. Here, guideline-based care can be instituted by the healthcare organization by specifying, for example, that any discharge of a patient with a myocardial infarction will include a prescription for a beta blocker. Thus, rather than rely on the physician having read the CPG, the systematic review, and the most recent articles confirming the effectiveness of such prescribing; rather than rely on the physician remembering this effectiveness at the time of discharge; and rather than rely on the physician ordering it, the system provides a checkbox for the physician; checking that box represents the entire evidence search and evaluation cycle. The challenge is for the system to know that the specific patient had a myocardial infarction at the time of discharge and to make sure that the physician is using the computer system to enter discharge orders.

Customized guided choice is possible as well but is generally not available. Here, the system composes a checklist, say, for the specific patient. While composing a checklist from a union of other checklists is clearly easily done, checking for interferences, dependencies, and other interactions is much less so.

The third class of decision support is knowledge-based prompts; these are the classic alerts, where the physician has ordered something and the machine responds that that order is in error, or the physician has not ordered something and the computer recommends an action. The knowledge behind these alerts is generally framed as rules, and these rules are usually referenced to the literature. While the knowledge of effectiveness would seem to be the same across institutions, the ideal of sharing rules has not been borne out by the realities of system implementation because of the variety of ways in which different systems store the information needed by the rules. Thus, each institution is left to vet its own rules on its own. In addition, commercial entities that sell knowledge bases, such as those containing evidence-based drug-drug interactions, are concerned with their own risk profile and so include a wide range of interactions that make the systems generally unusable, leaving institutions, again, to face the decisions themselves over what alerts to keep and what not even to show the physician.

The evidence on all such systems is mixed. Kawamoto and colleagues' systematic review showed the systems to have a positive impact 68% of the time and confirmed the factors most likely to lead to success: providing decision support within the context of the workflow at the place and time the action was needed, providing action items (not just assessments), and using a computer-based system. The harms that provider-order entry systems have demonstrated recently have not been related to evidence-based decision support. However, too much experience shows that the low specificity and high sensitivity of the alerts leads to "alert fatigue" and inattention when the system cries wolf.

The Future

Interventions for evidence-based practice are based on the experience of EBM but with application to different domains. Evidence-based nursing has led to specific resources for nurses but not the depth of computer-based support that clinicians have available to them. Evidence-based public health has focused on clinical issues and not on the more systemic interventions that public health practitioners must effect nor on the more global concerns that affect their work. There are some generic and guided-choice-based tools for decision support, but outside of biosurveillance, there is little decision support based on knowledge-based prompts, and in biosurveillance, the alerts are not necessarily based on research evidence. Each of these areas will likely grow in the future.

The National Institutes of Health's initiative regarding Clinical and Translational Science Awards will push innovation to the "left" side of the translation and evidence-generation process. The new innovations may aggravate matters by generating too many technologies to accommodate—or may induce a new attention to the entire translation process on the "right"-hand side. Such attention jibes well with the new attention given to the care provider system itself. Computer-based decision support systems seem to be the best bet for bringing evidence into practice. A further source of evidence will be the electronic patient record itself, as the data from operational use are stored in clinical data warehouses for mining and local research. Such research will overcome several of Roger's barriers:

1. Relative advantage could be assessed directly or modeled, based on local data.

2. Compatibility could be assessed by reviewing the number and types of patients to whom the new evidence (technology) applies.

3. Complexity could be assessed through an environmental scan of clinic, unit, and staff capabilities.

4. Trialability could be assessed through pilot projects whose data are made available in a regular manner.

5. Observability could be achieved by review of the data warehouse data of patients treated with the new technology.

It may just require linking the workaday, sloppy observational data of routine care with the pristine results of carefully constructed studies to achieve the long-wished-for goal that patients receive the best care that science says they should receive. This possibility provides researchers with further challenges in providing healthcare institutions and clinicians the new tools they need to achieve this synthesis.

Harold Lehmann

See also Clinical Algorithms and Practice Guidelines; Computational Limitations; Evidence-Based Medicine; Randomized Clinical Trials

Further Readings

Avorn, J., & Soumerai, S. B. (1983). Improving drug-therapy decisions through educational outreach: A randomized controlled trial of academically based "detailing." *New England Journal of Medicine, 308*(24), 1457–1463.

Berwick, D. M. (1975). Disseminating innovations in health care. *Journal of the American Medical Association, 289*(15), 1969–1975.

Cabana, M. D., Rand, C. S., Powe, N. R., Wu, A. W., Wilson, M. H., Abboud, P.-A. C., et al. (1999). Why don't physicians follow clinical practice guidelines? A framework for improvement. *Journal of the American Medical Association, 282*(15), 1458–1465.

Cimino, J. J., Aguirre, A., Johnson, S. B., & Peng, P. (1993). Generic queries for meeting clinical information needs. *Bulletin of the Medical Library Association, 81*(2), 195–206.

Cochrane Database of Systematic Reviews: http://www.cochrane.org

Greenhalgh, T., Robert, G., Macfarlane, F., Bate, P., Kyriakidou, O., & Peacock, R. (2005). Storylines of research in diffusion of innovation: A meta-narrative approach to systematic review. *Social Science & Medicine, 61*(2), 417–430.

Grimshaw, J. M., Thomas, R. E., MacLennan, G., Fraser, C., Ramsay, C. R., Vale, L., et al. (2004). Effectiveness and efficiency of guideline dissemination and implementation strategies. *Health Technology Assessment, 8*(6), iii–iv, 1–72.

Kawamoto, K., Houlihan, C. A., Balas, E. A., & Lobach, D. F. (2005). Improving clinical practice using clinical decision support systems: A systematic review of trials to identify features critical to success. *British Medical Journal, 330*(7494), 765.

Institute of Medicine. (2001). *Crossing the quality chasm: A new health system for the 21st century.* Washington, DC: National Academy Press.

McGlynn, E. A., Asch, S. M., & Adams, J. (2003). The quality of health care delivered to adults in the United States. *New England Journal of Medicine, 348,* 2635–2545.

National Guideline Clearinghouse: http://www.guideline.gov

Perreault, L. E., & Metzger, J. (1999). A pragmatic framework for understanding clinical decision support. *Journal of Healthcare Information Management, 13*(2), 5–21.

PubMed: http://www.ncbi.nlm.nih.gov/sites/entrez?db=pubmed

Rogers, E. M. (1995). *Diffusion of innovations* (4th ed.). New York: The Free Press.

University of Alberta, Evidence Based Medicine Toolkit: http://www.med.ualberta.ca/ebm

Williamson, J. W., German, P. S., Weiss, R., Skinner, E. A., & Bowes, F. (1989). Health science information management and continuing education of physicians: A survey of U.S. primary care practitioners and their opinion leaders. *Annals of Internal Medicine, 110,* 151–160.

EVALUATING CONSEQUENCES

Decisions in medical contexts have immediate and obvious consequences in terms of health and sometimes death or survival. Medical decisions also have less obvious and less immediate consequences, including effects on the long-term physical and mental well-being of patients, their families, and caregivers, as well as on the distribution of scarce medical resources. Some of these consequences are hard to measure or estimate. Even harder, perhaps, is the determination of the relative value of different consequences. How should consequences be evaluated? How do uncertainties and biases affect our evaluations? What influence should our evaluations of consequences have on our actions? These questions are all philosophical in nature.

Consequences and Value

To evaluate something is most basically to determine its value or to determine its effect on that which has value. The positive value of health may be taken as a given in medical decision making. Sometimes, however, it is not clear what concrete outcomes contain more health. Will a patient in chronic pain be more healthy taking opiates that reduce her mental abilities and may create dependency, or will she be more healthy without opiates but with more pain? Will an elderly patient with myeloma enjoy better health after treatment with cytostatics that pacify the disease but weaken the immune system, or will his health be better without the treatment? Depending on the details of the case, the answers to these questions are far from obvious, showing that the concept of health is complex and will sometimes stand in need of specification.

Health may be defined biomedically as the absence of disease and infirmity. This is the common definition in medical practice, though seldom explicitly stated. Alternatively, health may be defined biopsychosocially, which is common in theoretical contexts. The 1946 constitution of the World Health Organization (WHO) states that health is "a state of complete physical, mental and social well-being." Several recent definitions aim to avoid the somewhat utopian character of the WHO definition and to shift focus from outcome to opportunity, by defining health in terms of potential or ability rather than well-being.

Quantitative measurements of health have increasingly been made in terms of quality-adjusted life years (QALYs), that is, the number of person life years adjusted by a factor representing the quality of the person's life. Like health, quality of life may be defined biomedically or biopsychosocially, and more or less broadly. What will be said in the following about values in general and health in particular holds equally for quality of life. Regardless of how exactly quality is defined, evaluating consequences in terms of QALYs incorporates a richer understanding of why we value life, as opposed to measuring only years of life of whatever quality or only death or survival. A strategy of QALY *maximization* has the further advantage of allowing quantitative comparisons of different alternatives, such as treatment programs, but has the disadvantage that other values may be disregarded, such as equity and autonomy.

Like any value, the value of health may be final and/or instrumental. Health is obviously instrumental to other values such as happiness and achievement. In other words, we need health to promote or protect these other values. In addition, however, health may also be of final value—of value in itself, independently of its impact on other values. Whether or not health has final value becomes important in conflict cases, where it must be balanced against other values. If, for example, health, defined biomedically, is important only because of its instrumental contribution to the higher value of happiness, a healthy life without happiness has no value. This conclusion may have direct relevance for important medical decisions concerning life and death, including the issue of euthanasia.

Values may be subjective or objective. That the value of health is subjective would mean that health is of value only to the extent that the individual patient considers it to be of value or to the extent that she desires it. That the value is objective, on the other hand, would mean that health may be of value despite the fact that the patient does not subjectively value it. That a value is objective does not mean that it is insensitive to individual preferences, since objective values depend on individual preferences indirectly. Even if happiness, for example, is objectively valuable, what makes people happy depends on their preferences. Similarly, even if health is objectively valuable, what makes people healthy will depend on their physical constitution and individual character, including preferences. Whether values are subjective or objective naturally affects how we should treat each other in medical and other contexts.

Beyond the somewhat related values of health, quality of life, well-being, and happiness, autonomy is arguably the main value relevant for medical decision making. This value is institutionalized through the practice of informed consent, but it may be affected also in other ways. For example, addictions may be considered to decrease autonomy, and so treatment of addiction may promote autonomy. Further values of possible relevance include dignity, equity, personal relationships, and perfection or excellence. Dignity may be relevant to hospice care and other care of dying patients, equity to any decision affecting the distribution of scarce medical resources, relationships to how families are treated and to decisions affecting the patients' potential to uphold personal relationships after treatment, and perfection to neonatal screening and genetic and medical enhancement.

Which things have objective value, if any, is a fundamental philosophical question, and opinions and theories diverge. Lacking agreement, we may look to social value as determined by willingness to pay or stated preference; to politically, ideally democratically, determined values; to expert judgment; or to our own judgment. Again, opinions and theories diverge. The consequences of decisions should be evaluated in terms of those things that are determined to have value.

If more than one value is affected by a decision, as seems likely for most medical decisions, we must determine how these values relate to each other. Most fundamentally, values may or may not be commensurable. If the value of health and the value of autonomy are incommensurable, we cannot weigh one against the other and so must make decisions that affect both values without guidance from such weighing. If the values are commensurable, they may be more or less open to comparison. At one end of the spectrum, we may know only that a little health is less important than a lot of autonomy, but we may not know how to compare much of each or little of each. At the other end of the spectrum, any amount of each value may be represented by a number and the values aggregated in multi-attribute utility analysis. The very different character of some values may make them seem incommensurable, while the need to make decisions that affect more than one value forces us to compare them, or at least to act as if we had compared them.

Uncertainties and Biases

In evaluating consequences, we are inescapably faced with a number of uncertainties and biases. It is widely recognized that we do not even know if established medical practice on the whole efficiently promotes best outcomes (though the growing field of outcomes research aims to address that question). The uncertainty is naturally greatest for consequences of decisions not yet made. We often do not know what consequences will follow from alternative courses of action. In evaluating possible future consequences, these uncertainties can to some extent be handled by decision theoretical methods. If we are uncertain about what consequences will follow, we may at least know, or be able to estimate approximately, the probabilities of different possible outcomes, each with a set of consequences. Given these probabilities, we may estimate the expected value of different alternatives. To a large extent, however, uncertainty about the future must simply be accepted as a fact of life.

Uncertainty does not pertain only to future consequences but also to the value of consequences, future as well as past and present. Even if we know that we value health and we know the consequences of a certain decision, we might not know to what extent those consequences further our values. This may be because we are not certain how exactly our values should be specified or because we are not certain how much the concrete consequences contribute to our values, however thoroughly specified. For example, if health is defined in terms of ability, we may not know to what extent successful treatment of radical mastectomy will contribute to this value. A person's overall ability depends partly on her attitudes, and patients may react differently to this medical procedure even when the physical outcome is the same.

Uncertainty about the value of consequences is increased by different sorts of biases. We tend to exaggerate the impact of certain things and belittle the impact of others. Some biases concerning our own well-being have been rather straightforwardly proven by psychological research. For example, we tend to overvalue variation in our consumption in the sense that we opt beforehand for variation but regret this once we get it. Other biases are harder to prove. For example, we value good things in the near future higher than similarly good things in the more distant future, and the reverse for bad things. This means, for example, that the social value of QALYs in the distant future is much lower than the social value of the same number of life years and QALYs in the near future. Whether this is an irrational bias that should be compensated for or an indication of our true values is a matter of controversy.

Uncertainties about consequences introduce another level of value—it requires us to determine how much we value certainty. A program of maximization of expected QALYs presumes that 1 QALY for sure is as good as a one-in-two chance of 2 QALYs. This is not so if we are risk-averse, that is, if we value goods that we are certain to get higher than goods we may or may not get, even when the expected value is the same. In fact, people tend to be risk-averse. However, this may be considered an irrational bias.

Consequences and Principles

In bioethics, principles are often understood as nonrigid rules and recommendations that must be interpreted in concrete cases with a large dose of moral judgment. Such principles are essentially statements of what has value, with the add-on that we have a duty to promote or protect that value. The question of which bioethical principles there are and how they should be understood corresponds to the question of what values there are and how they should be understood. Whether one prefers duty talk or value talk depends on whether one finds duty or value to be the more fundamental moral category. This is another matter on which opinions or sentiments diverge.

There are other kinds of principles, however, that do not as closely resemble values but that rather regulate the evaluation of consequences. Some of these principles are rules of thumb, stating that for practical reasons such as time constraint and limited information and information processing capacity, we should restrict our evaluation of consequences in different ways. A rule that the most severely injured should be treated first may be such a rule. It is not a deep moral truth that the most severely injured deserves the first treatment, but in most cases, the rule is fair and efficient and reasonably easy to follow without time-consuming judgment. That this is a rule of thumb rather than a fundamental principle is shown by our reactions to the hypothetical case where there are obvious reasons to diverge from the rule, for example, when it is clear that the most severely injured will not benefit from quick treatment while others will. If diverging from the rule in such circumstances is morally unproblematic, then the rule is one of thumb. In contrast, while a moral principle may be overridden, this is not unproblematic but normally gives cause for regret and may give rise to residual obligations.

Rules of thumb replace or restrict evaluations of consequences for practical reasons. Moral principles do so for moral reasons. There are essentially two sorts of moral principles. Action-focused principles, or side constraints, state that certain things must or may not be done, regardless of other considerations. Examples include general principles such as "never lie" as well as specific medical principles such as "never force medical care on a patient against her explicit wish." Reason-focused or value-focused principles, in contrast, state that certain reasons or values should be disregarded in the molding of various considerations into an all-things-considered judgment of what should be done. An example is the principle that a patient's estimated future contribution to society should not influence our medical treatment of the patient.

Many principles are tied to our social and legal roles, for example, as medical practitioners.

These roles come with social expectations, rules, and laws, which regulate how and to what extent we may consider certain consequences of our actions. If such role principles are motivated only by expedience, they may be seen as rules of thumb. However, if they become ingrained in the culture of a society, they acquire the status of moral principles. Even as rules of thumb, role principles are unusually rigid, because they are motivated by practical reasons on a collective or system level. While individual practitioners may on occasion have the time and capacity to judge a case on its own merits, they may be obliged to follow rules nonetheless, because this makes for stability and transparency in the medical system as a whole. The rigidity of role principles should not be exaggerated, however. The social and legal frameworks rarely, if ever, determine in detail how we should act and think. Even in applying well-defined rules, we need value judgments to guide our application of those rules to particular circumstances. Furthermore, as rational and moral beings, we can always question the social and legal framework within which we live and work.

A Model for Evaluating Consequences

The different aspects of evaluating consequences covered above may be captured in the following model. This somewhat novel model incorporates a series of not-so-novel considerations. The model does not describe how evaluations are performed in practice but rather proscribes what steps should be taken in order that all the aspects of evaluation discussed above be considered. In other words, the model is not psychological but philosophical. If implemented in practice, the steps of the model should not necessarily be taken in strict order. In particular, Steps 2, 3, and 4 may all require glancing ahead to subsequent steps.

1. Determine which things have value—that is, which values there are. This includes deciding whether values are subjective or objective, and final or instrumental.

2. Determine the available alternatives.

3. Decide whether an alternative is demanded by principle. If so, act.

4. Decide whether some alternatives are forbidden by principle. If so, exclude them from further consideration. If only one alternative is not forbidden, act.

5. Estimate for each alternative the possible outcomes and the (approximate) probability of each outcome.

6. Estimate the consequences of each outcome in terms of each value; adjust for bias.

7. Decide whether the consideration of some values is forbidden by principle, and if so, disregard these values.

8. Estimate the expected consequence of each alternative in terms of each value.

9a. If values are commensurable, estimate or decide the overall value of each alternative and act on the best alternative.

9b. If values are incommensurable, act on the alternative with the most appealing or most acceptable mix of expected consequences.

Kalle Grill

See also Bioethics; Construction of Values; Decision Rules; Expected Utility Theory; Health Outcomes Assessment; Moral Factors; Multi-Attribute Utility Theory; Outcomes Research; Protected Values; Quality-Adjusted Life Years (QALYs); Quality of Well-Being Scale; Risk Aversion; Values; Willingness to Pay

Further Readings

Beauchamp, T. L., & Childress, J. F. (2001). *Principles of biomedical ethics* (5th ed.). Oxford, UK: Oxford University Press.

Bircher, J. (2005). Towards a dynamic definition of health and disease. *Medicine, Health Care and Philosophy, 8,* 335–341.

Griffin, J. (1986). *Well-being: Its meaning, measurement and moral importance.* Oxford, UK: Oxford University Press.

Hastie, R., & Dawes, R. M. (2001). *Rational choice in an uncertain world.* Thousand Oaks, CA: Sage.

Kane, R. L. (2006). *Understanding health care outcomes research.* Sudbury, MA: Jones & Bartlett.

O'Neill, O. (2001). Practical principles and practical judgment. *Hastings Center Report, 31*(4), 15–23.

Raz, J. (2003). *The practice of value.* Oxford, UK: Oxford University Press.

Savulescu, J., Gillon, R., Beauchamp, T. L., Macklin, R., Sommerville, A., Callahan, D., et al. (2003). Festschrift edition in honour of Raanan Gillon. *Journal of Medical Ethics, 29,* 265–312.

Schroeder, M. (2008). Value theory. In E. N. Zalta (Ed.), *The Stanford encyclopedia of philosophy* (Spring 2008 ed.). Retrieved February 2, 2009, from http://plato.stanford.edu/archives/spr2008/entries/value-theory

World Health Organization. (1946). Constitution of the World Health Organization. In *Basic documents.* Geneva, Switzerland: Author.

EVIDENCE-BASED MEDICINE

Evidence-based medicine (EBM) is the judicious application of the best, relevant clinical study results to patient care. EBM is not a new form of medical practice. It neither replaces medical expertise nor ignores patient preferences. EBM is a tool to enhance medical practice. While it is axiomatic that clinicians are interested in using the results of clinical studies for their patients' benefit, until recently, lack of access, limited critical analysis skills, and overreliance on expert opinion, personal experience, and clinical habit have hampered the rapid integration of high-quality clinical study evidence into clinical practice. This entry discusses how EBM and the EBM process address this issue and reviews the origins of EBM and its scope, resources, and role in modern clinical practice.

Origins

The term *evidence-based medicine* was coined in 1990 by Gordon Guyatt. While there have been many contributors to the development of EBM, Guyatt and his colleagues at McMaster University—principal among them David Sackett and Brian Haynes—have played major roles in developing the principles of EBM and have been instrumental in popularizing it throughout the world. In 1985, Sackett, Haynes, and Guyatt, together with Peter Tugwell, published the book *Clinical Epidemiology: A Basic Science for Clinical Medicine.* In this book, the authors explained, simplified, and organized the basic EBM principles (though not yet referred to as EBM) for the practicing clinician. In essence, this was the first EBM book, which served as the basis for their later books and articles that generated and developed the EBM approach to clinical practice.

Scope

EBM was developed for practicing physicians. However, over the past decade, it became increasingly clear that many other professions participating in patient care would benefit equally from the EBM approach. In recent years, dentistry, nursing, pharmacy, physical therapy, occupational therapy, public health, library sciences, and other disciplines have developed a strong interest in EBM. With this broadened focus, the term EBM is slowly being replaced with EBP, evidence-based practice.

The past decade also has seen the rapid spread of EBM learning in all aspects of medical training. It is routine now in medical schools and residency programs in North America, Europe, and elsewhere to include EBM as a standard part of their curriculum. The acquisition of skills of critical judgment is a requirement of the Liaison Committee on Medical Education (accreditation committee for medical schools) in the United States. EBM learning is explicitly mentioned in the standards of the Accreditation Council for Graduate Medical Education and is included among the subcategories of their six core competencies for residency programs in the United States.

One remarkable corollary of EBM's increasing popularity has been the encouragement and expectation of scientific rigor in clinical research. This has led to the ubiquitous use of statistical methods to evaluate results, the rise of the randomized controlled trial as the standard for determining therapeutic benefit, and greater attention generally to methodological validity across all areas of clinical investigation.

Finally, the emergence of EBM has brought about a changed relationship of the practicing clinician to the medical literature. Previously, the busy clinician was forever attempting to catch up on journal reading—most poignantly represented by unread stacks of journals lying forlorn in the corner of one's office. The EBM process has encouraged decreasing catch-up journal reading and increasing patient-focused journal reading. The patient encounter has become the catalyst of learning about new treatments, diagnostic tests, and prognostic indicators and the focus of a personal program of continuing medical education.

Process

The EBM process begins and ends with the patient. The patient is the impetus for and genesis of a four-step approach to knowledge acquisition, ending in application of that new knowledge to the care of the patient. The four steps include (1) formulating the clinical question, (2) searching for and acquiring evidence from the medical literature, (3) assessing that evidence for methodological validity and analyzing the study results for statistical significance and clinical importance, and (4) applying, where appropriate, the valid important study results to the patient.

Formulating the Clinical Question

The first step in the process is recognizing that one has a knowledge gap in some aspect of a specific patient's management and to craft this knowledge gap into a focused question. One of the more popular approaches is the PICO (patient/problem, intervention, comparison, outcome) format. An example of this type of format is as follows. P: In otherwise healthy infants with presumed herpetic gingivostomatitis, I: what is the therapeutic efficacy of acyclovir, C: compared with placebo, O: in reducing the time to resolution of symptoms. The PICO format helps clarify and focus the clinician's specific evidence needs as well as to suggest an evidence search strategy, employing the terms in the question as online literature search terms. Carl Heneghan and Douglas Badenoch reviewed the mechanics of using the PICO approach in their book *Evidence-Based Medicine Toolkit*. A useful tool is the PICOmaker from the University of Alberta (www.library.ualberta.ca/pdazone/pico), which provides a palm-based platform for developing and saving clinical questions.

Searching for the Evidence

Primary Evidence

The next step in the EBM process is to look for an answer. Brian Haynes has suggested an *information hierarchy* to assist clinicians in their search

for evidence. There are five levels in the hierarchy (from lowest to highest): primary studies, syntheses, synopses, summaries, and systems—the assumption being that the higher one ascends the hierarchy, the more reliable and applicable the evidence. It follows that one would begin an evidence search at the highest level. However, in practice, the systems level of evidence is rarely encountered. Summaries are more commonly found, synopses even more common, and so on. At the lowest level are primary studies. These are the individual clinical investigations that form the corpus of the clinical scientific literature. In many instances, one's search for evidence will end here as the other levels of the hierarchy are not available. The two most commonly employed search engines for identifying primary studies include PubMed and Ovid, the former being free. PubMed searches the U.S. National Library of Medicine online medical database MEDLINE. Ovid can search other databases as well (such as the European-based EMBASE). Methodological quality filters, designed to identify only the highest-quality studies, have been incorporated into PubMed, under the "Clinical Queries" section, and are available for Ovid as well.

Syntheses

The next level up in the information hierarchy is syntheses, including systematic reviews and meta-analyses. A systematic review is a study that answers a focused clinical question using all relevant primary research studies. When appropriate, these results may be mathematically combined, resulting in a new, combined estimate of the outcome. This last step is termed *meta-analysis*. The assumption underlying placing systematic review/meta-analysis at this level of the hierarchy is that consideration of results from multiple studies is more reliable than consideration of the results of any one individual study.

Systematic reviews and meta-analyses are increasingly popular in the medical literature. They are indexed in the clinical databases, and there are specific search engines to help locate them, including one in PubMed. A key source for these types of studies is the Cochrane Collaboration, named in honor of Archie Cochrane, a British physician and researcher who, in 1979, challenged the medical community to critically summarize—by specialty and with periodic updates—all relevant scientific literature. The Cochrane Collaboration is a fellowship of volunteers from around the world who produce systematic reviews following the exacting Cochrane guidelines. In addition to the collection of systematic reviews, the Cochrane Collaboration Web site is home to a listing of hundreds of thousands of controlled therapeutic trials. Cochrane reviews are listed in PubMed, but the full review is available only by subscription.

Synopses

The next level up on the information hierarchy is the synopsis. A synopsis is a brief review of a primary study or systematic review, summarizing the key methodological issues and results, as well as pointing out areas of concern and caution. The purpose of this type of resource is to free the clinician from the bother of critically appraising the methodology and results of a study. Synopses come in many shapes and sizes, ranging from high-quality, peer-reviewed sources, such as ACP Journal Club, Bandolier, DARE, and Evidence-Based Medicine, to private online collections of study reviews of questionable quality.

Summaries

Summaries are reviews of all the methodologically sound evidence on a medical topic. An example of a topic would be "the treatment of asthma with bronchodilators," in contrast to a question relating to a specific outcome and a specific bronchodilator. Summaries allow for comparison of various competing therapeutic options for a specific problem, all evaluated using the analytical tools of EBM. Sources for summaries include clinical evidence and PIER (Physicians' Information and Education Resource; http://pier.acponline.org/index.html).

Systems

The highest level in the information hierarchy is systems. The most sophisticated of these would be a computerized decision support system, linking a patient's specific medical characteristics and preferences to the best available evidence and then recommending a specific management approach. These are not widely available. Included in this category, though much less sophisticated, are clinical guidelines. However, a note of caution is in order. Similar to the situation mentioned above with regard to synopses, the quality of guidelines varies. Guyatt and others have developed a grading system (the GRADE approach) for assessing the quality of a guideline based on methodological validity and the results of the guideline's evidence base.

Analyzing the Evidence

This is the EBM step that has been called "critical appraisal." If one has found a piece of evidence in the synopsis, summary, or systems categories above, this step should have been completed by the authors. If not, the methodology and results require critical analysis. Medical schools, residencies, and other clinically oriented programs are now providing instruction in EBM, much of which focuses on critical appraisal. There are many online and print resources that can aid in critical appraisal of a study and in critical appraisal skill learning. This is the crucial step in the EBM process determining whether the results of the study are reliable and important and therefore worthy of consideration in the management of one's patient. This is also the point at which one may decide that the study validity is insufficient and therefore one should look for other evidence.

Applying the Results

This is the final step of the EBM process—bringing the results of the EBM analysis back to the patient. At times, this step may be very straightforward—when benefits clearly outweigh costs, such as vaccination against pneumococcal infection and IVIG treatment in Kawasaki disease. At other times, the decision is not straightforward, even when the results of a study are highly valid, such as surgery versus medical treatment for prostate cancer. In all cases, patient peculiarities and preferences need to be factored into the medical decision. There is an entire discipline, medical decision making, which is dedicated to aiding clinicians and their patients in making medical management choices. The field is still relatively new, and results from research are only beginning to be applied in the clinical setting.

Future Directions

The rise of EBM has changed the way clinicians approach patient management problem solving, medical education at all levels, and the scientific basis for clinical investigations. There is a significant amount of work currently under way to simplify the EBM process, automate it, and generally make it more user-friendly for the clinical consumer. On the horizon are the decision systems discussed above that will link high-quality, current research with specific patient characteristics and preferences. Given the remarkable ascendancy of EBM in a relatively short period of time and its broad acceptance, the demand among clinicians for such systems will likely spur their rapid development.

Jordan Hupert and Jerry Niederman

See also Diagnostic Tests; Number Needed to Treat

Further Readings

ACP Journal Club: http://www.acpjc.org

Bandolier: http://www.jr2.0x.ac.uk/Bandolier

Clinical Evidence: http://clinicalevidence.bmj.com/ceweb/index.jsp

Cochrane Collaboration: http://www.cochrane.org

CRD database—DARE: http://www.crd.york.ac.uk/crdweb

Evidence-Based Medicine: http://ebm.bmj.com

GRADE Working Group. (2004). Grading quality of evidence and strength of recommendations. *British Medical Journal, 328,* 1490–1497.

Guyatt, G., & Drummond, R. (2002). *Users' guides to the medical literature.* Chicago: AMA Press.

Heneghan, C., & Badenoch, D. (2006). *Evidence-based medicine toolkit* (2nd ed.). Malden, MA: Blackwell.

PICOmaker, University of Alberta Libraries: http://www.library.ualberta.ca/pdazone/pico

PIER: http://pier.acponline.org/index.html

Schwartz, A. (2006). *Evidence-based medicine (EMB) decision tools.* Retrieved February 2, 2009, from http://araw.mede.uic.edu/~alansz/tools.html

Straus, S. E., Richardson, W. S., Glasziou, P., & Haynes, R. B. (2005). *Evidence-based medicine. How to practice and teach EBM* (3rd ed.). Edinburgh, UK: Elsevier.

University of Illinois, Library of the Health Sciences, Peoria. (2008). *Evidence-based medicine.* Retrieved February 2, 2009, from http://www.uic.edu/depts/lib/lhsp/resources/ebm.shtml

EVIDENCE SYNTHESIS

There is a plethora of information in almost every area of healthcare. For example, a search of MEDLINE (the U.S. National Library of Medicine's bibliographic database) using only the terms *depressed, depressive,* or *depression* yields more than 3,000 hits of articles published since 1980—and MEDLINE is only one of many health-related electronic bibliographic databases. The same terms on the search engine Google on the World Wide Web yield upward of 84,000,000 hits. Yet informed health-related decision making is dependent on having access to current knowledge. Without some help in assembling, organizing, and summarizing this information, the patient, healthcare practitioner, or policy maker would be at a loss to navigate through this mass of information. The vast amount of information available gives rise to the need for literature reviews that synthesize the available evidence to provide an overall reflection of the current knowledge base. Yet evidence synthesis itself is not a simple or straightforward task. There are many different factors that should be considered and many different views on how evidence synthesis should be conducted.

Types and Sources of Evidence

One of the important factors to be considered in both carrying out and making use of a synthesis is the tremendous diversity in the types and sources of evidence that a synthesis might potentially consider. Most current evidence syntheses restrict themselves to research studies published in peer-reviewed journals. Yet even this restriction can yield an overwhelming amount of evidence, given the numerous electronic biographic databases that can be searched (of which MEDLINE, PubMed, PsycINFO, and EMBASE are only a few examples) and the number of languages in which health research studies are published. Other evidence synthesis methodologies also strive to include "fugitive" literature, that is, the search for evidence is expanded to include unpublished studies through searching conference proceedings and the Internet, by including relevant government reports and unpublished studies conducted by pharmaceutical companies, and by using personal networking to identify other studies that may not have been submitted to or published by peer-reviewed journals. The main advantage of this strategy is that there is still a bias on the part of journals to publish studies that report positive findings. However, an important limitation of including these reports is that they have not undergone (or passed) a peer review process. Plus, attempting to include all published and unpublished studies can become an overwhelming task because of the sheer volume of information.

Still other evidence syntheses draw on professional expertise and opinion. Although professional expertise must surely be considered a form of evidence, good research studies, where they are available, should take precedence in an evidence synthesis. However, professional expertise and expert consensus can be especially useful when there are few studies available, and they are invaluable in helping interpret the meaning of and importance of study findings where they do exist. Issues of practicality and evidence of public acceptance of a particular practice (e.g., a particular prevention or intervention strategy) should also be important considerations, although not all evidence syntheses attend to these issues. However, in using an evidence synthesis to aid in clinical or policy decision making, these are important issues to consider.

Currently, most evidence syntheses combine evidence from quantitative studies only, and most synthesis methodologies do not consider the role of theoretical frameworks or the context in which a particular study (with its particular findings) was conducted. This may be of more relevance in reviews of some health issues (such as the prognosis in whiplash-associated disorders or most effective strategies for prevention of teen pregnancies) and of less relevance in reviews of other health issues (such as the efficacy of a particular medication for treating a particular disease). A recently emerging area, requiring a very different synthesis methodology, is the synthesis of evidence from qualitative studies. The combination of evidence from both quantitative and qualitative studies is even less well developed but would conceivably yield a rich and more complete understanding of many health concerns.

Considerations for Users of Syntheses

Even where the primary source of information is published quantitative studies, there is a great diversity in the particular questions addressed in those studies. For example, when synthesizing information from published intervention studies, there are a number of different questions that the study might address. Among others, these questions might include the following: Can an intervention be effective? What happens when a particular intervention is used on a widespread basis with the "usual" patient in the "usual" clinical setting? What interventions do patients prefer? Is that intervention *cost-effective* when used on a large-scale basis? In studies of a single intervention strategy, these questions might yield very different answers. An evidence synthesis is useful to a particular reader only when it addresses the same question that concerns the reader and where the study participants and clinical care providers are similar to those of the reader's interest. For example, a particular procedure carried out on the "ideal" patient by a highly specialized healthcare provider may yield very different results when carried out on "usual" patients (who may have comorbid conditions that are different or more serious than those in the studies included in the evidence synthesis). Similarly, some procedures have a higher success rate and lower complication rate when carried out at highly specialized and selected facilities than at facilities providing more varied and generalized care. The reader of an evidence synthesis needs to ensure that the synthesis is relevant to the particular decisions that he or she needs to make.

The reader of an evidence synthesis should also keep in mind that different research questions require different research designs. For example, wherever possible, questions about the effectiveness of a particular intervention strategy are best answered using a randomized controlled trial (RCT). Most Cochrane Collaboration reviews and evidence syntheses are of this sort, and many such reviews exclude observational studies. However, designs other than RCTs are better suited to answering other important clinical questions. In particular, RCTs are rarely the design of choice to assess diagnostic techniques and have little to offer us when studying the usual course and prognosis of a health condition. The types of evidence needed to develop an evidence synthesis and the methods employed to synthesize the information once the evidence is assembled are highly dependent on the particular question being asked.

Another important source of diversity in evidence syntheses relates to the methodological quality of that evidence. Some synthesis procedures, but not all, evaluate the methodological quality of the studies included. Moreover, some methodological quality assessments use rating scales (and may or may not use these ratings for establishing weights for each study in developing their conclusions). Others use dichotomous criteria by which only those studies judged to have adequate methodological soundness are included in the synthesis. Still others use combinations of these strategies. An important consideration is that the conclusions in the synthesis have been shown to differ depending on which method is used to appraise the quality of the evidence. Even in peer-reviewed publications, the methodological quality of studies varies widely. Generally, an evidence synthesis that does not consider the methodological quality of the evidence it combines should be viewed with caution. The evidence synthesis should alert the reader to the strength of the findings so that the reader can assess how much confidence he or she should place on the synthesis conclusions and what populations these findings might apply to. As stated previously, a crucial consideration in interpreting evidence from studies is whether the findings from a series of carefully selected participants and settings can be generalized to the wider clinical setting or population.

Different stakeholders also have different needs from a synthesis of evidence. For example, a policy maker and a clinician may have different requirements in an evidence synthesis, since the types of decisions to be made are quite different. The healthcare provider is responsible for considering his or her patient's individual needs and ensuring that his or her patient receives the most appropriate diagnostic and treatment options. A policy maker must consider the needs not only of healthcare patients but also of the community in general. Decision making in this situation considers not only efficacy of clinical practice but also allocation of resources; the general values, standards, and beliefs of the community; and the practicality of incorporating, on a larger scale, what the evidence tells us. This has implications for the type of evidence required for the synthesis, how the synthesis is interpreted, and even the makeup of the group doing the evidence synthesis. The creators of the evidence synthesis should alert the reader as to the

target audience of their synthesis; in addition, readers should consider for themselves whether the evidence synthesis is appropriate for their own particular needs.

Combining the Evidence

Once a researcher has addressed these important questions and has a well-formulated question, has clarified the target audience, has adequately searched for evidence, and has appraised the quality of the study (or has decided against such appraisal), he or she comes to the issue of how to perform the actual synthesis of the evidence. What then? How does one combine the evidence? In an ideal world, the researcher would have a substantial number of studies of excellent methodological quality, all with consistent findings. These would provide sufficient variability in the populations studied to assure him or her that the findings can confidently be generalized to the broader population with that particular health problem. Outcomes considered would cover the range of relevant outcomes and would provide the researcher with confidence that the findings are robust. Where this is the case, the evidence is clear, unambiguous, and strong. The researcher knows what the evidence shows and how strong the associations are: The particular strategy used for combining the evidence becomes largely irrelevant.

However, that scenario is the exception for most areas of medical research. More frequently, the researcher has many studies of (at best) moderate-quality evidence, which may or may not contradict each other; one or two studies of adequate methodological quality, which may or may not contradict other studies of poor methodological quality; or many studies of poor methodological quality, which may or may not contradict each other. Even studies examining the same research question, using the same research design, and of similar methodological quality may have widely diverse findings and come to different conclusions. And where the available studies are all methodologically strong, they may lack relevance in real-world settings because all include only highly selected patients, who may not reflect the usual clinical practice.

This is one of the main challenges in developing a useful and valid evidence synthesis. There are two main ways of combining evidence. These are meta-analysis, whereby findings from the relevant studies are combined statistically to yield an overall direction and size of an effect, and a more narrative, descriptive approach to synthesizing the information from the relevant studies.

A meta-analytic approach is most often seen in evidence syntheses that address issues of intervention effectiveness—for example, many Cochrane Collaboration reviews. To be valid and useful, this approach requires that the studies be reasonably homogeneous, that is, similar with respect to the particular intervention assessed, the population being studied, the context or setting in which the intervention is being assessed, the nature of the outcomes of interest, the measures used to assess those outcomes, and the follow-up time—when the outcomes are assessed. This, of course, requires that the studies to be included report this information in sufficient detail and that the findings (the estimate and variability of the effect) are reported clearly and in a manner that permits statistical combination of these effects. Where these conditions are present, this strategy can overcome some of the limitations of multiple small, underpowered studies that fail to achieve statistical significance because of low sample size. It should be remembered, however, that small RCTs may not only lack statistical power, but they are also at greater risk that random group allocation may have failed to equalize groups, thus introducing confounding. This problem is not necessarily eliminated by pooling studies in a meta-analysis. In addition, where an "overall effect size" is reported, some important explanations for differences among the individual studies might be neglected. For example, differences in patient characteristics among study settings might be responsible for differences in the effectiveness of a particular treatment. If these issues are not explored, the user of the synthesis may miss some important information necessary for successful implementation of the intervention with individual patients.

However, in many cases, there is too much heterogeneity in the studies to justify statistical pooling of study findings. In this case, a qualitative (rather than a quantitative) synthesis of the available evidence must be employed. It is important to distinguish this from a traditional, narrative review. In a traditional, narrative review, the search for studies is neither comprehensive nor systematic,

nor is there a systematic critical appraisal performed. Although traditional narrative reviews can be useful sources of information, they are often based on a selected number of studies, which may reflect the biases of the author. Even when a meta-analysis cannot occur because of heterogeneity in the studies, a qualitative synthesis (such as a best-evidence synthesis) based on studies ascertained using a comprehensive and systematic search and a thorough critical review of the studies' methodological soundness can be an important strategy for summarizing the available literature. A sound, informative qualitative analysis of the literature can be a complex and challenging task, since not only similarities but also dissimilarities in studies (e.g., study populations, context and setting, exact nature of the intervention, type and timing of outcomes measured) need to be described and explored as they relate to similarities and differences among study findings.

Where meta-analytic techniques can be employed, they can provide very important information to the clinician and policy maker. Meta-analytic techniques are relatively well standardized and codified. However, meta-analyses rarely explore theoretical or conceptual issues and generally do not address the mechanisms through which the intervention has its effect. A qualitative analysis of the evidence produced by a systematic search and critical review of the literature requires more judgment, and the procedures are less codified. Such approaches lend themselves more easily to an exploration of theoretical issues and of the mechanisms of the intervention, although not all qualitative analyses address these issues.

Whichever approach is used in the evidence synthesis, the reader should have access to a description of each study included in the synthesis, preferably in tabular form so that the studies can be easily compared. At a minimum, this should include a description of the research design used (if more than one research design is included in the synthesis), the study setting, the study sample (source of sample, sample characteristics, number in each group at inception and at follow-up), a summary of the intervention (if more than one is included in the synthesis), the outcomes assessed, their timing and measures used, and the findings (estimates and the variability around those estimates, e.g., confidence intervals). This allows readers to determine for themselves how closely the study samples and settings relate to their own patient populations and healthcare settings, whether the outcomes being assessed are of relevance in their own particular circumstances, and how much variability there is in the literature.

Finally, it should always be remembered that no matter how the evidence is combined in an evidence synthesis, both the individual studies and the synthesis of these studies report average, not individual, risks and benefits. Whether the decisions being made are policy decisions or clinical decisions, the quality of the decision depends on having access to both good evidence and good judgment.

Linda Jean Carroll

See also Meta-Analysis and Literature Review; Qualitative Methods; Randomized Clinical Trials

Further Readings

Altman, D. G., Schulz, K. F., Moher, D., Egger, M., Davidoff, F., Elbourne, D., et al. (2001). The revised CONSORT statement for reporting randomized trials: Explanation and elaboration. *Journal of the American Medical Association, 134,* 663–694.

Forbes, A., & Griffiths, P. (2002). Methodological strategies for the identification and synthesis of "evidence" to support decision-making in relation to complex healthcare systems and practices. *Nursing Inquiry, 9,* 141–155.

Slavin, R. E. (1995). Best evidence synthesis: An intelligent alternative to meta-analysis. *Journal of Clinical Epidemiology, 48,* 9–18.

Starr, M., & Chalmers, I. (2003). *The evolution of the Cochrane library, 1988–2003.* Oxford, UK: Update Software. Retrieved February 2, 2009, from http://www.update-software.com/history/clibhist.htm

Van der Velde, G., van Tulder, M., Côté, P., Hogg-Johnson, S., Aker, P., Cassidy, J. D., et al. The sensitivity of review results to methods used to appraise and incorporate trial quality into data synthesis. *Spine, 32,* 796–806.

EXPECTED UTILITY THEORY

Expected utility theory (EUT) states how an EUT decision maker makes choices among options that have specified characteristics. Each option is in some sense viewed by the EUT decision maker as beneficial to the EUT decision maker, but the option also has risks associated with the benefits and the EUT decision maker must bear the adverse outcomes associated with these risks should they occur. In addition, both the benefits and the risks of the options are uncertain, hence EUT decision makers must consider a set of uncertainties of benefits and risks among options (or alternatives) as they make their way through the decisions they face. Compared with other types of decision makers who pursue different routes in coming to a choice among alternatives with trade-offs, the EUT decision maker makes his or her choice in one way: by comparing the weighted sums of the options that are open to him or her. The weighted sums of options are obtained by adding the utility values of each of the outcomes multiplied by each outcome's respective probability of occurrence across the set of outcomes open to the EUT decision maker.

The origins of the EUT can be traced back to 1738, when Daniel Bernoulli wrote what he described as a new theory of the measurement of risk. But what assumptions was Bernoulli coming up against that required a "new" formulation?

Floris Heukelom traces the history of the mathematics of rational behavior to 1654, when Chevalier de Méré instigated Blaise Pascal, and therewith Pierre Fermat, to consider gambling problems. Heukelom notes that from an examination of a large body of literature on Enlightenment mathematicians who were interested in probability, it seemed as if these mathematicians were not making a real distinction between the determination of what they considered to be an answer to the question "What should the rational solution to the problem be in situations of uncertainty?" and the question "What would a rational person actually do (or how would a rational person act) in those same situations of uncertainty?" For these mathematicians, the two questions were one and the same.

One such construction of a gamble is the St. Petersburg game that came under the scrutiny of Bernoulli. Chris Starmer notes the following about EUT as it was first proposed by Bernoulli to the St. Petersburg game. Starmer notes that Bernoulli proposed EUT in response to an apparent puzzle surrounding what price a reasonable person should be prepared to pay to enter a gamble. It was the conventional wisdom at the time that it would be reasonable to pay anything up to the expected value of a gamble. But Bernoulli proposed making a game out of flipping a coin repeatedly until a tail is produced, and let us make a game of this situation. The game rules are as follows: If one is willing to participate in the game, one will receive a payoff of, say, 2^n, where n is the number of the throw producing the first tail (T). If one goes about looking for players for this game, one finds that people do not want to get involved in this game, where, in fact, the expected monetary payoff is infinite. In fact, and to the surprise of theoretical mathematicians, people are only prepared to pay a relatively small amount to even enter the game. Bernoulli argued that the "value" of such a gamble to an individual is not, in general, equal to its expected monetary value as theoretical mathematicians believe. Rather, Bernoulli argued and proposed a theory in which individuals place subjective values, or *utilities*, on monetary outcomes. Here, for Bernoulli, the value of a gamble is the expectation of these utilities.

Heukelom notes that instead of the "objective value of the monetary gain" being taken as the expectation in people, the "subjective value of the utility" should be taken as the mathematical expectation of a game or gamble. Here, when considering the subjective value of the utility, the St. Petersburg paradox does not go to infinity but, depending on the exact parameters of Bernoulli's equation, will asymptotically go to a number that is in fact quite reasonable.

Bernoulli's Theory of the Measurement of Risk

Bernoulli's first paragraph of his formulation of the St. Petersburg game, translated from Latin into English by Louise Sommer, notes that ever since mathematicians first began to study the measurement of risk, there has been general agreement on the proposition that "expected values" are computed by multiplying each possible gain by the number of ways in which it can occur and then dividing the sum of these products by the total number of possible cases where, on this theory, the consideration of cases that are all of the same probability is insisted on.

Bernoulli then notes that the proper examination of the "numerous demonstrations of this proposition" all rest on one hypothesis: Since there is no reason to assume that of two persons encountering identical risks, either should expect to have his or her desires more closely fulfilled, the risks anticipated by each must be deemed equal in value.

Bernoulli then focuses in on the term *value* above and argues that the determination of the *value* of an item must not be based on its *price* but rather on the *utility* it yields. The price of the item depends only on the thing itself and is equal for everyone; the utility, however, depends on the particular circumstances of the person making the estimate. Bernoulli concluded by making explicit the point that there is no doubt that a gain of 1,000 ducats is more significant to a poor person than to a rich person, although both the poor person and the rich person gain the same amount.

For Bernoulli, what becomes evident is that no valid measurement of the value of a risk can be obtained without consideration being first given to its utility, that is, the utility of whatever gain accrues to the individual or how much profit is required to yield a given utility.

Exceedingly Rare Exceptions

Bernoulli, however, was quick to recognize that he needed to consider the case of what usually happens and not place his focus solely on the case of exceedingly rare exceptions. The exceedingly rare exception referred to was the case of a prisoner. For although a poor person generally obtains more utility than does a rich person from an equal gain, it is nevertheless conceivable, for example, that a rich prisoner who possesses 2,000 ducats but needs 2,000 ducats more to repurchase his freedom will place a higher value on a gain of 2,000 ducats than does another person who has less money than he.

Bernoulli's Risk Aversion

Excluding these rare exceptions, Bernoulli argued that we should consider what usually happens and assume that there is an imperceptibly small growth in the individual's wealth, which proceeds continuously by infinitesimal increments. For Bernoulli, it is highly probable that *any increase in wealth, no matter how insignificant, will always result in an increase in utility, which is inversely proportionate to the quantity of goods already possessed.*

Daniel Kahneman notes that Bernoulli suggested that people do not evaluate prospects by the expectation of their monetary outcomes but rather by the expectation of the subjective value of these outcomes. This subjective value of a gamble is again a weighted average, but now it is the subjective value of each outcome that is weighted by its probability. Kahneman then argues that to explain "risk aversion" within this framework, Bernoulli had to propose that subjective value, or utility, is a concave function of money. Hence, the concavity of the utility function entails a risk-averse preference for the sure gain over a gamble of the same expected value, although the two prospects have the same monetary expectation.

Commentary on Bernoulli's Work

Heukelom gives Bernoulli credit for successfully introducing a theory of maximizing expected utility (EUT) as the basis for the study of rational decision behavior under uncertainty and adds that—as anachronistic as it may seem—what is being seen in these discussions is the beginnings of today's decision theory.

Writing on the early history of experimental economics, Alvin E. Roth considers Bernoulli's work on the St. Petersburg paradox as perhaps the best candidate for the *first* economic experiment. Roth is referring here to Bernoulli's paper "Exposition of a New Theory on the Measurement of Risk." For Roth, Bernoulli did not simply rely on and attempt to publish only his own intuitions but rather adopted the practice of asking other famous scholars for their opinions on difficult choice problems. Here, Bernoulli is argued by Roth to be using a similar information report methodology to what is now being used in the hypothetical choice problems that generate hypotheses about individual choice behaviors today, and furthermore, it can be argued that this can be seen as a continuum from Bernoulli's work to the work of theorists of individual choice behavior in cognitive psychology today.

In this history of experimental economics, Roth gives credit to L. L. Thurstone's 1931 experiment on

individual choice and the problem of experimentally determining an individual's indifference curves. Here, Roth argues that Thurstone was concerned with testing the indifference curve representation of preferences and with the practicality of obtaining consistent choice data of the sort needed to estimate these indifference curves.

Kahneman also traces the psychophysical approach to decision making to this essay by Bernoulli on risk measurement.

Starmer considers Bernoulli's theory the first statement of EUT with his solution to the St. Petersburg puzzle but asserts that modern economists in the 1950s only discovered and built on Bernoulli's insight. Here, Starmer argues that a possible explanation for this time delay in theory development is at least partly explained by the fact that the form of Bernoulli's theory presupposes the existence of a cardinal utility scale. And this assumption about cardinal utilities did not sit well with the more modern theorists' drive toward ordinalization in the first half of the 20th century. John von Neumann and Oskar Morgenstern revived interest in Bernoulli's approach and showed that the expected utility hypothesis could be derived from a set of apparently appealing axioms on preference.

Paul J. H. Schoemaker notes that $U(x)$, the utility function proposed by Bernoulli, was logarithmic and thus exhibited diminishing increases in utility for equal increments in wealth. However, Schoemaker notes that Bernoulli did not explicitly address the issue of how to measure utility, nor did Bernoulli address why his expectation principle should be considered as rational. Without such further exploration, Shoemaker argues that Bernoulli's theory may only be interpreted as a "descriptive model" by some commentators, even though the expectation principle at the time may have enjoyed face validity as a "normative model."

Medical Decision Making

Today, in the area of medical decision making, the following questions regarding work like Bernoulli's on risk are still being asked: Is expected utility theory supposed to describe individuals' choices? Is it supposed to be prescriptive for medical decision making? Is it supposed to be normative for medical decision making? Is it normative or just simply practical? These challenges to expected value theory's strengths and further defining of expected values theory's weaknesses have followed expected value theory since its early formulation by Bernoulli, and these perspectives continue to challenge ethicists, researchers, and theorists in medical decision making, economics, and EUT today.

Dennis J. Mazur

See also Nonexpected Utility Theories; Risk Aversion; Subjective Expected Utility Theory

Further Readings

Bernoulli, D. (1954). Exposition of a new theory on the measurement of risk (Trans. L. Sommer). *Econometrica, 22,* 23–26. (Original work published 1738)

Cohen, B. J. (1996). Is expected utility theory normative for medical decision making? *Medical Decision Making, 16,* 1–6.

Heukelom, F. (2007). *Kahneman and Tversky and the origin of behavioral economics* (Tinbergen Institute Discussion Paper No. 07-003/1). Retrieved February 2, 2009, from the SSRN Web site: http://ssrn.com/abstract=956887

Kahneman, D. (2007). Preface. In D. Kahneman & A. Tversky (Eds.), *Choices, values, and frames* (pp. ix–xvii). New York: Cambridge University Press.

Roth, A. E. (1993). On the early history of experimental economics. *Journal of the History of Economic Thought, 15,* 184–209.

Samuelson, P. A. (1977). St. Petersburg paradoxes: Defanged, dissected, and historically described. *Journal of Economic Literature, 15,* 24–55.

Schoemaker, P. J. H. (1982). The expected utility model: Its variants, purposes, evidence, and limitations. *Journal of Economic Literature, 20,* 529–563.

Starmer, C. (2000). Developments in non-expected utility theory: The hunt for a descriptive theory of choice under risk. *Journal of Economic Literature, 38,* 332–382.

Thurstone, L. L. (1931). The indifference function. *Journal of Social Psychology, 2,* 139–167.

von Neumann, J., & Morgenstern, O. (1944). *Theory of games and economic behavior*. Princeton, NJ: Princeton University Press.

Expected Value of Perfect Information

Simply basing decisions on expected cost-effectiveness or, equivalently, net health or monetary benefit will ignore the question of whether the current evidence is a sufficient basis for adopting or reimbursing a health technology. It would fail to address the question of whether further research is needed to support such a decision in the future. The value of evidence or the health costs of uncertainty can be illustrated using a simple example as shown in Table 1. Each row represents a realization of uncertainty, that is, the net health benefit (commonly measured in quality-adjusted life years, or QALYs) that results when all the parameters that determine expected costs and effects each take one of their many possible values. These realizations may be generated by probabilistic sensitivity analysis, which commonly randomly samples (Monte Carlo simulation) from each of the distributions assigned to parameters. Therefore, each row can be thought of as representing one of the ways things could turn out given our current uncertainty. The expected net benefit for Treatments A and B is the average over all these possibilities (in this example, the range of potential values is simplified to only five possibilities).

On the basis of current evidence, we would conclude that Treatment B was cost-effective, and on average we expect to gain an additional 1 QALY per patient treated compared with Treatment A. However, this decision is uncertain, and Treatment B is not always the best choice (only 3 times out of 5), so the probability that B is cost effective is .6. For some realizations (2 out of 5), Treatment A would have been the better choice. Therefore, a decision to adopt B based on current evidence is associated with an error probability of .4. This is substantially greater than the traditional benchmarks of statistical significance, such as .05. But whether or not this level of uncertainty "matters" depends on the consequences, that is, what improvement in net benefit (or avoidance of harm) could have been achieved if this uncertainty had been resolved.

The decision maker is faced with three choices: (1) adopt Technology B based on current evidence, (2) adopt the technology now but conduct further

Table 1   Expected value of perfect information

How Things Could Turn Out	Net Health Benefit			Best We Could Do if We Knew
	Treatment A	Treatment B	Best Choice	
Possibility 1	9	12	B	12
Possibility 2	12	10	A	12
Possibility 3	14	17	B	17
Possibility 4	11	10	A	11
Possibility 5	14	16	B	16
Average	12	13		13.6

research so that this initial decision can be reconsidered once the new evidence is available, or (3) withhold approval until further research resolves some of the uncertainty. Therefore, some assessment of whether uncertainty matters and of the value of additional evidence is required.

For example, if uncertainty could be completely resolved, that is, through complete evidence or perfect information about effect and cost, then we would know the true value of net health benefit before choosing between A and B. Therefore, with perfect information, we should be able to adopt whichever technology provided the maximum net benefit for each realization of uncertainty (the fifth column in Table 1). Of course, we can't know in advance which of these values will be realized, but on average (over the fifth column) we would achieve 13.6 rather than 13 QALYs—a gain of .6 QALYs. It should be clear that the cost of uncertainty or the value of evidence is just as "real" as access to a cost-effective treatment, as both are measured in terms of improved health outcomes for patients. In principle, evidence can be just as, or even more important than, access to a cost-effective technology. In this case, the expected value of perfect information is .6 QALYs, which is more than half the value of the technology itself, that is, 1 QALY gained by adopting B.

Additional evidence can be used to guide the treatment of all other current and future patients. Therefore, the maximum value of evidence to the healthcare system as a whole requires estimates of this current and future patient population (where the population expected value of perfect information [EVPI] is the discounted sum). This requires a judgment to be made about the time over which additional evidence that can be acquired in the near future is likely to be useful and relevant. Generally, fixed time horizons of 10, 15, and 20 years have commonly been used in the health literature as well as the environmental risk and engineering literature. There is some empirical evidence that suggests that clinical information may be valuable for much longer (a half-life of 45 years). However, any fixed time horizon is really a proxy for a complex and uncertain process of future changes, all of which affect cost-effectiveness and the future value of evidence. In health, some future changes can be anticipated (a new technology will be launched, a trial that is recruiting will report, or a branded drug will go generic), and differing judgments about time horizons in different contexts might be appropriate.

As well as a simple metric of the relative importance of uncertainty across different clinical decision problems, the population EVPI can be expressed as net monetary benefit and compared with the expected cost of additional research, which includes the net benefit forgone if conducting research requires delaying approval of a technology that appears to be cost-effective based on current evidence. If these expected opportunity costs of research exceed the population EVPI (maximum benefits), then the research is not worthwhile—the resources could generate more health improvement by being used elsewhere in the healthcare system, and coverage should be based on current estimates of expected cost-effectiveness. Therefore, EVPI provides a necessary condition for conducting further research and a means to start to prioritize the allocation of research and development resources within the healthcare system.

Expected Value of Perfect Partial (Parameter) Information

If further research is potentially worthwhile (EVPI exceeds the expected cost of research), it would be useful to have an indication of what type of additional evidence might be most valuable. This can inform the decision of whether approval should be withheld until the addition research is conducted or whether a "coverage with evidence development" would be appropriate.

The analysis of the value of information associated with different (groups of) parameters is, in principle, conducted in a very similar way to the EVPI for the decision as a whole. The expected value of perfect information for a parameter or group of parameters (EVPPI) is simply the difference between the expected net benefit when their uncertainty is resolved (and a different decision can be made) and the expected net benefit given the existing uncertainty.

EVPPIs can be used as a simple metric of the relative importance (sensitivity) of different types of parameters and sources of uncertainty in contributing to the overall EVPI. As a simple measure of sensitivity, it has a number of advantages: (1) It combines both the importance of the parameter (how strongly it is related to differences in net benefit) and its uncertainty; (2) it is directly related to whether the uncertainty matters (whether the decision changes for different possible values); and (3) it does not require a linear relationship between inputs and outputs. In addition, it can be expressed in health or money values and either per patient or for the population of current and future patients.

When population EVPPI is expressed in monetary terms, it can be directly compared with the expected opportunity costs of the type of research that might be needed to provide the evidence.

This is important as some uncertainties are relatively cheap to resolve (in terms of time and resource) compared with others (e.g., an observational study to link a clinical end point to quality of life compared with a randomized clinical trial of long-term relative treatment effect). Which source of uncertainty is most important requires a comparison of these benefits and opportunity costs.

Evaluating EVPPI often comes at a computational cost. For linear models, each estimate of EVPPI requires some additional computation (the manipulation of the simulated values rather than repeated simulations). When the model itself is not computationally expensive, it is a generally manageable expense. However, if the model is nonlinear, EVPPI may require many repeated runs of the same probabilistic model, which can become prohibitively expensive. Therefore, the computational expense of EVPPI needs to be justified, that is, if the analysis of population EVPI suggests that additional evidence might be required. It is also more efficient and more informative to first consider a limited number of groups of parameters, informed by the types of research required, for example, randomized clinical trial, survey of QALYs, or an observational epidemiological study. If there is substantial EVPPI associated with a particular group, only then conduct additional analysis to explore which particular source of uncertainty within the group matters the most.

Expected Value of Sample Information

The EVPI and EVPPI place an upper bound on the returns to further research so can only provide a necessary condition for conducting further research. To establish a sufficient condition, to decide if further research will be worthwhile and identify efficient research design, estimates of the expected benefits and the cost of sample information are required.

The same framework of EVPI analysis can be extended to establish the expected value of the sample rather than perfect information. For example, a sample from a particular type of study that provides information about some or all parameters will generate a sample result that can be used to update the parameter estimates and recalculate net benefits of the alternative treatments. Once the result of this sample is known, then the decision maker would choose the alternative with the maximum expected net benefit when those expected net benefits are averaged over the posterior distribution (the combination of sample result and prior information). Of course, there are many possible results that might occur, so the range of possible sample results from the sample must be evaluated, that is, similar to the realizations in Table 1 but now realization of the sample results rather than uncertainty itself. Which particular sample result will occur should the sample be taken is unknown, so the expected value of a decision taken with the sample information is the average over all the possible predicted results and predicted posteriors, that is, similar to averaging over Column 5 in Table 1. The difference between the expected net benefits with sample information and expect net benefit with current information is the expected value of sample information (EVSI).

This type of calculation would provide the EVSI for a single study design and only one sample size. To establish the optimal sample size for this particular type of study, these calculations would need to

be repeated for a range of possible sample sizes. The difference between the EVSI for the population of current and future patients and the costs of acquiring the sample information (Cs), which should include both resource and opportunity costs, is the expected net benefit of sample information (ENBS) or the societal payoff to proposed research. The optimal sample size for a particular type of study is simply the sample size that generates the maximum ENBS. This is illustrated in Figure 1 and shows how the EVSI will increase with sample size but at a declining rate (it will approach the relevant EVPI or EVPPI in the limit). In this case, the costs of sampling increase at a constant rate and the ENBS reached a maximum at $n = 1,100$.

There are usually a number of different ways in which a particular type of study could be designed. For example, a randomized clinical trial can be designed to collect information on limited clinical end points or include quality of life and costs. A range of follow-up periods is also possible, providing information on either short- or long-term effects. Patients recruited to the trial can also be allocated in different ways to the different arms. The efficient design of a

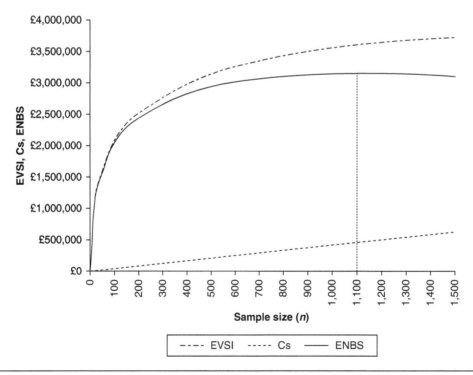

Figure 1   Expected value of sample information (EVSI), costs of acquiring the sample information (Cs), and expected net benefit of sample information (ENBS)

particular type of study will be one that provides the maximum ENBS. However, in most decision problems, a range of different types of study can be conducted at the same time to provide information about different types of parameters, for example, a randomized clinical trial to inform relative effect, a survey of the quality of life associated with a clinical end point, and an epidemiological study to inform other events. The problem is now to evaluate each possible portfolio of research, including the optimal allocation of sample (patients) to these different types of study. Of course, these dimensions of design space become even larger once the sequence in which studies might be conducted is considered. In principle, a measure of societal payoff to research provides a means to explore this design space and identify efficient research design and optimal portfolios of research.

Karl Claxton

See also Decision Trees: Sensitivity Analysis, Basic and Probabilistic; Expected Value of Sample Information, Net Benefit of Sampling; Managing Variability and Uncertainty; Net Benefit Regression

Further Readings

Ades, A. E., Lu, G., & Claxton, K. (2004). Expected value of sample information in medical decision modelling. *Medical Decision Making, 24*(2), 207–227.

Briggs, A., Claxton, K., & Sculpher, M. J. (2006). *Decision analytic modelling for the evaluation of health technologies.* Oxford, UK: Oxford University Press.

Claxton, K. (1999). The irrelevance of inference: A decision making approach to the stochastic evaluation of health care technologies. *Journal of Health Economics, 18,* 341–364.

Claxton, K., & Sculpher, M. J. (2006). Using value of information analysis to prioritise health research: Some lessons from recent UK experience. *Pharmacoeconomics, 24,* 1055–1068.

Pratt, J., Raiffa, H., & Schlaifer, R. (1995). *Statistical decision theory.* Cambridge: MIT Press.

Yokota, F., & Thompson, K. M. (2004). Value of information literature analysis: A review of applications in health risk management. *Medical Decision Making, 24,* 287–298.

Expected Value of Sample Information, Net Benefit of Sampling

Information has a value in utility terms. Consider a diagnostic test. It provides *data*, which, *when duly interpreted*, become *information* that may allow treatment to be individualized and expected outcome utility to increase. Three qualifications include the following:

First, a test may be too uninformative to influence treatment: VOI (*value of information*) = 0. However, expected utility cannot decrease: VOI is never negative.

Second, these are average statements. New diagnostic tests, even when correctly interpreted, will often cause outcome utility to decrease for *some* patients. When population screening is introduced, false positives pay a price.

Third, *misinformation* does carry negative value. Utility may suffer when decisions rest on biased research or when diagnostic test results are wrongly interpreted, for example, due to overly optimistic ideas concerning sensitivity or specificity.

In this clinical, single-case illustration, the *expected value of (perfect) test information* is the expected utility gained by a (perfect) diagnostic or therapy-guiding test. Analogous concepts find application in the collection of data to inform clinical policies. Complete elimination of uncertainty or biased opinions by means of properly conducted research offers a benefit, called the *expected value of perfect information* (EVPI), which ideally should outweigh research costs. Once again, however, *some* may pay a price. Suppose a vigorously promoted new drug is proven dangerous. However welcome this result may be—misinformation carries a negative value!—the result may deprive an unrecognized minority of the only drug that would save their lives.

A Pared-Down Example

Consider patients with a complaint that may signal a special endocrine disorder. The composition of the case stream is known (Table 1a), except that the sensitivity (Se) of a relevant imaging test is uncertain: It may be .60 or .80, giving rise to the question-marked numbers. The specificity (Sp) is .90.

Decisions have good and bad consequences. Here, we focus on human costs and, more specifically, on regret, that is, the "cost" of not treating the patient as one would were his or her condition fully known. As PVneg is high anyhow, the test negatives will always be treated by the wait-and-see policy, and either 16 or only 8 false negatives (out of 1,000 patients) will incur a regret B associated with a delayed clarification of their condition. There are 96 false positives that pay C units; this is the human cost of the invasive tests they must undergo. Obviously, this leaves two promising policies: W = wait and see (no need to test) or F = follow the test's advice.

Experts and ex-patients reach a consensus on C and B: C = 1 month (= 1/12 quality-adjusted life year, or QALY), B = 3.5 months. As an unfortunate result, the optimal policy depends on the unknown Se (see Table 1b): If Se is only .60, PVpos is too low to have any consequences, and W is

optimal (as its cost of 140 is less than 152). If Se = .80, F is optimal (as 124 < 140).

Now assume that the endocrinologists after studying the literature decide that the two values for Se are equally likely: This gives rise to an a priori mean number of (16 + 8)/2 = 12 false negatives (see the third row of Table 1b marked "F (average)"), so F beats W with a narrow margin of 2 months (= 140 − 138).

This was an assessment based on a priori hunches. What is the expected value of perfect information about Se? With prior probability .5, the Se proves to be .60, causing a change of policy from F to W for a mean regret of 140; with probability .5, the Se proves to be .80, in which case one sticks to F for a mean regret of 124. This *pre-posterior assessment* (we are guessing the situation that will prevail after obtaining some hoped-for information) leads to an average of (140 + 124)/2 = 132. That is, the EVPI = 138 − 132 = 6 months per 1,000 cases.

The situation, one may say, involves 6 units of uncertainty due to "cross-case" uncertainty concerning the performance of a clinical tool—and 132 (either 140 or 124, or the average of the two)

Table 1a   Composition of case stream (1,000 cases with prompting complaint)

Image Test	If Se Equals	Diseased	Healthy	Total
Positive	.60	(Se) × 40 = 24?	96	120? PVpos = .20
	.80	32?		128? PVpos = .25
Negative	.60	(1 − Se) × 40 = 16?	864 (as Sp = .90)	880? PVneg > .98
	.80	8?		872? PVneg > .98
Total	Total	40	960	1,000

Table 1b   Choosing a management policy (Wait and see vs. Follow test result)

Policy	Se	Regret (per 1,000 Cases)	Regret (per 1,000 Cases) With Consensus Values for B and C (Low Value Desirable)
W	.60 or .80	40B	140 months
F	.60	16B + 96C?	56 + 96 = 152 months?
	.80	8B + 96C?	28 + 96 = 124 months?
F	(Average)	12B + 96C	42 + 96 = 138 months

units of uncertainty that can only be eradicated by introducing a perfect diagnostic test, not by learning more about the present diagnostic tool ("intra-case" uncertainty due to an imperfect tool). The 132 units constitute an immutable dead weight in the calculations.

One starts out with either $C = 1$ or $B = 3.5$ months at stake per patient and ends up concluding that improved knowledge of the situation can only save 6/1,000 month, or 4 hours, per patient. Clearly, this is because everything is known apart from a minor uncertainty as to the Se. Ceteris paribus, Se will therefore have low research priority. Perhaps one should rather try to eat into the 132 months load by perfecting the imaging procedure.

Expected Value of (Research) Sample Information (EVSI)

Suppose a patient presents with verified disease. Hoping to benefit future patients, we seize the opportunity to obtain an improved Se estimate by testing this sample of $n = 1$ case.

If the patient proves test positive, it only reinforces the high-Se alternative and hence the prior decision in favor of F. Actually, the expected regret drops from its prior value of 138 to 136; this happens with prior probability .7 (the calculations in Table 1c). With probability .3, the patient will be test negative. This is the interesting case because it favors the low-Se alternative and hence W. Will it prompt a policy change to W? Yes. If the negative result materializes, the expected regret on Policy F increases (deteriorates) from its prior value of 138 to 142.67 (Table 1c), which is >140, so W now beats F.

Overall, what does the prior distribution predict the world to look like once the patient has been tested (pre-posterior assessment)? Foreseen is an expected regret of .7 × (updated consequences of F) + .3 × (consequences of W (which happen to be unchanged)) = .7 × 136 + .3 × 140 = 137.2, and EVSI is the gain from the prior level of 138 to 137.2, that is, .8 month.

The EVSI/EVPI fraction is here (.8 month)/ (6 months) = .13, so the very first patient with the

---

Table 1c   Updated consequences of Policy F in light of data from a single verified case

Unknown Parameter	Se = .60	Se = .80	Probability Sum
Parameter-dependent mean regret on Policy F	152[a]	124[a]	..
Prior probabilities	.5	.5	1
Prior mean regret	152 × .5 + 124 × .5 = 138		
Data = "Test is positive" with probability	.60 × .5 = .3	.80 × .5 = .4	.7[b]
Mean regret if positive	(152 × .3 + 124 × .4)/.7 = 136[c]		
Data = "Test is negative" with probability	(1 – .60) × .5 = .2	(1 – .80) × .5 = .1	.3[b]
Mean regret if negative	(152 × .2 + 124 × .1)/.3 = 142.67		

a. From Table 1b.

b. Bayes's denominator.

c. Quick route to this result: The odds of high versus low Se change from prior odds {1:1} to posterior odds = (prior odds) × (likelihood ratio) = {1:1} × {.80:.60} = {4:3}; that is, the updated chance that Se is .80 is 4/7. The expected regret associated with Policy F is the correspondingly weighted average of *152* and *124* (months per 1,000 cases).

disease that one gets a chance to study will eliminate 13% of the overall uncertainty.

Theoretical Formulation

Proper management of a prospectively delimited class of cases depends on some unknown parameter(s) θ (for notation, see Table 2), such as Se in the example. Had the true value of θ, $\theta°$, been known, there would be complete elucidation of the decision task; expected utility would attain the best possible level attainable with $\theta°$, and there would be 0 expected regret, because regret, by definition, is utility deficit relative to optimal handling of whatever happens to be the latent truth. The clinician's job is to minimize expected regret.

Before sampling, only the policy maker's prior knowledge is available, and the resulting expected regret is the deficit that perfect knowledge of θ would eliminate and thus constitutes the EVPI. It is 0 only if there is no residual uncertainty as to how to act. As defined in the table, $R(a|\theta)$ is the (expected) regret of action a when $\theta° = \theta$, and $A(\theta)$

is the prior probability that $\theta° = \theta$, so the ensuing optimal policy, $a*(A)$, is the a that minimizes $\sum_{\theta} A(\theta)R(a|\theta)$, and the minimum expected regret thus attained, symbolically $R*(A)$, is also the EVPI, as just explained. In sum,

$$\text{EVPI} = R*(A) = \sum_{\theta} A(\theta)R(a*(A)|\theta)$$
$$= \min_{a} \left\{ \sum_{\theta} A(\theta)R(a|\theta) \right\},$$

which is ≥ 0 because all terms are.

In the example above, policy a may be W or F; and θ, that is, Se, has two equally likely values: $A(\text{Se} = .60) = A(\text{Se} = .80) = .5$. So

$$\text{EVPI} = \min\{.5 \times R(W|.60) + .5 \times R(W|.80),$$
$$5 \times R(F|.60) + .5 \times R(F|.80)\}.$$

Now, $R(W|.60)$ is 0 because, if we knew that Se = .60, we could do nothing better than adopt Policy W, whereas F would be an inferior choice. Key figures from Table 1b tell us that its use would entail an unnecessary loss of 152 − 140 months per 1,000

Table 2	Notation and probability model
θ	parameter, or vector of parameters, describing a clinical population
$\theta°$	the true value of θ
$R(\ldots)$	the expected regret associated with . . .
a	available policy options
$R(a|\theta)$	expected regret, given θ, were option a to be chosen
$a*(\ldots)$	optimum policy choice based on . . .
$R*(\ldots)$	the expected regret when . . . is optimally responded to

Standard Bayesian data model

A	the policy maker's prior distribution of θ
x	observed study data
$Q(x|\theta)$	probability of observing x given θ, when
	$\text{Prob}_{AQ}(\theta, x) = A(\theta)Q(x|\theta),$
	$\text{Prob}_{AQ}(x) = \sum_{\theta} A(\theta)Q(x|\theta).$
B	posterior distribution based on prior A, observation x, and model Q:
	$B(\theta) = \text{Prob}_{AQ}(\theta|x) = \text{Prob}_{AQ}(\theta, x)/\text{Prob}_{AQ}(x)$

cases. That is, $R(F|.60) = 152 - 140 = 12$. By analogous arguments, $R(F|.80) = 0$, while $R(W|.80) = 140 - 124 = 16$. Substituting these figures, we have

$$\text{EVPI} = \min\{.5 \times 0 + .5 \times 16, .5 \times 12 + .5 \times 0\}$$
$$= \min\{8, 6\} = 6 \text{ months,}$$

as previously calculated in a more transparent way; and $a^*(A) = F$ as F beats W with a margin of $8 - 6 = 2$ months, again confirming the original analysis.

Once a data set x is available, the Bayesian policy maker's updated θ distribution $B(\theta)$ can be calculated the standard way (Table 2); the letter B is short for "Based on A, Q, and x." Proceeding as before, the data-conditional best action, $a^*(B)$, and associated expected regret are given by

$$R^*(B) = \sum_\theta B(\theta) R(a^*(B)|\theta) = \min_a \left\{ \sum_\theta B(\theta) R(a|\theta) \right\},$$

This quantity may be larger than $\text{EVPI} = R^*(A)$ because an outlying x may discredit θ° vis-à-vis other θs, but on average, sample information will hold a regret reduction, alias the EVSI:

$$\text{EVSI} = \text{EVPI} - \text{E}_{AQ}\{R^*(B)\} = R^*(A)$$
$$- \sum_x \text{Prob}_{AQ}(x) R^*(B).$$

The right-hand term is ≥ 0 and reflects the mean uncertainty left after observing the sample, proving $\text{EVSI} \leq \text{EVPI}$.

Note 1. In the example, x took two values (the only patient studied was positive or negative). It was natural to calculate $\text{EVSI} = .8$ as $138 - (.7 \times 136 + .3 \times 140) = 138 - 137.2$, but both terms contain the deadweight of 132 units, so a strict application of the formula above would pass via: $\text{EVSI} = (138 - 132) - (137.2 - 132) = 6 - 5.2 = .8$ units. The deadweight term is innocuous because it involves the "intracase" burden of diagnostic imperfection, represented by the figures 140 and 124 from Table 1b only, which the policy maker cannot change (though he or she may gradually learn which of them applies). Formally, a term $f(\theta)$ that only depends on θ may be added to each $R(a|\theta)$ without affecting optimal actions or EVSI-type regret differences (as both terms change by $\text{E}_A\{f(\theta)\}$).

Note 2. One may dissect the EVSI to prove that it, too, is ≥ 0:

$$\text{EVSI} = \min_a \left\{ \sum_\theta A(\theta) R(a|\theta) \right\} - \sum_x \text{Prob}_{AQ}(x) R^*(B).$$
$$= \min_a \left\{ \sum_x \left\{ \sum_\theta A(\theta) Q(x|\theta) R(a|\theta) \right\} \right\}$$
$$- \sum_x \left\{ \min_a \left\{ \sum_\theta A(\theta) Q(x|\theta) R(a|\theta) \right\} \right\}.$$

That this difference is ≥ 0 follows from "the fundamental trick of utility analysis," namely, that a sum of minima is smaller than, or equal to, the minimum of a sum: You save something by being allowed to minimize each term separately.

Note 3. Like the EVPI, the EVSI is *subjective*, as both depend on the point of departure, namely, the policy maker's prior for θ. The EVSI also depends on the design of the empirical study and on sample size(s).

Note 4. With its focus on Bayesian prediction of the situation that may prevail, or *on average will prevail*, once a planned data collection is completed, this is an instance of *pre-posterior analysis*.

Expected Value of (Partial, Alias) Parameter Information

When several clinical parameters are unknown, separate calculations can be made for each parameter or group of parameters, the uncertainty concerning the other parameters being handled as before. The expected value of perfect parameter information (EVPPI) for any one parameter is the EVSI of an imaginary study that reveals the true value of that parameter (without providing further empirical information). It is therefore $\leq$ the overall EVPI but $\geq$ the information afforded by real studies (*partial, parameter, EVSI*).

Clearly, a parameter that is inexpensive to investigate and also has a high EVPPI should receive high research priority.

Sample Planning: Expected Net Benefit of Sampling

Given an exchange rate between utilities and research expenses, the design and dimensions of the planned sample can be optimized. When sample size, n, is the issue, the *expected net benefit of sampling* (ENBS) becomes

$$\text{ENBS}(n) = \text{EVSI}(n) - \text{Cost}(n).$$

A Standard Example

If no research is undertaken, everything is zero. Otherwise, one faces an initial cost, C, and a cost per observation, c. Regrets may be roughly proportional to the squared standard error of the θ estimation and therefore inversely proportional to n, at least for large n. The regret expectation that remains after n observations is then Z/n, where the constant Z subsumes some variance and regret factors. So one gains $\text{EVSI}(n) = \text{EVPI} - Z/n$ by sampling. Combining the elements, one gets

$$\text{ENBS}(n) = [\text{EVPI} - Z/n] - [C + cn]$$
$$\text{for reasonably large } n.$$

A small study is never profitable because of the initial cost. As n grows beyond limits, costs also become prohibitive. The optimal sample size is $n* = \sqrt{Z/c}$, and sampling is profitable if the resulting $\text{ENBS}(n = n*)$ is positive, thus beating the no-research option.

Qualitative Policy Selection

When it suffices to document that θ lies right or left of a clinical decision boundary, $\text{EVSI}(n)$ usually approaches EVPI exponentially fast, and the required sample becomes small and less cost dependent than when the actual value of θ matters.

Interpersonal Aspects

Multiple Decision Makers

EVSI (and similar) calculations based on "an average policy maker's prior" may not match a sophisticated analysis that acknowledges differences of prior belief. However, even if rational experts start out with different prior beliefs, sound data collection will eventually bring about numerical agreement on parameters; and prior to that, it will induce a qualitative consensus about patient management policies. Lack of consensus implies regret (when two camps recommend different interventions, they cannot both be right), but a Bayesian formalization of the notion of *value of professional consensus* is difficult.

Ethics

Cool calculi face ethical obstacles. Informed consent is problematic toward the end of a randomized trial, when strict equipoise is impossible to maintain. What kinds of appeal to altruism are justifiable? Can skewed randomization be used in the trade-off between the interests of current and future patients? To benefit the former, "play the winner"; to benefit the latter, maximize VOI, which typically means playing the least explored alternative.

Jørgen Hilden

See also Economics, Health Economics; Expected Value of Perfect Information, Net Benefit Regression; Regret; Subjective Expected Utility Theory

Further Readings

Brennan, A., Kharroubi, S., O'Hagan, A., & Chilcott, J. (2007). Calculating partial expected value of perfect information via Monte Carlo sampling algorithms. *Medical Decision Making, 27,* 448–470.

Claxton, K., Ginnelly, L., Sculpher, M., Philips, Z., & Palmer, S. (2004). A pilot study on the use of decision theory and value of information analysis as part of the NHS Health Technology Assessment programme. *Health Technology Assessment, 8,* 1–103.

Claxton, K., & Posnett, J. (1996). An economic approach to clinical trial design and research priority-setting. *Health Economics, 5,* 513–524.

Eckermann, S., & Willan, A. R. (2008). Time and expected value of sample information wait for no patient. *Value in Health, 11,* 522–526.

Hilden, J., & Habbema, J. D. (1990). The marriage of clinical trials and clinical decision science. *Statistics in Medicine, 9,* 1243–1257.

Philips, Z., Claxton, K., & Palmer, S. (2008). The half-life of truth: What are appropriate time horizons for research decisions? *Medical Decision Making, 28,* 287–299.

Welton, N. J., White, I. R., Lu, G., Higgins, J. P., Hilden, J., & Ades, A. E. (2007). Correction: Interpretation of random effects meta-analysis in decision models. *Medical Decision Making, 27,* 212–214.

EXPERIENCE AND EVALUATIONS

The manner by which individuals evaluate how good or bad it is to be in a health state is central to reaching an informed medical decision. Evidence has shown that personal experience with illness, such as being diagnosed with cancer, leads to a more positive evaluation of that health state than the general public's perception. This disparity has been attributed to a focusing bias on the part of the general public—the tendency to focus too narrowly on a single event, for example, cancer, while forgetting all the other aspects of life that will remain unaffected. One potential means for overcoming such a bias is to ask the public to imagine standing in the shoes of the patient. This perspective-taking exercise might be achieved through exposure to a vicarious illness experience, though further research is needed to test this hypothesis.

Personal Illness Experience

Researchers have consistently found that the general public gives lower evaluations of a particular health state, such as having chemotherapy to treat cancer, compared with individuals who have had personal experience with that health state. This has been described as the distinction between predicted utility, people's predictions about what they think chemotherapy *would* be like (i.e., unimaginably horrible), versus experienced utility, how the experience of chemotherapy actually *is* like for cancer patients (i.e., not as bad as they expected).

Discrepancy Between Patients' and Public's Evaluations

In trying to understand how health state evaluations are affected by personal experience (or the lack thereof), researchers seem to have converged on a single explanation: focusing bias. This is the tendency for the general public to focus too much on a particular event (i.e., the cancer diagnosis) and not enough on the consequences of other new and ongoing future events that will compete for one's attention. For example, the general public may evaluate health states as worse than patients do because the general public focuses too narrowly on the (a) illness, forgetting that other facets of life will be unaffected; (b) immediate loss of health, forgetting patients' ability to adapt; (c) intense negative emotions aroused by the diagnosis, forgetting that extreme emotions tend to dissipate over time; and so on.

If the general public's inability to predict the effect of illness is due to focusing too narrowly, the question then becomes "What can broaden this narrow perspective individuals bring to the medical decision-making process when they have no personal experience?"

Vicarious Illness Experience

To broaden the general public's perceptions, they could be asked to imagine what it is like to live with a long-term, chronic illness. One means for achieving this perspective-taking task could be through exposure to a second type of illness experience: the vicarious experience (VE) of illness. For clarity, it is necessary to define the terminology used here. Firsthand personal experience is when A has been diagnosed with cancer; secondhand experience is when A tells B about his cancer diagnosis; and thirdhand experience is when B tells a third party, C, about A's cancer. Of course, one may have multiple types of experiences simultaneously, as when a man's father is diagnosed with cancer. The son has his own experience of being with his father while he is treated (firsthand) and also hears from his father what the experience of being diagnosed with and undergoing treatment for cancer was like for him (secondhand). Here, VE is defined as secondhand, being directly told about another's experience.

Why VE? When patients are newly diagnosed with cancer, they are faced with decisions about health states they typically have no real understanding of. Therefore, many actively seek out others with expertise, particularly former cancer patients. When former patients vicariously share their experiences, they may help newly diagnosed patients (a) broaden their focus by stepping back from their immediate, narrow fears and, consequently, (b) develop more informed expectations of how treatment will (and will not) change their lives, but this proposition has not yet been tested.

Theoretically, VE could have a positive impact because it provides information typically unavailable to individuals for two reasons. First, from an information-processing perspective, learning from VE is rational and adaptive for events that are rare but of high consequence, such as cancer, because direct experience may be fatal. It is not adaptive to have to wait until one has a cancer scare to learn the importance of, and be motivated to undergo, screening for cancer.

Second, real-world personal experiences are idiosyncratic and asymmetric in nature. Individuals only learn about the outcomes of the particular choices they make. They get no information, and therefore learn nothing, from the alternatives they did not choose. If they develop false beliefs based on these experiences, such as the belief that cancer treatment is useless, these false beliefs cannot be disconfirmed if they do not change their behavior and experience different outcomes. However, they *can* learn from the experience of others that treatment may increase the chances of survival.

This is not to imply VE is always beneficial. As with anything, if implemented poorly or if inaccurate information is conveyed, it can have suboptimal results. Accordingly, one may also learn from others that cancer treatment does not lead to survival. A poignant example exists in African American communities, where many believe that cancer is a death sentence. Because of the fear and stigma surrounding cancer, neither cancer patients nor survivors feel free to discuss their experiences. Therefore, the VE most individuals have is attending the funerals of those who have died from cancer.

Real-World Example

There is a real-world experiment that provided evidence that being exposed to a positive VE could both (a) improve noncompliant individuals' evaluations of an invasive and uncomfortable cancer-screening test and (b) motivate them to undergo screening. One of the most efficacious and least used cancer-screening tests is colonoscopy to detect and treat colorectal cancer. In March 2000, the NBC anchor Katie Couric underwent a live, on-air colonoscopy on the *Today* show to screen for colon cancer, a cancer that had led to the death of her husband. Researchers compared colonoscopy utilization rates before and after this powerful VE. They found that colonoscopy rates significantly increased after Couric's program, whereas there

was no concomitant increase in other cancer-screening tests.

Vicarious Illness Experience Remains Poorly Understood

To an extent, the gap in our knowledge about VE reflects the fact that much experimental research in psychology has focused on intraindividual factors. Therefore, it has been necessary to experimentally control potentially confounding factors, such as the influence of others' experiences. Further research is needed to draw a more complete picture of the role that personal experience and VE play in the evaluation of health states in medical decision making.

Julie Goldberg

See also Biases in Human Prediction; Cognitive Psychology and Processes; Construction of Values; Context Effects; Decision Making in Advanced Disease; Decision Psychology; Expected Utility Theory; Health Outcomes Assessment; Hedonic Prediction and Relativism; Judgment; Managing Variability and Uncertainty; Subjective Expected Utility Theory

Further Readings

Cram, P., Fendrick, A. M., Inadomi, J., Cowen, M. E., Carpenter, D., & Vijan, S. (2003). The impact of a celebrity promotional campaign on the use of colon cancer screening: The Katie Couric effect. *Archives of Internal Medicine, 163*(13), 1601–1605.

Hagen, K., Gutkin, T., Wilson, C., & Oats, R. (1998). Using vicarious experience and verbal persuasion to enhance self-efficacy in pre-service teachers: "Priming the pump" for consultation. *School Psychology Quarterly, 13*(2), 169–178.

Llewellyn-Thomas, H. A., Sutherland, H. J., & Thiel, E. C. (1993). Do patients' evaluations of a future health state change when they actually enter that state? *Medical Care, 31*(11), 1002–1012.

Ubel, P. A., Loewenstein, G., Hershey, J., Baron, J., Mohr, T., Asch, D. A., et al. (2001). Do nonpatients underestimate the quality of life associated with chronic health conditions because of a focusing illusion? *Medical Decision Making, 21*(3), 190–199.

Wilson, T. D., Wheatley, T., Meyers, J. M., Gilbert, D. T., & Axsom, D. (2000). Focalism: A source of durability bias in affective forecasting. *Journal of Personality and Social Psychology, 78*(5), 821–836.

EXPERIMENTAL DESIGNS

As in other branches of science, the time-honored method of research in the realm of medicine is one factor at a time. This practice of minimizing or eliminating changes in all factors of interest and then, one by one, changing the levels of each factor and recording the responses to those changes has been and continues to be used for the simple reason that it works and because most researchers do not realize that better methods exist. From the standpoint of efficiency with respect to time, money, effort, and quality of results, one-factor-at-a-time research is a failure.

A factor is any variable whose changes might result in responses of interest to an investigator. Factors include, but are not limited to, things such as dosage levels of one or more medicines, exercise regimens, types of sutures, mechanical properties of prosthetic devices, and material compositions of any medically implanted item or device.

The most efficient method for investigating the effects of variables over which an investigator has a degree of control is that of experimental design. The first work on experimental designs was done by R. A. Fisher at the Rothamsted Experimental Station in Hertfordshire, England, in the early 1920s. Work on the development of new designs and methods for their analysis continues to the present day.

To provide a basic understanding of the concepts of experimental designs, the discussion will be limited to the most elementary types of design, where the factors are limited to two levels, and the discussion will focus only on the assessment of single-factor effects.

For the purposes of this discussion, the levels of the factors in the design will be referred to as "absent" or "present"; however, designs are not limited to this simple dichotomy. In most designs, "absent" and "present" are usually a "low" and a "high" level of some property of a given factor.

Experimental Designs

An experimental design is, at the most basic level, nothing more than carefully organized one-factor-at-a-time experimentation. For example, let us assume we have two factors that we need to test on a sample population. The simplest basic *ideal* set of one-at-a-time experiments in this case would be that of Table 1.

For purposes of illustration, assume that we are interested in studying the effects of medicine and exercise on the speed of recovery following a surgical procedure. If Factor 1 was a dose level of a given medicine and Factor 2 was the number of minutes of treadmill walking at a given speed, then the experimental design from Table 1 would look like that of Table 1a. Thus, a patient assigned to receive the treatment of Experiment 1 would be the control—no medicine or exercise, and the patient assigned to the treatment of Experiment 4 would be given medicine and assigned 15 minutes of exercise on the treadmill.

Table I   Matrix of experiments for ideal one-factor-at-a-time experimental design for two factors

Experiment	Factor A	Factor B
1 (Control)	Absent	Absent
2	Present	Absent
3	Absent	Present
4	Present	Present

Table Ia   Illustrated examples of actual factor names and levels

Experiment	Dose Level	Minutes of Walking
1 (Control)	None	None
2	10 mg	None
3	None	15
4	10 mg	15

This set of experiments is identical to an experimental design of two factors at two values (levels). In this case, the values are the simple presence or absence of the factor of interest.

For three factors, the basic ideal one-factor-at-a-time list of experiments would be those in Table 2.

Table 2 Matrix of experiments for ideal one-factor-at-a-time experimental design for three factors

Experiment	Factor A	Factor B	Factor C
1 (Control)	Absent	Absent	Absent
2	Present	Absent	Absent
3	Absent	Present	Absent
4	Present	Present	Absent
5	Absent	Absent	Present
6	Present	Absent	Present
7	Absent	Present	Present
8	Present	Present	Present

This list of experiments is identical to a three-factor design, where each factor has two values (levels). This kind of a design is called a *full factorial*. Thus, for one to truly adhere to the principle of one factor at a time, an investigator would need to run eight experiments to properly identify the effects of three factors.

If the only concern is the ability to assess the effects of the three factors and assess them independently of one another, then it is possible to use the methods of experimental design and fractionate the above design so that the three factors can be assessed using only four experiments:

Table 3 Fractionated design

Experiment	Factor A	Factor B	Factor C
1 (Control)	Absent	Absent	Absent
4	Present	Present	Absent
6	Present	Absent	Present
7	Absent	Present	Present

If the third factor was the application of heat for 10 minutes to the area of repair, then the final fractionated design for three variables would be that of Table 3a.

The methods used to fractionate a design will not be discussed here. However, the interested reader is referred to the Further Readings at the end of this entry.

Table 3a Fractionated design

Experiment	Dose Level	Minutes of Walking	Minutes of Heat
1 (Control)	None	None	None
4	10 mg	15	None
6	10 mg	None	10
7	None	15	10

One-Factor-at-a-Time Design Matrix

The design matrices in Tables 1 through 3 are, as mentioned, the ideal one-factor-at-a-time design matrices. In reality, the *typical* one-factor-at-a-time design matrix for three factors is that of Table 4.

Table 4 Typical design of a one-factor-at-a-time matrix

Experiment	Factor A	Factor B	Factor C
1 (Control)	Absent	Absent	Absent
2	Present	Absent	Absent
3	Absent	Present	Absent
4	Absent	Absent	Present

Or we could express the matrix in terms of our three hypothetical factors (see Table 4 [Modified]).

Table 4 (Modified) Typical design of a one-factor-at-a-time matrix

Experiment	Dose Level	Minutes of Walking	Minutes of Heat
1 (Control)	None	None	None
2	10 mg	None	None
3	None	15	None
4	None	None	10

At first glance, a simple count of experiments in the design tables would seem to suggest that the design of Table 4 is superior to that of Table 2 and equal to the design of Table 3. However, Table 4 only lists the *basic combinations* an experimenter would need to run in a typical one-factor-at-a-time experiment involving three factors, whereas Tables 2 and 3 list the *total number* of experiments needed for a single run of an experimental design.

For a typical one-factor-at-a-time experiment to have the same precision of estimate of the effects of the factors that would be achieved by a single run of the experiments in Table 2, the investigator would need to run each of the low and high settings of each of the three variables in Table 4 four times for a total of 8 runs per factor and a total experimental effort of 24 runs. Thus, the true matrix of experiments for a typical three-factor one-factor-at-a-time experiment would be that of Table 4a.

In some cases, where all the experimentation was performed during a short period of time (a day or two) and the factors were all biological in nature, it might be possible to run a single control group of four animals. This would result in some decrease in the precision of the estimates of the effects, and it would reduce the above matrix from 24 to 16 runs. However, this would still be twice as many experiments as Table 2, and it would have the additional assumption that over the ranges of the factors of interest, the effect of any given factor would be the same regardless of the settings of the other variables—that is, over the ranges of the factors of interest, the effect of the factors on the response is that of simple addition. If this is not the case, then in addition to better precision with fewer experiments, the design in Table 2 will also provide the means to detect and estimate the interactions (synergistic effects) that measure this non-additive behavior.

The reason for the differences in the number of experimental runs needed for a one-factor-at-a-time versus a factorial design is due to the way in which the two methods compute the mean estimates of the factor effects.

For the one-factor-at-a-time matrix in Table 4, the effect of Factor A is computed by taking the sum of the responses to Experiments 1, 3, 5, and 7 and subtracting this from the sum of the response values to Experiments 2, 4, 6, and 8. This result is then divided by 4, the number of measurements at each of the two values of Factor A (absent and present). The result is the average effect of Factor A. This same procedure must then be carried out

Table 4a   Typical design of a one-factor-at-a-time matrix: Three factors

Experiment	Factor A	Factor B	Factor C
1 (Control)	Absent	Absent	Absent
2	Present	Absent	Absent
3 (Control)	Absent	Absent	Absent
4	Present	Absent	Absent
5 (Control)	Absent	Absent	Absent
6	Present	Absent	Absent
7 (Control)	Absent	Absent	Absent
8	Present	Absent	Absent
9 (Control)	Absent	Absent	Absent
10	Absent	Present	Absent
11 (Control)	Absent	Absent	Absent
12	Absent	Present	Absent
13 (Control)	Absent	Absent	Absent
14	Absent	Present	Absent
15 (Control)	Absent	Absent	Absent
16	Absent	Present	Absent
17 (Control)	Absent	Absent	Absent
18	Absent	Absent	Present
19 (Control)	Absent	Absent	Absent
20	Absent	Absent	Present
21 (Control)	Absent	Absent	Absent
22	Absent	Absent	Present
23 (Control)	Absent	Absent	Absent
24	Absent	Absent	Present

for the eight experiments for Factor B and the eight experiments for Factor C.

In the full-factorial experimental design in Table 2, the effect for Factor A is computed by taking the sum of the responses of the experiments where Factor A was absent and subtracting them from the sum of the responses of the experiments where Factor A was present and dividing this difference by 4. To compute the effect for Factor B, the same strategy is followed, only now we are adding and subtracting the responses based on the values of Factor B.

If you are accustomed to thinking in terms of one-factor-at-a-time experimentation and analysis, the explanation of the computation of the effect of Factors A and B in the above paragraph would appear to be complete and utter rubbish. How is it possible to take the same eight experiments where both Factors A and B (and C!) are changing at the same time and independently identify the effects of these three factors?

The key to understanding this is to visualize the sentence "The effect for Factor A is computed by taking the sum of the responses of the experiments where Factor A was absent and subtracting them from the sum of the responses of the experiments where Factor A was present and dividing this difference by 4" in tabular form. If this is done, then for Factor A, Table 2 will be modified as shown in Table 5.

If we add up Experiments 1 to 8 according to the coefficients in the column for Factor A, we will have the following:

$$1 \times \text{Present} + 1 \times \text{Present} + 1 \times \text{Present}$$
$$+ 1 \times \text{Present} - 1 \times \text{Absent} - 1 \times \text{Absent}$$
$$- 1 \times \text{Absent} - 1 \times \text{Absent},$$

which reduces to

$$4 \times \text{Present} - 4 \times \text{Absent}.$$

This divided by 4 will give us the average effect of Factor A.

If we apply this same pattern of $\pm$ values to the column for Factor B, we will have Table 6.

If we add up Experiments 1 to 8 according to the coefficients in the column for Factor B, we have the following:

$$1 \times \text{Present} - 1 \times \text{Present} + 1 \times \text{Present}$$
$$- 1 \times \text{Present} + 1 \times \text{Absent} - 1 \times \text{Absent}$$
$$+ 1 \times \text{Absent} - 1 \times \text{Absent},$$

which reduces to

$$2 \times \text{Present} - 2 \times \text{Present} + 2 \times \text{Absent}$$
$$- 2 \times \text{Absent} = 0.$$

Table 5   Illustration of Factor A level coding for purposes of computing Factor A effects

Experiment	Factor A	Factor B	Factor C
1 (Control)	−1 × Absent	Absent	Absent
2	1 × Present	Absent	Absent
3	−1 × Absent	Present	Absent
4	1 × Present	Present	Absent
5	−1 × Absent	Absent	Present
6	1 × Present	Absent	Present
7	−1 × Absent	Present	Present
8	1 × Present	Present	Present

Table 6   Illustration of Factor A and Factor B level coding for purposes of computing Factor A and Factor B effects

Experiment	Factor A	Factor B	Factor C
1 (Control)	−1 × Absent	−1 × Absent	Absent
2	1 × Present	1 × Absent	Absent
3	−1 × Absent	−1 × Present	Absent
4	1 × Present	1 × Present	Absent
5	−1 × Absent	−1 × Absent	Present
6	1 × Present	1 × Absent	Present
7	−1 × Absent	−1 × Present	Present
8	1 × Present	1 × Present	Present

In other words, the computation of the average effect of Factor A results in the simultaneous elimination of the effect of Factor B (Factor B's average effect when computed in this manner is 0). If the same set of coefficients is applied to the column for Factor C, it too will disappear. The same thing occurs when you compute the effect of Factor B—Factors A and C disappear, and similarly for the computation of the effect of Factor C.

The computation of factor effects outlined above is the key to understanding the power and utility of experimental designs. All experimental designs, regardless of the name, are based on this method of determining factor effects.

Table 7   Number of experiments needed to investigate a given number of factors using fractional-factorial, full-factorial, and one-factor-at-a-time methods of experimental design

Number of Factors	Fractional Design	Ideal One-Factor-at-a-Time (Full Factorial)	Typical One-Factor-at-a-Time
2	4	4	12
3	4	8	24
4	8	16	64
5	8	32	160
6	8	64	384
7	8	128	896
8	16	256	2,048
9	16	512	4,608
10	16	1,024	10,240

Reduction of the Experimental Effort

This ability to fractionate a design means that it is possible for an investigator to independently examine the effects of large numbers of factors on one or more measured responses. Table 7 illustrates the savings in experimental effort that can be achieved with this method.

Since biological units (patients and lab animals) typically exhibit more natural unit-to-unit variation than units in an engineering setting (e.g., machines, processes), an investigator will want to run more than one unit with each experimental condition. If one runs as few as four animals per experimental condition and is interested in the effects of just three factors, the total number of animals required to measure the effects of those factors using one-at-a-time methods versus that of fractional-factorial experimental designs is 16 versus 96—a sixfold difference. It is easy to see that the differences in total number of animals and total number of experiments translate into large differences in time, effort, and cost.

Benefits

Experimental designs are the most efficient methods available for identifying significant relationships between factors and responses. They avoid the serious methodological problems of one-factor-at-a-time experimental efforts, and they allow the investigator to independently assess the significance of the effects of multiple factors on any measured response.

Robert S. Butler

See also Equivalence Testing; Hypothesis Testing; Statistical Testing: Overview

Further Readings

Box, G. E. P., Hunter, W. G., & Hunter, J. S. (1978). *Statistics for experimenters: An introduction to design, data analysis, and model building.* New York: Wiley.

EXPERT OPINION

Expert opinion is a judgment that applies knowledge to a domain-specific problem by a person with superior knowledge in that domain. The term therefore involves two concepts, domain specificity and superiority of knowledge—called expertise. Both are necessary for one to be in a position to offer expert opinion.

Expert opinion is based on judgment. Judgment is an integration task, integrating relevant available cues while excluding irrelevant cues and inferring unavailable information. Judgment becomes opinion with the inference of the unavailable information.

Expertise

Domain specificity means that expertise in one domain does not necessarily transfer to another. An expert in medicine does not likely possess expertise in law. Although there are a few individuals who have training and experience in both domains, whether or not they maintain expertise in both is open to question. Furthermore, within a broad domain such as medicine, expertise is generally limited to subsets of domain knowledge. Thus, an expert in orthopedic surgery would not likely possess expertise in vascular surgery, nor would the expert be likely to have expertise in internal medicine. That does not mean that an individual with expertise in a specific domain would not have useful knowledge of other domains. It merely means that, generally, an individual possesses expertise in only a narrow subset of domain-specific knowledge.

Superior knowledge entails a number of prerequisites. Experience is a necessary, but not sufficient, prerequisite for expertise. Experience can allow an individual to develop schema for domain-specific problems. Schemata are mental representations of a situation. For instance, an internist specializing in infectious tropical disease would likely have a schema for schistosomiasis. A general practitioner practicing in the rural United States would not be likely to have such a schema.

Experience may further elaborate schemata through feedback and allow for the development of ability to discriminate between similar schemata. For instance, a specialist with extensive experience in tropical infectious disease should be able to differentiate between schistosomiasis, Chagas disease, and malaria. Other physicians likely would not. Experience and the feedback that is gained through experience allows for the development of scripts to match specific schema. Scripts are behavioral protocols that are appropriate for specific schemata. With experience, discrimination of the script that accompanies a schema becomes increasingly automatic. This is why experts often have difficulty

articulating their thoughts; the schema and scripts have become so automatic that they are processed rapidly without conscious awareness. Thus, experts may be able to offer an expert opinion more easily than they can explain how they reached that opinion. However, if one is not organizing experience into schemata, attending to feedback, developing scripts to accompany specific schema, and continually updating these memory structures, one may have experience without expertise.

As is implied by the need to update memory structures, expertise must be continuously updated. Domain knowledge in many fields, medicine being a prime example, is not static. An individual who is an expert in orthopedic surgery at one point in time, but who does not continually update and expand his or her knowledge, loses expertise. This is why expertise is often found in academic arenas. To teach, one must continually update knowledge to maintain and further develop schemata and scripts.

Level of expertise in making judgments in any specific domain is related to how much knowledge is available about how that domain operates and is structured and how much feedback is available from decisions previously made in that domain. People are more likely to become expert if they operate in fields where much is known and feedback from previous decisions is consistent and relevant. Those who practice without these environmental elements are handicapped in their ability to develop expertise.

Experts need not and often don't agree. Although on the surface, this seems like an oxymoron, it follows from two facts. First, if two people provide opinions that disagree, one may later be found to be correct, and the other by elimination would be incorrect. However, which is correct may not be known at the time a decision must be made. Sometimes, the correct opinion is not known until after the decision is made. Second, since judgment is an integration of known information to infer otherwise unavailable information, agreement between judges does not imply that an agreed-on opinion is correct. At one time, experts agreed that the sun revolved around the earth.

Types of Expertise

Within a domain, information and performance can be separated into three kinds of mental models. This delimitation of expertise is the work of Jens Rasmussen. Expertise can be described as skill based, rule based, and knowledge based. Skill-based mental models allow for the ability to physically manipulate the environment within a spatial and temporal frame of reference, based on superior sensory motor skill. Skill is useful for many domains and necessary for some, for example, surgery. Skill qualifies one as an expert in a domain of physical practice, such as surgery. Skill-based expertise allows one to physically intervene in a situation where skill is required. However, superior skill does not qualify one to offer an expert opinion on the domain.

Rule-based mental models involve knowledge of relationships between cues that activate familiar schemata and scripts. Superior skill and superior rule-based knowledge may be found in the same individual. Recognition-primed decisions are rule based. An expert in rule-based decision making can quickly identify the schema and scripts that are appropriate to a familiar situation. A person who has superior rule-based expertise is in a position to offer an opinion about which rule should be applied to situations for which there are established rules, but this person does not necessarily have the ability to offer an expert opinion about novel situations.

Mental models based on knowledge involve understanding of the organization and operation of domain phenomena and of relationships between structures and concepts within the domain. Knowledge-based mental models allow novel situations to be understood and appropriate responses to be developed. It is possible to have all three levels of expertise, but this is not always the case. A unique trait of knowledge-based decision makers is the ability to know when a rule does not cover a situation and to develop novel alternatives.

Well-developed knowledge-based mental models allow one to offer an opinion about how to respond to a novel situation for which the rules are unclear or for which rules do not exist. Knowledge-based decision making is not restricted to the ability to diagnose but rather includes the ability to recognize what information is demanded by the situation and what tests and procedures will clarify that information. Knowledge-based decision making includes the ability to select the best treatment and to know how to monitor that treatment so that it can be evaluated and adjustments made.

Measurement of Superior Knowledge

One measure of expertise is to survey those in the domain for which one requires expert opinion and choose the person whom most peers judge to be the most expert. This approach is likely to confuse skill-, rule- and knowledge-based expertise. It has the added limitation of a halo effect: Those who are most likeable are often judged as more expert. Still another method of establishing expert knowledge is to develop a panel of people with domain experience and assume that the points on which the panel agrees can be considered expert opinion. Guidelines for clinical practice often encapsulate a consensus view from professionals designated as experts. This approach is based on two assumptions: first, that experience, and often hierarchical position, captures expertise and second, that consensus captures truth. Both assumptions have been shown to be invalid, as noted above.

There is no way to measure superior knowledge directly. Expert opinion involves making a judgment rather than acting on that judgment. Since judgment is necessary prior to decision and action, expert opinion involves the knowledge from which to make a judgment but does not necessarily involve decision making. However, performance implies knowledge and can be objectively measured.

The best way to identify expert performance is to identify those who exhibit the ability to discriminate relevant cues in a domain of practice and do so consistently. The focus on the ability to discriminate relevant cues from irrelevant ones taps into cognitive elements underlying performance. The focus on consistency in this ability eliminates performance that is effective only part of the time because the individual does not have a thorough grasp of the knowledge necessary to make a consistent decision. Expert opinion might be available from those who are able to consistently discriminate what is important to decisions in a particular practice domain.

Application

Expert opinion is often used to provide guidance when more objective guidance, such as testing, is unavailable or equivocal or in decisions for which the rules are unclear. Therefore, expert opinion usually refers to knowledge-based expertise. It is not surprising to see much of the literature on expert opinion aimed at forensic decisions, such as likelihood to reoffend. However, some use of expert opinion may involve providing information on the correct rules that should be applied, such as when an expert is asked to state the standard of practice for a given situation.

Selection Criteria

When selecting someone from whom to obtain an expert opinion, the selection criteria should include the following: (a) The experts must be knowledgeable, not just skilled, in the specific domain about which they are to express an opinion; (b) they should understand the rules of that domain as well as possess an in-depth understanding of the mechanisms that underlie the operation of that system; (c) they should have shown that they are able to make accurate judgments within that domain on the task for which they will offer an opinion; and (d) they should have done this with a high level of consistency. Nowhere in these criteria is there a direct requirement for experience; however, most, if not all, of the criteria imply experience as a prerequisite.

James Shanteau and
Alleene M. Ferguson Pingenot

See also Expert Systems; Judgment

Further Readings

Ericsson, K. A., Charness, N., Feltovich, P. J., & Hoffman, R. R. (Eds.). (2007). *The Cambridge handbook of expertise and expert performance*. New York: Cambridge University Press.

Rasmussen, J., Pejtersen, A. M., & Goodstein, L. P. (1994). *Cognitive systems engineering* (Wiley Series in Systems Engineering). New York: Wiley.

Weiss, D. J., & Shanteau, J. (2003). Empirical assessment of expertise. *Human Factors, 45*(Spring), 104–114.

EXPERT SYSTEMS

The concept of expert medical systems has changed over several decades from that of a system that would replace human decision making with machines modeled on the behavior of experts to that of software systems that provide information and support to human decision makers. Expert medical systems are computer systems that facilitate the work of clinical decision makers, increasing their efficiency and accuracy while remaining responsive to changes in knowledge and flexible in response to clinical needs. Despite progress in design, recent systems still experience failure more often than is acceptable, and performance is suboptimal in many cases.

It was easy, in the rush to capitalize on the ability to store information in computers, to design what some considered expert medical systems without first gaining a thorough understanding of the concepts integral to expertise in medicine. Furthermore, knowledge in medicine is always expanding. Any system designed without a mechanism for continual review and updating of information quickly becomes out of date and is hence worse than useless. A system that does not consider the needs of all users is an error-prone system.

Researchers have gained insights into how effective human decision makers think as well as knowledge of what machines do best and what humans do best. They also are learning about how the two, man and machine, interact. These are tools necessary to accomplish the goal of designing functional and reliable expert medical systems.

Human Decision Behavior

It is not necessary to have an exact model from which to design a functional system. Rather, it is important to identify information that is critical to effective decisions in the targeted situations. The ability to design a system that includes critical information, but is inexact otherwise, allows for the development of adaptive systems.

Research on human experts can identify information needed for effective decision making. Human experts do not use all available information. Rather, they use information relevant to the decision at hand. They know what information is missing and look for disconfirming as well as confirming evidence. Experts use feedback from each small, incremental decision to adjust their understanding of the situation before making the next decision. This approach allows for both flexibility and recovery from error.

Interaction of Human and Machine

The interaction of human and machine (computer) can be conceptualized as similar to two individuals working on a joint project. That is, the human and the machine are part of a decision-making dyad. Machines can only do what they are programmed to do. The human part of the dyad must be able to perceive whether and how some action might be best accomplished using the machine. This means that the interface must be designed to be intuitive to the user.

The work of humans interacting with machines is supervisory. Machines do some things well, such as retrieving stored information, conducting complex operations, performing repetitive or routine tasks, and maintaining archives. The human decides what information to provide to the machine, uses information retrieved from storage, directs computations to be performed, and updates evidence for practice.

Safety

Keeping the human decision maker in charge is especially important when exceptions arise or the situation changes—circumstances that machines are not designed to accommodate. Experts have knowledge of the situation and the goals to be accomplished, and can devise novel approaches to solve unusual problems that arise.

Change in system state must be collaborative between the human user and the machine. Without feedback, the behavior of the human user can be irrational, even dangerous. Accident investigations often reveal that lethal errors occured when a human user misunderstood what a machine was doing, for example, when the interface did not provide information in a way that was intuitive to the user. As a result, the human made erroneous decisions. Feedback from the machine is important even when a program does most of the work because when the human takes over, he or she needs to know what has happened in the system prior to making a decision and taking action.

Constraints should be built into the system. Constraints are identified by a thorough understanding of the work as a whole, including the specific goals, tasks, and options of the operator. Constraints identify behaviors that *can't* be done; for example, one should not order incompatible drugs. A well-designed expert system would notify the user of drug incompatibility rather than blindly documenting administration, as is the case with many existing systems. An expert system designed with constraints in mind, but that includes flexibility for situations when the built-in rules do not apply, is critical for success.

When expert decision systems are programmed with default settings, the default should be a safe setting. Fatalities have resulted from machines that were programmed for default settings that turned out to be lethal. To properly select a default setting, research should identify the typical or "normal" setting of the system and program that as the default, requiring the user to actively change the default settings if using other than typical values. Expert systems must never be programmed to perform outside the safe limits of operation. Any change to a setting outside safe operational range should require verification for the change.

The issue of locking out behavior that shouldn't be performed has generated lively debate. Decision aiding and warning flags should be viewed as information exchange between the machine and the human decision maker. Experienced clinicians can think of examples where exceptions must be made to the general rule or where a decision support simply does not have the relevant information. The ability to know when rules don't apply or when critical information is missing is a trait identifying human experts.

Flexibility in expert systems allows for human experts to modify the system's behavior based on experience or information not available to the machine. Clinicians should be able to override warnings by documenting their clinical reasoning and take responsibility for the decision. In addition, it would be useful for clinicians to supply a plan for identifying and responding to adverse outcomes to their decision. This approach preserves flexibility while demanding accountability. Design of warnings within decision aids is an area ripe for research.

Decision Support

The usefulness of decision support systems depends on how well they are designed. There are areas about which researchers have a great deal of prior knowledge and can therefore build "expert systems" using if-then rules. These systems are particularly useful for nonexperts, who must sometimes make decisions for which they lack the knowledge or skills. Also, such systems can be useful for training students.

Some machine behavior enhances human performance by accomplishing things that humans are physically or cognitively unable to perform, such as the precise serial radiography of a CT machine. However, these machine behaviors serve to enhance the behavioral response of the decision maker rather than replace the human. Although a CT machine incorporates an expert system, it must be programmed by humans using specific parameters to accomplish the task to be done.

There are a number of ways in which expert advice can be designed into medical systems to assist in accessing relevant information. Rather than simply adapting existing machine structures from other applications, such as business, it is imperative that clinical decision making be examined in terms of goals, the needs of the clinician, information flow, and a deep understanding of the clinical situation. When appropriately designed systems meet the needs of users, they will be used. However, evidence shows that decision support systems do not necessarily lead to better clinical decision making, nor do they necessarily increase patient safety or reduce costs. It is well known that well-intentioned decision support systems are often overridden by users.

There are areas where the knowledge needed to build an expert system simply doesn't exist (e.g., some complex treatment problems). In these decision contexts, it is more useful to produce probabilistic advice based on linear modeling of what is known, rather than outputting a single decision per se. The question to the decision support tool in some of these situations might be posed as "the probability of x happening if treatment regimen y is pursued, given the known facts of the patient situation." Such linear models have been shown to outperform human decision makers, particularly in situations where information is ill-defined and incomplete.

One area where decision supports are being developed is for aiding patients in their own healthcare decision making. Decision aids designed for the lay public are necessarily different in focus from those designed for clinicians. Research on these decision tools focuses on issues such as how best to display information, which information is most relevant on specific topics, and designs for ease of access and use. Interestingly, it appears that more research may be dedicated to the design of patient decision aids than to the design of clinical decision support for clinicians.

Innovative Uses of Machines to Manage Information

The availability of large clinical data sets led to research that identifies and categorizes information for the study of specific clinical problems. For such work (collection and organization of information), machine systems are invaluable. Research using large clinical data sets includes studies of adverse drug reactions and analysis of the relationship of cancer stages to other clinical information. In addition, computer systems assist with quality-of-care assessments by informing clinical decisions that improve delivery of care.

The complexity of medical data is at the root of many of the problems encountered in developing effective expert tools for supporting clinical decision making. Several research programs studying design of expert medical systems have explored the use of fuzzy logic systems as a way to model the complex flow of information required in medicine. This approach seems compatible with the fact that human experts use information in an incomplete but highly functional way, as was discussed above.

It is especially encouraging to find that expert system design innovations are now being more carefully evaluated than were early systems. However, many of these evaluations are based primarily on qualitative feedback from users. As research on the design of clinical systems matures, it is hoped that more objective measures, such as clinical outcomes and efficiency, will become standards of design excellence.

Future Directions

The outlook for expert medical systems is bright. However, the future belongs to systems that augment human decision making by performing simple repetitive activities and calculations that humans do poorly and providing critical information in a timely way. Once these systems become functional, they will likely be well accepted. It might be useful, however, to recognize that interacting with machines changes our behavior. It seems likely that the integration of expert medical systems has already and will continue to change the social environment in which medicine is practiced, perhaps in ways we can't imagine at present.

James Shanteau and
Alleene M. Ferguson Pingenot

See also Computer-Assisted Decision Making

Further Readings

Nelson, W. L., Han, P. K. U., Fagerlin, A., Stefanek, M., & Ubel, P. A. (2007). Rethinking the objective of decision aids: A call for conceptual clarity. *Medical Decision Making, 27*(5), 609–618.

Pingenot, A., Shanteau, J., & Sengstache, D. (2008). Cognitive work analysis of an inpatient medication system. In *Computers, informatics, nursing.* Hagerstown, MD: Wolters Kluwer/Lippincott Williams & Wilkins. Manuscript submitted for publication.

Shanteau, J. (1992). The psychology of experts: An alternative view. In G. Wright & F. Bolger (Eds.), *Expertise and decision support* (pp. 11–23). New York: Plenum Press.

Vicente, K. J. (1999). *Cognitive work analysis: Toward safe, productive and healthy computer-based work.* Mahwah, NJ: Lawrence Erlbaum.

Weir, C. R., Nebeker, J. J. R., Hicken, B. L., Campo, R., Drews, F., & LeBar, B. (2007). A cognitive work analysis of information management strategies in a computerized provider order entry environment. *Journal of the American Medical Informatics Association, 14*(1), 65–75.

Wright, G., & Bolger, F. (Eds.). (1992). *Expertise and decision support.* New York: Plenum Press.

EXTENDED DOMINANCE

The term *dominance* in the context of cost-effectiveness analysis refers to the situation in which two clinical strategies are being compared.

One strategy, Strategy X, is said to dominate another, Strategy Y, if either (a) the expected costs of Strategy X are less than the expected costs of Strategy Y and the expected benefits of Strategy X are at least as great as the expected benefits of Strategy Y or (b) the expected benefits of Strategy X are greater than the expected benefits of Strategy Y and the expected costs of Strategy X are not greater than the expected costs of Strategy Y. Usually, the dominant strategy is both more effective and less costly than the alternative. This concept of dominance is also referred to as *strong dominance* or *simple dominance.*

The *extended dominance principle* (also known as *weak dominance*) is applied in cost-effectiveness studies that compare mutually exclusive interventions. This is the situation where only one of the strategies is available to each participant.

The concept of extended dominance is applied in incremental cost-effectiveness analysis to eliminate from consideration strategies whose costs and benefits are improved by a mixed strategy of two other alternatives. That is, two strategies may be used together as a "blended" strategy, instead of assigning a single treatment strategy to all members of a population. Blending strategies only becomes relevant when the most effective strategy is too costly to recommend to all.

The concept may have been first suggested when a particular clinical strategy was "dominated in an extended sense," thus leading to the term *extended dominance.* Extended dominance rules out any strategy with a higher incremental cost-effectiveness ratio (ICER), which is greater than that of a more effective strategy. That is, extended dominance applies to strategies that are not cost-effective because another available strategy provides more units of benefit at a lower cost per unit of benefit.

Among competing choices, an alternative is said to be excluded by extended dominance if its ICER relative to the next less costly undominated alternative is greater than that of a more costly alternative.

Here is a simple example of a competing choice problem that can be evaluated for strong dominance and extended dominance. Table 1 shows costs and outcomes for standard of care and five hypothetical interventions.

From the comparison of costs and outcomes, we can rule out Intervention E because it is strongly dominated by Intervention D. Intervention D costs

Table I   Costs and outcomes for standard of care and five hypothetical interventions

Strategy	Cost ($)	Effectiveness (QALYs)
Standard of care	5,000	1
E	12,000	1.5
D	10,000	2
C	25,000	3
B	35,000	4
A	55,000	5

less and gives better outcomes than E. Having ruled out Intervention E, we can compare the remaining strategies based on their ICERs. This is where the principle of extended dominance comes in. Table 2 shows the remaining interventions listed in order of effectiveness. The ICER of each intervention is found by comparing it with the next most effective option.

We can now use the principle of extended dominance to rule out Intervention C. Intervention C has an ICER of $15,000 per quality-adjusted life year (QALY). To agree to use Intervention C, the deciding body would have to agree to adopt all interventions with ICERs up to $15,000 per QALY. If so, they would be much better off choosing Intervention B over Intervention C, since a greater number of QALYs can be obtained with this intervention at a lower cost per QALY. The logic goes thus: If one is willing to pay a smaller amount to gain a life year (or QALY or whatever unit of effectiveness) with the more expensive

strategy, then one should not choose the strategy with the higher ICER.

Table 3 shows the interventions and their ICERs after the extended dominance principle has been applied. It is now up to the decision maker to choose among the interventions based on how much they are willing to pay for a QALY.

If willingness to pay (WTP) is not even $5,000 per QALY, then none of the interventions generates sufficient worth to be adopted. If however, WTP is greater than $20,000 per QALY, then Intervention A would be adopted.

As mentioned above, when extended dominance exists, it is possible to create a mixed strategy of two alternatives (i.e., when one portion of the population receives one strategy and the remainder receives an alternative strategy) that can yield greater or equal benefits at an equal or cheaper cost than would a third alternative, if applied to all members of the population. For those strategies that were eliminated from consideration by extended dominance, a range of plausible mixed strategies that would dominate the eliminated alternatives can be computed.

The coefficient of inequity is defined as the minimum proportion of people receiving the worst strategy within a mixture of two strategies when invoking extended dominance. The coefficient of inequity represents a level of unfairness if a mixed strategy were ever to be implemented. Since in extended dominance, a linear combination of two strategies can be shown to dominate a third strategy, from a practical perspective, this may have ethical ramifications. It implies that a strategy is dominated because a given fraction of the population may be receiving an inferior strategy for the overall health of the population to be improved.

Table 2   Strategies after considering simple (strong) dominance

Strategy	Cost ($)	Effectiveness (QALYs)	ICER ($)
Standard of care	5,000	1	—
D	10,000	2	5,000
C	25,000	3	15,000
B	35,000	4	10,000
A	55,000	5	20,000

Table 3   Strategies after considering extended (weak) dominance

Strategy	Cost ($)	Effectiveness (QALYs)	ICER ($)
Standard of care	5,000	1	—
D	10,000	2	5,000
B	35,000	4	12,500
A	55,000	5	20,000

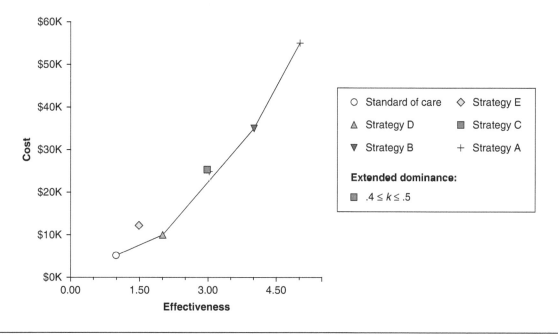

Figure 1   Example of extended dominance

The above example is graphically represented in Figure 1.

In the example, Strategy E is dominated by Strategy D (dominance). Strategy C is dominated by a blend of Strategy D and Strategy B (extended dominance), with a coefficient of inequity equal to .4. The coefficient of inequity is calculated as the difference of the cost of the more expensive strategy and the cost of the weakly dominated strategy divided by the difference of the cost of the more expensive strategy and the cost of the cheaper strategy; in this case, this is

$$(35,000 - 25,000)/(35,000 - 10,000)$$
$$= 10,000/25,000 = .4.$$

Lesley-Ann N. Miller and Scott B. Cantor

See also Cost-Benefit Analysis; Cost-Effectiveness Analysis; Cost-Utility Analysis; Dominance; Efficacy Versus Effectiveness

Further Readings

Cantor, S. B. (1994). Cost-effectiveness analysis, extended dominance and ethics: A quantitative assessment. *Medical Decision Making, 14,* 259–265.

Gold, M. R., Siegel, J. E., Russell, L. B., & Weinstein, M. C. (Eds.). (1996). *Cost-effectiveness in health and medicine*. New York: Oxford University Press.

Hunink, M. G. M., Glasziou, P. P., Siegel, J. E., Weeks, J. C., Pliskin, J. S., Elstein, A. S., et al. (2001). *Decision making in health and medicine: Integrating evidence and values*. Cambridge, UK: Cambridge University Press.

Johannesson, M., & Weinstein, M. C. (1993). On the decision rules of cost-effectiveness analysis. *Journal of Health Economics, 12,* 459–467.

Kamlet, M. S. (1992). *The comparative benefits modeling project: A framework for cost-utility analysis of government health care programs*. Washington, DC: U.S. Department of Health and Human Services.

Raiffa, H., Schwartz, W. B., & Weinstein, M. C. (1977). Evaluating health effects of societal decisions and programs. *Decision making in the environmental protection agency* (Vol. 2b, pp. 1–81). Washington, DC: National Academy of Sciences.

Stinnett, A. A., & Paltiel, A. D. (1996). Mathematical programming for the efficient allocation of health care resources. *Journal of Health Economics, 15,* 641–653.

Torrance, G. W., Thomas, W. H., & Sackett, D. L. (1972). A utility maximization model for evaluation of health care programs. *Health Services Research, 7,* 118–133.

Weinstein, M. C., & Fineberg, H. V. (1980). *Clinical decision analysis*. Philadelphia: W. B. Saunders.

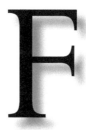

Factor Analysis and Principal Components Analysis

On the surface, the methods of factor analysis and principal components analysis (PCA) share similarities and common purposes. In particular, they both involve the characterization of multiple variables into components, or factors. However, factor analysis is much more ambitious than PCA in that it involves modeling assumptions, in particular the modeling of latent, unobservable factors.

Principal Components

PCA can be used to reduce the dimensionality of data in the sense of transforming an original set of variables to a smaller number of transformed ones. Such a purpose is desirable as it allows for the parsimonious explanation of the systematic variation of data with as few variables as possible. Obtaining parsimonious representations of data is especially useful when confronted with large numbers of variables, such as those found in survey data or genetics data. Socioeconomic variables have been combined into a smaller number through PCA as well. Furthermore, in regression analyses, multicollinearity can be a serious concern when there are a large number of variables to model. Reducing the number of variables used in an analysis or transforming the original variables to make them uncorrelated, as PCA does, can alleviate this problem.

PCA involves rotating multivariate data, which involves transforming the original variables into a new set of variables that are linear combinations of the original variables. This rotation process yields a new set of variables with desirable properties.

Let $X_1, \ldots, X_p$ (the Xs) denote the original variables. For instance, the Xs could be clinical variables, such as X_1 being weight measurements, X_2 being heights, X_3 being systolic blood pressure, and so on. Each X_i, $i = 1, \ldots, p$, is a vector with n elements, representing, for instance, n observations of the variable X_i from n subjects. A linear combination of the Xs would take the form $a_1 X_1 + \ldots + a_p X_p$, for some constant weights $a_1, \ldots, a_p$. Loosely speaking, one object of PCA is to find uncorrelated linear combinations of the Xs that maximize the variance, a measure of the variability in data. Weights for the linear combinations being considered are restricted so that the sum of their squared values is 1. This restricts possible solutions under consideration to be derivable from rotations. Based on elegant theories from linear algebra, a sketch of how they are derived is given below (for more details, see Tatsuoka, 1988).

Given variables $X_1, \ldots, X_p$, one can construct a $p \times p$ matrix $\mathbf{A}$ that is composed of sample covariances A, with the i,jth entry in $\mathbf{A}$ corresponding to the sample covariance between X_i and X_j. Covariances measure the degree to which two variables vary together, or are correlated. We can solve what is known as the characteristic equation for the matrix $\mathbf{A}$ and generate p nonnegative roots (although it is possible that some roots are equal, or even zero, depending on the rank of **A**). This equation is derived based on the objective of finding linear combinations of the Xs that maximize variance. These roots are known as the eigenvalues of the matrix **A**. Furthermore, given these eigenvalues, corresponding vectors, called eigenvectors, can be derived where the elements in the eigenvectors give the weights for the desired linear combinations. Moreover, the eigenvalues are equal to the corresponding variance of the linear combination of the Xs, with weights corresponding to the eigenvector. Hence, the eigenvalues and eigenvectors that are generated provide the essential practical information in attaining the objectives of PCA.

Denote the eigenvalues in descending order as $\lambda_1, \lambda_2, \ldots, \lambda_p$ so that $\lambda_1 \le \lambda_2 \le \ldots \le \lambda_p$. More explicitly, PCA will generate a new set of variables, or components, $Y_1, \ldots, Y_n$ (the Ys), with

$$Y_1 = a_{(11)} X_1 + \ldots + a_{(1n)} X_n,$$
$$Y_2 = a_{(21)} X_1 + \ldots + a_{(2n)} X_n, \ldots,$$

where $a_{(ij)}$ are constants such that the sum of the squared values of $a_{(ij)}$ is 1. Again, these constants are derived from the elements in the associated eigenvector. Importantly, the new components have conditionally maximal variances in the following sense: Y_1 has maximum variance among all such linear combinations of the Xs, Y_2 has maximum variance among all such linear combinations of the Xs that are uncorrelated with Y_1, Y_3 has maximum variance among all such linear combinations of the Xs uncorrelated with Y_1 and Y_2, and so on. Moreover, the variance of Y_1 is λ_1, the variance of Y_2 is λ_2, and so on.

An important result of this transformation is that the sum of the λs is equal to the sum of the variances of the Xs. Thus, the variation of the Xs can be viewed as "reshuffled" among the Ys, and this variation is concentrated on as few variables as possible. It is in this variation that the statistical information provided by the variables is contained. A subset of the Ys can be parsimoniously selected for subsequent analyses, and such a subset indeed does represent much of the variation in the Xs. We can determine this as follows.

If the Xs span a linear subspace with dimension r, with $r < p$, then PCA will find $(p - r)$ degenerate components (all zero weights for those components). While in practice, purely nondegenerate components

won't be found due to random variation, components nonetheless could appear to be "essentially" degenerate, for instance, as measured by relatively small associated eigenvalues. In such cases, the components with the larger associated eigenvalues would contain most of the variation in data across the X variables, and hence little information would be lost by retaining only those components.

So a key methodological issue in applying PCA involves determining which components to keep for an analysis and which to discard. There are many approaches and criteria in helping make this decision. Two basic rules of thumb for selecting components are as follows: (1) retain components with the highest associated variances (eigenvalues) such that the total variation ratio, which is equal to the ratio of the sum of eigenvalues associated with the retained components to the sum of all eigenvalues, is greater than .85 or .90, and (2) choose components with a corresponding eigenvalue of at least 1.0. Another approach is the scree test, where eigenvalues are plotted in order of magnitude and truncation of components is determined by identifying a cutoff for when the changes in associated eigenvalue magnitudes appear to begin leveling off as the eigenvalues get increasingly smaller. Components are truncated when associated eigenvalues that are of the smallest magnitude are deemed to be beyond the cutoff.

Importantly, for PCA, there are no distributional assumptions that have to be made about the Xs. Moreover, there are no modeling assumptions to validate either. PCA is thus a widely applicable statistical tool with a clearly defined and attainable purpose.

Factor Analysis

Factor analysis attempts to describe an observed set of variables (the Xs) in terms of a linear model of unobservable factors (the Ys), much as in a regression model. However, a key difference is that the Ys are latent and unobservable. Factor analysis can thus be used to explore or reveal an internal structure or hidden relationships between observable variables by linking them to underlying latent constructs. Because of the presence of latent factors and the key role they play, factor analysis presents a difficult and ambitious statistical modeling problem. Yet it is a commonly used method because there are a range of problems in which it is desirable to model observable phenomena as a function of unobservable factors.

For instance, in psychologically related applications, such as in psychiatry, quality-of-life measurement, and neuropsychological assessment, it is sometimes posited that underlying constructs are a driving force in the behavior of observed variables. For example, collections of neuropsychological measures (the Xs) could be employed to assess the impact of a treatment on cognitive functioning. Such measures could assess different aspects of cognition—for example, through tasks that require memory or strategizing. Factor analysis could be used to assess what types of underlying cognitive functions (the Ys), as represented by latent constructs, are in fact being tested. Examples of latent constructs that are identified in such applications include various types of memory functions, motor skills, and executive functions, which are posited as higher-order functions used to regulate other cognitive abilities.

A factor analysis model can be written as follows to relate the observable variables X_i, $i = 1, \ldots, p$, to unobservable factors Y_j, $j = 1, \ldots, k$:

$$X_i = a_{i1}Y_1 + \ldots + a_{ik}Y_k + d_iU_i,$$

where the $a_{(ij)}$, $j = 1, \ldots, k$, are called the factor loadings and are constants; U_i is a unique factor associated with X_i; and d_i is the factor loading for U_i. It is assumed that U_i are statistically independent from the Ys.

Note then that these models of the observable X variables have two components: (1) that which can be attributed to, or explained by the latent Y factors that are common among all observable X variables and (2) that which is unique to each variable, not part of the common-factor structure of the Ys. The uniqueness of each X_i is described by d_iU_i. Generally, it is assumed that X_i represents a standardized variable, in the sense that the mean of X_i is 0 and the variance is 1. This can be achieved by transforming the original variables through subtracting from each X_i variable its mean and then dividing this difference by the standard error of X_i.

For each variable X_i, the variance that is attributable to the common latent factors is known as its communality. Denote this communality by h_i^2.

Thus, $1 - h_i^2$ is the variance unique to the given X_i variable.

Since the unique factors are independent from the common factors, if the respective communalities can be substituted along the diagonal of the correlation matrix between the Xs, this modified correlation matrix thus represents the correlation between the common factors, given that the linear model is true. Such a modified matrix is called the reduced correlation matrix. Unfortunately, communalities are not known in advance and must be estimated.

Communalities must be estimated iteratively, since we must have an understanding of the factor structure (number of factors and loadings) first before estimating them. On the other hand, communalities must be known to create the reduced correlation matrix on which estimation of the factor structure depends. Generally, prior estimates of the communalities are made, then the factor structure is estimated, the communalities are then reestimated, and this process is iterated until convergence is met, as defined by some criteria that indicate that the estimates have stabilized from iteration to iteration.

Based on the reduced correlation matrix, the same matrix theory as the one used for PCA can be employed to derive uncorrelated factors and associated factor loadings. This is done by solving for eigenvalues and eigenvectors, as before. Again, the number of factors to keep in the model must be determined, by using the scree test or other methods.

Since factor analysis is used to assess the underlying latent structure and relationships between the observable variables, it is desired to understand and characterize the nature of the latent factors that are found. This is done by interpreting the sign and magnitude of the factor loadings and identifying the patterns that arise in terms of how the factor loadings are associated with the observable variables. Generally, though, the factors and their relationship to the observable variables do not easily lend themselves to interpretation. This drawback also is shared with PCA, which also can be used to assess if there is some pattern, or structure, between variables. Yet such interpretation is a major aim for many practitioners as they set out to conduct factor analysis. Interpretation can be improved through rotation, since rotations will change the factor loadings. Transformed factors may no longer be uncorrelated, but the reduced correlation matrix for the transformed factors remains unchanged, and hence the rotated factors are an equally plausible statistical formulation of the factor structure.

L. Thurstone described target criteria for selecting a rotation such that the transformed factors have certain characteristics that make interpretation easier. The main ones are roughly as follows: (a) each row should contain at least one zero so that not all variables are related to all factors; (b) each column should contain zeros as well so that each factor is not related to all variables; and (c) every pair of columns should contain rows whose loadings are zero in one column but nonzero in the other, so that factors are differentially related to the variables. Of course, no real-life factor-loading pattern will satisfy these criteria exactly, but it is certainly still desirable that they be approximately satisfied. There are a number of rotational techniques that have been developed to enhance interpretability of factor loadings, such as the varimax rotation.

As an example, using factor analysis, suppose two main underlying factors are identified among six measures, with the following factor loadings:

	Factor 1	Factor 2
Measure 1	0.8	0.05
Measure 2	0.9	0.05
Measure 3	−0.8	0.04
Measure 4	0.05	0.8
Measure 5	0.04	0.8
Measure 6	0.05	−0.9

The above factor structure approximately satisfies Thurstone's target criteria. Indeed, one could now attempt to identify an underlying common theme within the collection of the first three measures and within the collection of the last three measures in order to give interpretations to the two latent factors, respectively. Note that in practice, factor loadings can be negative. In terms of interpretation, this would imply that larger values of the observed factor are associated

with smaller values of the underlying associated factor.

Factor analysis is used in validating scales, where, for instance, certain questions are grouped together and the response scores are combined to generate a scale score. For instance, in the quality-of-life survey SF-36, subscales can be generated from subsets of questions relating to body pain, social functioning, physical functioning, mental health, and so on. Justification for such groupings is supported if grouped questions share similarly high factor loading values on the same factor relative to other variables. Of course, such groupings must also be justified clinically.

Factor analysis is dependent on the information provided by correlations to estimate underlying relationships and factor loadings. Correlations are suited for measuring the strengths of linear relationships. Hence, nonlinear relationships between latent factors and observable variables may not be modeled well. Interpretation of factors is not clear-cut, nor is the selection of an appropriate rotation. Another critical subjective decision that must be made concerns the number of factors to keep in the model. These ambiguities make the task of detecting underlying structure more difficult. Modeling latent factors is an ambitious endeavor, and hence, model fit must be validated in a thorough manner, such as through cross-validation. Replication of findings may be elusive given all these issues. In sum, one should be cautious in drawing conclusions through factor analysis.

Curtis Tatsuoka

See also SF-36 and SF-12 Health Surveys; Variance and Covariance

Further Readings

Catell, R. (1966). The scree test for the number of factors. *Multivariate Behavioral Research, 1,* 245–276.

Kaiser, H. (1958). The varimax criterion for analytic rotation in factor analysis. *Psychometrika, 23,* 187–200.

Kaiser, H. (1960). The application of electronic computers in factor analysis. *Educational and Psychological Measurement, 20,* 141–151.

Tatsuoka, M. (1988). *Multivariate analysis: Techniques for educational and psychological research* (2nd ed.). New York: Macmillan.

Thurstone, L. (1947). *Multiple factor analysis.* Chicago: University of Chicago Press.

FEAR

Fear and anxiety can alter decision making in a wide range of domains, not least of all decisions about one's own health or the health of patients under a physician's care. Past research has demonstrated this influence, including in medicine. Understanding the impact that these basic emotions have on medical decisions, particularly those involving risky and uncertain options, is essential to understanding medical decision making and building accurate predictive models of choice. Traditional economic models of decision making, such as expected utility theory, propose that patients and physicians weigh decision options rationally and choose an action based on the likelihood and the payoff of outcomes. These models rarely include psychological influences on behavior, particularly the emotional ones. In the medical context, an important omission from these models is the effect of patients' and physicians' emotions as they weigh the options associated with treating a serious medical condition and choose an action.

Patients and physicians must consider the possible consequences of treatment decisions, and how likely these would be to occur. Decisions involving risky, uncertain outcomes are especially susceptible to the influence of emotions such as anxiety. Anxiety is common in patients with serious illness who must make risky treatment decisions with major consequences: death, functional disability, diminished quality of life and psychological well-being. Their fear and anxiety can significantly alter their decisions. Both patients and physicians can be affected by fear and anxiety when making these decisions.

Influence on Decision Making

Fear and anxiety are related emotions that can influence decision making in multiple ways. Two potential formulations for the role of anxiety are that (1) anxiety and fear about risks alter the evaluation process (such as probability assessments) and (2) anxiety and fear lead to seeking relief from the state. There appears to be a curvilinear relationship between escalating anxiety and performance. Under this conception, anxiety is emotional arousal, and it places a load on central cognitive processing, so that anxious decision makers evaluate evidence differently than nonanxious ones. At low levels, arousal can improve task performance, likely by recruiting additional cognitive resources, initiating coping strategies, and increasing motivation for success. However, when arousal becomes sufficiently high to be appreciable anxiety and fear, it then exceeds the cognitive analytic capacities and leads to greater use of problem simplification. This is most problematic if the decision maker has limited information, as many patients do, or if one has many complex problems and uncertain factors to consider, as many physicians do.

Additionally, immediate strong (negative) emotions (i.e., "hot states") can overwhelm cognitive goals and affect the way future dispassionate risks (i.e., "cold states") are evaluated. Initial, primitive reactions to personally relevant information consist of a rudimentary "good versus bad" interpretation. Fearful reactions to risk have been shown to cause decision making to diverge from cognitive-based assessments of risk. Anxiety is formulated as a psychic-physiologic state that one is highly motivated to alleviate and from which one wishes to return to a nonanxious, or less anxious, baseline.

Influence on Medical Decision Making

In the field of medicine, anxious individuals make decisions to alleviate existing anxiety states as well as to avoid new situations that cause anxiety. Although statistical odds might indicate that continuing watchful waiting, in lieu of initiating a risky treatment, is advisable at an early stage of a disease, patients and physicians may fear the consequences of not treating so acutely that the evidence-based statistical guidelines are overruled. Likewise, patients may avoid indicated treatment due to the anxiety that it evokes. Thomas Denberg and colleagues' investigation of men's treatment choices for localized prostate cancer yielded many cases where patients considered risky surgery as "dreadful" and associated with likely death.

William Dale and Joshua Hemmerich's work on watchful-waiting scenarios supports George Loewenstein's hypothesis that the vividness of an anxiety-provoking outcome increases the emotional response to like situations and changes physician behavior. Dale and Hemmerich investigated how a preceding premature abdominal aortic aneurysm rupture can influence vascular surgeons' and older adults' subsequent decisions about the timing of surgery. They found that experiencing a rupture during watchful waiting accelerated people's decision to end watchful waiting, even when statistical guidelines suggest patients should continue with watchful waiting. Laboratory-based follow-up studies show that participants in the simulation are significantly anxious following the rupture.

Detecting the presence of anxiety does not complete the task of explaining its influence on decision making. The locus of anxiety is another key determinant of how it will affect treatment decisions. Fear and anxiety can be tied to erroneous beliefs or realistic, well-founded concerns. The fear of treatment can be as influential as the fear of a disease, and it is possible that decision makers have multiple and potentially conflicting worries, anxieties, and fears. One must understand the specific sources of fear and anxiety if one is to intervene and manage the behavior they influence.

Another difficulty is that people have a poor appreciation for how emotions such as fear and anxiety can alter their decision making about the future; to put it succinctly, people are poor affective forecasters. People poorly predict what they would do when placed in a state of anxiety as an impending dreaded event approaches. It is important for medical-decision-making researchers to know what patients and physicians are afraid of and how afraid they are of it. Attempts to model treatment decisions where uncertainty and risk are involved will likely be inaccurate unless anxiety is appropriately incorporated into the model.

Fear and anxiety are underappreciated influences on medical decisions. Anxiety causes patients and physicians to make different choices about risky, uncertain decisions. Anxiety can distort decision makers' ideas of risk and valuation of possible options, and it is also a psychophysiological state that people take steps to avoid. Many medical decisions involve dreaded potential outcomes that provoke fear, leading to the avoidance of those situations. Understanding this influence is important for implementing evidence-based recommendations in practice.

William Dale and Joshua Hemmerich

See also Decision Making and Affect; Decision Psychology; Emotion and Choice; Mood Effects

Further Readings

Becker, G. S. (1976). *The economic approach to human behavior.* Chicago: University of Chicago Press.

Berns, G. S., Chappelow, J., Cekic, M., Zink, C. F., Pagnoni, G., & Martin-Skurski, M. E. (2006). Neurobiological substrates of dread. *Science, 312,* 754–758.

Dale, W., Bilir, P., Han, M., & Meltzer, D. (2005). The role of anxiety in prostate carcinoma: A structured review of the literature. *Cancer, 104,* 467–478.

Dale, W., Hemmerich, J., Ghini, E., & Schwarze, M. (2006). Can induced anxiety from a negative prior experience influence vascular surgeons' statistical decision-making? A randomized field experiment with an abdominal aortic aneurysm analog. *Journal of the American College of Surgeons, 203,* 642–652.

Denberg, T. D., Melhado, T. V., & Steiner, J. F. (2006). Patient treatment preferences in localized prostate carcinoma: The influence of emotion, misconception, and anecdote. *Cancer, 107,* 620–630.

Gilbert, D. T., & Ebert, J. E. J. (2002). Decisions and revisions: The affective forecasting of changeable outcomes. *Journal of Personality and Social Psychology, 82,* 503–514.

Hastie, R., & Dawes, R. M. (2001). *Rational choice in an uncertain world: The psychology of judgment and decision making.* Thousand Oaks, CA: Sage.

Kahneman, D., & Tversky, A. (2000). *Choices, values, and frames.* New York: Cambridge University Press.

Loewenstein, G. (1996). Out of control: Visceral influences on behavior. *Organizational Behavior and Human Decision Processes, 65,* 272–292.

Loewenstein, G. F., Hsee, C. K., Weber, E. U., & Welch, N. (2001). Risk as feelings. *Psychological Bulletin, 127,* 267–286.

FIXED VERSUS RANDOM EFFECTS

The terms *fixed* and *random* are commonly used in the regression modeling literature and pertain to whether particular coefficients in a model are treated as fixed or random values. A statistical model is classified as a fixed effects model if all independent variables are regarded as fixed, a random effects model if all independent variables are regarded as random, and a mixed effects model if the independent variables constitute a mix of fixed and random effects. Analytic methods vary depending on the model. The approach selected depends on the nature of the available data and the study objectives.

A fixed variable is one that is assumed to be measured without error. The values of the fixed variable from one study are assumed to be the same as the values in any attempted replication of the study; that is, they are the only levels of a factor that are of interest (hence the term *fixed*). Gender and marital status are examples of fixed variables because they have a small fixed number of categories (levels). There is no larger population of gender categories that the levels male and female are sampled from. Fixed effects regression and analysis of variance (ANOVA) refer to assumptions about the independent variable and the error distribution. The independent variables are assumed to be fixed, and the generalization of results applies to similar values of the independent variable in the population or in other studies.

A random variable is one whose levels are assumed to be a random sample from a larger population of levels for that variable. Subjects, hospitals, physicians, schools, and litters are examples of random factors since investigators usually want to make inferences beyond the particular values of the independent variable that were captured to a larger population. Designation of variables as fixed or random is not always straightforward. Some basic questions an investigator should ask are the following: (a) Is it reasonable to assume that the levels of an independent variable were randomly sampled from some population? (b) Is the goal to make inferences to a population from which the levels of the variable were selected or from the particular levels on hand? Treatments or drug doses from a clinical trial are usually considered fixed variables since they represent all levels of interest for a study; however, they can be considered as random if their levels are a subset of the possible values one wants to generalize to.

Random effects models are referred to as variance component models, hierarchical linear models, multilevel regression models, nested models, generalized linear mixed models, and random coefficient or mixed models (using both fixed and random effects). These models can be considered as extensions of linear models and have gained popularity with advances in computing and software availability.

Models

The underlying goal of much clinical research is to evaluate relationships among a set of variables. In an experiment, a change, or experimental condition, is introduced (the independent variable) to a subject or some experimental unit, and the effect of this change is studied on a characteristic of the subject (the outcome, dependent, or response variable). An experimental condition can be a treatment or combination of treatments or factors. Multiple factors are considered in the experimental design, such as the levels of treatment or experimental condition, patient population and selection of patients, assignment of treatment condition, and the response variable of interest.

A linear statistical model where the response variable (Y_i) is modeled as a function of the independent variables ($X_1, X_2, \ldots, X_k$) is given below:

$$Y_i = \beta_0 + \beta_1 X_1 + \beta_2 X_2 + \ldots + \beta_k X_k + \varepsilon_i,$$

where β_0, the intercept term, is a constant. $X_1, X_2, \ldots, X_k$ are fixed variables assumed to be observed without error. The β parameters are fixed effects of treatment or experimental condition on response and are regarded as constant, although unknown. The response variable is subject to error (denoted by ε_i) and is most often, but not necessarily, assumed to be normally distributed with zero mean and constant variance, σ^2. It represents unexplained variation in the dependent variable. The error terms are assumed to be uncorrelated for different subjects. The unknown parameters $\beta_0, \beta_1, \beta_2, \ldots, \beta_k$ characterize the relationship and are estimated from this equation to provide the best fit to the data. The method of least squares is used to obtain the best-fitting model. This is done by minimizing the sum of squares of the distances between the observed responses and those given by the fitted model. The least squares estimator is unbiased regardless of whether the error distribution is normally distributed or not. When the error distribution is normally distributed, the least squares estimates are equivalent to maximum likelihood estimates. The independent variables are also sometimes referred to as regressors, explanatory variables, exogenous variables, and predictor variables.

In a random effects model, an independent variable with a random effect has an infinite set of levels (a population of levels). The levels present in a study are considered a sample from that population. This induces random variation between subjects or experimental units. An investigator's interest is in drawing inferences that are valid for the complete population of levels. A specific example is patients treated in a multicenter study whereby a sample of hospitals across a region is studied as opposed to all hospitals in that region. The goal is to make inference on the population of hospitals from which the sample was drawn. This is a two-level data structure, with patients at Level 1 and hospitals at Level 2. In this setting, there are two kinds of random variation that need to be accounted for: (1) that between patients within a hospital and (2) that between different hospitals. Extending the notation from above, the random effects model that can account for the variability due to a single center can be expressed as follows:

$$Y_{ij} = \beta_0 + \beta_1 X_{1j} + \beta_2 X_{2j} + \ldots + \beta_k X_{kj} + t_j + \varepsilon_{ij},$$

where β_0 is an intercept that applies to all patients in the study, t_j is a random quantity for all patients in the jth hospital, and ε_{ij} is a random quantity for the ith patient in the jth hospital. In this model, it is assumed that the error and random effects (t_j) are independent and normally distributed with zero mean and constant variance, σ_j^2 and σ_e^2, respectively. Therefore, the residual variance is partitioned into two components: (1) a between-hospital component, the variance of the hospital-level residuals that represent unobserved hospital characteristics that affect patient outcomes, and (2) a within-hospital component, the variance of the patient-level residuals. The additional term for the random effect is what distinguishes this model from the ordinary regression model described earlier. If there is no hospital-to-hospital variation,

then the parameter estimates from the random effects model will be identical to those from the ordinary regression model. Inferences may be made on the fixed effects, random effects, or variance components using either least squares or maximum likelihood estimation and likelihood ratio tests. This model can also be fit with data from a repeated measures or longitudinal design, where random variation may be due in part to multiple measurements recorded on a single experimental unit or multiple measurements taken over time.

There are many extensions to the basic random effects model outlined above, including random intercept, random slope, nested, cross-classified, and generalized linear mixed models. A random intercept model would allow for the intercept term in the regression equation to vary randomly across hospitals (or higher-level units). The effects of the independent variables are assumed to be the same for each hospital. In this setting, a plot of the predicted hospital regression lines would show parallel lines for each hospital. If the assumption that the effects of explanatory variables are constant across hospitals does not hold, then one can fit a random slope model (also referred to as a random coefficient model), where the hospital prediction lines can have different slopes. A nested random effects model would be fit with data from three levels. For example, suppose one was interested in studying the outcomes of patients treated by surgeons in hospitals. If it is unreasonable to assume that the data are truly hierarchical, or nested—that is, if surgeons typically operate at more than one hospital—then surgeons and hospitals are non-nested. A cross-classified random effects model can be fit with an additional random effect for surgeon included in the model.

If the response or outcome is binary, the methods are somewhat less well developed and computationally more burdensome than for normally distributed data, primarily due to the lack of a discrete multivariate distribution analogous to the multivariate normal. An extension of the random effects model described above, proposed by Breslow and Clayton and by Wolfinger and O'Connell, which can accommodate random effects for a logistic model, can be used. Such a model is referred to as a generalized linear mixed model. Complex algorithms are required for estimation of the fixed and random effects; hence, these models are computationally burdensome and may be impracticable in some settings. For binary outcomes, a common estimation procedure is the quadrature method using numerical approximations. Different adaptations for binary data have been presented in the literature, such as those of Breslow and Clayton; Wolfinger and O'Connell; Stiratelli, Laird, and Ware; and Zeger and Karim.

Katherine S. Panageas

See also Logistic Regression; Ordinary Least Squares Regression; Report Cards, Hospitals and Physicians; Risk Adjustment of Outcomes

Further Readings

Breslow, N. E., & Clayton, D. G. (1993). Approximate inference in generalized linear mixed models. *Journal of the American Statistical Association, 88*, 9–25.

Kleinbaum, D. G., Kupper, L. L., & Muller, K. E. (1988). *Applied regression analysis and other multivariate methods.* Belmont, CA: Duxbury Press.

Searle, S. R., Casella, G., & McCulloch, C. E. (1992). *Variance components.* New York: Wiley.

Snijders, T., & Bosker, R. (1999). *Multilevel analysis.* London: Sage.

Stiratelli, R., Laird, N., & Ware, J. H. (1984). Random effects models for serial observations with binary response. *Biometrics, 40*, 961–973.

Verbeke, G., & Molenberghs, G. (2000). *Linear mixed models for longitudinal data.* Springer Series in Statistics and Computing. New York: Wiley.

Wolfinger, R., & O'Connell, D. (1993). Generalized linear mixed models: A pseudo-likelihood approach. *Journal of Statistical Computation and Simulation, 48*, 233–243.

Zeger, S. L., & Karim, M. R. (1991). Generalised linear models with random effects: A Gibbs sampling approach. *Journal of the American Statistical Association, 86*, 79–102.

FREQUENCY ESTIMATION

Frequency estimation is a judgment task in which one conceptualizes and conveys the anticipated likelihood of an event. It is often used to measure perceptions of personal risk of disease or benefits of treatment in quantitative terms and is therefore an important component of medical decision making. In this entry, a frequency format is distinguished from other formats used to present probabilistic information, the skills needed to estimate frequency are highlighted, and the following pertinent issues related to frequency estimation are discussed: (a) the reasoning strategies used to estimate frequency, (b) the biases associated with frequency estimation, and (c) the importance of response scale and format in frequency estimation.

Frequency Format

A frequency format is one way to represent a probabilistic statement. Other formats commonly used to represent the likelihood of an event are a percentage format (with a range of 0–100%) and a probability format (with a range of 0.0–1.0). Frequency estimation requires consideration of both a numerator (the anticipated number of times the event will occur) and a denominator (the total number of times at risk for the event to occur). Representing risk in a frequency format may be a more intuitive way to communicate risk information for certain types of judgment tasks than using other probability formats.

Needed Skills

Accurate frequency estimation requires some knowledge about the outcome being estimated and the ability to understand probabilistic information. Accurate frequency estimation also requires skills in numeracy, including a conceptual understanding of the concepts of probability. People are often inaccurate in frequency estimates of the likelihood of their developing or dying from a given disease or the benefit of a given treatment. For example, women tend to overestimate their personal risk of dying from breast cancer. In contrast, smokers tend to underestimate their risk of dying from lung cancer.

Types of Reasoning Used

There are two general types of reasoning used in frequency estimation: deliberative reasoning and experiential reasoning. In deliberative reasoning, people will attempt to integrate knowledge of relevant probabilities in formulating an estimation of frequency. In experiential reasoning, people will rely to a greater degree on intuition, emotion, and affect in formulating an estimate of frequency. One aspect of experiential reasoning is use of the availability heuristic. The availability heuristic incorporates personal experience and exposure to the outcome in question in making a frequency estimate. The use of a pictograph with a spatial array to convey frequency information has been found to decrease the bias that can be associated with anecdotal information presented alongside frequency information in the context of a medical decision. Frequency estimates may also be influenced by optimistic bias, which reflects people's tendency to view themselves as being at lower risk than others. One theory that explains how people formulate frequency estimates is fuzzy-trace theory. Fuzzy-trace theory holds that people will naturally conceptualize frequency estimates in the most general way possible in order to solve a problem or make a decision.

Importance of Response Scale and Format

Numeric estimates of frequency are influenced by additional factors including the magnitude of the risk assessed, the response scale used, and whether the frequency estimate is made in isolation or in comparison with other risks. There is a tendency to overestimate small-frequency occurrences and to underestimate large-frequency occurrences. One approach to assist people with estimates of small frequencies is the use of a scale that has a "magnifying glass" to represent probabilities between 0% and 1% on a logarithmic scale or to use other response scales with greater discrimination among smaller probabilities. The choice of response scale can influence the magnitude of the frequency estimates assessed. Specifically, frequency estimates have been found to differ when using a percentage versus frequency format scale. Frequency estimation can also be assessed using a scale with a $1/X$ format, with an increasing value of X indicating a lower frequency. However, the $1/X$ format has been found to be a more difficult format for judgment tasks in which a person is asked to compare risk magnitudes. In frequency judgments, people may find the task easier and be more accurate when comparing their risk with that of others versus providing a frequency estimate for their risk of a given outcome in isolation.

Conclusion

Frequency estimation is a judgment task that conveys perceptions of risk using quantitative terms. Accurate frequency estimation involves some knowledge as well as numeric skills, including knowledge of the concepts of probability. Frequency estimation is an important aspect of risk communication and decision making. However, when assessing frequency estimates or conveying frequency information, one must be cognizant of the role of critical and experiential reasoning in frequency estimation as well as the biases associated with response scales and numeric and graphic formats used to convey probabilistic information.

Marilyn M. Schapira

See also Biases in Human Prediction; Decision Making and Affect; Numeracy; Risk Perception

Further Readings

Ancker, J. S., Senathirajah, Y., Kukafka, R., & Starren, J. B. (2006). Design features of graphs in health risk communication: A systematic review. *Journal of the American Medical Informatics Association, 13,* 608–618.

Fagerlin, A., Wang, C., & Ubel, P. A. (2005). Reducing the influence of anecdotal reasoning on people's health care decisions: Is a picture worth a thousand statistics? *Medical Decision Making, 25,* 398–405.

Hoffrage, U., & Gigerenzer, G. (1998). Using natural frequencies to improve diagnostic inferences. *Academic Medicine, 73,* 538–540.

Lichtenstein, S., Slovic, P., Fischhoff, B., Layman, M., & Combs, B. (1978). Judged frequency of lethal events. *Journal of Experimental Psychology: Human Learning and Memory, 4,* 551–579.

Reyna, V. F., & Adam, M. B. (2003). Fuzzy-trace theory, risk communication, and product labeling in sexually transmitted diseases. *Risk Analysis, 23,* 325–342.

Slovic, P., Monahan, J., & MacGregor, D. G. (2000). Violence risk assessment and risk communication: The effects of using actual cases, providing instruction, and employing probability versus frequency formats. *Law and Human Behavior, 24,* 271–296.

Tversky, A., & Kahneman, D. (1982). Availability: A heuristic for judging frequency and probability. In D. Kahneman, P. Slovic, & A. Tversky (Eds.), *Judgment under uncertainty: Heuristics and biases* (Chap. 11, pp. 163–178). Cambridge, UK: Cambridge University Press.

FREQUENTIST APPROACH

The frequentist (or classical) approach is a branch of statistics that currently represents the predominant methodology used in empirical data analysis and inference. Frequentist statistics emerged as a prevailing method for inference in the 20th century, particularly due to work by Fisher and, subsequently, by Neyman and Pearson. Given that distinct differences exist between the research conducted by these authors, however, frequentist inference may also be subcategorized as being either Fisherian or Neyman-Pearson in nature, although some view the Fisherian approach to be a distinct philosophy apart from frequentist statistics altogether.

Frequentist methods are often contrasted with those of Bayesian statistics, as these two schools of thought represent the more widely considered approaches through which formal inference is undertaken to analyze data and to incorporate robust measurements of uncertainty. Although frequentist and Bayesian statistics do share certain similarities, important divergence between the approaches should also be noted. In this context, the central tenets that differentiate the frequentist paradigm from other statistical methods (e.g., Bayesian) involve (a) the foundational definition of probability that is employed and (b) the limited framework through which extraneous information (i.e., prior information) is assessed from sources outside of the immediate experiment being conducted. Ultimately, these characteristics affect the breadth of research design and statistical inference. By formally focusing primarily on data that emanate from an immediate experiment being conducted (e.g., a randomized clinical trial) and not on additional sources of information (e.g., prior research or the current state of knowledge), results of a frequentist analysis are essentially confined to an immediate study. Reliance is thus often placed on a more informal process to consider extraneous data from sources beyond the immediate study. Although this issue has, in part, led to its theoretic appeal among both regulatory agencies and scientists as being an "objective" method of inference (e.g., the conclusions of a single study do not allow for other findings to affect statistical inference), the frequentist approach has also been viewed as lacking a full rigor that parallels the comprehensive aspects of scientific inquiry and decision theory. Despite a lengthy debate concerning these philosophical issues, the frequentist approach remains the most commonly used method of statistical inquiry. When correctly applied and interpreted, frequentist statistics also represent a robust standard for point estimation, interval estimation, and statistical/hypothesis testing. Consideration of the frequentist approach is additionally important when addressing the overall study design, sample size calculations, and effect sizes.

Within the frequentist paradigm, *probability* is defined as a long-run expected limit of relative frequency within a large number of trials or via a *frequency concept of probability* that denotes the proportion of time when similar events will occur if an experiment is repeated several times. Hence, classical statistical analysis and inference yields interpretations only within a context of repeated samples or experiments. While the theory of infinitely repeatable samples may be viewed as a largely hypothetical issue for an analyst (i.e., because researchers typically obtain only one random draw from a population), the concept becomes of fundamental importance in interpreting results within the frequentist paradigm. Furthermore, the assumption of infinite repeated samples imparts asymptotic properties (e.g., the law of large numbers, convergence, the central limit theorem), which are required for robust inference under the frequentist approach.

Samples and populations are key concepts in frequentist statistics. Researchers use frequentist analysis and inference to generalize findings from a given sample to a broader population. In this context, research questions often focus on obtaining a point estimate, interval estimate, or statistical/hypothesis test concerning a population parameter whose value is assumed to be both fixed and unknown.

Point Estimation

Point estimation is undertaken to find a statistic that is calculated from the sample data and ultimately used for inference concerning the fixed, unknown population parameter. A common nomenclature for this research question involves denoting the population parameter θ and its estimator statistic $\hat{\theta}$. Importantly, the frequentist paradigm defines an *estimator* of the population parameter, $\hat{\theta}$, as a random variable that provides inference concerning the fixed, unknown population parameter θ under the assumption that infinite random samples are drawn from the population itself. The exact value that an estimator $\hat{\theta}$ takes for any given sample is termed an *estimate*. Procedures for obtaining point estimations of population parameters include methods of moments (MoM), maximum likelihood estimation (MLE), and ordinary least squares (OLS), among others. Also contingent on the assumption of infinite random sampling, a theoretical *sampling distribution* (i.e., the probability distribution of a statistic under repeated sampling of the population) exists for the estimator, $\hat{\theta}$, from which a researcher ultimately obtains a random draw. Figure 1 graphically presents the concept of an estimator, a likelihood function that may be estimated via maximum likelihood, and a sampling distribution that may be represented via infinitely repeated samples.

Robust results in frequentist point estimation are produced with minimal bias when the expected value of an estimator $\hat{\theta}$ equals the value of the population parameter, θ, via infinite repeated sampling. For an estimator to be deemed *unbiased*, the mean value of the sampling distribution would be equal to that of a true population parameter. In frequentist statistical theory, emphasis is placed on obtaining unbiased estimators because it is under these conditions that these statistics equal that of a true population parameter, specifically when its average value is found across an infinite random sampling of that population. Given that considerable difficulties may emerge in calculating a sampling distribution, it is also common to rely on asymptotics to approximate infinite sampling requisites in frequentist statistics.

Interval Estimation

In addition to point estimation, researchers often seek to obtain a *confidence interval* (CI) (i.e., a range of values represented by a lower and an upper bound) of estimators that have an a priori (i.e., "before the fact") probability of containing the true value of the fixed unknown population parameter. Based on a given a priori significance level chosen for an analysis, α, the straightforward "$(1 - \alpha) \cdot 100\%$" CI defined for a population parameter θ is

$$\Pr(L_{\text{bound}} < \theta < U_{\text{bound}}) = 1 - \alpha,$$

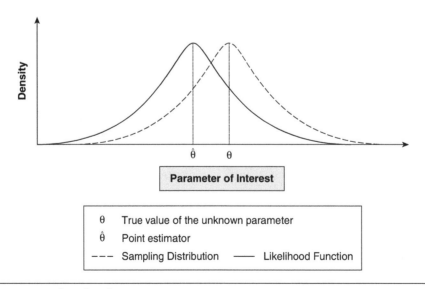

Figure 1   Frequentist sampling distribution

Sources: Skrepnek, G. H. (2007). The contrast and convergence of Bayesian and frequentist statistical approaches in pharmacoeconomic analysis. *PharmacoEconomics, 25,* 649–664. Kennedy, Peter. *A Guide to Econometrics, fifth edition,* figure 13.1, p. 231, © 2003 Peter Kennedy, by permission of The MIT Press.

where Pr denotes probability; L_{bound} and U_{bound} are the lower and upper bounds of the CI, respectively; θ is the population parameter being estimated; and α is the a priori significance level chosen for the analysis. Under conditions wherein a sampling distribution is approximately normally distributed, the CI is

$$\hat{\theta} = \pm c \times SE(\hat{\theta}),$$

where $\hat{\theta}$ is the coefficient estimate, c is the critical value obtained from a t or Z table (depending on sample sizes and adherence to a level of confidence and degrees of freedom), and $SE(\hat{\theta})$ is the standard error of the mean, equal to the standard deviation divided by the square root of the sample size. While the most typical CI in frequentist analyses is 95%, other CIs may be calculated for 90%, 99%, or 99.9%. In instances of large sample sizes, the critical values for 90%, 95%, 99%, and 99.9% CIs are approximately 1.645, 1.96, 2.58, and 3.27, respectively, from the standard normal distribution table (i.e., Z table). Thus, under the condition of a large sample size, the 95% CI would be

$$\hat{\theta} \pm 1.96 \times \sigma/-\sqrt{n},$$

where $\hat{\theta}$ is the coefficient estimate, 1.96 is the critical value for a 95% CI, and $\sigma/-\sqrt{n}$ is the standard deviation divided by the square root of the sample size (i.e., standard error of the mean). Figure 2 presents a graphical depiction of a 95% CI for a normal sample distribution whose mean value of the point estimate is 0.

An area of concern among researchers involves the correct interpretation of a CI. Importantly, it is *incorrect* to infer a probability statement concerning a calculated interval itself in that it might be a "probability that the true value of a parameter is contained within its lower and upper bounds." Rather, CIs are correctly interpreted in terms of a certain percentage of the intervals (e.g., 95%) that will contain the true parameter in the long run. Thus, for example, a 95% CI is properly presented as representing 95% of the intervals derived from infinite sampling of the underlying population of interest that would include the true value of the fixed unknown population parameter. The rationale

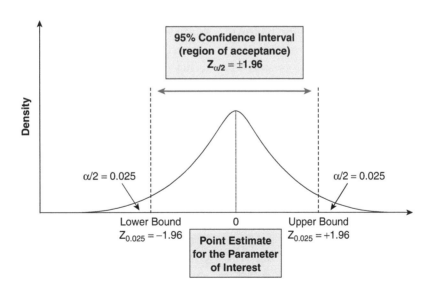

Figure 2 95% confidence interval

Source: Gujarati, D. N. (1995). *Basic econometrics* (3rd ed.). New York: McGraw-Hill. Reproduced with permission of The McGraw-Hill Companies.

behind this interpretation is that the probability level (e.g., .05) of a CI refers to the interval itself and not to the parameter, because the parameter is a fixed unknown and not a random variable. Furthermore, the lower and upper bounds of a CI are considered random only prior to sampling of the population. After sampling, the explicit values obtained for the CI are not random, and thus, it does not have a probability associated with it.

Several methods are available for calculating CIs, each of which may be appropriate for a particular sampling distribution. Researchers, for example, have developed methods to obtain exact CIs for linear functions of a normal mean and variance. Given the extensive requirements to calculate exact CIs, approximate CIs are often used wherein a strong reliance is placed on the assumptions of the law of large numbers and the central limit theorem.

Significance and Hypothesis Testing

Whereas Fisher developed and popularized *significance testing* to weigh evidence against a given hypothesis, Neyman and Pearson developed *hypothesis testing* as a method to assess two directly competing hypotheses. Central to these inferential techniques is the assessment of whether the findings observed within a given experiment were based on chance alone. Additionally, central to both significance and hypothesis testing is the concept of the null hypothesis H_0, which is used to describe the lack of a treatment effect. Importantly, frequentist approaches can never "accept" the null hypothesis. Rather, research can either "reject" or "fail to reject" the null, suggesting that a treatment effect either was or was not observed, respectively. The rationale for this decision rule concerning the null is one of rigorous scientific method—if an investigation fails to reject a null hypothesis, it cannot necessarily be concluded that the null is true under all circumstances.

Significance and hypothesis testing both require that an appropriate test statistic (e.g., t test, F test, regression) be employed to summarize the sample data relevant to the research hypothesis being evaluated. CIs are also related to hypothesis testing in that if the CI does not include a null hypothesis, then a hypothesis test will reject the null, and vice versa. Although significance and hypothesis testing are closely related, differences do exist between the concepts, so the two are not synonymous. Despite this, the term *hypothesis testing* is routinely used to describe the general process of testing for the presence of a treatment effect.

Initially, Fisher developed significance testing to assess the *direct probabilities* (i.e., changes in observed data $\hat{\theta}$ within an immediate experiment leading to rejection of a hypothesis H, or $\Pr(\hat{\theta}|H)$) rather than relying on the *indirect probabilities* (i.e., the probability of a hypothesis given observed data, or $\Pr(H|\hat{\theta})$). Neyman-Pearson hypothesis testing built on Fisher's work by explicitly formalizing the specification of a rival alternate hypothesis H_A, which had only been indirectly addressed in frequentist statistics until that point. The specification of an alternate hypothesis allowed Neyman and Pearson to formalize issues concerning sample size, power, and effect size. This occurred, in part, because the concepts of Type I and Type II errors complemented the development of a formal rival hypothesis against the null.

Type I and Type II errors involve the potential of either incorrectly rejecting or incorrectly failing to reject a null hypothesis, respectively, and are concepts that play an important role in the broader design and interpretation of experiments. The probability of committing a Type I error, represented as α, is the probability of a statistical test to incorrectly reject a null hypothesis when the null is actually true (i.e., committing a false positive). Conversely, the probability of a Type II error, denoted by β, is the probability of a statistical test to incorrectly fail to reject a null hypothesis when the null is actually false (i.e., committing a false negative). The *power of a test*, calculated as $1 - \beta$, is defined as the probability of rejecting a false null hypothesis when the null is actually false (i.e., a correct decision) or, stated differently, the ability of a test to detect a statistical relationship. In practice, the power of a test is often calculated prior to conducting an experiment to ascertain sufficient sample sizes. Alternatively, post hoc power analyses may be computed to determine if a sufficient sample size had been obtained and to determine effect sizes for interpretation of a study's results. Beyond establishing if the treatment effect is statistically significant, *effect sizes* are measures that represent the actual magnitude of a treatment effect. In describing the relationships between hypothesis testing, Type I and Type II errors, and power, Figure 3 graphically presents these aforementioned concepts relating to Neyman-Pearson hypothesis testing.

Importantly, the probabilities of committing a Type I or Type II error are inversely related (i.e., the smaller the probability of one, the higher the probability of the other). Thus, the smaller the significance level specified for an investigation, the greater the probability of failing to reject a false null hypothesis. As such, the researcher must weigh the importance of protecting from committing a false positive versus a false negative when establishing an appropriate significance level versus the power of a test. Depending on the research question being addressed, either a Type I or a Type II error may be considered to be the most important to avoid. To illustrate, a Type I error would occur if a research study concluded that the treatment was observed to yield a statistically significant effect compared with the placebo control when, in reality, there was no difference between them. Conversely, a Type II error would occur if no difference was observed in the study when a difference actually existed. Committing a Type I error in this instance concerning efficacy may result in the use of an ineffective therapy, while a Type II error would suggest that a potentially efficacious therapy would not be used. If the research question involved safety, however, it would be crucial to minimize the potential of committing a Type II error (i.e., suggesting that safety existed when it actually did not) rather than a Type I error. Pragmatic methods to reduce the probability of incurring either type of error emphasize following a robust study design with appropriate sample sizes. Figure 4 presents a graphical depiction of the relationship between a Type I error, a Type II error, and the power of a test for distributions of a null hypothesis H_0 and an alternate hypothesis H_A—noting that shifting the critical value ultimately affects each of the representative

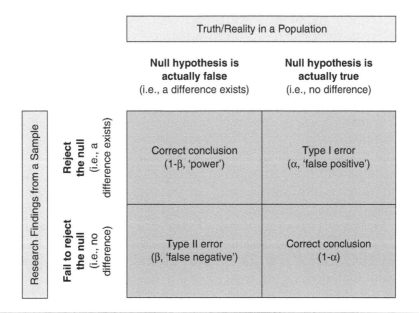

Figure 3   Neyman-Pearson hypothesis testing

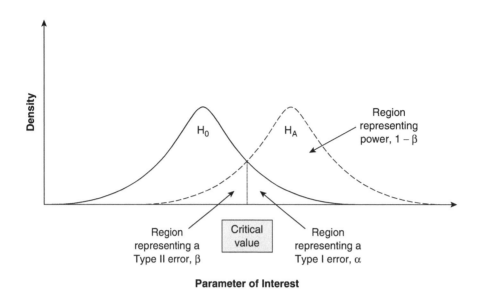

Figure 4   Type I and Type II errors in hypothesis testing

Source: From Hays, W. L. *Statistics,* 5th ed. © 1994 Wadsworth, a part of Cengage Learning, Inc. Reproduced by permission. www.cengage.com/permissions.

regions. Additionally, Figure 5 illustrates the concept of the inverse relationship between Type I and Type II errors according to the probability of rejecting a null hypothesis versus the ratio of the true variances among two populations, σ_x^2 / σ_y^2, noting again that power is the probability that a false null hypothesis will actually be rejected. Herein, the probability of rejecting the null increases when the probability of committing a Type I error, α, increases and the probability of a Type II error, β, decreases (i.e., with increasing power $1 - \beta$, there is an increasing ability for a statistical test to detect a difference when one truly exists).

In practice, significance and hypothesis testing both use p values, or probability values, to express the likelihood that results may have been observed by chance alone. A concept addressed extensively by Fisher, a p value may be formally defined as the probability of obtaining a test statistic at least as extreme as a calculated test statistic if a null hypothesis were true, and thus representing a measure of strength against the null itself. Stated differently, the p value is the probability that a result at least as extreme as that which was observed in an experiment would occur by chance alone. Notably, p values have been misinterpreted to

be "the probability that a null hypothesis is true." Overall, a p value is the lowest significance level wherein a null hypothesis can be rejected.

The p value or a priori α level of .05 as an acceptable value for significance or hypothesis testing remains a contentious area of discussion, albeit corresponding to the most commonly chosen figure used to designate statistical significance in scientific research. Furthermore, criticism concerning the reliance on p values or α levels for statistical testing appears in both a theoretical and an applied context, particularly concerning their association with sample size. Additionally, adjustments of p values or α levels to more conservative figures may be warranted in instances of sequential, subset, or multiple-comparison analysis (e.g., via Bonferonni, Holm, Sidak, or other corrections). Beyond these debates, results from an analysis wherein p values are calculated to be equal to or below an a priori α level chosen for significance suggest a statistically significant relationship concerning a treatment effect that is being researched. When reporting results, analysts may choose to explicitly present an exact value of a computed p value that is obtained from a statistical test or, alternatively, report whether a null hypothesis

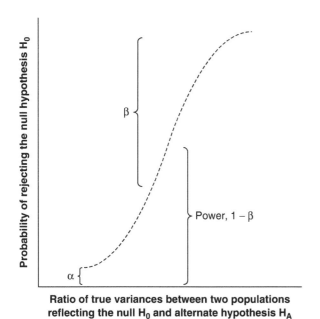

Figure 5 Relationship of the probability of rejecting a null hypothesis relative to the ratio of true variances between two populations

Source: Young, R. K., & Veldman, D. J. *Introductory Statistics for the Behavioral Sciences*, 4th ed. © 1981 Wadsworth, a part of Cengage Learning, Inc. Reproduced by permission. www.cengage.com/permissions.

is rejected based on an a priori α level chosen for statistical significance (i.e., $\alpha = .05$) and if the computed p value of that statistical test is below this α level.

Beyond the statistical significance of a test, assessing the *clinical significance* of a result is also warranted. To illustrate, when a statistic is found to be significant, it suggests that the statistic itself is a reliable estimate of the population parameter or that some treatment effect exists (i.e., that such a finding is unlikely due to chance alone). For example, an investigation may find a statistically significant difference of .5 mmHg between two groups. This in itself does not prove that the finding is relevant, important, or able to support final decision making. Determining clinical (or practical) significance involves assessing the broader aspects of clinical practice, the study design employed in a given investigation, and identifying the smallest magnitude of an effect that is typically associated for a clinically beneficial or harmful impact.

Conclusion

Frequentist methods currently constitute the most widely used approach to empirical data analysis and statistical inference. The hallmarks of this philosophy involve a definition of probability that emphasizes an interpretation over long-run, repeated trials and a focus on results that are confined to an immediate empirical investigation. While the foundation of frequentist statistics does allow for robust inference under several conditions, other statistical approaches may additionally offer sound frameworks with which to engage in scientific inquiry. To fully capture the positive elements of any statistical methodology, researchers must remain fully cognizant of the specific elements associated with each approach concerning appropriate application and interpretation.

Grant H. Skrepnek

See also Confidence Intervals; Hypothesis Testing; Maximum Likelihood Estimation Methods; Sample Size and Power; Statistical Testing: Overview

Further Readings

Berger, J. O., & Sellke, T. (1987). Testing a point null hypothesis: The irreconcilability of *p*-values with evidence (with discussion). *Journal of the American Statistical Association, 82,* 112–139.

Bloom, B. S., de Pouvourville, N., & Libert, S. (2002). Classical or Bayesian research design and analysis: Does it make a difference? *International Journal of Technology Assessment in Health Care, 18,* 120–126.

Cohen, J. (1988). *Statistical power analysis for the behavioral sciences* (2nd ed.). Hillsdale, NJ: Lawrence Erlbaum.

Cowles, M., & Davis, C. (1982). On the origins of the .05 level of significance. *American Psychologist, 37,* 553–558.

Cox, D. R. (2005). Frequentist and Bayesian statistics: A critique. In L. Lyons & M. K. Unel (Eds.), *PHYSTAT 05: Proceedings of statistical problems in particle physics, astrophysics and cosmology* (pp. 3–7). London: Imperial College Press.

Fisher, R. A. (1935). *The design of experiments.* Edinburgh, UK: Oliver & Boyd.

Goodman, S. N. (1999). Toward evidence-based medical statistics: 1. The *p*-value fallacy. *Annals of Internal Medicine, 130,* 995–1004.

Hays, W. L. (1994). *Statistics* (5th ed.). Austin, TX: Harcourt Brace.

Hubbard, R., & Bayarri, M. J. (2003). Confusion over measures of evidence (*p*'s) versus errors (α's) in classical statistical testing. *American Statistician, 57,* 171–182.

Kennedy, P. (2003). *A guide to econometrics* (5th ed.). Cambridge: MIT Press.

Neyman, J., & Pearson, E. S. (1933). On the problem of the most efficient tests of statistical hypotheses. *Philosophical Transactions of the Royal Society of London, Series A, Containing Papers of a Mathematical or Physical Character, 231,* 289–337.

Skrepnek, G. H. (2005). Regression methods in the empiric analysis of health care data. *Journal of Managed Care Pharmacy, 11,* 240–251.

Skrepnek, G. H. (2007). The contrast and convergence of Bayesian and frequentist statistical approaches in pharmacoeconomic analysis. *PharmacoEconomics, 25,* 649–664.

Sterne, J. A. C., & Smith, D. (2001). Sifting the evidence: What's wrong with significance tests? *British Medical Journal, 322,* 226–231.

Fuzzy-Trace Theory

Fuzzy-trace theory explains how people remember, reason, and decide. The theory has been applied to a variety of domains in health and medical decision making, including HIV prevention, cardiovascular disease, surgical risk, genetic risk, and cancer prevention and control. Within these domains, it explains the mysteries of framing effects, ratio bias, frequency-formatting effects, and base-rate neglect, among other classic phenomena. Fuzzy-trace theory has led to the discovery of new, counterintuitive effects too. For example, studies show that adolescents think about risks more logically and quantitatively than mature adults do, which, paradoxically, promotes risk taking—a surprising but predicted effect.

Fuzzy-trace theory has been applied to a variety of populations, including patients and physicians. As a developmental theory, it focuses on changes in memory, reasoning, and decision making with age (differences among children, adolescents, young adults, and the aged). It also specifies when age does not make a difference; for example, adolescents and expert physicians perform equally poorly on base-rate neglect problems involving medical diagnosis (underestimating the effects of prior probabilities of disease on subsequent probabilities once a diagnostic test result is known). Most recently, fuzzy-trace theory has been used to characterize the changes in cognition that accompany disease processes, such as in Alzheimer's and Parkinson's disease, as well as mild cognitive impairment.

The phrase *fuzzy trace* refers to a distinction between verbatim memory representations that are vivid and gist memory representations that are "fuzzy" (i.e., vague and impressionistic). The distinction between verbatim and gist representations was initially borrowed from psycholinguists, who had amassed substantial evidence for it and had applied it to the representation and retention of verbal materials. However, despite the continued use of the term *verbatim* in fuzzy-trace theory, these types of representations were extended to describe memories of nonverbal stimuli, including numbers, pictures, graphs, and events.

For example, if a physician tells a patient that she has a 22% chance of having a stroke in the next 3 years, she forms two kinds of memories for that information: (1) a memory of the precise details of what was said ("22% chance of stroke"), which fades rapidly and is subject to interference (e.g., from anxiety), and (2) a memory of the bottom-line meaning, or gist, of what was said (e.g., there is a good chance of having a stroke in the next few years). Multiple gist memories are typically encoded into memory for a single piece of information.

Research on the major paradigms of judgment and decision making and of developmental psychology have shown a common pattern of results with respect to verbatim and gist memories: Individuals encode parallel representations of information along a continuum of precision that is anchored at each end by gist and verbatim representations, or memory traces. Verbatim traces preserve veridical details at the precise end, and gist traces preserve extracted meanings and patterns at the fuzzy end. This first tenet of fuzzy-trace theory is not an assumption, in the usual sense of that term, but, rather, is based on the results of numerous experiments that tested alternative hypotheses regarding memory representations.

A second tenet of the theory, central to understanding reasoning, is the idea that retrieval of either verbatim or gist representations is cue dependent, a conclusion that is also based on empirical evidence. That is, the two types of traces are stored separately and retrieved independently, and their successful retrieval depends on cues, or specific reminders, in the environment. As many studies have demonstrated, two different cues presented to the same individual can elicit contradictory responses about what is stored in memory (such as those found in false-memory reports). Different values and reasoning principles are retrieved from memory, depending on cues in the environment, which helps explain why reasoning and decision making are so variable.

A number of factors conspire to make gist traces the default representations used in reasoning. Verbatim traces become rapidly inaccessible and are sensitive to interference. Reasoning therefore gravitates to using gist (or fuzzy) representations, which minimizes errors due to the fragile and cumbersome verbatim representations. Moreover, this adaptive tendency to use gist representations—the fuzzy-processing preference—increases with development as individuals gain experience at a task. Studies of children (comparing older with younger children) and of adults (comparing experts with novices in a domain of knowledge) have demonstrated that reliance on gist representations increases with development. For example, a study comparing medical students and physicians varying in expertise in cardiology showed that the more expert processed fewer dimensions of information and processed it in an all-or-none (gist based) manner (i.e., patients with chest pain were seen as either requiring intensive care or safely discharged with a 72-hour follow-up).

People think using simple gist representations of information, often processing them unconsciously, and engage in parallel rather than serial processing of that information (leaping ahead based on vague gist impressions of the relations and patterns in information without fully encoding details). This kind of thinking is what is meant by "gist-based intuitive reasoning." The third tenet of the theory is that people exhibit a fuzzy-processing preference (a preference for reasoning with the simplest gist representation of a problem). This preference produces more coherent thinking (because working with gist representations is easier and less error-prone) and more positive decision outcomes (e.g.,

less unhealthy risk taking in adolescents). Recent research has linked gist-based intuitive reasoning to lower HIV risk. The reliance on gist as a default mode of processing is associated with more adaptive responses to risk as people mature.

From these tenets, it can easily be seen why fuzzy-trace theory's prescriptions to improve health communication and medical decision making differ from those of standard utility or dual-process theories. The goal of informed consent, for example, is to reach an understanding of the bottom-line gist of risks and benefits (e.g., of surgery) rather than to regurgitate verbatim facts. Similarly, the goal of prevention programs in public health is to inculcate rapid and unconscious recognition of the gist of risky situations and to retrieve relevant values (e.g., involving unprotected sex) rather than to consciously deliberate about the details and degrees of risk. Thus, contrary to other dual-process theories, gist-based intuition is an advanced form of thought.

Valerie F. Reyna

See also Gain/Loss Framing Effects; Risk Communication; Risk Perception

Further Readings

Reyna, V. F. (2004). How people make decisions that involve risk: A dual-processes approach. *Current Directions in Psychological Science, 13*, 60–66.

Reyna, V. F., & Adam, M. B. (2003). Fuzzy-trace theory, risk communication, and product labeling in sexually transmitted diseases. *Risk Analysis, 23*, 325–342.

Reyna, V. F., & Brainerd, C. J. (2008). Numeracy, ratio bias, and denominator neglect in judgments of risk and probability. *Learning and Individual Differences, 18*, 89–107.

Reyna, V. F., & Farley, F. (2006). Risk and rationality in adolescent decision-making: Implications for theory, practice, and public policy. *Psychological Science in the Public Interest, 7*(1), 1–44.

Reyna, V. F., & Lloyd, F. (2006). Physician decision making and cardiac risk: Effects of knowledge, risk perception, risk tolerance, and fuzzy processing. *Journal of Experimental Psychology: Applied, 12*, 179–195.

Reyna, V. F., Lloyd, F., & Whalen, P. (2001). Genetic testing and medical decision making. *Archives of Internal Medicine, 161*, 2406–2408.

G

GAIN/LOSS FRAMING EFFECTS

Amos Tversky and David Kahneman's work in the 1980s on framing (presentation) effects was a stimulus for other researchers to examine how these effects affect medical decision making. Interestingly, the work by Tversky and Kahneman in framing effects was based on consideration of a transmissible infectious disease in a population.

Tversky and Kahneman's use of the term *frame* was in the arena of type of description applied to data. In its most basic sense, framing refers to the way in which medical decision making alternatives are presented. For example, in one frame, all data might be presented in terms of *survival*; in the second frame, all data could be presented in terms of *mortality*. Here, the term *framing effect* would be similar to the term *presentation effect*, where a frame is a type of presentation of data to study subjects in a research survey or research questionnaire. Presenting the data in terms of survival would be an example of gain framing; presenting the data in terms of mortality would be an example of loss framing.

Risky and Riskless Contexts

Tverksy and Kahneman describe this aspect of their work as research on the cognitive and psychophysical determinants in risky and riskless contexts. For these authors, framing refers to the cognitive point at which decision problems can be described (framed) in multiple ways, giving rise to different preferences being elicited that are dependent on the frame.

They further argue that framing effects can help explain some of the anomalies found in consumer behavior. Other researchers have extended their point to medical decision making in that caution needs to be used in deciding how decision problems are presented to patients.

Early Research in Framing

Attention to the use of data in decision making was brought into the medical-decision-making arena in a scientific article by Barbara J. McNeil, R. Weichselbaum, and S. G. Pauker appearing in the *New England Journal of Medicine* in 1978 on the fallacy of 5-year survival in lung cancer. McNeil and colleagues focused attention on the 5-year survival data in lung cancer. This article focused attention on the importance of choosing therapies not only on the basis of objective measures of survival but also on the basis of patient attitudes. However, while McNeil and colleagues derived their data from existing data on 5-year survival from the published medical literature, they did not present graphical displays of 5-year survival curves to study participants. Rather, McNeil and colleagues presented data derived from 5-year survival for lung cancer in terms of *cumulative probabilities* and *life-expectancy data* in this study.

In a subsequent article published in the *New England Journal of Medicine* in 1979, McNeil, Pauker, H. C. Sox, and Tversky asked study participants to imagine that they had lung cancer and to choose between two therapies on the basis of either cumulative probabilities or life-expectancy data. In this study, different groups of respondents received input data that differed in the following ways: whether or not the treatments were identified (as surgery and radiation therapy) and whether the outcomes were framed in terms of the probability of living or the probability of dying. The authors found that the attractiveness of surgery as a treatment choice, relative to radiation therapy, was substantially greater (a) when the treatments were identified rather than unidentified, (b) when the information consisted of life expectancy rather than cumulative probability, and (c) when the problem was framed in terms of the probability of living (survival frame) rather than in terms of the probability of dying (mortality frame). The authors in their conclusion suggest that an awareness of such influences among physicians and patients could help reduce bias and improve the quality of medical decision making.

Yet two questions can be asked of both studies: First, how useful did the study participants find cumulative probabilities and life-expectancy data? Second, are there other forms of data displays that patients may find as useful or more useful to consider for their own choice of therapy in cases where surgery is to be contrasted with radiation therapy? In the case of Stage 3 lung cancer, surgery has a better long-term (and worse short-term) survival than radiation therapy, while radiation therapy has a better short-term (and worse long-term) survival than surgery for the same Stage 3 lung cancer.

Graphical Displays Comparing 5-Year Survival Curves

In the 1990s, Dennis J. Mazur and David H. Hickam studied graphical displays of 5-year data as survival curves. These graphical displays and comparison of survival curves out to 5 years illustrate how framing effects can be illustrated in graphical displays of data.

In medical decision making, framing has been most typically depicted in comparisons of scenarios within which the data are depicted in one of two frames, Frame 1 or Frame 2. Frame 1 depicts all outcomes in terms of survival, and the other frame, Frame 2, depicts all outcomes in terms of mortality.

The time line over which the survival data and the mortality data are typically provided to volunteers in these research studies goes from the time of the initial treatment with a medical intervention (T_0) to a time 5 years after the initial treatments (T_5). Five-year survival data are a common form of data used by physicians in oncology, and the first types of medical conditions (disease processes) studied to look for framing effects were more aggressive cancers, for example, Stage 3 lung cancer. The 5-year survival curve would not be appropriate for a cancer such as prostate cancer, where the chance of survival goes well beyond 5 years.

Underlying assumptions of the above study design include the point that patients cannot shift from one treatment to another and must remain with the treatment they choose throughout. For example, if the two time lines of treatment of Treatment 1 and Treatment 2 cross at some midpoint, the participant cannot shift from the treatment that has a better survival over the time line T_0 to the midpoint to the other treatment that has a better survival from the midpoint to the time T_5.

An example of two treatments where one treatment has a better short-term (T_0 to midpoint) survival and a worse long-term (midpoint to T_5) survival are surgery and radiation therapy for Stage 3 lung cancer. Here, with surgery, there is an initial chance of patients dying with a surgical intervention at time T_0 but a better chance of their still being alive at T_5; with radiation therapy, there is little to no chance of dying from the radiation therapy itself at time T_0, but fewer patients are alive at T_5 with radiation therapy than with surgery.

Here, the following assumptions come into play. First, there is the assumption that the patient will not die as a result of radiation therapy. In fact, a rare patient may die during radiation therapy; therefore, it is not necessarily guaranteed that all patients will survive the radiation therapy. Second, there is the assumption that the patient incurs a high risk of dying during surgery. In fact, the chance that a patient may die with a surgical intervention is highly dependent on the status of the individual patient's cardiovascular and respiratory condition. (The risk of dying from anesthesia is built into the surgical death rate, as a surgery cannot be performed without anesthesia.)

In a typical framing study in medical decision making, study participants are randomized to one of two frames, Frame 1 or Frame 2. Participants randomized to Frame 1 receive all data in terms of survival (number of patients alive after treatment); participants randomized to Frame 2 receive all data in terms of mortality (number of patients dead after each treatment).

In the typical verbal study of framing effects, the participant is provided information about the number of patients being alive after the initial intervention (surgery and radiation therapy) at T_0 and the number of patients still alive after surgery and radiation therapy 5 years later at T_5.

Researchers present data to the study participants in two distinct frames. Frame 1 depicts data to participants only in terms of survival (the chance of still being alive after the initial intervention and the chance of still being alive 5 years after that intervention); Frame 2 depicts data to participants only in terms of mortality (the chance of dying during the initial intervention and the chance of dying within 5 years after that intervention).

Framing Effects in Tabular and Graphic Displays

The initial framing study of McNeil and colleagues provided study participants with frames presented in terms of quantitative descriptions of data (cumulative probabilities and life-expectancy). Since that time in research on human study participants, such effects with framing have been demonstrated using tabular and graphic expressions of chance (likelihood) as well, where tabular or graphical expressions of chance or likelihood depict the survival and mortality data the participants are asked to consider.

The depiction of data in terms of *words and numbers*, as contrasted with *graphical data displays*, brings into play the following considerations. When attempting to see if framing effects are present in a particular study where data are provided to participants in terms of words and numbers, the researchers may simply provide participants with the number of patients alive after the surgical or radiation therapy interventions at time T_0 and time T_5 and ask each participant to choose which treatment he or she prefers.

However, if data are provided to participants in terms of graphical comparisons of two 5-year survival curves (one 5-year survival curve for surgery

and one 5-year survival curve for radiation therapy), the researchers are providing patients with much more data than simply the number of patients alive and dead at T_0 and T_5. The patients being provided the data in terms of 5-year survival curves are also being presented with midpoint data that can influence their choice.

The other point about the depiction of framing effects in terms of words and numbers as contrasted with graphical data displays is that even if a researcher devises a graphical display of only two sets of data (the number of patients alive at T_0 and the number of patients alive at T_5), there may well be a point where one survival curve crosses the other, and participants could use this point within their decision, making the interpretation of the graphical data comparison more complex than that of the choice depicted in terms of words and numbers at T_0 and T_5 only.

Yet, despite the above considerations, the results of such framing studies in medical decision making have shown a marked consistency.

Results of Typical Framing Studies

The results of typical framing studies in medical decision making are as follows: Participants who are presented with data framed solely in terms of survival choose the treatment that gives patients a better chance of being alive 5 years after the initial treatment (T_5), that is, the treatment with the better long-term (and worse short-term) result; participants who are presented with data framed solely in terms of mortality choose the treatment that has a better chance of being alive after the initial treatment at T_0, that is, the treatment with the better short-term (and worse long-term) result.

Graphical Displays Comparing Survival and Mortality Curves

Karen Armstrong and colleagues studied the effect of framing in terms of survival versus mortality on understanding and treatment choice, randomizing study participants to receive one of three questionnaires: one presenting survival curves, one presenting mortality curves, or one presenting both survival and mortality curves. Armstrong and colleagues found that study participants who received only survival curves or who received both survival and mortality curves were significantly more accurate in answering questions about the information than participants who received only mortality curves ($p < .05$). They found that participants who received only mortality curves were significantly less likely to prefer preventive surgery than participants who received survival curves only or both survival and mortality curves ($p < .05$).

As with the Mazur and Hickam studies with graphical displays of 5-year survival curves, Armstrong and colleagues' study participants who received information in terms of graphical displays of 5-year survival data preferred the long-term survival of surgery rather than the short-term survival advantage with radiation therapy. Armstrong and colleagues also showed that adding a graphical display of mortality curves to a survival curve comparison yields similar effects as those that result from providing study participants with survival curves alone. Here, the suggestion remains that a well-discussed graphical display of 5-year survival curves with appropriate information may provide useful information to patients in representing treatment decisions related to surgery versus radiation therapy for a disease entity such as lung cancer. The research question that remains about graphical displays using comparisons of survival curves alone (or survival curves and mortality curves together) is how to best provide that discussion and explanation to patients without unfairly influencing their choices about survival (mortality) in the short term, medium term, and long term.

Questions About Framing Effects

The main questions about framing effects today are not related to whether these effects are demonstrable in paper-and-pencil type research settings where study participants are asked to choose between or among treatments in hypothetical scenarios. Rather, the questions focus on the actual impact that frames have in advertising in general and in direct-to-consumer advertising of medical products (prescription medicines and medical devices).

Future Research on Framing

Further research on framing needs to focus on how to best present data to patients in ways that minimize the influence of framing on the choices they must make. Initial work on the control of framing effects has focused on tabular displays of data. This work needs to be extended to all verbal and graphical data displays and all presentation formats to offer patients the best display of data for their decision making with the minimum intrusion of influences on the choices they are considering at all times.

Dennis J. Mazur

See also Bias; Cognitive Psychology and Processes; Decision Psychology

Further Readings

Ancker, J. S., Senathirajah, Y., Kukafka, R., & Starren, J. B. (2006). Design features of graphs in health risk communication: A systematic review. *Journal of the American Medical Association, 13,* 608–618.

Armstrong, K., Schwartz, J. S., Fitzgerald, G., Putt, M., & Ubel, P. A. (2002). Effect of framing as gain versus loss on understanding and hypothetical treatment choices: Survival and mortality curves. *Medical Decision Making, 22,* 76–83.

Kahneman, D., & Tversky, A. (1984). Choices, values, and frames. *American Psychologist, 39,* 341–350.

Kahneman, D., & Tversky, A. (2007). *Choices, values, and frames.* New York: Cambridge University Press.

Mazur, D. J., & Hickam, D. H. (1990). Interpretation of graphic data by patients in a general medicine clinic. *Journal of General Internal Medicine, 5,* 402–405.

Mazur, D. J., & Hickam, D. H. (1990). Treatment preferences of patients and physicians: Influences of summary data when framing effects are controlled. *Medical Decision Making, 10,* 2–5.

Mazur, D. J., & Hickam, D. H. (1993). Patients' and physicians' interpretations of graphic data displays. *Medical Decision Making, 13,* 59–63.

Mazur, D. J., & Hickam, D. H. (1994). The effect of physicians' explanations on patients' treatment preferences: Five-year survival data. *Medical Decision Making, 14,* 255–258.

Mazur, D. J., & Hickam, D. H. (1996). Five-year survival curves: How much data are enough for patient-physician decision making in general surgery? *European Journal of Surgery, 162,* 101–104.

McNeil, B. J., Pauker, S. G., Sox, H. C., Jr., & Tversky, A. (1982). On the elicitation of preferences for alternative therapies. *New England Journal of Medicine, 306,* 1259–1262.

McNeil, B. J., Weichselbaum, R., & Pauker, S. G. (1978). Fallacy of the five-year survival in lung cancer. *New England Journal of Medicine, 299,* 1397–1401.

O'Connor, A. M., Boyd, N. F., Tritchler, D. L., Kriukov, Y., Sutherland, H., & Till, J. E. (1985). Eliciting preferences for alternative cancer drug treatments: The influence of framing, medium, and rater variables. *Medical Decision Making, 5,* 453–463.

Tversky, A., & Kahneman, D. (1981). The framing of decisions and the psychology of choice. *Science, 211,* 453–458.

GAMBLES

The standard gamble is a method for eliciting a person's preferences for different outcomes where an outcome may be a physical object, a monetary gain, a medical condition, or some other state of affairs. It uses simulated choices among various outcomes of known preference to quantify the value (or utility) of the target outcome.

To determine how much a myopic (nearsighted) patient values his or her vision, for instance, the following standard gamble may be presented: "Imagine that your doctor offers you a treatment that is known to always permanently reverse myopia with 100% effectiveness and safety. It would provide you with perfect vision without the need for corrective lenses. The treatment does not cause pain, have side effects, wear off, or cost money. Would you accept the treatment?" As most patients respond "yes" to this all gain/no risk scenario, an element of gambling is introduced: "Now imagine that the treatment is successful 50% of the time, but causes immediate painless death in the other half of patients. Your doctor cannot predict whether you will have a success or not. Would you accept this treatment?" If the patient says "yes," the probability of success is decreased (and the complementary probability of death is increased) and the gamble re-presented. If the patient says "no," the probability of success is increased. The gamble is repeatedly presented with new probabilities until the patient is indifferent between the two choices.

The probability of success at which the patient is indifferent is a quantitative expression of the patient's value for his or her vision on a scale that is anchored by death at 0.0 and perfect vision at 1.0. The patient who is willing to accept a treatment with 95% efficacy and 5% chance of death, but not at a higher probability of failure, is said to have a utility of .95 for their vision deficit. Another patient willing to accept a 60% chance of death to attain perfect vision has a utility of .40 for their current vision.

Uses

Preferences (also called values or utilities) are one of the critical aspects of a decision that must be specified for decision analysis or cost-effectiveness modeling. (The others are the choices that are under consideration, their potential outcomes, and the probabilities of those outcomes.) The standard gamble is one of several methods for eliciting preferences.

For instance, the decision to undergo laser eye surgery to repair myopia can be modeled as a choice between continued use of corrective lenses and surgery. Each choice is associated with different monetary costs and different probabilities of achieving perfect vision, requiring lenses into the future, and experiencing complications (including pain, blindness, and, rarely, death). These outcome states and their probabilities may be more or less accurately described by an expert such as a physician. However, some patients will place a greater value on some of the outcomes than other patients will. A myopic actor with a tendency to eye infections from contact lenses and the need to eschew eyeglasses on stage may value achieving perfect vision more than a graduate student on a limited budget. The way people feel about the outcomes is important to understanding both how they behave when faced with decisions and how medical providers might advise them.

Utilities are the gold standard measure of quality of life; combined with life-expectancy, they are used to calculate quality-adjusted life years (QALYs).

Assumptions

Standard gambles are derived directly from the assumptions of John von Neumann and Oskar Morgenstern's expected utility theory, which asserts that decision makers must be able to express a preference (or indifference) among any two health states; preferences are transitive (if $A > B$ and $B > C$, then $A > C$); if $A > B > C$, there is a probability p such that the decision maker is indifferent between B for certain or A with probability p and C with probability $1 - p$; the decision maker must prefer the gamble with the highest probability of attaining the preferred health state; and the decision maker is indifferent among results attained through any combination of simultaneous gambles.

Assume that A is perfect vision without spectacles, B is current vision with spectacles, and C is total binocular blindness. If we can assign a numeric value to perfect vision (A = perhaps 1.0) and to blindness (C = 0.0), the assumptions allow us to estimate the value of spectacles. (Remember that B must lie between A and C.) The gamble is a choice between keeping the status quo (B) for sure or accepting the chance of getting either A or C. If $p = .95$, there is a 95% chance of achieving perfect vision, but a 5% chance of death. Certainly, some, but not all, eyeglass wearers would accept that gamble. They are willing to accept at least a 5% mortality to improve their vision. Some would be willing to accept a higher mortality (perhaps 10% or 20%), and some would refuse the gamble unless p were higher (perhaps .99) and the chance of mortality ($1 - p$) correspondingly lower (.01). The lowest p that the subject is willing to accept is called the utility. A subject who is willing to accept a 90% chance of success, but not 89%, has a utility for spectacles of .90.

Standard gambles assume that the target health state lies on a coherent number line between the two anchor states. If the target is much disfavored (perhaps persistent vegetative state), some subjects may value it less than 0 on a scale anchored by death and perfect health. Standard gamble values less than 0 (or greater than 1) are not easily interpretable.

Standard gambles further assume that the value of a health state is independent of the time spent in that state ("constant proportional trade-off"). A headache is no more or less severe for lasting 1 hour or 1 month. (The effect of duration is modeled independently and combined with the utility to generate the expected utility.)

Limitations

The standard gamble actually measures two values that are conflated in the single result. In addition to the value of the health state itself, the patient must deal with loss of control and other risky aspects inherent to the gamble. Some patients avoid risk so assiduously that they cannot be made to assign a utility less than 1.0 to any health state, no matter how dire. Others seem to have the attitude of inveterate gamblers or adolescents and seek out risky alternatives out of all proportion to the benefits, apparently because they desire the risk itself.

Some investigators feel that the standard gamble is difficult for subjects to complete. It is not clear if this is an accurate representation. If so, the difficulty may stem from dealing with the concept of death or the necessity to carefully consider their values when answering. In fact, many subjects report stopping to think about family obligations, personal aspirations and goals, and other essential issues during the standard gamble exercise. Although emotionally and intellectually challenging, it is unlikely that "easier" methods that avoid such introspection yield results that are as valid.

Some subjects (about 3% to 7% in most studies) fail to rank health states in an apparently rational order. For instance, in assessing various vision states, some subjects place a higher standard gamble value on binocular (total) blindness than blindness in one eye. In fact, some assessors use these two health states to introduce the method to subjects and test comprehension of the task. If the utility of binocular blindness is greater than the utility of monocular blindness, all the other standard gamble results for that subject are considered invalid.

In common with other methods of eliciting utilities, the standard gamble is subject to *framing effects*. People tend to be risk-averse when considering gains but risk tolerant when avoiding equivalent losses. For instance, many people are willing to take a higher risk of death to prevent becoming blind than to cure existing blindness.

Alternative Approaches

Utilities can be assessed in a number of ways. The most straightforward methods, such as asking the patients directly or having them mark a visual analog scale, tend to be subject to a remarkable number of cognitive biases. Perhaps chief among these is that patients don't seem to know their preferences, at least in quantitative form. Of course, they know what they like and what they don't like, but putting numeric utility values on these preferences is not part of their everyday experience. Therefore, the answers they give to direct assessments are often grossly misleading when used in formal models.

Observing real-world choices is limited by the difficulties and expense of data collection and by the fact that people often get bargains. A patient who is bothered by corrective lenses a great deal will make the same observable decision (to have surgery) as one who has only a moderate distaste for glasses as long as the risks and costs of surgery are low enough. In this case, the first patient is getting more value for the same risk as the second, but an observer cannot discern the difference.

Simulated decisions, such as the standard gamble, allow the decision to be repeated multiple times with slight variations in the conditions of the choices until the pattern of decisions reveals the underlying value trade-offs. Other approaches to utility assessment that take advantage of the simulated trade-off use different anchors to frame the decision. For instance, the time trade-off replaces the varying risk of death in the standard gamble with varying survival times. Rather than "What risk of death would you accept to improve your health?" the question is "What reduction in length of life would you accept to improve your health?" Because the time trade-off specifies the time of death, it avoids the probabilistic or risky aspects of the standard gamble. This has the advantage of eliminating risk tolerance from the assessment but the disadvantage that the outcomes are delayed. Many decision makers value postponed outcomes less than current outcomes of similar value. This discounting effect, like the risk-tolerance effect in the standard gamble, may partially obscure the value of the underlying health state.

Willingness-to-pay methods express utilities in monetary terms. "How much money would you pay to avoid the health state?" Unfortunately, it is difficult to compare the values derived from a multibillionaire with those from an indigent farm laborer.

Benjamin Littenberg

See also Chained Gamble; Disutility; Expected Utility Theory; Quality-Adjusted Life Years (QALYs); Utility Assessment Techniques; Willingness to Pay

Further Readings

Gafni, A. (1994). The standard gamble method: What is being measured and how it is interpreted. *Health Services Research, 29,* 207–224.

McNeil, B. J., Weichselbaum, R., & Pauker, S. G. (1978). Fallacy of the five-year survival in lung cancer. *New England Journal of Medicine, 299,* 1397–1401.

Pauker, S. G., & Kassirer, J. P. (1987). Decision analysis. *New England Journal of Medicine, 316,* 250–258.

Sox, H. C., Blatt, M. A., & Higgins, M. C. (2007). *Medical decision making.* Philadelphia: ACP Publications.

Torrance, G. W., & Feeny, D. (1989). Utilities and quality-adjusted life-years. *International Journal of Technology Assessment in Health Care, 5,* 559–575.

Genetic Testing

Genetic testing includes prenatal and clinical diagnosis or prognosis of fetal abnormalities, predicting risk of disease, and identifying carriers of genetic disorders. Genetic testing is distinguished from genetic screening, which is offered to healthy people who might benefit from more information about their genetic risk profile. In this context, the initiative for a genetic test comes from the healthcare professional and not from the counselee. Learning about the perceptions of genetic risks and the way people make decisions with regard to these risks is becoming increasingly relevant, given the rapidly growing knowledge about the human genome. Recent developments in molecular genetics have led to speculations that we are moving into a new era of predictive medicine in which it will be possible to test for a variety of genes to determine the chances that an individual will at some point in the future develop a disease. At this moment, genetic counseling mostly takes place in clinical genetic centers. In the future, this will probably be done in other settings, and clinicians, primary care physicians, and other healthcare professionals will be more and more often confronted with persons seeking advice about their genetic risks. Furthermore, an increasing number of tests will be available for screening for genetic diseases (self-help kits are already being offered on the Internet).

The aim of individual genetic counseling, but also of population genetic screening, is to provide people with information about (future) diseases or possible diseases in their offspring and help them process the information in such a way that they can make informed decisions or take some action, for example, therapy or preventive measures. In this view, providing probability information in an understandable way is one of the most essential components of genetic education and counseling. An accurate risk perception is assumed to be an important determinant for taking preventive measures, or it may provide a basis on which counselees can make informed decisions about important personal matters such as childbearing. However, inaccurate perceived risk may also lead to unwanted behavior, such as excessive breast self-examination in case of heritable breast cancer, and an increased vulnerability to worry and distress or an unhealthy lifestyle; or it may lead to false reassurance. The underlying assumption that accurate perception of risk could help counselees make informed and individual decisions seems to be based on the principle of the autonomous and rational decision maker. However, the characteristics of genetic risk information as well as of the decisions to be made complicate a rational trade-off of pros and cons of genetic testing.

Genetic Risk Perception

Genetic risk information is often complex and replete with uncertainties, associated not only with the hereditary nature of the disease but also with the informativeness of the test results, the effectiveness of possible preventive measures, and the variability of expression of the disease. The uncertainties involved in genetic information differ between different genetic testing settings. The following examples illustrate the complexity of genetic risk information and the many ways in which these risks can be expressed.

Genetic counseling for hereditary cancer, such as hereditary breast cancer, includes education regarding the genetics of cancer; the probability of developing cancer and of carrying a genetic mutation; the benefits, risks, and limitations of genetic susceptibility testing; and prevention strategies. A woman who wants to have a DNA test for hereditary breast cancer may receive a nonconclusive test result, meaning that although she has a family history of breast cancer, a genetic disposition is not found. If, on the other hand, she receives a positive test result, she knows for certain that she is a carrier of a mutant breast cancer gene, but she is not certain about the chance (between 45% and 65%) of developing breast cancer during her life. She also does not know when she may get breast cancer. If she decides for a prophylactic breast amputation to prevent the development of breast cancer, she is not even certain that this drastic intervention will reduce her chances of developing breast cancer to zero. Besides, she has to consider the potential impact that the information about hereditariness of breast cancer might have on her family.

Different uncertainties are involved in prenatal testing. Pregnant women have to make a decision whether or not to have a prenatal screening test on congenital disorders, in particular, Down syndrome. There are many probabilities that a woman might consider before making this decision. If she is 36 years old, she has an increased age-related chance of having a child with Down syndrome of 1 out of 250. A woman of her age has a large chance (about 20%) of receiving a positive test result if she opts for screening, that is, an increased risk of larger than 1 out of 250 of having a child with Down syndrome. However, a negative—favorable—test result does not mean that she is not carrying a child with Down syndrome. If she decides not to have prenatal screening, her chance of being pregnant with a child with Down syndrome is based on her age. This chance is quite large compared with younger women. In case the test result is positive, she must also decide whether or not she wants to have an amniocentesis, which has a risk of 1 out of 300 of inducing an abortion of either an affected or a healthy fetus. In addition to this information, she might also consider the severity of the handicap of a child with Down syndrome. The severity of mental retardation cannot be predicted. However, it is known that about 40% of children with Down syndrome experience heart problems. Deafness and other health problems are also possible.

Multifactorial diseases such as type 2 diabetes and cardiovascular disease are caused by a complex interplay of many genetic and nongenetic factors. Although genetic testing for susceptibility genes for many multifactorial diseases, such as type 2 diabetes, is not yet warranted in clinical practice, an increased susceptibility can be determined using family history information. Family history is an important risk factor that may be used as a surrogate marker for genetic susceptibility and is seen as a useful tool for disease prevention in public health and preventive medicine. Family history reflects the consequences of a genetic predisposition, shared environment, and common behavior. Based on family history and other factors such as lifestyle, an individual's risk of disease can be determined. The information may be used either to identify high-risk groups or as an intervention tool to tailor behavioral messages. For an individual with an increased susceptibility for cardiovascular disease, for example, a healthy diet, physical exercise, and not smoking are even more important than for a person with a population risk of disease.

Research has shown that the perception of genetic risks tends to be inaccurate. Genetic counseling for hereditary cancer, for example, has been shown to improve accurate risk estimation in some women with a family history of breast cancer, although the majority of women still have an inaccurate perception of their lifetime risk after counseling. Meta-analysis of controlled trials showed that genetic counseling improved knowledge of cancer genetics but did not alter the level of perceived risk. Prospective studies, however, reported improvements in the accuracy of perceived risk. Studies about risk perception and prenatal screening showed that pregnant women do not have an accurate perception of their risk of being pregnant with a child with Down syndrome, which is assumed to be important for the decision to have the prenatal testing performed. Research showed that the decision to undergo prenatal screening for Down syndrome was mainly determined by the woman's attitude toward undergoing prenatal screening and not her perceived risk of having a child with Down syndrome. The increased risk due to family history of, for example, type 2 diabetes, is also underestimated. Recent studies indicate that fewer than 40% of people with a positive family history of type 2 diabetes actually perceive themselves to be at risk.

Genetic Decisions

Genetic testing may enable early disease detection and surveillance leading to effective prevention strategies, among other benefits. Genetic decisions are decisions for which informed decision making is seen as particularly important due to the lack of

curative treatment for certain conditions. However, in reality this aim is not always achieved. A Dutch study in which prenatal screening for Down syndrome was offered in an experimental setting showed that only 51% of the pregnant women made an informed and reasoned choice despite detailed information leaflets. Studies in other countries have shown even more pessimistic results. Informed decision making in the context of genetic testing for monogenetic diseases or diseases caused by specific genes, such as hereditary breast and colon cancer, has not been studied. For these settings, it is even unclear whether knowing one's risk really increases the freedom of choice or the rationality of a decision. It has been argued that counselees are not really interested in knowing the probability of getting the genetic disease. Traditionally, genetic counseling has been concerned with communicating information about risk largely within the context of reproductive decision making, and risk was seen as a stimulus that elicited a largely predictable response. It was assumed that counselees given risk information would make reproductive plans that reflect the risk level of the birth defect. Investigations of outcomes of genetic counseling, however, have not consistently supported these expectations. Research confirmed that it was not the risk factor that influenced reproductive decisions but the burden of risk to that family and the personal experience with the disorder. The magnitude of the genetic risk was of relative importance only.

Knowledge of genetic risk for multifactorial diseases, that is, susceptibility to a disease, may motivate people to engage in risk-reducing behaviors and might be more motivating than other types of risk information because of its personalized nature. On the other hand, a genetic susceptibility may be perceived as a fixed, unchangeable self-attribute, especially when it is established by DNA testing, and may trigger feelings of fatalism, the belief that little can be done to change the risk, and may adversely affect motivation to engage in risk-reducing behavior. Evidence concerning responses to this kind of genetic risk information is limited and inconclusive. Some studies show that genetic risks are perceived as less controllable and less preventable, while others find no support for this.

For genetic information for risk of disease, whether it is hereditary breast cancer, Down syndrome, or familial diabetes, dilemmas that generally are not part of patient decision making in many nongenetic contexts play a role. The familial quality of genetic information may raise ethical dilemmas for physicians, particularly related to their duty of confidentiality, especially when multiple family members are seen at the same clinic. It is therefore important to use careful procedures to ensure that results and other sensitive information are not inadvertently communicated to a third party. The principle of confidentiality can expand to the social level as well, given the potential for genetic discrimination. Testing for multifactorial diseases implies different dilemmas. Genetic prediction of disease is based on testing for multiple genetic variants. A person's risk of disease will be based on this genetic profile and may have a range of different probabilities, mostly associated with an increased risk for more than one disease. Because multiple genes are involved, family members most likely will not share the same profile and their susceptibility to diseases will probably differ.

Because of the far-reaching consequences of genetic information, it is particularly important that decisions be autonomous decisions, that clients make an informed, noncoerced testing decision, and that they understand the benefits, risks, and limitations of testing. Informed decision making presupposes adequate knowledge and should be based on the participants' values. Decision aids are a promising type of intervention to promote informed decision making, although research is not conclusive about whether they indeed lead to better-informed decisions. For multifactorial diseases, providing genetic information about an increased susceptibility for disease is not enough to motivate behavioral change to reduce this risk, and tailored education strategies might be needed.

Danielle R. M. Timmermans and
Lidewij Henneman

See also Informed Decision Making; Patient Decision Aids; Shared Decision Making; Uncertainty in Medical Decisions

Further Readings

Bekker, H., Thornton, J. G., Airey, C. M., Connolly, J. B., Hewison, J., Robinson, M. B., et al. (1999). Informed decision making: An annotated bibliography and systematic review. *Health Technology Assessment, 3,* 1–156.

Berg, M., Timmermans, D. R. M., Ten Kate, L. P., Van Vugt, J. M., & Van der Wal, G. (2006). Informed decision making in the context of prenatal screening. *Patient Education and Counseling, 63,* 110–117.

Braithwaite, D., Emery, J., Walter, F., Prevost, A. T., & Sutton, S. (2006). Psychological impact of genetic counselling for familial cancer: A systematic review and meta-analysis. *Familial Cancer, 5,* 61–75.

Burke, W. (2002). Genetic testing. *New England Journal of Medicine, 347,* 1867–1875.

Collins, R. S. (1999). Shattuck lecture: Medical and societal consequences of the human genome project. *New England Journal of Medicine, 341,* 28–37.

Emery, J. (2001). Is informed choice in genetic testing a different breed of informed decision-making? A discussion paper. *Health Expectations, 4,* 81–86.

Green, J. M., Hewison, J., Bekker, H. L., Bryant, L. D., & Cuckle, H. S. (2004). Psychosocial aspects of genetic screening of pregnant women and newborns: A systematic review. *Health Technology Assessment, 8*(33), 1–109.

Heshka, J. T., Palleschi, C., Howley, H., Wilson, B., & Wells, P. S. (2008). A systematic review of perceived risks, psychological and behavioral impacts of genetic testing. *Genetics in Medicine, 10,* 19–32.

Khoury, M. J., McCabe, L. L., & McCabe, E. R. B. (2003). Population screening in the age of genomic medicine. *New England Journal of Medicine, 348,* 50–58.

Yoon, P. W., Scheuner, M. T., Peterson-Oehlke, K. L., Gwinn, M., Faucett, A., & Khoury, M. J. (2002). Can family history be used as a tool for public health and preventive medicine? *Genetics in Medicine, 4,* 304–310.

GOVERNMENT PERSPECTIVE, GENERAL HEALTHCARE

The perspective of the decision maker is a very important element of the decision-making process. Awareness of the decision maker's perspective can help guide the decision prior to it being made or understand the decision after it has been finalized. This is especially important for the decisions made by government agencies because of the important role that those agencies assume with respect to healthcare.

The emphasis here is on government agencies rather than the government as a whole because, contrary to what some believe, governments are usually not monolithic entities with a single societal perspective. Rather, they are collections of individual organizations, each with a distinct role (or set of roles) and, hence, perspective. The U.S. government is a good example, as it has multiple agencies with unique, and sometimes conflicting, roles and perspectives. Understanding "the government's position" requires one to first determine which agency is involved and what role it is assuming with respect to the issue at hand. That role then determines its perspective—the primary viewpoint that goes along with that role.

When it comes to healthcare, the federal government has several different roles that it fills through its various agencies. It is a driver of innovation, a protector of public health, a regulator, a payer, a payer-provider, and a stimulator of system change and quality improvement. In what follows, these different roles and the perspectives that they imply are discussed. Although this entry focuses on the federal government, similar examples could be taken from state and local governments as well as from large, democratically elected governments in other countries.

Driver of Innovation

The federal government drives innovation in a few different ways. First, it awards patents to the developers of new technologies, such as new drugs and new medical devices. This process is handled by the U.S. Patent and Trademark Office (USPTO). The perspective of the USPTO focuses on getting potentially useful inventions to market as quickly as possible so that society can benefit from the new innovation. It is also focused on the protection of intellectual property so as to maintain the incentives for innovation.

The second way the government stimulates innovation is through the conduct and sponsoring of basic research. Consider, for example, the U.S. National Institutes of Health (NIH), a research organization that is primarily focused on conducting basic research aimed at understanding diseases and identifying potential biologic interventions that could eliminate or reduce the burden of those diseases. As such, the perspective of the NIH

revolves around the generation of new information about the biologic causes of disease. Because this frequently takes a lot of time, its perspective is also more long term in nature.

Protector of Public Health

The federal government also acts as a protector of public health. One of the lead agencies in this role is the U.S. Centers for Disease Control and Prevention (CDC), which investigates disease outbreaks, sponsors programs to improve the health of populations, and conducts applied research that is focused on specific interventions that are known to reduce the burden of a disease—especially those that are concerned with behavior.

Another example of a government agency that acts as a protector of public health is the U.S. Food and Drug Administration (FDA). Specifically, the FDA regulates healthcare technologies, especially when they are first being introduced to the healthcare marketplace. Its goal is to ensure that those technologies are safe and effective, and its perspective toward healthcare is centered on that goal.

Because of their roles as protectors of public health, the perspectives of these two agencies are centered on the health of populations rather than the health of single individuals. They also tend to value safety above all other concerns.

Regulator

Regulation is an important part of government business, and healthcare is one of the areas subject to government regulation. The role of the FDA as a protector of public health has already been discussed. Unlike the CDC, though, the FDA also has a major role in regulation, with the authority to deny market access to drugs and medical devices that it deems unsafe.

The USPTO in its role as a driver of innovation has also been discussed. Like the FDA, it also has regulatory power insofar as it can grant or deny patents to the inventors of new technologies. This implies that the USPTO acts to regulate the competitiveness of healthcare markets that are created by new innovations.

Another example of an agency that assumes the role of regulator in the healthcare marketplace is the U.S. Federal Trade Commission (FTC). The

FTC works to ensure that markets remain competitive (except for those protected by a patent). It tries to prevent one firm or a set of firms from gaining market power—the power to set prices at a higher level than one would otherwise expect in a competitive marketplace. This applies to the market for healthcare just as it does to other industries. An example would be the prevention of anticompetitive mergers, such as those involving hospital chains or healthcare plans. The FTC perspective is focused on ensuring a competitive marketplace, even if that means denying mergers that could generate efficiencies that lower healthcare costs.

Payer and Payer-Provider

The U.S. Centers for Medicare and Medicaid Services (CMS) is an example of a government agency that takes on the role and perspective of a payer, as it has assumed financial responsibility for the healthcare given to older citizens (Medicare) and those living in poverty (Medicaid). Thus, unlike some of the other agencies, CMS is very concerned with the cost and quality of healthcare, particularly that given to its beneficiaries. This is especially true for new technologies that have received a patent from the USPTO and been approved for use by the FDA. As these new innovations are adopted as part of routine care, CMS (and its financial backer, the U.S. Congress) must be concerned with the impact the new technologies have on its overall budget.

Another agency that shares the payer perspective is the U.S. Office of Personnel Management (OPM), the organization that is responsible for overseeing the Federal Employee Health Benefit Program (FEHBP). As with CMS, it also has a keen interest in the cost and quality of healthcare given to its "members"—federal employees and their families.

The U.S. Department of Defense (DOD) and the U.S. Department of Veterans Affairs (VA) also have a payer perspective, with a strong focus on the cost and quality of healthcare. However, these two agencies also play the role of provider insofar as they have clinics, hospitals, and personnel who actually provide some of the care to their members. This allows them to directly control some of the cost and quality of healthcare—an element of control that CMS and OPM do not have.

Stimulator of System Change and Quality Improvement

Several of the agencies discussed above have some role in stimulating system change and quality improvement. For example, CMS has pilot projects that are meant to determine whether the current healthcare system and the level of quality created by it could be improved. However, these kinds of efforts are not the focus of those agencies. One agency that does have this as its primary focus is the U.S. Agency for Healthcare Research and Quality (AHRQ). AHRQ is committed to help improve the U.S. healthcare system, primarily through health services research that evaluates the quality, effectiveness, and efficiency of specific medical interventions targeted to individual patients. As such, its perspective reflects an interest in the care received by individual patients, with less emphasis on the health of populations.

Edward C. Mansley

See also Government Perspective, Informed Policy Choice; Government Perspective, Public Health Issues; Medicaid; Medicare

Further Readings

Agency for Healthcare Research and Quality. (n.d.). *About AHRQ*. Retrieved August 29, 2008, from http://www.ahrq.gov/about

Centers for Disease Control and Prevention. (n.d.). *About CDC*. Retrieved August 29, 2008, from http://www.cdc.gov/about

Centers for Medicare & Medicaid Services. (n.d.). *About CMS*. Retrieved August 29, 2008, from http://www.cms.hhs.gov/home/aboutcms.asp

Federal Trade Commission. (n.d.). *About the Federal Trade Commission*. Retrieved August 29, 2008, from http://www.ftc.gov/ftc/about.shtm

National Institutes of Health. (n.d.). *About NIH*. Retrieved August 29, 2008, from http://www.nih.gov/about/index.html

U.S. Department of Veterans Affairs. (n.d.). *About VA Home*. Retrieved August 29, 2008, from http://www.va.gov/about_va

U.S. Food and Drug Administration. (n.d.). *About the Food and Drug Administration*. Retrieved August 29, 2008, from http://www.fda.gov/opacom/hpview.html

U.S. Office of Personnel Management. (n.d.). *Federal Employees Health Benefits Program*. Retrieved

September 2, 2008, from http://www.opm.gov/insure/HEALTH/index.asp

U.S. Patent and Trademark Office. (n.d.). *Introduction.* Retrieved August 29, 2008, from http://www.uspto.gov/main/aboutuspto.htm

GOVERNMENT PERSPECTIVE, INFORMED POLICY CHOICE

Governmental perspectives on the individual's right to choice in healthcare and, in particular, the concept of informed choice, are relatively recent. Choice is now seen as being integral to healthcare reforms (patient-led care) taking place in the United Kingdom, the United States, and elsewhere. These policies contrast with some previous policies in which the government made choices on behalf of the population. Current government policy toward informed choice, in countries such as the United States and the United Kingdom, is based on the premise that people have an individual responsibility for their own health and are able to make their own choices. The provision of information (particularly evidence-based information) is viewed as being the key to enabling people to make rational choices.

Responsibility for Health

Individual choice in modern health policy in the West has its origins in the intellectual and economic revolutions of the 18th century. Before industrialization, attitudes on health and disease were largely defined by religion. The effect of the Enlightenment and the scientific revolution was to replace this with reason. At the same time, the industrial revolution brought with it a new wave of disease and death related to rapid urbanization. Liberal, laissez-faire economic theory initially influenced thinking on health, which as a result was seen as the responsibility of the individual rather than the government. However, investigations and a report by British politician Edwin Chadwick in 1842 linked ill health to water, overcrowding, and other environmental problems. Thereafter the U.K. government took greater responsibility for the health of the population, particularly the sick poor. Public health measures included centralization of the provision of drainage, water, and sanitary regulations. Such centralization was also seen in parts of Europe but took longer to happen in the United States.

Responsibility by the government for the health of the population was to achieve its greatest expression in the United Kingdom with the creation of the National Health Service (NHS) in 1946. By the 1970s, however, the triumph of neoliberal ideology within the leadership of the Conservative Party led to the primacy of ideas of competition, deregulation, and individual choice, ideas that were to continue to influence the new Labour governments from 1997 onward and to become the dominant ideology across the political spectrum. Their application to health meant that users of health services were seen as individualized consumers who (it was assumed) would place a high value on choice and particularly the concept of informed choice.

Informed Choice and Informed Consent

The concept of informed choice is largely based on the principles of informed consent, but there are significant differences between the two concepts. Informed choice usually (although not always) implies the stage before a decision has been made and concerns providing information for people to make rational choices, for example, about the place of care, whether to have health screening, or what type of treatment to have. Informed consent implies that a decision has already been made and concerns the disclosure of the risks involved in, for example, undergoing surgery or an invasive procedure. Both informed choice and informed consent in medical care (and in research), however, have one overarching principle: promoting patient autonomy by providing information on risks and benefits of a healthcare choice, intervention, or treatment.

The doctrines of informed consent and informed choice have ethical, legal, and clinical interpretations. It has been argued that medicine has long been committed to ethics and morality when dealing with the patient, although this commitment may be incomplete at times. Ethical concerns over informed consent have been around since the early 20th century. However, it was not until the mid-1950s that an autonomy model rather than a beneficence model (which depicts the physician's primary obligation as providing medical benefit) governed the justifications for informed consent.

Legal interest in informed consent and the rights of patients has been evolving alongside the ethical interest. Initially, this concerned consent to treatment, however uninformed. However, it became recognized that patients are autonomous human beings with rights and interests independent of the medical profession. The judicial doctrine of informed consent in healthcare is based primarily on decisions about treatments.

The doctrine of informed consent in clinical care emerged to some extent because of the perception that patients were uninformed and thus powerless in healthcare (i.e., without autonomy). Informed consent was developed in clinical care from an obligation by doctors to disclose information on the risks of procedures and to act with beneficence and nonmalfeasance. One way to redress the imbalance of power between patient and clinician is to inform the patient. The concomitant of the doctrine of informed consent is therefore the right to refuse treatment. Thus, there was necessarily a shift (in theory), away from paternalism and beneficence in medicine (however benign), toward a partnership between patient and physician, with the transference of information playing a crucial role. However, what the information should comprise, and how best to inform people (or make them informed), is the subject of a large body of research.

Information Required to Make an Informed Choice

As an ethical principle, provision of unbiased information is seen as being the key to respecting patient autonomy. However, it has been recognized that the provision of information alone will not necessarily ensure that people become autonomous or fully informed; the information also needs to be evidence-based, understandable, unbiased, and relevant. Research indicates that people still lack knowledge in certain areas, despite information given to them. Although policy makers cannot assume that the provision of information necessarily results in an informed (i.e., knowledgeable) population, they still have a responsibility to provide such information and ensure that it is the

information that the population wants and needs to make an autonomous choice.

There is also debate and uncertainty as to what constitutes "sufficient" information to make someone informed. Recent research suggests that people want information through which to contextualize their choices, not just information on risks and benefits. In addition, many of the organizations that develop information resources are the same organizations that are involved in delivering the services. This may mean that the information is highly regulated or that it lacks independent scrutiny.

Informed choice is gaining prominence in two particular areas of government health policy making: giving patients choice about the location or types of care (e.g., Hospital A or Hospital B) and encouraging healthy choices (e.g., going for health screening, exercising more).

Choice of Location of Care

In the United Kingdom, for example, the government's policies are increasingly aimed at offering, and expecting, people to make choices about the location of their care (e.g., choice of hospital). Choice is promoted as being a positive element of the health services experience, something that all patients want. In 2004 and 2005, a number of U.K. government policies were set out that required NHS organizations to offer a choice of four to five hospitals to patients requiring elective care ("choose and book"). The aim of this policy was to achieve one of the standards set out in the NHS Improvement Plan. This policy of choice of hospital was thought to benefit both patients and the NHS. For the patients, it was viewed as a way of providing them with more personalized, flexible, convenient care. For the NHS, it was viewed as reducing administrative bureaucracy and patient cancellations and providing a more standardized and improved service.

The policy makers recognized that people would need support to make informed choices about which hospital to choose and identified four key areas of information that they would need. These were waiting times, location and convenience of the hospital, patient experience, and clinical quality.

Although such government policies involve encouraging people to make informed choices about various aspects of their healthcare, it is not clear as to what extent people are able, or indeed want, to make rational, informed choices about their place of care at times when they may be already overwhelmed with other information about their disease or condition. There is some evidence to suggest that not all people see choice as a positive element of healthcare, as it can create stress and anxiety, especially if the choice that they make is later deemed to be the "wrong" choice. Also, the choices that they are being offered (e.g., choice of hospital) do not necessarily reflect the choices that they want (e.g., care at home). There is also scant evidence for the impact of choice policies on other issues such as equity—for example, some people may be more likely than others to get their hospital of choice or the maternity service that they request.

Informed Choice for Health Screening

Until recently, the focus of health screening programs and policies has been to maximize cost-effectiveness by achieving the highest coverage and uptake possible. The benefits of screening for cancer were deemed to be so great that any potential harm or limitations were given little attention. However, there is increasing recognition by U.K. government policy makers that, even when it is accepted that screening has a net beneficial effect (to the population), one of the inherent limitations is that some individuals will be harmed. In the United Kingdom, screening policy makers now, in principle, at least, consider informed choice alongside more conventional screening parameters such as quality assurance procedures and improvements in survival. The reasons given by the U.K. National Screening Committee in 2000 for promoting informed choice were the recognition of change in social attitudes and the acknowledged risks and consequences. It was observed that the advantage of increasing informed choice is that it prevents people feeling coerced. It was also seen as having economic advantages in that an informed choice policy may create opportunities for selective screening based on individual risk profiles. However, there may be conflicting or even contradictory motives at work among those involved in screening. For example, although an informed choice policy may be presented as one that promotes individual choice and autonomy, other factors (such as

target payments for uptake of cervical screening) may discourage health professionals from actively implementing the policy. Therefore, policy makers in cancer screening may need to decide whether they really want to increase and promote informed choice, or whether they want to increase informed participation—the choice to decline screening is neither promoted nor endorsed.

Informing Healthier Choices

Government policies toward public health may involve a combination of encouraging the population to take responsibility for their own health by making informed, healthier choices (e.g., using health promotion initiatives to tell people to stop smoking) and the government taking responsibility for health (e.g., through legislation and regulation). For example, policies in the United Kingdom include "Informing Healthier Choices: Information and Intelligence for Healthy Populations." These policies encourage informed choice, but the overarching aim is population health improvement by people choosing to live a healthier lifestyle.

One of the difficulties for government policies promoting individual informed choice is that there is only one "choice" that the government wants: people choosing healthy lifestyles. As in health screening, it is unlikely that the government actually wants people to exercise autonomous choices that result in nonparticipation in screening or to choose unhealthy lifestyles. However, as mentioned previously, the concept of informed choice is based on the premise that both choices are equal and people can make an autonomous choice. If the principles of informed choice are considered valid by policy makers, then the implication is that people should be able to choose not to take up the healthy living advice if they are informed and autonomous.

Current increases in mortality and morbidity attributable to unhealthy behaviors (e.g., rise in heart disease, diet-related cancers) suggest that people are not making healthy choices even when informed by mass media campaigns. One way that government policies try to respond is to take back responsibility for health and try and enforce healthy behaviors by, for example, banning smoking in public places. However, this approach results in people losing their autonomy in exercising choice.

Tensions Between Informed Choice and Public Health Policies

Public health policies such as health screening, immunization, and health promotion initiatives are often only effective if a high percentage of the population complies with the government policies and directives. Tensions and dilemmas arise when the government is trying to implement policies at a population level (e.g., health screening) in tandem with policies aimed at individuals within that population (e.g., promoting informed choice and autonomous decision making). What is not clear is whether a policy of informed choice can operate within a structure where both information and choice are, to some extent, regulated by the need to benefit populations (the public good) rather than individuals. The central issue is whether government-sponsored health initiatives are compatible with the concept of respect for individual autonomy. Many public health policies, such as health screening, are grounded in positions based on outcomes (the theory of utilitarianism). Thus, there may be a tension between policies aimed at the benefit of the population and other policies promoting individual autonomous decision making.

Government policies designed to increase (informed) choice are difficult to reconcile with policies aimed at improving the health of populations. Those aimed at promoting choice will not ensure that desired population health outcomes are achieved. Those designed to benefit populations will mean that a degree of individual choice is lost.

Ruth Jepson

See also Government Perspective, Public Health Issues; Informed Consent; Informed Decision Making

Further Readings

Faden, R. R., & Beauchamp, T. L. (1986). *A history and theory of informed consent.* New York: Oxford University Press.

Jepson, R. G., Hewison, J., Thompson, A., & Weller, D. (2005). How should we measure informed choice? The case of cancer screening. *Journal of Medical Ethics, 55,* 20–25.

Mazur, D. J. (2003). Influence of the law on risk and informed consent. *British Medical Journal, 27,* 731–734.

National Screening Committee. (2000). *Second report of the National Screening Committee.* Retrieved January 8, 2009, from http://www.nsc.nhs.uk/library/lib_ind.htm

O'Neill, O. (2003). Some limits of informed consent. *Journal of Medical Ethics, 29,* 4–7.

Petersen, A., & Lupton, D. (1996). *The new public health: Health and self in the age of risk.* London: Sage.

Porter, R. (1997). *The greatest benefit to mankind: A medical history of humanity from antiquity to present.* London: HarperCollins.

GOVERNMENT PERSPECTIVE, PUBLIC HEALTH ISSUES

The perspective of any decision-making entity determines which costs and outcomes will be included in a decision and is determined by who the audience to the decision is and how that audience will use the information contained in the decision or disseminated as a result of the decision. In questions of government or public health policy, it is usually most appropriate to adopt a societal perspective, because a more narrowly defined perspective will lead to an inefficient allocation of scarce public resources. A government public health perspective, therefore, would include an audience that tends to be society in general, including those who do and those who do not benefit from a program, policy, or intervention and including those who do and those who do not pay for the program, policy, or intervention. Therefore, from the government public health perspective, all benefits and costs, regardless of those to whom they accrue, would be included in the decision-making process. For example, when assessing costs of a mandatory human papillomavirus (HPV) screening program, a public health perspective would include not just the costs to deliver the screening but the losses in productivity associated with the persons receiving the immunization or experiencing illness and the long-term costs to society for transmission of disease in the absence of disease prevention. Society will use information stemming from government public health decision making to decide how to improve community-level health with societal resources.

Decision making from the government perspective is often based on interventions that are population based rather than individual based. For example, suppose that the outcome of interest is a reduction in lung cancer. Individual interventions to reduce the incidence of lung cancer could include a decision between therapeutic nicotine patches, gums, or lozenges. Public health interventions from the government perspective, however, could consider such population-based policies as requiring designated smoking spaces within public buildings or banning smoking in public buildings altogether. Thus, interventions, programs, or policies considered from a government public health perspective, by definition, are intended to provide a positive return to the population, in general, and not to just one individual at a time. In the smoking example, the public health intervention is designed to limit the smoking opportunities of the individual and reduce the secondhand smoke affecting the nonsmokers in society.

Decision making from a government public health perspective may also include community-based rather than clinical interventions. Community-based interventions are those interventions intended to promote the community's health and prevent disease and include decisions about interventions typically delivered in states or provinces, local agencies, healthcare organizations, worksites, or schools. Examples of community-based interventions designed to increase physical activity and reduce obesity include the promotion of school-based physical activity programs, urban design and land use policies, and social support services in community settings. Examples of community-based interventions designed to prevent violence include early home visitation to prevent violence against the child, school-based programs to prevent violent behavior, and group-based cognitive behavior therapy to reduce the harmful effects of traumatic events.

Guidance on how to deliver evidence-based community interventions often complements the evidence-based guidance available for clinical settings. For example, evidence-based community interventions that have been recommended to reduce tobacco use initiation include increasing the unit price for tobacco units, restricting access for minors, and conducting mass media campaigns combined with clinical interventions and community mobilization campaigns combined with clinical interventions.

Regardless of intervention setting, the value of government perspective decision making in public health is a focus on prevention versus treatment in promoting health. In an entirely systematic way, the public health perspective examines the effectiveness, economic efficiency, and feasibility of interventions to combat risky behaviors such as tobacco use, physical inactivity, and violence; to reduce the impact of specific conditions such as cancer, diabetes, vaccine-preventable diseases, and motor vehicle injuries; and to address social determinants of health such as education, housing, and access to care.

A focus on prevention, however, makes public health decision making often incommensurate with clinical decision making. Prevention efforts typically result in costs that occur in the short term, while benefits occur in the longer term. For example, the benefits of a nutrition and exercise program may not be realized until many years later, with future reductions in cardiovascular disease and diabetes, whereas clinical decisions often pertain to interventions whereby both the costs and benefits are realized in the short term: for example, statin treatment to lower cholesterol level and reduce the incidence of coronary heart disease and vascular events such as heart attack and stroke. When considering the present value of future costs and outcomes, treatment efforts will always appear more favorable than prevention efforts, if benefits are realized in different time frames.

Another important consideration in public health decision making is the challenge of establishing a causal link between intervention and outcomes because of a lack of longitudinal data to show future outcomes or sustained outcomes. For example, without longitudinal data, it may be difficult to establish the long-term benefits to a community that may result from an environmental improvement plan to provide more green space and exercise facilities for its residents. Thus, decision making from a public health perspective may need to be considered separately from decision making in a clinical setting, where the value of the decision-making information serves different purposes.

Phaedra Corso

See also Government Perspective, General Healthcare; Moral Choice and Public Policy; Trust in Healthcare

Further Readings

Owens, D. K. (2002). Analytic tools for public health decision making. *Medical Decision Ma king, 22*(5), S92–S101.

Schneider, M. (2006). *Introduction to public health* (2nd ed.). Sudbury, MA: Jones & Bartlett.

ZaZa, S., Briss, P., & Harris, K. (Eds.). (2005). *The guide to community preventive services: What works to promote health?* New York: Oxford University Press.

H

HAZARD RATIO

The hazard ratio in survival analysis is the effect of an explanatory variable on the hazard or risk of an event. In this context, the hazard is the instantaneous probability of the event (such as death) within the next small interval of time, assuming that one has survived to the start of that interval. The hazard ratio then compares the hazard of the event under one condition (e.g., treatment for a disease) with the hazard of the same event under a second (baseline) condition (e.g., placebo) by taking the ratio of one hazard over the other. A hazard ratio greater than 1 indicates an increase in the hazard of the event under the first condition over the hazard of the event under the second condition.

Survival Analysis

Survival analysis is a class of statistical methods that deals with the timing of the occurrence of particular events. These methods focus on modeling the *time* to an event such as onset of a particular disease. Survival analysis methods were originally designed to study death, hence the name. However, an event can be defined as the first diagnosis of cancer, the failure of a manufacturing machine, the progression of disease from one stage to another, and attrition times among criminals. An event can also signify a positive occurrence such as marriage, pregnancy, or cure from a disease. Survival analysis is also termed *reliability*

analysis or *failure time analysis* in engineering, *duration analysis* or *transition analysis* in economics, and *event history analysis* in sociology. In general, survival analysis involves the modeling of time-to-event data.

Survival Data

Since survival analysis deals with data collected over time until an event occurs, the time origin and event or end point of interest need to be clearly defined. In clinical research, the time origin is typically the time at which a patient is recruited into a study. The event or end point would then be the occurrence of a particular condition such as an adverse event or even death. In another such study, the event of interest could be being cured of the disease. In general, an event is a clearly definable transition from one discrete state to another. Examples of these transitions include the following: from being in pain to pain relief, from being disease-free to having a disease, or from being free to being incarcerated. However, in survival analysis, it is not sufficient to know only who is disease-free and who is not; one also needs to know *when* the transition occurred. Exact times of the event are sometimes known, but often, the timing of an event may only be known within a range. For example, in a well-monitored clinical trial, the onset of an adverse event may be pinpointed to a particular day (e.g., 10 days after study entry). On the other hand, in a study of menarche, only the year (e.g., age 13) of first menstruation may be collected.

There are several reasons why survival data cannot be suitably analyzed by standard statistical methods. First, survival data are typically not symmetrically distributed. For example, in a study of actual death times, the distribution of time to death will often be positively skewed (a histogram of the data will have a long tail to the right of where the majority of observations lie). Hence, those data are not readily amenable to standard statistical procedures that require data to have a normal distribution. Second, many variables that may influence the event or outcome of interest may change over time. These are called time-varying covariates. For example, a patient's increase in blood pressure over time may affect his or her risk of cardiovascular disease. These changes in the blood pressure variable can be easily accommodated in survival analysis models. Finally, and most important, survival analysis methods can deal with censored observations that are described next.

Censoring

One primary feature of survival data that is difficult to deal with using conventional statistical methods is censoring. The survival time of an individual is said to be censored when the end point of interest has not been observed for that individual. If the end point of interest is death, then an individual's survival time may be censored because that individual has been "lost to follow-up." For example, a patient participating in a clinical trial may unexpectedly move to another city before the end of the study and may no longer be contacted. The only survival information that would be available on that patient is the last date that that patient was known to be alive, which may be the date that the patient was last seen at the clinic. On the other hand, an individual's survival time may be censored because the patient is still alive at the end of the study period and his death date is not observed. An observed survival time (i.e., time to death) may also be regarded as censored if the death is known to be unrelated to the treatment under study. For example, a person's death due to a car accident is most likely unrelated to the chemotherapy that the patient was receiving in a clinical trial. However, in instances where it is not clear whether the death is unrelated to the treatment under investigation, it is more appropriate to consider survival time until death due to all causes; or it may be of interest to analyze the time to death from causes other than the primary condition for which the patient was being treated.

There are three primary types of censoring: right censoring, left censoring, and interval censoring. If we let T be a variable that represents the time of occurrence of a particular event, then T is said to be right censored if the only information we have on T is that it is greater than some value, c. For example, if T represents age at death, but a patient was lost to follow-up at age 65, then for that patient we only know that $T > 65$, in which case the patient's event time is right censored at age 65. The right-censored survival time is less than the actual, but unknown, survival time (the censoring occurs to the right of the last known survival time). Left censoring occurs when the actual survival time is less than that observed. One example in which left censoring may occur is in a follow-up study of cancer recurrence in which patients are seen by their oncologist 6 months after their initial treatment for their primary cancer. At the 6-month visit, a patient is examined for disease recurrence. Some patients will have evidence of recurrence at that visit, but the recurrence may have occurred at any time prior to that clinic visit. Hence, the recurrence time is said to be left censored (the censoring occurs to the left of the known examination time). Interval censoring is a combination of both right and left censoring. Revisiting the cancer recurrence example, if patients are followed by their oncologist every 6 months, and cancer recurrence is detected at their third follow-up visit but not at prior visits, then we know that the actual recurrence time is between their second and third clinic visit. The observed recurrence time is said to be interval censored. Right censoring is the most common type of censoring and is handled more readily than other types of censoring when using standard analytic software packages.

Because censored observations are a common occurrence in time-to-event data, all survival analysis approaches provide ways to deal with these types of observations. The most commonly used survival analysis model that allows for censored observations is the proportional hazards model described next.

Estimating the Hazard Ratio

Often, the objective of a survival analysis study is to compare two groups (e.g., those who are given a treatment for a disease vs. those who are administered a placebo) on their risk or hazard of death. The hazard is defined as the instantaneous probability of death within the next small interval of time, assuming that one has survived to the start of that interval. When comparing the hazards of two groups, an assumption is commonly made that the ratio of the hazards (the hazard of death in those treated divided by those given placebo) is the same at all possible survival times. This is called the *proportional hazards assumption*. If the hazards in the two groups at time t are denoted as $h_0(t)$ and $h_1(t)$, then proportional hazards implies that $h_1(t)/h_0(t) = \varphi$ at all survival times, t, and where φ is a constant that does not change over time. This constant is called the *hazard ratio*. Since hazards are always positive, the hazard ratio can conveniently be expressed as $\varphi = e^\beta$, where β is a parameter that can be positive or negative. For two individuals who differ only in their group membership (e.g., treatment vs. placebo), their predicted log-hazard will differ additively by the relevant parameter estimate, which is to say that their predicted hazard rate will differ by e^β, that is, multiplicatively by the antilog of the estimate. Thus, the estimate can be considered a hazard ratio, that is, the ratio between the predicted hazard for a member of one group and that for a member of the other group, holding everything else constant.

Proportional Hazards Regression Models

The parameter β can be estimated by regression models that treat the log of the hazard rate as a function of a baseline hazard $h_0(t)$ and a linear combination of explanatory variables. Such regression models are classified as proportional hazards regression models and include the Cox semiparametric proportional hazards model and the exponential, Weibull and Gompertz parametric models. These models differ primarily in their treatment of $h_0(t)$. The proportional hazards model first introduced by Cox in 1972 is the most widely used regression model in survival analysis. The main advantage to this model is that it does not require a particular form for the survival times; specifically, the baseline hazard does not need to be specified.

Interpretation

Statistical software packages used to fit a proportional hazards model will generally provide point estimates of the hazard ratio and of the parameter β. A hazard ratio with a value of 1 (corresponding to a value of 0 for β) can be interpreted to mean that there is no apparent difference in hazard of death under the treatment versus the placebo. A hazard ratio less than 1 indicates that the treatment group has a reduced hazard of death over the placebo group, and a hazard ratio greater than 1 indicates an increased hazard of death for those in the active treatment group. In addition to a point estimate, statistical packages will also provide standard errors that allow one to better access the accuracy of the hazard ratio estimate. These standard errors can be used to obtain approximate confidence intervals for the unknown β parameter. In particular, a $100(1 - \alpha)\%$ confidence interval for β is the interval with limits $\hat{\beta} \pm z_{\alpha/2} SE(\hat{\beta})$ where $\hat{\beta}$ is the estimate of β and $z_{\alpha/2}$ is the upper $\alpha/2$ point of the standard normal distribution. If the confidence interval (usually a 95% confidence interval) for β does not include 0, then this is evidence that the value of β is nonzero. The corresponding confidence interval for the hazard ratio can be found simply by exponentiating the confidence limits of β. If the 95% confidence interval for the true hazard ratio does not include 1, then one can be fairly confident that the value of the hazard ratio is not 1. One can also test the hypothesis that there is no difference in hazards between two groups by testing the null hypothesis that $\beta = 0$. This can be tested using the statistic $\hat{\beta}/SE(\hat{\beta})$, whose value can be compared with the percentage points of the standard normal distribution to obtain the corresponding p value. This corresponds directly to testing whether the hazard ratio is equal to 1.

Nandita Mitra

See also Cox Proportional Hazards Regression; Log-Rank Test; Parametric Survival Analysis; Survival Analysis

Further Readings

Collett, D. (2003). *Modelling survival data in medical research* (2nd ed.). London: Chapman & Hall.

Cox, D. R., & Oakes, D. (1984). *Analysis of survival data*. London: Chapman & Hall.

Hosmer, D. W., Lemeshow, S., & May, S. (2008). *Applied survival analysis: Regression modeling of time to event data* (2nd ed.). New York: Wiley.

Kalbfleisch, J. D., & Prentice, R. L. (2002). *The statistical analysis of failure time data* (2nd ed.). New York: Wiley.

Klein, J. P., & Moeschberger, M. L. (2005). *Survival analysis: Techniques for censored and truncated data*. New York: Springer.

Kleinbaum, D., & Klein, M. (2005). *Survival analysis: A self-learning text*. New York: Springer.

Therneau, T. M., & Grambsch, P. M. (2001). *Modeling survival data: Extending the Cox model*. New York: Springer.

HEALTH INSURANCE PORTABILITY AND ACCOUNTABILITY ACT PRIVACY RULE

Protections in health and medical care are not limited to the protection of an individual's right to make decisions about his or her own body and mind. Protections also extend to the release of an individual's privacy-protected information in medical care and medical research settings. An example of such an extension of protection is the Health Insurance Portability and Accountability Act of 1996 (HIPAA) in the United States.

HIPAA (Public Law 104-191), as enacted in the United States on August 21, 1996, required the Secretary of the Department of Health and Human Services (HHS) to issue privacy regulations governing individually identifiable health information if Congress did not enact privacy legislation within 3 years of the passage of HIPAA.

Since Congress did not enact privacy legislation within that time frame, HHS developed a proposed rule and released it for public comment on November 3, 1999. After review of 52,000 public comments, the final regulation—the Privacy Rule— was published on December 28, 2000. The Standards for Privacy of Individually Identifiable Health Information (Privacy Rule) established for the first time in the United States a set of national standards for the "protection" of all "individually identifiable health information" held or transmitted by a covered entity or its business associate in any form or medium (electronic, paper, or oral).

Distinctions in Data Identifications

When considering issues of identification, one must distinguish among the following concepts. First, one must distinguish between "anonymous data" and "nonanonymous data." Second, in the area of nonanonymous data and individual identification, one must distinguish between two types of individual identification: nonunique versus unique.

Anonymous Versus Nonanonymous Data

Anonymous data are data from which all unique identifiers have been removed. Ideally, it should be impossible to identify a unique individual from a data set composed of anonymous data. However, what may appear on the surface to be an example of anonymous data may become problematic after further examination, as is illustrated later in this entry.

Nonanonymous data are data where individual identifiers have not been removed, and therefore, the data can be traced back to individuals. Sometimes this tracing back will yield one individual; sometimes several; sometimes many.

All individual identifiers are not necessarily unique identifiers. Individual identifiers in HIPAA include the following:

- Names
- All geographic subdivisions smaller than a state, including street address, city, county, precinct, zip code, and their equivalent geocodes, except for the initial three digits of a zip code if, according to the publicly available data from the Bureau of the Census,
  - The geographic unit formed by combining all zip codes with the same three initial digits contains more than 20,000 people and
  - The initial three digits of a zip code for all such geographic units containing 20,000 or fewer people are changed to 000.
- All elements of dates (except year) for dates directly related to an individual, including birth

date, admission date, discharge data, and date of death; and all ages over 89 and all elements of dates (including year) indicative of such age, except that such ages and elements may be aggregated into a single category of age 90 or older

- Telephone numbers
- Fax numbers
- Electronic mail addresses
- Social Security numbers
- Medical record numbers
- Health plan beneficiary numbers
- Account numbers
- Certificate/license numbers
- Vehicle identifiers and serial numbers, including license plate numbers
- Device identifiers and serial numbers
- Web Universal Resource Locators (URLs)
- Internet Protocol (IP) address numbers
- Biometric identifiers, including finger and voice prints
- Full-face photographic images and any comparable images
- Any other unique identifying number, characteristic, or code

Unique Versus Nonunique Individual Identifiers

An individual identifier can be used to link an individual with a piece of health or medical information contained, for example, in a larger data set of health information, but this individual identifier may not be able to identify the individual uniquely. Thus, there are unique identifiers and nonunique identifiers and a range of identifiers in between.

For example, a visual illustration of an individual identifier is a full-face photograph of a patient. While the photo may be an individual identifier, it may not be a unique identifier. In the case of identical twins, the full-face photograph may be able to reduce the number of possibilities in the world to two candidates for the identity of the individual in the photo—that is, the twin or his or her identical sibling. However, someone examining the full-face photograph may not be able to distinguish between the two identical twins. A unique identifier would be able to pick out one or the other of the two twins on the basis of a property held by one twin but not by his or her identical sibling.

Why the Need to Identify Individuals Uniquely?

Why is there a need to identify individuals uniquely as associated with a data set based on a blood or tissue sample and/or a study test result? A data set can contain a result or a set of study results from a test or set of tests used to screen for disease in an asymptomatic patient or to diagnose disease in a symptomatic patient (in medical care) or results obtained after an individual has agreed to participate in a research study and is studied before and then again after a research intervention. In both settings, test results (especially abnormal test results) need to be traced back to the donor of the blood or tissue sample or the individual who agreed to participate in the study. If a blood sample yields a markedly abnormal result, the blood sample will (1) need to be repeated to check the accuracy of the first specimen and then (2) acted on as quickly as possible.

The following is an example. A high serum lead level in an infant being cared for by a provider or participating in a research study needs to be acted on immediately to prevent further damage to the infant from the lead. This requires being able to identify the individual uniquely so that the infant's parents can be told about the abnormality, to remove the infant from continued exposure, and to get the infant into a medical care facility to be treated.

Why the Need to Protect Individuals From Unique Identification?

Why is there a need to protect individuals from unique identification in medical care or medical research? First, there are ways to inappropriately use data derived from blood and tissue specimens to stigmatize individuals as having a specific disease. Individuals and families (in the case of a genetically linked condition) need to be protected in society from such stigmatization. HIPAA attempts to eliminate (reduce) harm to individuals based on misuse of individually identifiable health information, including attempts to exclude individuals from job and employment opportunities and attempts to exclude individuals from present and future entitlements within society.

Second, there are economic uses of blood and tissue samples derived from humans (which include the development of medical products). While individuals may be willing to provide specimens for their own medical care, they may not be willing to donate a sample for research purposes. Or if they are willing to donate a sample for research purposes one time, they may not be willing to be pursued by a researcher or product manufacturer over time to provide additional specimens.

Third, by being uniquely identified as having a specific disease, an individual may be targeted for advertising related to medical products that can be used in managing and treating his or her disease. While certain individuals consider the receipt of such new product advertising an opportunity, other individuals may not want to be so targeted.

Finally, in the medical research setting, although an individual may be willing to allow his or her blood or tissue samples to be used in a study to test a particular scientific hypothesis or to donate blood or tissues to a data bank for future research (whose scientific hypotheses have not even been conceived of today), that individual may be willing to donate his or her specimen only if it is labeled in such a way that the data cannot be traced back to that donating individual (completely anonymous data).

Genetically Identifiable Health Information

This entry so far has considered the types of decisions that decisionally capable individuals are able to make on their own: the decision to participate in medical care and the decision to volunteer to participate in a research study. However, in the case of data of genetic origin, while the individual may not care about protecting himself or herself from possible harm related to data release and while the individual may be willing to donate a specimen for a present or future research study, the individual does not have the right, with only his or her own permission, to donate materials whose release could damage other genetically linked family members, even if the individual possesses decisional capacity. Those individuals genetically linked to one another can have this linkage identified on the basis of examination of DNA, RNA, unique proteins, and other biologic materials with the same shared characteristic. In research that requires as its substrate genetically linked material, the major question in need of clarification is the

following: How does anyone secure the relevant informed consents from all relevant genetically linked individuals to allow this genetically based study to start up and then continue over time (or to allow specimens to be banked over time to allow future research on the specimens)? This key question still remains unanswered and open for continued debate and research.

Difficult De-Identification

Perhaps the most difficult case in which to attempt to de-identify data with respect to an individual involves clinical care of the one patient with a rare medical condition who is followed in one medical center. Here, simply the labeling of the individual with the name of the rare medical condition or disease process he or she has is enough to label that individual within that medical center uniquely. If that individual is the only individual with that rare disease in the town, city, county, state, or nation in which he or she lives, the problem of de-identification (nonuniquely identifying the individual) will remain with that individual throughout his or her life.

Dennis J. Mazur

See also Decisions Faced by Institutional Review Boards; Informed Consent

Further Readings

Charo, R. A. (2006). Body of research: Ownership and use of human tissue. *New England Journal of Medicine, 355,* 1517–1519.

GAIN Collaborative Research Group. (2007). New models of collaboration in genome-wide association studies: The Genetic Association Information Network. *Nature Genetics, 39,* 1045–1051.

Ginsburg, G. S., Burke, T. W., & Febbo, P. (2008). Centralized biorepositories for genetic and genomic research. *Journal of the American Medical Association, 299,* 1359–1361.

Kauffmann, F., & Cambon-Thomsen, A. (2008). Tracing biological collections: Between books and clinical trials. *Journal of the American Medical Association, 299,* 2316–2318.

Mazur, D. J. (2003). Influence of the law on risk and informed consent. *British Medical Journal, 327,* 731–734.

Mazur, D. J. (2007). *Evaluating the science and ethics of research on humans: A guide for IRB members.* Baltimore: Johns Hopkins University Press.

Milanovic, F., Pontille, D., & Cambon-Thomsen, A. (2007). Biobanking and data sharing: A plurality of exchange regimes. *Genomics, Society, and Policy, 3,* 17–30.

Moffatt, M. F., Kabesch, M., Liang, L., Dixon, A. L., Strachan, D., Heath, S., et al. (2007). Genetic variants regulating ORMDL3 expression contribute to the risk of childhood asthma. *Nature, 448,* 470–473.

Summary of the HIPAA Privacy Rule. (2003). Retrieved June 5, 2008, from http://www.hhs.gov/ocr/privacy/hipaa/understanding/summary/privacysummary

Topol, E. J., Murray, S. S., & Frazer, K. A. (2007). The genomics gold rush. *Journal of the American Medical Association, 298,* 218–221.

Yuille, M., van Ommen, G. J., Bréchot, C., Cambon-Thomsen, A., Dagher, G., Landegren, U., et al. (2008). Biobanking for Europe. *Briefings in Bioinformatics, 9,* 14–24.

HEALTH OUTCOMES ASSESSMENT

Have population-wide death rates and disability levels attributable to disease X declined over the past decade? In a randomized clinical trial comparing drug Y with standard therapy, is there a clinically important difference in patient survival or in patient-reported outcomes (PRO) such as symptom bother? In an economic evaluation of screening for disease Z annually rather than semi-annually, what are the estimated differences in quality-adjusted life years (QALYs) per dollar spent? If a patient, working closely with her physician, is considering two therapies with similar projected survival benefits, how might she determine which provides the better health-related quality of life (HRQOL)? These quite diverse queries share a central common feature: They involve health outcomes assessment.

Health outcomes assessment (HOA) is a systematic and frequently multistep analytical *process* that may entail (1) identifying the health-related issue or problem to be investigated and the relevant audiences for the assessment (which may or may not be an identified decision maker); (2) selecting health outcome measures applicable to the problem at hand; (3) establishing an appropriate study design and collecting and analyzing the health outcomes data, often in conjunction with additional data deemed necessary for the particular assessment being done (e.g., one may want to draw inferences about the potential determinants of health outcomes); and (4) translating findings from (3) into information useful to the audiences identified in (1). By implication, health outcomes *measurement* is an essential step in health outcomes assessment but is not synonymous with health outcomes assessment. The health outcomes of interest pertain generally to quantity of life (mortality, survival, disease-free survival), quality of life (to encompass a range of PROs, including HRQOL and symptom bother), or both (as indexed, say, by the QALY).

As thus defined, health outcomes assessment may be viewed as a central task of health outcomes research, which, according to the U.S. Agency for Healthcare Research and Quality, "seeks to understand the end results of particular health care practices and interventions." Such end results are to be distinguished from "intermediate" outcomes (e.g., disease-screening rates) and "clinical outcomes" (e.g., changes in the individual's underlying medical condition). To be sure, medical interventions are very frequently aimed at improving such clinical or intermediate outcomes; health outcomes assessment asks the bottom-line question of whether such improvements translate into a longer life or better health.

The sections that follow discuss the health outcomes assessment process, with particular attention to linkages between the purpose of the assessment, the selection of specific outcome measures, and the translation of findings into useful information for the intended audience. That said, it is not the intent here to provide a detailed examination of each of the components of the multistep HOA process but rather to indicate how these considerations can be jointly brought to bear in the conduct of an assessment.

Areas of Application

Most health outcome assessments are designed to inform decision making in one of five areas of application: (1) population-level health surveillance, (2) randomized controlled trials, (3) observational (nonrandomized) studies of intervention effectiveness, (4) cost-effectiveness analyses, and (5) patient–clinician deliberations about interventions and outcomes.

Population-Level Health Surveillance

This includes international, national, or subnational (e.g., state, regional) studies of health outcomes, either at the individual disease level or across diseases. Depending on the purpose of the study and the data available, the focus may be on trends in mortality, survival, or various PRO measures, including morbidity levels, symptoms, functional status, or HRQOL. The primary purpose of such surveillance studies, which are conducted routinely in some form by most developed nations and by international organizations such as the World Health Organization, is to inform policy discussions and the research agenda by revealing successes, shortcomings, and issues requiring more intensive investigation.

Considerable progress has been achieved in North America and Europe in the calculation of mortality and survival rates in a consistent fashion and in the application of multidimensional HRQOL instruments. For example, the SF-12 instrument is routinely administered as one component of the U.S. Medical Care Expenditure Panel Survey (MEPS), while variants of the SF-36 instrument are used in the ongoing Health Outcomes Survey of enrollees in Medicare managed care plans, conducted by the U.S. Centers for Medicare & Medicaid Services. The EQ-5D, a HRQOL measure designed to incorporate population preferences for health outcomes, has been used in several representative surveys of the U.K. population by Kind and colleagues. The Health Utilities Index, another preference-based HRQOL measure, is being applied on an ongoing basis across Canada and also in the Joint Canada-U.S. Survey of Health (JCUSH).

Regarding the HOA process delineated earlier, most population-level assessments focus on Steps 1, 2, and 4; historically, there has typically been less emphasis on sorting out the determinants of variations in population health. However, there is a growing interest in identifying disparities in health (and access to healthcare) across population subgroups defined by race/ethnicity, demographics, or geography.

Randomized Controlled Trials

The purpose of health outcomes assessment in most experimental studies of drugs, devices, biologics, or other interventions is clear: to generate evidence on safety, efficacy, and clinical benefit to inform regulatory decisions about product approval and labeling and (subsequent) decision making by purchasers, providers, and patients.

Recent developments in oncology offer a particularly rich opportunity for examining these issues in a concrete way. As officials of the U.S. Food and Drug Administration have written, approval of cancer drugs is based on "endpoints that demonstrate a longer life or a better life." From these officials' published reviews of cancer regulatory decisions spanning the period 1990 to 2006 in total, clinical outcomes (primarily tumor response) clearly played an important role in the majority of approval decisions, although patient-reported outcome measures—particularly symptom relief—provided critical or supplementary support in a number of instances. These officials report, however, that in no case was a cancer drug approval based on a HRQOL measure.

In 2006, the FDA issued its own draft "guidance to industry" on the use of PRO data (including HRQOL) in medical product development to support labeling claims generally. In 2007, the National Cancer Institute (NCI) fostered the publication of a series of papers (in the *Journal of Clinical Oncology*) assessing the state of the science of PRO application in cancer trials supported through the NCI. Also in 2007, a series of papers interpreting and evaluating the FDA PRO draft guidance appeared in another scholarly journal (*Value in Health*).

In sum, this is an era of intense debate about health outcomes assessment in clinical trials, particularly regarding the choice of appropriate end points and the closely related issues of study design, data collection, and analysis (corresponding to Steps 2 and 3 in the HOA process). While oncology studies have been very much in the spotlight, similar issues arise in any clinical trial where the patient's own perspective is regarded as an essential element in the outcomes assessment. Moreover, these issues have received analogous critical attention outside the United States.

Observational Studies of Intervention Effectiveness

There is a vast literature examining the impact of interventions—ranging from prevention activities, to disease screening, to treatments that may be surgical, medical, or radiological, or other—on health outcomes in the real-world practice of medicine. Depending on the disease and the purpose of the study, the focus may be largely on survival outcomes (e.g., do AIDS patients receiving a certain drug cocktail have a longer life expectancy?); HRQOL outcomes (e.g., do rheumatoid arthritis patients receiving a new disease-modifying agent report better functioning and less pain than before?); or both (e.g., do patients with two-vessel heart disease have better quality-adjusted survival with angioplasty or with coronary artery bypass surgery?).

Still relatively rare are longitudinal health outcomes assessments to track over time the impact of interventions on HRQOL, satisfaction with care, and other PROs, in addition to survival. A noteworthy example is the NCI-supported Prostate Cancer Outcomes Study, which has followed more than 3,500 newly diagnosed patients for up to 60 months, attempting to survey each at four different time points regarding symptom bother, functional status, and other aspects of HRQOL as well as about satisfaction with care and with the outcomes being experienced.

Because the validity of such observational (non-randomized) studies may be threatened by selection effects (i.e., the subjects choosing Intervention A may not be comparable to those choosing Intervention B, in ways that may not be observable to the analyst), certain statistical correctives are increasingly being applied. These include both instrumental variable and propensity scoring techniques, two approaches in pursuit of a common aim: namely, to permit valid inferences about the impact of some hypothesized causal factor (e.g., a healthcare intervention) on a dependent variable of interest (e.g., a health outcomes measure) when it is likely that the variables are codetermined (mutually causal).

In general, the steps within the HOA process requiring the greatest attention here are the choice of outcomes measure(s) and study design and data analysis issues (i.e., Steps 2 and 3). In contrast to most clinical trials, the majority of such nonrandomized intervention studies inform decision making (if at all) in a generally more indirect or diffused way.

Cost-Effectiveness Analyses

In economic evaluations of whether a candidate intervention (e.g., individualized smoking cessation therapy) offers good value for the money compared with some alternative (e.g., an anti-smoking ad campaign), health outcomes assessment plays a pivotal role. This is because the "value" component of the cost-effectiveness analysis (CEA) is measured in terms of health outcomes improvement—for example, life-years gained or (most commonly now) QALYs gained. To carry out the CEA, therefore, requires sound statistical evidence on the health impact of each competing intervention, as would typically be derived from randomized or observational studies. Also required is information on the associated costs of each intervention and on a host of other factors (covariates) that allow the health and cost calculations to be tailored to specific population subgroups.

A prominent example of such a CEA, carried out in close conformance to the recommendations of the U.S. Panel on Cost-Effectiveness in Health and Medicine, is the study by Ramsey and colleagues comparing lung volume reduction surgery with medical management for elderly emphysema patients. CEA ratios in terms of dollars per QALY gained were computed for patients at varying degrees of clinical severity and under a variety of other clinical, economic, and statistical assumptions. This CEA and the randomized clinical trial on which it was based were sponsored by the U.S. Centers for Medicare & Medicaid Services (CMS), which covers virtually all Medicare-eligible patients and had a direct interest in the findings. Following publication of the trial and CEA findings, CMS approved coverage of lung volume reduction surgery for Medicare-eligible patients meeting specific clinical and behavioral criteria.

Frequently, such CEAs are conducted to inform public- or private-sector clinical policies relating to practice guidelines development or coverage decisions. In these instances, the process of health outcomes assessment feeds into the larger process of health economic evaluation.

Patient-Clinician Decision Making

There is growing interest, experimentation, and real-world application of health outcomes assessment to enhance the substantive content and overall quality of communications between patients and their healthcare providers. The aim is to strengthen shared decision making about intervention strategies and, ultimately, to improve patient outcomes. In most applications to date, patients complete questionnaires—focusing typically on aspects of their health-related quality of life—and the information is fed back to clinicians to inform healthcare management decisions.

Compared with the other areas of application, this use of health outcomes assessment is still in its infancy. There are promising results from some studies, including at least one randomized, controlled trial, indicating that providing clinicians with feedback on the patient's HRQOL status can favorably influence the perceived quality of communications and the patient's subsequent HRQOL. However, for this application of health outcomes assessment to realize its potential, several challenges must be confronted. These include strengthening the theoretical basis for anticipating and interpreting the impact of PRO measurement on decision making in routine clinical practice; understanding better how HRQOL measures developed originally to assess the impact of interventions on *groups* of patients can be informative for *individual-level* decision making; identifying targeted, patient-appropriate interventions based on responses to HRQOL questionnaires; and developing more user-friendly software to facilitate data collection and sharing. Progress on all fronts is expected to accelerate in the years ahead.

Informing Decision Making

Health outcomes assessment may be viewed as a multistep process, which progresses through identifying the decision problem to be addressed, the selection of appropriate outcomes measures, and the design and execution of the assessment itself, to the translation of findings to the intended audience(s) of analysts and decision makers. An assessment that carefully considers these steps in turn has the highest likelihood of successfully informing decision making.

*Joseph Lipscomb, Claire F. Snyder,
and Carolyn C. Gotay*

See also Cost-Effectiveness Analysis; Mortality; Oncology Health-Related Quality of Life Assessment; Outcomes Research; Propensity Scores; Quality-Adjusted Life Years (QALYs)

Further Readings

Agency for Healthcare Research and Quality. (2000). *Outcomes research fact sheet.* Retrieved January 20, 2009, from http://www.ahrq.gov/clinic/outfact.htm

Clauser, S. B. (2004). Use of cancer performance measures in population health: A macro-level perspective. *Journal of the National Cancer Institute Monograph, 33,* 142–154.

Greenhalgh, J., Long, A. F., & Flynn, R. (2005). The use of patient reported outcome measures in routine clinical practice: Lack of impact or lack of theory? *Social Science & Medicine, 60,* 833–843.

Lenderking, W. R., & Revicki, D. A. (Eds.). (2005). *Advancing health outcomes research methods and clinical applications.* McLean, VA: Degnon.

Lipscomb, J., Gotay, C. C., & Snyder, C. (Eds.). (2005). *Outcomes assessment in cancer: Measures, methods, and applications.* Cambridge, UK: Cambridge University Press.

Patrick, D. L., Burke, L. B., Powers, J. H., Scott, J. A., Rock, E. P., Dawisha, S., et al. (2007). Patient-reported outcomes to support medical product labeling claims: FDA perspective. *Value in Health, 10*(Suppl. 2), 125–137.

Shortell, S. M., & Richardson, W. C. (1978). *Health program evaluation.* St. Louis, MO: C. V. Mosby.

Tunis, S., & Stryer, D. (1999). *The outcomes of outcomes research at AHCPR: Final report.* Retrieved June 30, 2008, from http://www.ahrq.gov/clinic/out2res

HEALTH PRODUCTION FUNCTION

The health needs of any population will be considerable, and there will never be enough resources to meet them all. As resources are scarce in relation to needs, they must be allocated by some mechanism, driven by the government or the private market.

To understand the results of the various ways that resources can be allocated, economists have developed a concept called the production function.

A production function is a mathematical concept that expresses a relation between resources and the outputs which the resources produce. The venue of the production can be a department, a plant, or a business firm. An economic "actor" or "manager" is responsible for combining the resources so they yield the outputs. An exemplified expression for a production function is $Q(L, K, t)$, where Q is an output (e.g., bushels of wheat), L represents the quantity of labor input, and K represents the quantity of capital equipment. The term t represents the stage of technological knowledge, which generally changes over time.

Hypotheses

The production function was initially used to predict how resources were combined to produce physical outputs of plants or firms, such as steel producers, shoe manufacturers, or agricultural firms. There are four primary hypotheses that can be generated from this concept. These are as follows:

1. As one resource increases while the others are held constant, the additional output from this increase will eventually decline. As an example, successive increases in receptionist time in a clinic (with other resources such as physician time and equipment held fixed) will initially lead to increased clinic output (visits). But this will happen only up to a point. Beyond that level, as more receptionist time is successively added, the increase in visits will become smaller.

2. As all resources increase together, in equal proportions, the *additional* output resulting will initially increase in a greater proportion ("economies of scale"), level off ("constant economies"), and then decrease ("diseconomies of scale"). For example, a moderate size clinic will have a greater productivity (in terms of visits per resource unit) than will a very small one. However, there are limits to which the productivity will increase with expansions in clinic size.

3. Over time, the entire curve will increase, indicating that more output can be achieved with the same quantity of resources ("technological change"

or "increases in productivity"). In recent years, the mechanization of lab services has led to a reduction in the total resources that are used to produce lab tests. This means an upward shift in the production curve that relates outputs (lab tests) to inputs. It should be noted that quality of care is a component of output, though one that is difficult to measure.

4. The incorporation of one set of resources in two different applications within the same organization (a nursing home and a hospital), rather than in separate organizations, can result in economies (or diseconomies) of scope. For example, if we divide the hospital into distinct diagnostic units (pediatric, geriatric, cancer care), then economies of scope will be evidenced if a multiservice unit that incorporates many of these is less costly than a series of separate specialized hospitals.

Application to Medical Care

The production function concept has been used to explain how changes in the use of resources can yield different volumes of output (i.e., services produced) of *medical care*. Thus, John Cawley has examined how the use of specific types of capital-intensive services or equipment (catheters, tube feeding, psychotropic drugs), when used in nursing homes, will influence the use of labor (nurses' time) per resident day. That is, the capital equipment can be substituted for labor, keeping the amount of services produced at the same level. Production functions can also be used to explain factor substitution in health maintenance organizations, physicians' offices, and hospitals.

In 1965, Gary Becker published an article on the allocation of time within the household. The production function, formerly used to analyze how business firms combined resources, could now be used to analyze how households could combine resources, including purchased inputs and personal time, to produce activities that yield consumer benefits. Michael Grossman used this model in 1972 to examine how persons could use resources such as time and medical care to produce the output "health."

The first empirical studies of health production functions used mortality rates as a measure of health output (now called outcomes). A 1971 study by Charles Stewart characterized resources in four groups: treatment, prevention, information, and research. In estimating the production function, Stewart showed that in developed countries, physician inputs, when increased, had an insignificant impact on life expectancy. The statistical procedure used in this model was challenged by Edward Meeker and Ronald Williams; when population health status and more appropriate statistical measures were taken into account, the statistical models showed a statistically significant impact of physician density on mortality, though not a large one.

The most influential studies associated with health production come from longitudinal analyses of mortality by David Cutler and Frank Lichtenberg. Responding to the noticeable improvements in mortality rates of selected groups since the 1970s, Cutler conducted several analyses of health production for people with different health conditions, including heart attacks and lung cancer. The findings are that trends in medical care for heart attacks in the past 30 years have resulted in improvements in health productivity. The same has not been true for lung cancer. Lichtenberg analyzed the impact of new drugs on mortality with positive findings as well.

In the studies discussed, outcomes were expressed in physical units, such as years of life or age-adjusted mortality: Production functions are concepts that relate physical units of resources to physical measures of outputs. Some analysts have put a dollar value on the changes in mortality. Using results obtained from estimating the value that people put on changes in mortality from other studies, the investigators have compared the value of increased longevity with the costs of the resources. Valuations placed on changes in mortality do indicate what people are willing to pay for the increases in life spans, but they are not necessarily the same valuations that will be used for making policies, because they place a low value on the health of the poor and destitute. In addition, analysts have attached prices to individual resources, which has yielded measures of the cost of production. Behind the money cost and benefit measures that are obtained from these calculations lie the more fundamental measures of physical relationships between physical inputs and health states. That is, cost and benefit calculations are derivative from the production function.

Recently, investigators have extended the health production function by examining outcomes that are reflective of changes in health status, not only in mortality. Among the measures of health status that have been used are time spent working and health-related quality of life (HRQOL). Not all the studies have related the changes in resources during a time span (e.g., a year) with changes in health status over the same time span; some have measured a relation between the health status at the beginning, or end, of a period with the quantities of resources used during the same period. While the use of personal and medical resources during a given year can indeed have an impact on health status after (or before) the year is over, the use of the health status at the end of the period as an outcome measure is not an appropriate indicator to use in the health production function. The use of health resources will have an impact on *changes* in health status during the year or afterwards. The health status at the start of the year, in addition to how health status changes during the year, will affect the health status at the year's end. To get around this problem, investigators who use the health status at the end of the period in their studies have used the starting health status as an independent variable in their statistical analyses (e.g., Hakkinen, Jarvelin, Rosenqvist, & Laitinen, 2006; Lu, 1999).

Influence

The health production function has been widely used to conceptualize the impact of resources or changes in health states. The results of research inform, and probably influence, policy decisions. Earlier studies in this area raised skepticism about the overall effectiveness of adding more medical resources to the healthcare system. Policy makers and policy analysts were influenced by these results, and terms such as "flat of the curve medicine" became popular as descriptions of the state of use of health (and especially physician) services. More recent studies have shown that medical, pharmaceutical, and personal resources all have impacts on health status. If further studies corroborate these results, policy decisions will be influenced by this information.

Philip Jacobs

See also Cost-Effectiveness Analysis; Economics, Health Economics; Efficacy Versus Effectiveness; Efficient Frontier

Further Readings

Becker, G. (1965). The theory of the allocation of time. *Economic Journal, 299,* 493–517.

Cawley, J., Grabowski, D. C., & Hirth, R. A. (2006). Factor substitution in nursing homes. *Journal of Health Economics, 25,* 234–247.

Cutler, D. M., & McClellan, M. (2001). Is technological change in medicine worth it? *Health Affairs, 20,* 11–29.

Grossman, M. (1972). On the concept of health capital and the demand for health. *Journal of Political Economy, 80,* 233–255.

Hakkinen, U., Jarvelin, M. R., Rosenqvist, G., & Laitinen, J. (2006). Health, schooling and lifestyle among young adults in Finland. *Health Economics, 15,* 1201–1216.

Kenkel, D. S. (1995). Should you eat breakfast? Estimates from health production functions. *Health Economics, 4,* 15–29.

Lichtenberg, F. R. (2003). The economic and human impact of new drugs. *Clinical Psychiatry, 64*(Suppl. 17), 15–18.

Lu, M. (1999). The productivity of mental health care: An instrumental variable approach. *Journal of Mental Health Policy and Economics, 2,* 59–71.

Meeker, E. (1973). Allocation of resources to health revisited. *Journal of Human Resources, 8,* 257–259.

Rosen, A. B., Cutler, D. M., Norton, D. M., Hu, H. M., & Vijan, S. (2007). The value of coronary heart disease care for the elderly: 1987–2002. *Health Affairs, 26,* 111–123.

Stewart, C. T. (1972). Allocation of resources to health. *Journal of Human Resources, 6,* 103–122.

Williams, R. L. (1975). Explaining a health care paradox. *Policy Sciences, 6,* 91–101.

Woodward, R. M., Brown, M. L., Stewart, S. T., Cronin, K. A., & Cutler, D. M. (2007). The value of medical interventions for lung cancer in the elderly: Results from SEER-CMHSF. *Cancer, 110,* 2511–2518.

HEALTH RISK MANAGEMENT

Decision making is a critical element in the field of medicine that can lead to life-or-death outcomes, yet it is an element fraught with complex and conflicting variables, diagnostic and therapeutic uncertainties, patient preferences and values, and costs. Judgments and decisions made daily in clinical work necessitate the assessment and management of risks. The physician must determine what may be wrong with a patient and recommend a prevention or treatment strategy, generally under less-than-optimal circumstances and time frames. A patient decides whether or not to follow this recommendation and, once under care, may or may not faithfully pursue a recommended strategy. Health policy makers and insurers must decide what to promote, what to discourage, and what to pay for. Together, such decisions determine the quality of healthcare, quality that depends inherently on counterbalancing risks and benefits and competing objectives such as maximizing life expectancy versus optimizing quality of life, or quality of care versus economic realities.

Therefore, diagnostic reasoning and treatment decisions are a key competence of physicians and have been attracting increasing interest. Reasoning skills are imperfect in many clinical situations, and it has been found that diagnostic errors are more frequently a result of failure to properly integrate clinical data than of inaccurate data. Diagnostic experts use relatively few clinical data, with modes of reasoning sometimes oversimplified. These limitations are connected to several aspects of clinical decision making; one of these aspects is to acknowledge components of knowledge used in clinical practice.

Moreover, the literature on the reasoning process is often unfamiliar to physicians, and studies of diagnostic reasoning are often simpler than the diagnostic reasoning in real-life situations. Although studies provide information about the outcomes of decisions, they provide little or no information about the process of the decision.

How are sound treatment decisions determined? Are they based on the value of the outcome or the probability of the outcome? Are judgments and decisions based on both variables, or are the simplifying strategies employed by experts based on only one of the variables? Judgments and decisions are made daily in clinical work, where the assessment of risk is necessary. Risk is involved in the choice of tests to use in reaching a diagnosis. There is also uncertainty and risk in interpreting test results. With lab tests indicating an infection, what level of antibiotics should be used in treatment? What other factors should a doctor consider in a diagnosis and treatment?

With this uncertainty taken into consideration, how should information from clinical and biomedical knowledge be combined to reach a diagnosis? Is there an additive relationship between different sources of information, or is there a multiplicative relationship? That is, is the interpretation of risk dependent on risk in still another variable? A high temperature can be interpreted in a certain way in one context, but given another picture of symptoms, it is interpreted another way. With a diagnosis obtained with some certainty, what treatment should be chosen? In all these cases, there is risk involved for multistage decision problems.

Modeling and Risk

Mathematical modeling is used widely in economic evaluations of pharmaceuticals and other healthcare technologies. Clinical decision making may benefit from the same modeling approach, since the task of the healthcare provider is to provide care and to incorporate the probability of obtaining certain health outcomes, whether explicit or implicit; the latter varies with providers and in many cases may not be done at all. Weighting the value of an outcome by the probability of its occurrence provides both patient and provider with information about decision making.

A model based on values and beliefs provides a conceptual framework for clinical judgments and decisions; it also facilitates the integration of clinical and biomedical knowledge into a diagnostic decision. From this perspective, decision research in health has increasingly recognized evaluated value and probability of outcome in explaining judgments and decisions in various domains, seeing them as based on the product of these two parameters, termed *expected value*. This is a prescription approach, however, and is often inconsistent with how people generally make decisions.

In clinical decision making, the values are healthier outcomes in various variables. The outcome assessment variables in rheumatoid arthritis have been pain, disability, and overall health. These variables are assessed by the patient. For the

patient with a heart attack, one assessment variable could be decreased pain and normalized electrocardiography another.

The probability for a certain outcome to occur will also have to be estimated in these diagnostic and treatment decisions.

Both value and probability are usually estimated values in clinical decision making. Therefore, model assumptions and parameter estimates should be continually assessed against data, and models should be revised accordingly. Estimated values and probabilities are involved sequentially for every step in the decision-making process. However, a dichotomous decision will have to be performed to reach a diagnosis and a treatment option. Moreover, there might be many differential diagnoses to exclude and also many treatment options. The number of differential diagnoses considered, and what they are, might have an influence on the diagnosis finally selected. The availability of treatment options might also affect what treatment is chosen.

Risk and Errors

One issue is the way clinical inferences generally are arrived at in making judgments and decisions. Theories have been provided about how doctors could include relevant information to improve decision making. Nonetheless, a reasoning error could be made in clinical inference, as it is characterized by backward reasoning, where diagnosticians attempt to link observed effects to prior causes. In contrast to this post hoc explanation, statistical prediction entails forward reasoning, because it is concerned with forecasting future outcomes given observed information.

Clinical inference uses information from prior periods to make a statement about today and tends to consider error as a nuisance variable. The statistical approach, on the other hand, accepts error as inevitable and, in so doing, probably makes fewer errors in prediction for periods extending over a relatively long time. Moreover, the statistical approach uses group data to arrive at a conclusion. The situation is different in clinical inference and decision making, where group data concerning risk constitute the basis for diagnostic and treatment choices regarding the individual patient.

It has also been found that doctors exhibit interindividual as well as an intra-individual variation in judgments. One example in practical work is the outcome of clinical examinations, which may vary between doctors. Another example is the interpretation of radiological pictures, which may exhibit a variation between doctors.

Many people tend to overestimate how much they know, even about the easiest knowledge tasks. Overconfidence (i.e., greater certainty than circumstances warrant) leads to overestimating the importance of occurrences that confirm one's hypothesis. This impedes learning from environmental feedback, resulting in deleterious effects on future predictions. In many decision settings, inexperienced practitioners and even naive laboratory subjects perform as well (or as poorly) as performers with more experience. The performance of the patient could be as good or as bad as these subjects.

Daily work with patients implies considering risks at many stages of the decision process. How does one convey to patients this information about risk and error as an unavoidable condition in clinical work to reach a mutual agreement on treatment judgments and decisions? Through an awareness of errors that can be made, some errors can be counteracted. Thus, a challenge for clinical practice is to include different features of risk.

Shared Decision Making by Doctors and Patients

The application of evidence-based medicine requires combining scientific facts with value judgments and with the cost of different treatments. This procedure can be approached from the perspective of doctors or of individual patients. Doctors may not value various aspects of health the same way patients do, and studies on patient control have found that patients generally respond positively to increased information.

However, research in cognitive psychology has shown that people are quickly overwhelmed by having to consider more than a few options in making choices. Therefore, decision analysis, based on the concepts of value and risk, might be expected to facilitate clinical judgments and shared decision making by providing a quantifiable way to choose between options. Overall, likelihood of a specific adverse outcome should be one parameter affecting the estimate of future risk and its

consequences. Risk estimates of future outcomes could be based on an outcome in the future having less importance than one in the present, where the adverse outcome may have different values for doctor and patient. Another parameter is that temporal distribution of risk is not homogeneous throughout the life span of the individual. Specific individual factors modify the risk for a specific person, and person-specific modifiers are likely to be distributed differently in time.

Patients dealing with chronic illness are increasingly knowledgeable. They must make multiple and repetitive decisions, with variable outcomes, about how they will live with their chronic condition. With rheumatoid arthritis, for instance, that demands lifelong treatment, doctor and patient share not one single decision but a series of decisions concerning treatment. Furthermore, in current healthcare, several doctors may be involved in the treatment.

Risk levels are adopted in a context, and their impact on decisions may be arbitrary when the norm for decisions involving risk is being set. With an uncertainty in diagnosis, at what risk level will treatment be chosen by both the doctor and the patient? How do patients and doctors estimate different variables? Psychological factors such as personal versus general risk, where personal risk relates to oneself and general risk to others and policy approaches, may have an impact on decisions. In a clinical decision-making situation, personal risks can be assumed to relate to the patient, while the doctor has a general perception of risk.

Perhaps patients might give a higher estimation of risk, being more conservative because the outcomes of decisions are more significant for them; it is their bodies and their lives that are affected. On the other hand, it is well-known that personal risks are underestimated; people judge their own risks from adverse health behaviors as smaller than the same risks for people in general. People's opinions about personal risk are generally too optimistic, whereas the perceived risk for others is more adequate.

In a study by Ayanian and Cleary, most smokers did not view themselves as being at increased risk of heart disease or cancer. The low perceived personal risk could tentatively be explained by risk denial. It has also been found that, in individual decision making, there is a preference for the low-risk treatment. In societal choices, however, treatment of the high-risk patient groups is preferred. Social framing may therefore induce a propensity to prefer interventions that target high-risk populations. These preferences were performed by healthy individuals.

Patient Satisfaction

There is an increased awareness of patients' involvement in the clinical decision process, where patients and providers consider outcome probabilities and patient preferences. Assessing health values and beliefs may help providers understand their patients' treatment behavior and increase patients' satisfaction with services and their motivation to comply with treatment regimens.

With chronic conditions, patients are increasingly knowledgeable about their medical condition. The challenge is to balance advocacy for an active patient role with the preferences of individual patients concerning participation. Agreement between physicians and patients regarding diagnosis, diagnostic plan, and treatment plan has been associated with higher patient satisfaction and better health status outcomes in patients.

To be effective, the clinician must gain some understanding of the patient's perspective on his or her illness. Introducing decision-analytic modeling provides a more complete picture of variables that influence the decisions performed by doctor and patient and can contribute to skillful counseling around unhealthy or risky behaviors, an important aspect of the communication that should be part of healthcare visits.

Monica Ortendahl

See also Applied Decision Analysis; Errors in Clinical Reasoning; Risk-Benefit Trade-Off; Risk Communication; Shared Decision Making

Further Readings

Ades, A. E., Lu, G., & Claxton, K. (2004). Expected value of sample information calculations in medical decision modeling. *Medical Decision Making, 24,* 207–227.

Ayanian, J. Z., & Cleary, P. D. (1999). Perceived risks of heart disease and cancer among cigarette smokers. *Journal of the American Medical Association, 281,* 1019–1021.

Groves, M., O'Rourke, P., & Alexander, H. (2003). The clinical reasoning characteristics of diagnostic experts. *Medical Teacher, 25,* 308–313.

Kempainen, R. R., Migeon, M. B., & Wolf, F. M. (2003). Understanding our mistakes: A primer on errors in clinical reasoning. *Medical Teacher, 25,* 177–181.

Klayman, J., Soll, J. B., Gonzales-Vallejo, C., & Barlas, S. (1999). Overconfidence: It depends on how, what and whom you ask. *Organizational Behavior and Human Decision Processes, 79,* 216–247.

Slovic, P. (2000). *The perception of risk.* London: Earthscan.

Teutsch, C. (2003). Patient-doctor communication. *Medical Clinics of North America, 87,* 1115–1145.

Weinstein, M. C., O'Brien, B., Hornberger, J., Jackson, J., Johannesson, M., McCabe, C., et al. (2003). Principles of good practice for decision analytic modeling in health-care evaluation: Report of the ISPOR Task Force on Good Research Practices—Modeling Studies. *Value in Health, 6,* 9–17.

HEALTH STATUS MEASUREMENT, ASSESSING MEANINGFUL CHANGE

Sensitivity is the ability of an instrument to measure change in a state irrespective of whether it is relevant or meaningful to the decision maker. Responsiveness is the ability of an instrument to measure a meaningful or clinically important change in a clinical state. Responsiveness, like validity and reliability, is not necessarily a generalizable property of an instrument and should be assessed for each population and for each purpose for which it is used. *Sensitivity* and *responsiveness* can refer to assessments of groups or individuals. Responsiveness is equivalent to longitudinal construct validity, where the ability of an instrument to measure a clinically meaningful change is evaluated. Sensitivity to change is a necessary but insufficient condition for responsiveness. Some dislike using *sensitivity* because it might be confused for terms often linked to sensitivity, such as specificity, positive predictive value, and negative predictive value, used in the description of diagnostic test performance. However, health status questionnaires are analogous to diagnostic tests in that they can be used in medical decision making to determine whether an individual has a condition or disease; to screen individuals for incipient disease, disability, or risk of either; and to monitor the course of a disease or the response to treatment.

Measures of generic and disease-specific health status are sensitive to changes in clinical status when applied to groups of patients. They are as sensitive as or more sensitive than many traditional measures, such as performance tests and laboratory evaluation of disease activity. However, it is unclear whether these instruments can capture meaningful changes in subgroups or in individuals. Indeed, most instruments show that data cannot take on a value higher than some "ceiling" (ceiling effect) or lower than some "floor" (floor effect), which indicates that they cannot be used for the entire continuum of patients seen. Controlled studies evaluating the utility of providing health status data do not show that outcomes, health resource use, or costs are affected. A number of explanations are possible: (1) Physicians are not trained to interpret such data or to determine what should be done to improve function, (2) the information was not provided in a timely manner, (3) diminished function and well-being are distal end points in the chain of causation and present fewer opportunities to affect their course, or (4) measures used to assess groups of individuals are imprecise, insensitive, and unresponsive to clinically important changes.

Studies show that patients and their healthcare providers may disagree about health priorities, quality of life, functional ability, psychological state, and the importance or magnitude of the change captured by questionnaires. Patients can mean different things when they say they are "better." Response-shift or instrumentation bias, recall bias, and amnestic bias can also affect the measurement and the perception of change.

A clinically meaningful or important change can be defined and therefore evaluated from the perspective of the patient, his or her proxy, society, or the health professional. It implies a change that is noticeable, appreciably different, that is of value to the patient (or physician). This change may allow the individual to perform some essential tasks or to do them more efficiently or with less pain or difficulty. These changes also should exceed variation that can be attributed to chance.

Some investigators have defined a clinically significant change as a return to usual functioning, but this is a stringent criterion for many chronic conditions. Others have defined "clinically meaningful" as whether an individual has surpassed some absolute criterion, but this definition does not permit one to document a change that is important but is short of the absolute criterion. Roman Jaeschke and colleagues suggested that a clinically meaningful change could be defined as the minimal important difference. This could be defined as the smallest difference in score in the domain of interest that a patient perceives as a change and that would mandate, in the absence of side effects and excessive costs, modification in the patient's management. Others have advocated that the maximum improvement is more important clinically.

Methods for Evaluating Sensitivity

Statistical techniques to estimate the sensitivity of an instrument vary, and there is no apparent consensus regarding the preferred technique. Many are variants of the effect size statistic and resemble the F statistic in analysis of variance (see Table 1).

It is not clear that the methods would show the same rank order of sensitivity when different instruments are compared or whether the observed findings might have occurred by chance.

If all measures of sensitivity rank an instrument high or low relative to other instruments, then one may be relatively confident that that instrument is the most sensitive. In this case, the question of which method is best is moot because all agree. If instruments change their rank order depending on which measure of sensitivity is used, then the instruments are probably roughly equivalent. Which method is best must be determined by other means.

Methods for Evaluating Responsiveness

In contrast to the methodologic work evaluating sensitivity, the significance of these changes and the techniques for evaluating responsiveness to clinically important or meaningful change have received little attention. No one technique has been established as being superior. In fact, different methods for the assessment of responsiveness may lead to different conclusions.

One way to study "meaningfulness" is to ask the subject, the person's provider, or both

Table I   Approaches to statistical evaluation of sensitivity

Effect size

Effect size index

Guyatt's method

F ratios, comparison of

Measurement sensitivity

Receiver operator characteristics

Relative change index

Responsiveness coefficient

Standard error of measurement

Standardized response mean (relative efficiency)

(a) whether a change has occurred ("transition question"), (b) how large the change is, (c) how important or relevant the change is, and (d) how satisfied the subject is with the change. The judgment of any or all of these could be done by patients, by an external judge, or by the use of a related construct. If patients are asked about a meaningful change, the framing and timing of the questions in relation to the intervention need careful consideration, because the extent of recall bias is unknown. An external judge could be a healthcare professional uninvolved with the subject's care, or a caretaker such as a family member or significant other, when the subject may be unreliable. Related constructs, such as patient satisfaction with the change or a change that allows resumption of normal work or necessitates assistance, are also possibilities. A problem for all methods is that a change in a state (e.g., function) derives its significance and meaning to the subject or to a proxy from the starting state as much as anything else.

Researchers have generally chosen test items appropriate to the content domain (domain sampling method) for the construction of health status in an attempt to maximize overall internal reliability (Cronbach's coefficient [alpha] of tests). This strategy tends to maximize reliability at or near the center of a scale, often by having more items with an average level of difficulty than items with very great or very slight difficulty on a test. With this, a test may not discriminate equally across its whole range. Thus, a subject who is near the middle of the range may change a small amount on true ability and yet change more than 1 point on the scale score because there are many items in the region where the subject is making the change. However, a subject who is at the high or the low end of a scale, where there are fewer items, may actually make a much larger or clinically meaningful change and not have it captured on the scale or have a small change as compared with the subject who started at the center. For example, in the Health Assessment Questionnaire, a measure of physical function, a subject with severe rheumatoid arthritis may rate all tasks as being maximally difficult; and yet this subject can still worsen to the point of being confined to home or completely dependent on others. An uncritical adoption of classic psychometric techniques for scale construction to maximize overall internal reliability has led to scales that may be more responsive in group applications (clinically meaningful) at the ends of the scale but more sensitive to change (statistically) at the center of the scale.

Developing a scale where items are equally spaced in terms of difficulty across the entire range of the scale (equidiscriminating) is one focus of item response theory, of which Rasch models provide a one-dimensional approach. With an equidiscriminating scale, when a patient moves a particular number of points, one can be relatively sure that he or she has moved the same distance on some true scale of difficulty.

A problem for both types of scales is that the perception of change in a state, such as health status, derives its significance and meaning in comparison with the starting state as much as any other referent. Studies suggest that perceived change of physical and sensory states may be a power function. For instance, persons who start at a low level of function on a scale and change a relatively small distance along the dimension may perceive the change as clinically significant. However, persons who start with much higher physical function may view the same size change as a trivial improvement and would need a much larger change to judge it as clinically significant. Thus, even "equidiscriminating" scales beg the question of whether the same amount of change in an underlying dimension is clinically significant at all levels or a function of the level at which one starts. An inherent limitation in scales measuring health status is that one cannot collapse all the subtleties of change into a single linear scale. For instance, a patient with arthritis can have a change in pain and a change in mobility, but each patient may attach a different utility to these changes. Collapse of these different utilities into one scale often compromises the individual utility functions. This is important because classic domain sampling assumes a single dimension along which persons are being measured, but most health status instruments actually measure several dimensions.

Potential assays for the evaluation of what constitutes a meaningful change on an instrument might involve the measurement of states in certain clinical situations: (a) in clinical trials or cohorts where the intervention has varying effectiveness, such as the surgical and conservative management of lumbar spinal stenosis or total joint arthroplasty; (b) after an effective medication is stopped; and (c) during the washout period in crossover studies.

Kirshner and Gordon Guyatt suggested an examination of the response of patients to a treatment of known efficacy and a comparison of the responses of patients who had and had not responded by the physician's judgment. Mark Lipsey recognized the logistical difficulties in this. He suggested identifying a group whose average response would be approximately the same as the desired detectable

change and administering the instrument just once to estimate the change in variance.

No single standard exists for the evaluation of responsiveness. The point of view from which responsiveness is being evaluated should be specified. Patients' judgments are influenced by their baseline health status, expectations and goals, illness duration, and actual need to perform some functions, as well as other factors. These judgments vary as compared with results of standardized measures of function. The physician's judgment usually includes knowledge of other patients with the same problem, knowledge of what domains are potentially treatable, and an appreciation for the significance of physiological (e.g., creatinine clearance) or physical findings that may not be symptomatic or apparent to the patient. Proxies, such as caretakers or significant others, may be preferred when the respondent or patient's status may not be reliably or validly reported. For measures of function and quality of life, responsiveness should be based on the subject's valuation of the magnitude and its importance. For measures of impairment or disease activity, the physician is the best judge.

Allen J. Lehman and Matthew H. Liang

See also Health Outcomes Assessment; Health Status Measurement, Floor and Ceiling Effects; Health Status Measurement, Minimal Clinically Significant Differences, and Anchor Versus Distribution Methods; Health Status Measurement, Responsiveness and Sensitivity to Change

Further Readings

Beaton, D. E., Tarasuk, V., Katz, J. N., Wright, J. G., & Bombardier, C. (2001). "Are you better?" A qualitative study of the meaning of recovery. *Arthritis Care and Research, 45,* 270–279.

Daltroy, L. H., Larson, M. G., Eaton, H. M., Phillips, C. B., & Liang, M. H. (1999). Discrepancies between self-reported and observed physical function in the elderly. *Social Sciences and Medicine, 48,* 1549–1561.

Fitzpatrick, R., Ziebland, S., Jenkinson, C., Mowat, A., & Mowat, A. (1993). Transition questions to assess outcomes in rheumatoid arthritis. *British Journal of Rheumatology, 32,* 807–811.

Hollon, S. D., & Flick, S. N. (1988). On the meaning and methods of clinical significance. *Behavioral Assessment, 10,* 197–206.

Kirshner, B., & Guyatt, G. (1985). A methodological framework for assessing health indices. *Journal of Chronic Disease, 38,* 27–36.

Liang, M. H., Larson, M. G., Cullen, K. E., & Schwartz, J. A. (1985). Comparative measurement efficiency and sensitivity of five health status instruments for arthritis research. *Arthritis and Rheumatism, 28,* 542–547.

Liang, M. H., Lew, R. A., Stucki, G., Fortin, P. R., & Daltroy, L. H. (2002). Measuring clinically important changes with patient-oriented questionnaires. *Medical Care, 40,* II45–II51.

Lipsey, M. W. (1993). A scheme for assessing measurement sensitivity in program evaluation and other applied research. *Psychological Bulletin, 94,* 152–165.

Redelmeier, D. A., & Lorig, K. (1993). Assessing the clinical importance of symptomatic improvements: An illustration in rheumatology. *Archives of Internal Medicine, 153,* 1337–1342.

HEALTH STATUS MEASUREMENT, CONSTRUCT VALIDITY

Just as it is important to ascertain that a measurement instrument produces reliable results across different situations, it is crucial to assess whether it measures what it is intended to measure—its validity. In the area of health status measurement, construct validation of measurement instruments underlies sound medical decision making. Validity is established through a process involving a series of experiments designed to test various relevant hypotheses about the structure and nature of the construct and its logical manifestations. The results of these experiments inform the level of confidence with which researchers make conclusions about the persons under study and the interpretation of instrument scores.

Early measurement of health focused heavily on disease and mortality rates for populations and on clinical variables representing disease activity for individuals. Over time, with the mounting challenges presented by chronic diseases and disorders, many health interventions have focused more on levels of physical, mental, and social functioning than on length of life. Under these circumstances, sound medical decision making about the value of healthcare interventions depends increasingly on the validity of instruments for measuring health status. The impact of validity on interpretation of clinical trials has been demonstrated empirically in psychiatry, with evidence that clinical trials using unvalidated measurement instruments were more likely to report treatment effectiveness than those employing validated measures. This entry describes the specific challenges involved in assessing the construct validity of health status measures, addresses the evolving conceptual framework for validity and associated taxonomy, explains the main approaches used, and provides additional resources for more in-depth discussion of theory and methods.

Challenges in Validation of Health Status

As compared with the measurement of physical attributes such as height and weight, the measurement of health status comes with special challenges because it is not a directly observable quantity but a construct; a variable that must be defined to be measured. The definition of the construct may originate from theory, clinical or empirical observation, or a combination of the two. Essentially a construct is itself a theory about what makes up the construct and how its component parts relate. Based on the definition, instrument developers decide what attitudes, behaviors, or characteristics would be the best indicators of the construct. For example, it is widely accepted that health status is a multidimensional construct that includes at least physical status, emotional or mental status, and symptoms. Potential indicators can be observable manifestations of the construct, such as behaviors, or they can be attitudes. Measurement may be conducted by observation of behaviors through performance tests or by eliciting subjects' reports of their behaviors. The measurement of attitudes requires posing questions that represent the attitude in question. For many constructs, including health status, self-report is the preferred approach to measurement; therefore, questions are used to tap aspects of each of the dimensions of health status, and responses are provided to allow numerical description or scaling. In the case of physical status, developers ask themselves, "What behaviors would represent a lot of (or little) physical function?" An ideal measurement instrument would cover the full range of relevant functional activities, with a sufficient number of increments in response categories to measure differences across the functional continuum.

Because there is no gold standard for the definition or measurement of health status, there is not one definitive test for the construct validity of a health status measure. Rather, construct validation is a process of accumulating evidence from empirical tests of hypotheses. These hypotheses rest fundamentally on the definition of the construct, the structure and relationships of its components, and relationships to other relevant concepts. There are many hypotheses that can be constructed about the structure or behavior of a construct; therefore, the validation process is incremental, requiring evidence from various studies to provide a reasonable level of confidence about the validity of conclusions made using the instrument. On the other hand, one sound negative validation study can put the validity of the construct in question. Using a hypothetical physical function scale *X* as an example, we might hypothesize that physical function would decline with increased health problems and test the correlation between scores on Scale *X* and those of a previously validated index of comorbid health problems. If a meaningful association between the two measures could not be demonstrated, this would be considered a negative study. Under these circumstances, the validity of physical function as a construct would be questioned, and the definition and theory underlying it would be reassessed. However, interpretation of construct validation studies is complicated by the fact that these empirical tests examine the validity of the construct *and* the validity of the measure itself in the application under study. In this example, perhaps physical function was a valid construct, but the instrument did not adequately represent it. Therefore, a negative study may mean that (1) the construct is not valid, (2) the construct is valid but the instrument is inadequate to measure it under the circumstances, or (3) both.

Validity and the Three Cs: Content, Criterion, and Construct Validity

The literature on validity contains references to many types of validity, which can cause confusion about the fundamental concepts involved. Historically, validity was often viewed as a characteristic of the measurement instrument, having three separate components: content, criterion, and construct validity. Criterion and construct validity have been further divided into several categories, with various naming conventions depending on study designs employed. *Content validity* addresses the degree to which the questions included in the instrument sample the full range of the attribute of interest. For example, for physical function, one would ask whether the instrument of interest provides questions at the lowest level of function and at the highest possible level, with adequate sampling in between. *Criterion validity* refers to the process of validation when there is a gold standard against which the instrument of interest can be compared. In contrast, *construct validity* refers to when there is no gold standard, and the measured variable is a construct. Finally, *face validity* is a term readers may find in validity studies, which refers to whether the instrument measures what it is meant to measure "on the face of it." Face validity can be placed within the realm of content validity. It usually signifies that researchers or instrument developers elicited the opinion of experts in the field on whether the instrument represents key components of the construct of interest.

More recently, there has been a shift toward viewing validity in terms of the inferences to be made from the data produced by an instrument. Ultimately, the goal of construct validation is to establish the level of confidence with which inferences can be made using the instrument. Therefore, the purpose of the application must be considered in developing hypotheses for testing validity. It is common for instruments to be applied for different purposes than those for which they were originally intended, and the evidence for the validity of inferences made for novel applications must be assessed.

Approaches to Assessing Construct Validity

Extreme Groups

One approach to assessing the construct validity of an instrument is to test it on two groups chosen for their divergent characteristics relative to the construct. This can be called *extreme groups, known groups,* or *discriminative validity testing.* In the case of health status measures, one group would be chosen for its low level of health relative to a second group. The research question would be whether the scores for each group were different, indicating that the measure could discriminate between the two groups. A range of indicators can be used to define the two groups, such as the presence of a particular diagnosis, number of comorbidities, or level of healthcare utilization. It is worth emphasizing that a negative study may mean that (a) the construct is not valid, (b) the instrument is not valid applied under these circumstances, or (c) both. These possibilities underline the need to consider the validity of inferences from an instrument relative to the range of evidence in support of its use for a particular purpose.

Convergent Validity

Hypotheses are developed to test whether the instrument of interest correlates with other measures of the same construct. For example, in assessing the validity of a generic health index for cost-utility analysis in spine disorders, a study was conducted to test correlations between several of the most widely used instruments for this purpose, finding correlations ranging from .57 to .72. In this case, the research hypothesis was that the instrument of interest would demonstrate a positive correlation with other instruments designed for the same general purpose. Do correlations from .57 to .72 support the validity of inferences made for medical decision making using these instruments among persons with spinal disorders? It is important to consider and explicitly address the acceptable range of correlation necessary to support validity when designing construct validation studies. The possible range of correlation coefficients is from −1, indicating perfect inverse relationship, through 1, indicating perfect positive relationship and includes 0, which indicates no association. Due to the existence of measurement error, the coefficient estimate must be less than 1. Furthermore, when correlating two measurement instruments, the maximum value for the correlation coefficient is given by the square root of the product of their reliabilities. In other words, the maximal correlation between two measurement instruments is likely to be meaningfully lower than 1.0. For example, for two instrument reliabilities of .88 and .90, the maximum correlation possible

between them would be .89. For instruments designed for the same general purpose, such as health indexes for cost-utility analyses, differences in construct definition or conceptual frameworks underpinning the design would contribute to diminution of correlation from this maximal value. With this in mind, the correlations noted above between health indexes could be considered moderate to strong evidence of construct validity. In the case of testing a new instrument, extremely high correlations may be evidence of redundancy and require revisiting the rationale for the creation of a new instrument. Under these circumstances, the new instrument should provide important practical advancements or meaningful improvements in face or content validity.

Experiments are also conducted to assess correlations of the instrument of interest with measures of other related constructs. For example, it may be hypothesized that a generic health index applied among persons with spine disorders would correlate with a disease-specific disability index. Both of these approaches are called convergent validity, and in practice, multiple measures are used for comparison. Depending on the construct used for comparison, the degree of correlation expected will vary.

Discriminant Validity

To be a valid measure of health status, a new instrument not only should correlate with measures of similar and related constructs, but should not correlate with unrelated variables. Investigators ask, "What variables or constructs should not be correlated with the measure in question?" and design experiments to assess the relationship between the instrument and a seemingly unrelated variable. An unanticipated association may guide instrument developers to areas of potential improvement in the instrument.

Assessing the Internal Structure of the Construct

Assessing the internal structure of an instrument in relation to the theoretical framework for the construct can make important contributions to evidence for construct validity. Factor analysis is a key analytic tool that is used to describe the relationships between questions or items in an instrument. For example, factor analysis can be used to test whether a health status measure designed to represent five dimensions of health (e.g., physical function, symptoms, mental health, self-care, and usual activities) actually represents five separate dimensions. If the questions within the instrument are found to aggregate in three major groupings, this would call into question the five-dimension definition of the construct. Alternatively, for measurement instruments designed to tap only one dimension, factor analysis can be used to confirm that only one dimension is included in the construct.

Christine M. McDonough

See also Health Outcomes Assessment; Health Status Measurement, Floor and Ceiling Effects; Health Status Measurement, Generic Versus Condition-Specific Measures; Health Status Measurement, Minimal Clinically Significant Differences, and Anchor Versus Distribution Methods; Health Status Measurement, Reliability and Internal Consistency; Health Status Measurement, Responsiveness and Sensitivity to Change; Health Status Measurement Standards

Further Readings

Aday, L. A., & Cornelius, L. J. (2006). *Designing and conducting health surveys* (3rd ed.). San Francisco: Jossey-Bass.

American Psychological Association. (1985). *Standards for educational and psychological testing.* Washington, DC: Author.

Bowling, A. (1997). *Measuring health: A review of quality of life measurement scales* (2nd ed.). Philadelphia: Open University Press.

Cronbach, L. J., & Meehl, P. E. (1955). Construct validity in psychological tests. *Psychological Bulletin, 52,* 281–302.

Health Outcomes Methodology Symposium Proceedings. (2000). *Medical Care, 2000, 38*(9 Suppl. II).

McDowell, I. (2006). *Measuring health: A guide to rating scales and questionnaires* (3rd ed.). New York: Oxford University Press.

Nunnally, J. C. (1978). *Psychometric theory* (2nd ed.). New York: McGraw-Hill.

Streiner, D. L., & Norman, G. R. (2003). *Health measurement scales.* New York: Oxford University Press.

HEALTH STATUS MEASUREMENT, FACE AND CONTENT VALIDITY

Health status measurement is a fundamental part of healthcare disciplines, for example, medicine, nursing, and clinical psychology. Health status refers to the perceptions of a person with respect to his or her health condition. Measuring health status is really a process in which a systematic and standardized attempt is made to observe an often complex clinical phenomenon. Health status measurement instruments are essential for this purpose. Instruments of health status measurement predominantly focus on overall well-being, functional status, symptom status, disease burden, health-related quality of life, psychological well-being, or satisfaction with care. Health status measurement has a significant impact on medical decision making. It provides important data and a platform for clinicians to monitor health conditions, predict clinical outcomes, assess the burden of a disease condition, and evaluate treatment effects. All health status measurements, from clinician-rated to patient-reported outcomes, should require convincing evidence that the clinical judgments or inferences drawn from scores on measurement instruments are valid and clinically useful.

Face and content validity are part of instrument development and validation, which provides theoretical support and some sorts of evidence about the validity of a health status measurement. *Content validity* refers to the degree to which the content and structural format of a health status measurement instrument are relevant to and representative of the intended construct (an abstract or a general idea, e.g., health-related quality of life) for particular characteristics of the client and purposes of the measurement. *Face validity* is a component of content validity that provides an additional attribute of the health status measurement instrument. It pertains to whether the content domains or items in a scale and their relation to the measurement purpose look valid to target respondents. Ensuring face validity is a minimum prerequisite for acceptance of a health status measurement instrument for target respondents.

Significance in Validity

The term *validity* refers to the degree to which a test or a measurement instrument measures what it purports to measure. *Test validity* encompasses reliability, validity, sensitivity, and responsiveness to change, which are interrelated and mutually inclusive to contribute to different aspects of evidence of the validity of a measurement instrument. Such lines of evidence include numerical analysis of internal structure of the instrument by correlating scores among items and with external criteria (other established instruments).

Face and content validity comprises a category of validity. The concept of face and content validity was first introduced into the literature of educational and psychological testing in the early 1940s. Face and content validity involves not only a qualitative process but also a numerical analysis to ensure that the measurement instrument as a whole has enough items and adequately covers the domain of content as well as having suitable structural format in the earliest stage of instrument development and validation. David Streiner and Geoffrey Norman, in 2003, pointed out the importance of face and content validity in measuring validity, in which the higher the content validity of an instrument, the broader are the inferences that can validly be drawn about the client under a variety of conditions and in different situations. Face and content validity is a fundamental requirement of all health status measurement instruments and is a prerequisite for establishing other types of validity. This initial stage of instrument development and validation is the most crucial, and no amount of psychometric analyses can transform an ill-conceived instrument into a good one.

Aspects of Face and Content Validity

There are several aspects of face and content validity: content domains, structural format, and target population. A content domain comprises the definition and dimension of the measurement of construct as well as the content items that are specific to the characteristics of the client and purposes of the measurement. The structural format includes the instructions to respondents, item wording, item format (question vs. statement) and item response form (ordinal vs. interval scale), temporal parameters of responses (timed vs. untimed), item weighting (equal vs. different weight in contributing to the total score), and scoring methods (summative score vs. transforming the raw score). *Target population* refers to the population for whom the instrument is to be applicable or to the patients who have a particular health condition or illness. All these aspects can affect the degree to which the observed data tap into the intended construct and the interpretation of the observed scores. Most important, they can influence the clinical judgments or inferences drawn from scores on the instrument and, thus, medical decisions.

Methods

Content validation occurs throughout the development of a health status measurement instrument. The ultimate goal of content validation is to maximize item coverage and relevancy so as to ensure that the health status measurement instrument comprises items that are relevant to and representative of the intended construct for the particular characteristics of the client and purposes of the measurement. It should be borne in mind that the content domains and items generated in content validation may change after other types of validity testing.

Item Coverage

Content coverage refers to the degree to which the content is adequate and representative for the intended construct and the purpose of the measurement. The extent of item coverage is not amenable to exploration by numerical analysis. It depends largely on the process of item generation. Subject-matter expert (e.g., clinician's) judgment, the patient-as-expert method, clinical observation, theoretical modeling, and literature review are the most commonly used approaches to item generation. Expert judgment is formed on the basis of a clinician's years of experience in the subject area. Clinicians who have extensive experience with the subject matter can explain the health status of particular salience to the intended construct from their perspective. The patient-as-expert method fulfills a basic requirement of patient-reported outcome instruments (e.g., condition-specific health-related quality-of-life instruments), in which the content should be generated from relevant patients. Patients can articulate what they feel and can explain the areas of salience and concern associated with their health conditions. Clinical observation in a systematic manner helps suggest items. Theoretical modeling provides a conceptual foundation underlying the development of a measurement instrument and helps inform the hypothesized dimensions of the measurement construct so as to guide the development of the content domain. A review of published literature (subject-area research and previous measurement instruments) provides additional items to avoid possible omission of items that could be clinically significant. These methods are not mutually exclusive but depend on the nature of measurement instruments.

Exploratory in-depth qualitative interviews and focus group discussions with subject-matter experts and patients suffering from the illness and/or their families are the most efficient techniques to generate items. There are no hard rules governing the use of expert judgments and the patient-as-expert method, such as how many experts or patients to use, or how to handle differences among the experts or patients. The criterion often used in qualitative interviews is *sampling to redundancy*; that is, interviewing people until the point at which no new significant themes emerge. Normally, two or three focus groups with 6 to 12 informants and a facilitator in each group are needed. It should be borne in mind that the informants should represent the full diversity of subject-matter experts and patients with illness to minimize bias elicited from underrepresented or overrepresented samples.

Item writing and structural format planning are essential to content validation, which should include input from subject-matter experts, linguistic experts, and psychometricians. The characteristics of the target population, including age and reading comprehension level, are the major considerations in self-reported instruments. Focus group discussion with members of the target population can be used to assess the face validity of the instrument. In focus groups, participants can comment on the clarity, understandability, and appropriateness of all instructions and content items and check on the most appropriate wording.

Item Relevancy

Content relevance refers to the congruence between the measurement content and the purpose of the measurement. All the items that are included should be relevant to the construct being measured, and any irrelevant items should be excluded. Items that are not related to the construct could introduce errors in the measurement. A health status measurement instrument aiming to assess sore mouth, for example, should include items relating to all relevant issues associated with sore mouth, such as mouth pain and difficulty in eating. Irrelevant items, such as headache, should be excluded. Otherwise the instrument would discriminate among the patients on some dimension (headache) other than the one purportedly tapped by the instrument (sore mouth), and this has implications for medical decision making.

Item relevance is commonly approached by using several reviewers to critically evaluate whether individual items and the entire instrument are relevant to the construct being measured. Irrelevant, redundant, and ambiguous items should be excluded. Reviewers also comment on other aspects of content validity (e.g., item formats and response forms, item weighting, and scoring). Reviewers should be chosen to include subject-matter experts, psychometricians, and the target population (e.g., patients). A minimum of five reviewers are needed to provide a sufficient level of control of error variance resulting from chance agreement. The underlying measurement construct and the general goal for measurement should be provided to the reviewers. This information allows the reviewers to have the necessary theoretical background to provide a comprehensive review of the construct and to determine whether the proposed format and wording yield the appropriate level of validity. The interrater agreement (IR) and content validity index (CVI) are commonly used to check the relevancy of items by the degree of agreement among the reviewers in evaluations of the measurement content. IR and CVI calculations should apply to both individual items and the entire instrument. CVI is derived from the rating of the content relevance of the items on an instrument using a 4-point ordinal rating scale: 1, *not relevant*; 2, *somewhat relevant*; 3, *relevant*; and 4, *very relevant*. The actual CVI is the proportion of items rated 3 or 4 by the reviewers. IR is computed by adding the number of agreements among the reviewers (all items rated 1 or 2 by all reviewers, plus all items rated 3 or 4 by all reviewers) and dividing by the total number of items.

Alternatively, the entire instrument can be administered to a group from the target population as a pretest. All the participants are then interviewed to determine whether they find the items to be relevant and important.

Karis K. F. Cheng

See also Health Status Measurement, Construct Validity; Health Status Measurement, Reliability and Internal Consistency; Health Status Measurement Standards

Further Readings

Burns, W. C. (1996). *Content validity, face validity, and quantitative face validity*. Retrieved January 20, 2009, from http://www/burns.com/wcbcontval.htm

Davis, L. L. (1992). Instrument review: Getting the most from a panel of experts. *Applied Nursing Research, 5,* 194–197.

Fayers, P. M., & Machin, D. (2001). *Quality of life: Assessment, analysis and interpretation*. New York: Wiley.

Haynes, S. N., Richard, D. C. S., & Kubany, E. S. (1995). Content validity in psychological assessment: A functional approach to concepts and methods. *Psychological Assessment, 7,* 238–247.

Lynn, M. R. (1986). Determination and quantification of content validity. *Nursing Research, 35*(6), 382–385.

Nunnally, J. C., & Bernstein, I. H. (1994). *Psychometric theory* (4th ed.). New York: McGraw-Hill.

Sireci, S. G. (1988). The construct of content validity. *Social Indicators Research, 45,* 83–117.

Streiner, D. L., & Norman, G. R. (2003). *Health measurement scales: A practical guide to their development and use* (2nd ed.). Oxford, UK: Oxford University Press.

Vogt, D. S., King, D. W., & King, L. A. (2004). Focus groups in psychological assessment: Enhancing content validity by consulting members of the target population. *Psychological Assessment, 16,* 2231–2243.

HEALTH STATUS MEASUREMENT, FLOOR AND CEILING EFFECTS

Floor and ceiling effects refer to specific limitations encountered when measuring health status scores. Floor effects occur when data cannot take on a value lower than some particular number; ceiling effects occur when data cannot take on a value higher than an upper limit. Health status instruments or surveys that are used to assess domains or attributes of health status use a rating scale. This is commonly a Likert scale with rating scales between 1 and 10, for example. There are limitations to the use of such instruments when measuring health status for either evaluative or discriminative purposes. An awareness of these limitations is important because of the problems that can occur in the interpretation of the results obtained when measuring health status, regardless of the domain being measured or the instrument that is being used. In interventional clinical trials, the degree to which health status changes is an important outcome; and the results of a study can be affected by floor and ceiling effects. In cost-effectiveness evaluations, the denominator of the ratio reported could be higher or lower than anticipated if there is a floor or ceiling effect. Therefore, recognizing ceiling and floor effects, and doing the best to minimize or eliminate these limitations, is important for studies that affect medical decision making. This entry further defines floor and ceiling effects, discusses how these effects are typically detected and potentially accounted for, provides examples of ways researchers try to minimize these scaling effects, and discusses the implications of floor and ceiling effects on randomized clinical trials and policy decisions. Finally, newer psychometric methods that are emerging to minimize such effects are briefly discussed.

Definitions

A ceiling effect occurs when the majority of scores are at or near the maximum possible score for the variable that the health status survey instrument is measuring. The survey instrument cannot measure scores above its ceiling. If a high percentage of people score at the top of a scale, it is impossible to detect an improvement in health for that group. Measures of activities of daily living (ADL) often have ceiling or floor effects in certain populations. For example, some individuals with specific chronic diseases such as stroke may exhibit high ceiling effects on more general surveys of health status, thus limiting the ability to distinguish certain aspects of health status between individuals scoring at the ceiling. Ceiling effects are particularly important limitations when researchers are looking for the impact of treatment interventions on changes in health status. A floor effect occurs when the majority of scores are at or near the minimum possible score for the variable that the health status survey instrument is measuring. If a high percentage of people score at the bottom of a scale, it is impossible to detect a decline in health for that group. In clinical trials, for example, floor effects occur when outcomes are poor in the treatment and control conditions.

There are numerous health status measurement survey instruments that are generally divided into generic and disease-specific measures. Common examples of generic health status questionnaires for individuals with chronic diseases include several iterations of the Medical Outcomes Study survey and the EuroQol (EQ-5D). Some examples of disease-specific health status questionnaires include the Chronic Heart Failure Questionnaire (CHQ) and the Peripheral Artery Questionnaire.

Effects can vary by instrument. For example, comparative examinations of the SF-6D and EQ-5D across seven patient/population groups (chronic obstructive airways disease, osteoarthritis, irritable bowel syndrome, lower back pain, leg ulcers, postmenopausal women, and the elderly) revealed evidence of floor effects in the SF-6D and ceiling effects in the EQ-5D. This suggested that the SF-6D tended to discriminate better at higher levels of function and had heavy floor effects, while the EQ-5D performed in the opposite manner—it did well at lower levels of function, but had high ceiling effects. The choice of an instrument depends on what one wishes to measure. If the population has considerable morbidity, the EQ-5D may be a better choice. For a generally healthy population, the SF-6D may be the better choice. Another illustrative example is that of the problems encountered in the Veterans Health Study that used the MOS-VA. The VA had to extend the MOS SF-12/36 to include some instrumental activities of daily living (IADL)/ADL type times because of floor effects that occurred with the standard MOS. The pervasiveness of ceiling and floor effects has prompted the quest for a more appropriate approach to health status questions to accurately assess the health status of individuals and populations.

Detecting Ceiling and Floor Effects

Traditionally, classical test theory (CTT), a type of psychometric theory that analyzes measurement responses to questionnaires, has been used to evaluate the psychometric properties of health. Determining if a floor or ceiling effect exists requires an examination of the acceptability of the distribution of scores for the health domains obtained from the health status instrument. Measures of central tendency of the data, including mean and median, as well as the range, standard deviation, and skewness are used for such purposes. A score would generally be considered acceptable if the values are distributed in a normal or bell-shaped curve, with the mean near the midpoint of the scale. Floor effects can be determined by examining the proportion of subjects with the lowest possible scores. Similarly, ceiling effects are calculated by determining the proportion of subjects who achieved the highest possible score. Criteria for defining floor and ceiling effects are controversial. Some recommend a skewness statistic between −1 and +1 as acceptable for eliminating the possibility of a floor or ceiling effect.

Dealing with scales where the distribution is skewed, that is, where there is a ceiling or floor effect, is most problematic when comparing groups, as many statistical procedures rely on scores being evenly distributed. Making comparisons between groups in a clinical trial, or testing the effect of an intervention, may require additional advanced statistical techniques to adjust or account for the skewness of the data.

Minimizing Ceiling and Floor Effects

There are considerable conceptual and methodological challenges that confront users of health status instruments. Some individuals believe that ceiling and floor effects can be managed with statistical techniques. Others believe that these effects can be avoided or minimized by using disease-specific health surveys. Other options are to begin with a generic survey and use the disease-specific survey only if a ceiling or floor effect is observed. Still others believe that valuable information about the quality of life for individuals can be obtained by using both types of surveys.

Implications in Clinical Trials

Increasingly, researchers believe that measures of health status should be included in clinical trials. Historically, clinical research has focused on laboratory outcomes such as blood pressure, cholesterol, HgbA1C, morbidity, and/or mortality. These have been the outcomes measures of greatest interest to researchers, clinicians, and patients.

It is now necessary to employ health status measures to obtain a comprehensive assessment of practical health outcomes for individuals enrolled in clinical trials. The selection of the survey depends on the objectives of the evaluation, the targeted disease and population, and psychometric characteristics. Many of the disease-specific health status measures are sensitive to the occurrence of clinical symptoms or relatively small differences between treatment interventions—in particular, those studies examining the effect of medications—thus reducing the possibility of ceiling effects. Detecting worsening health among people who are already ill presents a different challenge. Low baseline scores make it difficult to detect health status decline, arguing again for disease-specific measures to avoid floor effects. In general, if one encounters a floor or ceiling effect in a study using a general health status measure, then a disease-specific measure, which is purposefully designed to be responsive to disease progression and/or treatment responsiveness issues, should be administered as well.

Disease-specific measures are believed to be more sensitive to treatment effects; however, a number of generic health status measurement scales have demonstrated the ability to discriminate between groups and clinical responsiveness. Thus, while many argue for the exclusive use of disease- and domain-specific measures for different disease conditions, the general recommended approach in randomized clinical trials of new medical therapies is to incorporate both generic and specific instruments to comprehensively assess health status. It may be worthwhile to pilot measures in the type of population to be studied, thus establishing that the measures adequately represent the health of the population before using them to establish the effectiveness of interventions. There is general agreement on the need for more comprehensive measures with multiple domains and multiple items to detect subtle changes in both healthy and severely ill populations.

Policy Implications

Because health status measures can provide comparisons across conditions and populations, they are of interest to policy and decision makers. Such information has the potential to improve the quality of care and establish reasonable reimbursement practices.

These measures are also of interest to clinicians because they help to determine the impact of therapeutic interventions and quality of life in their particular patient populations. Health status measures may provide clinicians with information not otherwise obtained from patient histories. Surveys can be self-administered, scanned, and used to provide rapid feedback of health status data—a phenomenon already occurring in many parts of the United States.

However, these measures must also be interpretable by policy and decision makers, and challenges exist in ensuring that decision and policy makers and clinicians understand these more complex scaling issues with health status measures. Without a full understanding of the concepts and methods, results could impart an incorrect message to a clinician or policy maker and ultimately discourage continued use of the measure. Strategies to make scores interpretable have been described. For an evaluative instrument, one might classify patients into those who experienced an important improvement, such as change in mobility, and those who did not and examine the changes in scores in the two groups. Data suggest that small, medium, and large effects correspond to changes of approximately 0.5, 1.0, and greater than 1.0 per question for instruments that present response options on 7-point scales.

Item Response Theory

CTT remains the dominant theory of measuring health status by researchers and clinicians. However, in the field of psychometrics, CTT is becoming outdated and replaced by more sophisticated, complex models. Item response theory (IRT) potentially provides information that enables a researcher to improve the reliability of an assessment beyond that obtained with CTT. Although both theories have the same aims, IRT is considered to be stronger in its ability to reliably assess health status. IRT allows scaling of the level of difficulty of any item in a domain (e.g., physical function). Thus, theoretically, an item bank could have hundreds or thousands of survey questions covering a huge range of capabilities in a domain. Computerized adaptive testing (CAT) is a way of iteratively homing in on a person's level of ability in a particular domain by selectively asking questions across the broad domain and narrowing the estimate of ability by selecting new items to ask the person based on his or her responses to previous items. For example, if a person has told you that he or she can run a mile, there is no need to ask if he or she can walk one block. CAT could potentially eliminate floor and ceiling effects by having an item bank so broad that all meaningful levels of ability are covered.

However, the newer models are complex and spreading slowly in mainstream research. It is reasonable to assume that IRT will gradually overtake CTT, but CTT will likely remain the theory of choice for many researchers, clinicians, and decision makers until certain complexity issues associated with IRT can be resolved.

Barbara A. Bartman

See also Decision Making in Advanced Disease; Decisions Faced by Nongovernment Payers of Healthcare: Managed Care; EuroQoL (EQ-5D); Government Perspective, Informed Policy Choice; Health Outcomes Assessment; Health Status Measurement, Generic Versus Condition-Specific Measures; Health Status Measurement, Minimal Clinically Significant Differences, and Anchor Versus Distribution Methods; Health Status Measurement Standards; Measures of Central Tendency; Outcomes Research; Randomized Clinical Trials; Scaling; SF-6D; SF-36 and SF12 Health Surveys

Further Readings

Brazier, J., Roberts, J., Tsuchiya, A., & Busschbach, J. (2004). A comparison of the EQ-5D and SF-6D across seven patient groups. *Health Economics, 13*(9), 873–884.

Guyatt, G. H., Feeny, D. H., & Patrick, D. L. (1993). Measuring health-related quality of life, *Annals of Internal Medicine, 118,* 622–629.

Kazis, L. E., Miller, D. R., Clark, J. A., Skinner, K. M., Lee, A., Ren, X. S., et al. (2004). Improving the response choices on the veterans SF-36 health survey role functioning scales: Results from the Veterans Health Study. *Journal of Ambulatory Care Management, 27*(3), 263–280.

Kind, P. (2005). *EQ-5D concepts and methods: A developmental history.* New York: Springer.

McDowell, I. (2006). *Measuring health: A guide to rating scales and questionnaires.* Oxford, UK: Oxford University Press.

Mesbath, M. (2002). *Statistical methods for quality of life studies: Design, measurements, and analysis.* New York: Springer.

HEALTH STATUS MEASUREMENT, GENERIC VERSUS CONDITION-SPECIFIC MEASURES

Many measures of health status have been developed in the past decade for describing health outcomes and quantifying the changes. The term *health status measure* is often used interchangeably with other terms such as *health measure, health-related quality of life,* or *quality-of-life measure* even though the scope and definition of each term might not be the same. *Health status measurement* is defined as an instrument used to describe an individual's health state as defined by the descriptive system developed for each instrument.

Health status measurement can be classified into two main categories: generic measure and condition-specific measure. A generic measure is designed for use across a wide range of conditions, treatments, and populations. It is applicable to different subgroups in the general population or patient groups with various conditions or interventions. In contrast, a condition-specific measure is designed for measuring outcomes affected by a given condition only, for instance, lung cancer or arthritis. A condition-specific measure is tailor-made and is not supposed to be used for other conditions/diseases or the general population. A generic measure is designed to be applicable to any population; thus, it allows for meaningful comparisons between healthcare programs or interventions even if the involved patients or treatments may be different. In general, a generic measure has a descriptive system covering common domains of health so as to be relevant to everyone. Such core domain design, however, might be inappropriate or insensitive for some specific conditions. On the other hand, a condition-specific measure is more sensitive to the degree of severity of condition and change over time, since the measure can focus on the most important domains affected by the condition. It can also include domains that are relevant to the condition but that are often missed by generic measures so that the relevant consequences of the condition can be captured. However, the condition-specific measure, which focuses on domains of interest or importance affected by the condition, does not allow comparison between different conditions.

For any measurement, there are two principle elements—the description and valuation. In a health status measure, the description is based on establishing a nominal descriptive system with which the defined health may be expressed in terms of key domains of interest. In other words, the descriptive system comprising chosen domains reflects the health definition adopted by the instrument developers. There exist discrepancies between measures in terms of their health domains of interest, and, as a consequence, the descriptive system varies among measures. For instance, some measures have taken a broader approach toward health, including the aspect of participation in society as one of the health domains even though it is arguable that social activities or role performance are not matters of health, per se. Others have chosen the "within skin" approach, focusing on impairment or inability of the individual only. A health status measure in which health itself is expressed as the domain of interest is also called a *multi-attribute health status measure*. Again, the definition of health varies from one measure to another and it should be borne in mind that there is no single measure with a descriptive system that captures all aspects of health.

Another key component for measurement is valuation. To perform valuation is to determine a set of weights associated with elements of a descriptive system. Thus, with this set of weights (commonly known as the scoring system for an instrument), scores can be calculated for domains or health states defined by the descriptive system. Various methods exist for eliciting weights, such as category scaling, visual analogue scale (VAS), time trade-off (TTO), standard gamble (SG), and paired comparison. Different eliciting methods generate different values. For instance, the VAS value of a given health state is generally lower than the TTO score of the same state. In most measures of health status, however, all items score equally, with equal weight for each response level in an item and with all items of equal importance.

Generic Measure

Generic measures can be further divided into two categories: one is the preference-based measure, also known as the index-based measure, and the other is the profile measure, also known as the non-preference-based measure. A preference-based measure offers a single summary numerical score for each health state defined by the instrument. This form of presenting a health outcome is particularly useful in economic evaluation, where a single index of health-related quality of life that summarizes health status utilities is needed. This is unlike a profile-based measure, which describes a health outcome by several different domains/dimensions in such a way that it is presented as a profile with several scores.

Preference-Based Measure

Due to the growth of economic evaluation, the popularity of the preference-based measure that provides a single summary score as a health-related quality of life for quality-adjusted life year (QALY) calculation has boomed. Its ease of use and its off-the-shelf service, providing a ready-made questionnaire and a set of weights, has led it to be widely adopted in cost-effectiveness studies. There are many index-based measures available, and the most commonly seen include the Quality of Well Being (QWB) scale, the Health Utility Index Mark 2 and 3 (HUI2/3), the EQ-5D, and the SF-6D. The following sections give a brief introduction to the EQ-5D and the HUI2/3. The interested reader can refer to additional sources, such as the books by McDowell and by Brazier and his colleagues, as listed in the Further Readings. It should be noted that each measure varies considerably in several aspects, such as the chosen domains in the descriptive system, the eliciting method, and the sample population for conducting the valuation. Therefore, the values obtained by each measure do not necessarily agree with one another.

EQ-5D

The EQ-5D is a generic preference-based measure of health status developed by the EuroQol Group. Established in 1987, this group of multidisciplinary researchers from Europe designed the EQ-5D as a simple and generic measure to be used alongside other generic or condition-specific measures. Nowadays, the EQ-5D is one of the most widely used generic measures and has more than 100 official translations available.

The EQ-5D has two main components—the EQ-5D descriptive system and the EQ visual analog scale (EQ VAS). The EQ-5D descriptive system comprises the following five dimensions: (1) mobility, (2) self-care, (3) usual activities, (4) pain/discomfort, and (5) anxiety/depression. Each dimension has three levels: (1) no problems, (2) some problems, and (3) severe problems. The respondent is asked to choose the most appropriate statement in each of the five dimensions. The EQ VAS is a vertical 20-centimeter-long thermometer with the lower and upper end points valued at 0 and 100 and labeled as "Worst imaginable health state" and "Best imaginable health state," respectively. The respondent rates his or her current health state on the EQ VAS.

A total of 243 (3^5) possible health states is defined by this five-dimensional, three-level descriptive system. Each health state can be assigned a single summary index score on what is known as the EQ-5D index by applying a scoring algorithm that essentially attaches values (also called weights) to each of the levels in each dimension. An algorithm normally is derived from the valuation of a set of EQ-5D health states in general population samples. The most widely used value set (EQ-5D index scores for each of 243 health states) is the TTO-based set of values obtained from the Measurement and Valuation of Health (MVH) study in the United Kingdom, for which a representative sample consisting of 3,395 subjects from the general population was interviewed. Many other country-specific value sets have been developed, including ones for the United States, the Netherlands, Japan, and so on. There are three ways of reporting EQ-5D results: (1) the EQ-5D health state, a profile reporting the problem level in each dimension; (2) the EQ-5D index score, representing social preference for the health state defined in the descriptive system; and (3) the EQ VAS score, a self-rated health score based on a VAS.

The EQ-5D is designed for self-completion by respondents and can also be interviewer administered in person or over the phone. More information can be obtained from the official EQ-5D Web site.

HUI2/3

The Health Utility Index Mark 2 and 3 (HUI2/3) are generic preference-based health status measures. HUI instruments are designed to provide utility scores for health outcomes evaluations. The first version of a HUI instrument (HUI Mark 1) was created in the 1970s to evaluate the outcomes of neonatal intensive care. HUI measures have continued to develop, and there are now two versions available: HUI2 and HUI3. The HUI2 was initially designed for measuring long-term outcomes of treatment for children with cancer and now can be used as a generic measure. The latest version, HUI3, was developed to address some issues of the HUI2 by extending and altering the attributes of its predecessor version.

Based on survey results from parent and child pairs and a literature review, the HUI2 consists of seven attributes (domains), such as (1) sensation, (2) mobility, (3) emotion, (4) cognition, (5) self-care, (6) pain, and (7) fertility. Each attribute has three to five levels of function, and therefore, the HUI2 defines up to 24,000 unique health states. Removing attributes of fertility, replacing self-care with dexterity, and adding distinct components of sensation to the HUI2, the attributes addressed in the HUI3 are vision, hearing, speech, ambulation, dexterity, emotion, cognition, and pain; each attribute has five to six levels. As stated above, the HUI2 is a generic measure for adults; it can also apply to child populations after removing the attribute of fertility. In total, the HUI3 defines 972,000 unique health states. The choice of attributes in the HUI has been based on the "within the skin" approach—focusing on the most fundamental and important attributes of physical and emotional health status, and excluding aspects of participation in society, such as social activity or role performance.

The HUI2 scoring algorithm was developed from the valuation of a random sample of 293 parents of schoolchildren in Hamilton, Ontario,

Canada. Both VAS and SG methods were adopted to elicit values from the sample. The scoring system was developed based on the multi-attribute utility theory, where utility function for each attribute was estimated separately and multiplicative function form was adopted in the final scoring formula. A power transformation was developed to convert values of health state measured by a VAS into utility as elicited by the SG method. The scoring formula of the HUI3 uses a similar approach based on responses from a representative sample of 504 adults from Hamilton, Ontario.

Further information on the HUI instruments can be found at the Health Utilities Inc. Web site.

Profile Measure

Several generic health profile measures have been developed and are available in the literature, such as the Sickness Impact Profile, Nottingham Health Profile, Short Form 36, Short Form 12, WHOQOL-BREF, and so on. Following is a brief introduction to the Sickness Impact Profile and Short Form 36. The interested reader can refer to additional sources, such as the book by McDowell or the one by Bowling, as listed in Further Readings.

Sickness Impact Profile

The Sickness Impact Profile (SIP) is a landmark instrument in the development of outcomes measurement. Its design had great influence on later measures such as the Nottingham Health Profile. The great care and thoroughness that went into its development are noteworthy. It was originally designed as a generic measure intended for use across different conditions and populations. The SIP can be either self- or interviewer-administered.

The SIP is a behaviorally based measure of dysfunction focused on assessing the way in which sickness changes daily activities and behavior. The development of its descriptive system took a bottom-up approach, collecting statements for change in behavior attributable to sickness both from patients and individuals and from the literature. A total of 312 unique statements were identified and sorted into 14 categories by the research team. The final version contains 136 items in 12 categories, including ambulation (12 items), mobility (10), body care and movement (23), communication (9), alertness behavior (10), emotional behavior (9),

social interaction (20), sleep and rest (7), eating (9), work (9), home management (10), and recreation and pastime (8). Respondents choose/check the items in each category that describe and are related to their health.

The score can be presented by category, by physical and psychosocial dimensions, or by a single overall score within a range of 0 to 100. A lower score indicates better health. The overall score for the SIP is calculated as the sum of the weights of items checked across all categories divided by the sum of the weights for all items multiplied by 100. The same principle is used for calculating two-dimensional scores by limiting checked items to relevant categories only. Ambulation, mobility, and body care and movement form the physical dimension, while communication, alertness behavior, emotional behavior, and social interaction constitute the psychological dimension. The weights were developed using equal-appearing interval scaling procedures involving more than 100 judges.

More information can be obtained from the Medical Outcomes Trust Web site.

Short Form 36

One of the most widely used health profile measures is the Short Form 36 (SF-36) questionnaire. The SF-36 originated from the Medical Outcome Study (MOS), initially designed to evaluate health utilization of different health delivery systems in the United States. The 36 items comprising the SF-36 were derived from long-form measures of general health embodied in the MOS. Since its inception, the SF-36 has been continually developed by Ware and coworkers, being used for collecting data from several U.S. national surveys to develop social norms. There are several available versions of this 36-item questionnaire, and variation exists among their scoring systems. There are, for instance, the SF-36 by QualityMetric, the RAND 36-Item Health Survey 1.0 by RAND, and the RAND-36 HIS by the Psychological Corporation. There is also the SF-36v2, the latest version of the SF-36. This questionnaire, developed by QualityMetric, is demonstrated here as an example.

Like its predecessor, the SF-36, the SF-36v2 contains 36 items. Thirty-five items of the SF-36v2 cover eight health domains, such as (1) physical functioning (PF), (2) role-physical (RE), (3) bodily pain (BP), (4) general health (GH), (5) vitality (VT), (6) social functioning (SF), (7) role-emotional (RE), and (8) mental health (MH) scales. These domains are constructed with 2 to 10 items each, and each item has response levels ranging from three to five categories. The only item that does not contribute to any domain is the one measuring perceived health change. There are two forms available with different recall periods: standard (past 4 weeks) and acute (past 1 week). The questionnaire can be either self-completed or interviewer-administered in person or over the phone. The differences between Versions 1 and 2 of the SF-36 include a layout improvement, the wording of the items, and an increase in the response categories of 7 items from either dichotomous or six-category to five-category.

Item responses for each domain are summed and transformed (using a scoring algorithm) into a scale of 0 to 100, with a higher score representing better health. Apart from the domains of body pain and general health, the scoring algorithm for the rest of the domains assumes equal weights for each response level in an item and between items. The score can be further standardized into a mean of 50 and a standard deviation of 10 based on the U.S. population norm. Thus, a score above or below 50 is interpreted variously as above or below average. The 8-domain score can be further summarized into a physical and a mental component summary (PCS and MCS) using the algorithm developed from the 1990 U.S. general population survey with factor analysis and the orthogonal rotation method.

Currently, there are several different lengths and versions of Short Form questionnaires available, including the SF-12 and SF-8. More information can be obtained from the QualityMetric Web site.

Condition-Specific Measure

As described earlier, the emphasis of condition-specific measures is on aspects of health affected by a condition. There might be some overlapping between generic and condition-specific measures, but the latter have domains not included in generic measures or domains with more detailed scopes. For instance, condition-specific measures might include domains measuring particular treatment effects or symptoms or focus greatly on some domains such as mobility or dexterity, depending on what is of interest in the condition. Recently, there has been growing attention placed on developing preference-based, condition-specific measures. The rationale is that the generic measure might not be appropriate for a given condition, and most condition-specific measures do not provide a summary score weighted by social preference for use in economic evaluation. Here, this entry introduces the Functional Assessment of Cancer Therapy (FACT) and briefly discusses its development into a preference-based measure as an example.

Functional Assessment of Cancer Therapy

The FACT is a cancer-specific measure designed for use in the evaluation of intervention in various types of cancers. The FACT consists of a core set of items applicable to all types of cancer and cancer-specific supplements. The instrument has evolved, and its applications have been expanded to different chronic illnesses and conditions. Since 1997, it has been renamed the Functional Assessment in Chronic Illness Therapy (FACIT). The FACT-L, for lung cancer, is explained here.

The core set of 27 items applicable to all types of cancer is known as the FACT-General and comprises four domains: physical well-being (7 items), social/family well-being (7), emotional well-being (6), and functional well-being (7). These domains were identified using factor analysis. Each item in the FACT-General has a five-level response. The 10 items specific to lung cancer are labeled as additional concerns, assessing coughing, breathing, smoking, and so on.

The Trial Outcome Index (TOI) can be computed for any FACT measure. It is the sum of physical well-being and functional well-being, plus additional concerns subscales. In the FACT-L, a total of 21 items is used to calculate the TOI score. Like most condition-specific measures, the FACT assumes that there is equal weight for each level in an item and equal importance among items. Such a scoring system might be sensitive enough for clinical purposes. However, it does not have the necessary properties required by economic evaluation.

The development of the preference-based FACT-L is aimed at addressing the above issue. A study conducted by Kind and Macran developed a set of social preference weights for the FACT-L. The approach adopted consisted in first revising items in the FACT-L through both quantitative and qualitative methods to be amenable for valuation. The health states defined by the revised items were then valued by a sample of the United Kingdom's general population using a VAS through a postal survey. Econometric methods were used to develop weights for 10 items of the FACT-L based on the collected data. Thus, the derived utility weights of the FACT-L can be used in cost-utility analysis legitimately.

More information about the FACT can be obtained from the FACIT Web site.

Choosing a Measure

Generic and condition-specific measures can be seen as complementary measures to each other. One provides information for comparison across different populations, and the other offers the most relevant information on a given condition. However, when making the choice of measures—whether to use generic with condition-specific measures or choosing between a profile-based or a preference-based measure—care must be taken with regard to the purpose of the measurement as well as the burden that this would represent for respondents. It should be borne in mind that there is no single measure with a descriptive system that captures all aspects of health, and the exclusion does count—elements missing from the descriptive system have an arbitrary zero weight.

Ling-Hsiang Chuang

See also EuroQoL (EQ-5D); Health Status Measurement Standards; Health Utilities Index Mark 2 and 3 (HUI2, HUI3); SF-36 and SF12 Health Surveys; Sickness Impact Profile

Further Readings

Bergner, M., Bobbitt, R., Carter, W., & Gilson, B. S. (1981). The Sickness Impact Profile: Development and final revision of a health status measure. *Medical Care, 19*, 787–805.

Bergner, M., Bobbitt, R., & Kressel, S. (1976). The Sickness Impact Profile: Conceptual formulation and methodology for the development of a health status measure. *Journal of Health Service, 6*, 393–415.

Bowling, A. (2005). *Measuring health: A review of quality of life measurement scales* (3rd ed.). Maidenhead, UK: Open University Press.

Brazier, J., Ratcliffe, J., Salomon, J. A., & Tsuchiya, A. (2007). *Measuring and valuing health benefits for economics evaluation.* Oxford, UK: Oxford University Press.

Brooks, R. (1996). EuroQol: The current state of play. *Health Policy, 37*, 53–72.

Cella, D. F., Bonomi, A. E., Lloyd, S. R., Tulsky, D. S., Kaplan, E., & Bonomi, P. (1995). Reliability and validity of the Functional Assessment of Cancer Therapy–Lung (FACT-L) quality of life instrument. *Lung Cancer, 12*, 199–220.

Cella, D. F., Tulsky, D. S., Gray, G., Sarafian, B., Linn, E., Bonomi, A., et al. (1993). The Functional Assessment of Cancer Therapy scale: Development and validation of the general measure. *Journal of Clinical Oncology, 11*, 571–579.

EQ-5D: http://www.euroqol.org

The EuroQol Group. (1990). EuroQol: A new facility for the measurement of health-related quality of life. *Health Policy, 16*, 199–208.

Feeny, D. H., Furlong, W. J., Torrance, G. W., Goldsmith, C. H., Zenglong, Z., & Depauw, S. (2002). Multiattribute and single-attribute utility function: The Health Utility Index Mark 3 system. *Medical Care, 40*, 113–128.

Functional Assessment of Chronic Illness Therapy (FACIT): http://www.facit.org

Health Utilities Inc.: http://www.healthutilities.com

Kind, P., & Macran, S. (2005). Eliciting social preference weights for Functional Assessment of Cancer Therapy: Lung health states. *PharmacoEconomics, 22*, 1143–1153.

McDowell, I. (2006). *Measuring health: A guide to rating scales and questionnaires* (3rd ed.). New York: Oxford University Press.

Medical Outcomes Trust—Instruments: http://www.outcomes-trust.org/instruments.htm

QualityMetric: http://www.qualitymetric.com

Torrance, G. W., Feeny, D. H., Furlong, W. J., Barr, R. D., Zhang, Y., & Wang, Q. (1996). A multi-attribute utility function for a comprehensive health status classification system: Health Utilities Mark 2. *Medical Care, 34*, 702–722.

Ware, J., Kosinski, M., & Dewey, J. E. (2001). *How to score Version 2 of SF-36 Health Survey.* Lincoln, RI: QualityMetric.

Ware, J., Kosinski, M., & Keller, S. D. (1994). *SF-36 physical and mental health survey scale: A user's manual.* Boston: Health Institute, New England Medical Center.

Health Status Measurement, Minimal Clinically Significant Differences, and Anchor Versus Distribution Methods

When measuring quality of life, patient preferences, health status, or other types of patient reported outcomes (PROs), the term *minimal clinically significant difference* (MCSD) indicates the smallest amount of meaningful change or difference that can be assessed by a PRO measure. The term *meaningful change,* in this context, refers to the smallest difference that is perceived by patients (or other stakeholders) as beneficial or harmful and that would lead to a change in treatment.

From this perspective, the MCSD is a numerical value, and PRO score differences that exceed this value are considered indicative of important or meaningful change. MCSDs vary across different PRO measures (i.e., a difference of 10 points may be indicative of meaningful change for one measure but not another) and different populations (i.e., the same measure may have different MCSDs depending on the patient group being assessed). In practice, because of the difficulties inherent in establishing MCSDs, exact values are rarely identified. More frequently, investigators specify a range of values within which the MCSD is likely to fall.

Investigators frequently emphasize that the MCSD does not necessarily correspond to the smallest detectable difference. In other words, not all improvements or declines that are noticeable are necessarily noteworthy. Despite consensus on this point, investigators often disagree as to which methods allow determination of whether a difference is minimally important versus minimally detectable. This disagreement, in turn, may be linked to the noticeable variation in terminology that characterizes the MCSD literature. For example, although the current report employs the term *minimally significant clinical difference*, this concept is frequently referred to as the *minimal important difference, the clinically important difference, the minimal difference, the important difference,* and other similar combinations of words and phrases.

Despite occasional disagreement over terminology, investigators have made significant progress toward developing MCSD methods, primarily because without some means to assess meaningful change, PRO data cannot be used effectively. For example, suppose in the context of a clinical trial that a group receiving a new drug scores a statistically significant 8 points higher on a PRO measure of pain relief as compared with a placebo control group. Because statistical significance does not necessarily imply clinical significance, the investigators will be unable to conclude that the new drug provided a nontrivial benefit. In other words, without insight into the MCSD, there is no way to determine whether the drug's ability to reduce pain is large enough to make a meaningful difference in patients' lives. Similar issues arise when PRO data are employed in clinical, administrative, policy-making, or regulatory settings.

Given the complexity involved in identifying MCSDs, the current lack of a gold standard method for doing so is not surprising, although the health sciences appear to be converging toward a set of best practices. Currently, two different approaches are usually employed when identifying MCSDs: anchor-based and distribution-based methods. Anchor-based methods rely on some external criterion of known significance against which changes in PRO scores can be calibrated. Distribution-based methods rely primarily on the statistical properties of PRO sample values or the reliability of the PRO measure itself. The anchor- and distribution-based approaches are described individually in the following sections, but many authors recommend that both should be employed when identifying MCSDs, as each method approaches the task from a conceptually distinct perspective.

Anchor-Based Approaches

The anchor-based approach relies on identifying an external criterion (i.e., an anchor) that is relatively interpretable, and then examining how differences in PRO scores map onto that anchor. Anchors can take many forms, including patients' self-reports of change, clinical outcomes or conditions, or other events.

Jaeschke and his colleagues were one of the first groups to demonstrate the use of self-reported change using transition assessment items. Transition assessments are typically used in longitudinal investigations, such as clinical trials, in which patients periodically complete a PRO measure as well as a self-report transition item assessing whether the patient has experienced no change, small but important change, moderate change, or large change on the PRO of interest since the last assessment. Investigators essentially derive an estimate of the MCSD by computing the average difference between consecutive PRO scores for the group reporting small but important change. This same approach also permits the identification of meaningful changes that are moderate to large in magnitude by computing the average difference score of the relevant groups. When transition assessment items are used, MCSDs for positive and negative change are sometimes derived separately, as some prior work has demonstrated asymmetries in the MCSD depending on whether a patient is improving or declining.

Although the anchor-based method is sometimes equated with the use of transition assessments, clinically based anchors are also frequently employed by MCSD researchers. For example, as part of a study intended to determine the MCSD of the Impact of Weight on Quality of Life–Lite (IWQL-L) instrument, the investigators categorized patients from several longitudinal studies into groups according to how much weight they had lost. To derive the MCSD, the investigators calculated the average difference score from the IWQL-L for the group that had lost from 5% to 9.9% of their original weight, the smallest amount deemed meaningful by the Food and Drug Administration.

Clinical anchors vary across studies, depending on the patient population. Investigators frequently advocate using multiple anchors, which are usually chosen because they are related conceptually and statistically to the PRO of interest. For example, when establishing MCSDs for some of the Functional Assessment of Cancer Therapy (FACT) scales, investigators used hemoglobin level, performance status, and response to treatment as anchors. All three predict and are clinically relevant to the cancer outcomes assessed by the FACT.

Anchors not only can be based on different criteria (e.g., patients' perceptions, clinical factors) but may also be derived from studies with different methodological designs. Although within-subject anchors are frequently used (e.g., transition assessments), anchors derived from between-subjects or cross-sectional comparisons are also possible. For example, the difference score between two groups that differ in clinically important ways (e.g., healthy individuals vs. hypertensives) has sometimes been used as an indicator of the MCSD for a given PRO measure.

Some authors have suggested that anchor-based methods are superior to distribution-based methods because only the former provide direct information about the importance or meaningfulness of a change. However, anchor-based methods have also been critiqued on several grounds. Because anchors are often themselves arbitrary, there is usually no way to verify empirically that the groups formed by anchors truly differ in important ways. Some authors have suggested that transition assessment anchors may be particularly problematic. Although self-reported change is the only way to directly incorporate the patient's perspective, transition assessments usually consist of a single item and are retrospective in nature, characteristics that could undermine their psychometric validity. Baseline status (e.g., poor health vs. good health) also appears to affect the size of MCSDs, a tendency that is likely to be more pronounced when anchor-based methods are used. For these reasons, and because different types of anchors tend to produce different MCSDs, most investigators recommend using multiple anchors. Typically, various types of anchors are explored over several studies to arrive at an MCSD or, more commonly, a range of values in which the MCSD is likely to fall.

Distribution-Based Approaches

As stated earlier, distribution-based approaches rely primarily on the statistical properties of sample data or the PRO measure itself. The chief value of distribution-based approaches is that, unlike anchor-based methods, they allow the identification of differences or changes that are essentially too large to have occurred by chance or from measurement error. Several of the more popular distribution-based methods are summarized in the following sections.

One of the most common distribution-based approaches relies on the effect size associated with a difference or change. Effect size can be computed by dividing the difference between two sample means (or the average difference in the case of a repeated measures design) by the sample standard deviation or the pooled standard deviation. The resulting proportion, which essentially redefines the difference in standard deviation units, can be interpreted according to the well-known guidelines proposed for the behavioral sciences by Cohen, who suggested that effect sizes of .20 to .49, .50 to .79, and .80 and above should be considered small, moderate, and large, respectively. Thus, from this perspective, any difference or change associated with an effect size of .20 or greater would be considered clinically meaningful.

The reliable change index provides an alternative distribution-based method to identify MCSDs at the individual level and is computed by dividing the difference or change between two PRO scores by the standard error of the difference between the scores. The index, which depends on the standard error of measurement, contrasts an observed change with the change that would be expected from chance or measurement error. Some authors suggest that reliable change has occurred as long as the index value exceeds 1.96. This would indicate that the likelihood of obtaining the observed difference is only about 5% or less if there has been no actual change, suggesting that the change or difference is "real" and not the result of chance variation.

The standard error of measurement (SEM) can also be used in its own right to help derive MCSDs. The SEM is the standard deviation of an individual's scores on a specific measure. Because all measures contain some error, an individual's score would vary to some extent if the same measure were to be repeatedly administered to that individual. The SEM indicates how much variation would occur, with more precise or reliable measures having a lower SEM. Thus, the greater a difference or change relative to the SEM, the more likely that difference or change is likely to be "real" and not the result of chance or error. How much greater than the SEM a meaningful difference should be is somewhat controversial, with suggestions ranging from 1 SEM to 1.96 SEMs to 2.77 SEMs. The SEM can be calculated by multiplying the sample standard deviation by the square root of one minus the reliability of the PRO measure. Because of the inverse relationship between sample variance and measure reliability, a measure's SEM should remain fairly stable across different samples.

Distribution-based methods are relatively easy to implement because they do not require anchor data and, as previously noted, provide the additional advantage of identifying MCSDs that exceed variation due to chance or measurement error. However, as several investigators have noted, this property by itself does not guarantee that the change or difference is necessarily large enough to be important from the perspective of the patient or other stakeholder. Conversely, some distribution methods may result in MCSD estimates that are too large. For example, some investigators have noted that the 1.96 criterion commonly used in conjunction with the reliable change index is fairly strict, resulting in conservative (i.e., large) MCSD estimates relative to other methods. In general, it is often not clear which standards to apply when establishing MCSDs using distribution-based methods. For example, the number of SEMs that a difference or change has to exceed to be considered meaningful tends to vary across disciplines.

Distribution-based approaches, especially those involving effect size and the SEM, have received increasing attention over the past decade, largely due to the work of Wyrwich and her colleagues. Using data from a variety of patient samples, Wyrwich and others have found that 1 SEM is frequently, though not always, equivalent to an effect size of approximately .50 when PRO measures with appropriate levels of reliability are used. These findings suggest that differences or changes that exceed 1 SEM may generally be large enough to be meaningful.

Additionally, MCSDs identified using anchor-based approaches are often associated with an effect size approximating .50, although this phenomenon appears most robust in patients with chronic health conditions. Consequently, some authors have suggested that in the absence of other information, a difference or change associated with an effect size of .50 is likely to be clinically meaningful. However, as these and other authors have cautioned, some prior work has identified anchor-based MCSDs that are associated with effect sizes both smaller and larger than .50, thus highlighting the critical role that anchor-based methods can play.

Best Practices

Developing methods to identify MCSDs has proven a challenging and complex task. However, consensus is emerging over a set of best practices. Specifically, most investigators recommend triangulating on MCSDs using a combination of both distribution- and anchor-based approaches across multiple samples. Whereas distribution-based methods help ensure that MCSDs are large enough to exceed chance variation, anchor-based methods help ensure that MCSDs are properly sized to reflect truly meaningful and important change.

R. Brian Giesler

See also Health Status Measurement, Assessing Meaningful Change; Health Status Measurement, Responsiveness and Sensitivity to Change

Further Readings

Crosby, R. D., Kolotkin, R. L., & Williams, G. R. (2003). Defining clinically meaningful change in health related quality of life. *Journal of Clinical Epidemiology, 56,* 395–407.

de Vet, H. C., Terwee, C. B., Ostelo, R. W., Beckerman, H., Knol, D. L., & Bouter, L. M. (2006). Minimal changes in health status questionnaires: Distinction between minimally detectable change and minimally important change. *Health and Quality of Life Outcomes, 4,* 54–59.

Guyatt, G. H., Osoba, D., Wu, A. W., Wyrwich, K. W., & Norman, G. R. (2002). Methods to explain the clinical significance of health status measures. *Mayo Clinic Proceedings, 77,* 371–383.

Jacobson, N. S., & Truax, P. (1991). Clinical significance: A statistical approach to defining meaningful change in psychotherapy research. *Journal of Consulting and Clinical Psychology, 59,* 12–19.

Norman, G. R., Sloan, J. A., & Wyrwich, K. W. (2003). Interpretation of changes in health-related quality of life: The remarkable universality of half a standard deviation. *Medical Care, 41,* 582–592.

Revicki, D., Hays, R. D., Cella, D., & Sloan, J. (2008). Recommended methods for determining responsiveness and minimally important differences for patient-reported outcomes. *Journal of Clinical Epidemiology, 61,* 102–109.

Sloan, J. A., Cella, D., & Hays, R. D. (2005). Clinical significance of patient-reported questionnaire data: Another step toward consensus. *Journal of Clinical Epidemiology, 58,* 1217–1219.

Wyrwich, K. W., Bullinger, M., Aaronson, N., Hays, R. D., Patrick, D. L., Symonds, T., et al. (2005). Estimating clinically significant differences in quality of life outcomes. *Quality of Life Research, 14,* 285–295.

HEALTH STATUS MEASUREMENT, RELIABILITY AND INTERNAL CONSISTENCY

Reliability refers to the concept of consistency of measurement. Medical decision making is based on observations and measurements taken from the patient. For decision making to be based on the best possible information, such measurements should be both reliable and valid. Reliability of measurement is a necessary condition for a measure to be valid but is not sufficient to ensure validity. A psychometric test, attitude scale, or observational measurement may be reliable in that it can be consistently assessed over time but not valid in that it does not accurately reflect the construct it is designed to measure. In terms of statistical theory, reliability is defined as the ratio of the variation of the true score and the variation of the observed score.

Assessments of the reliability of a measure can be broadly split into two groups: (1) methods of determining the reliability of a test by repeated administration (e.g., test-retest reliability and inter-rater reliability) and (2) methods that require a single administration of the test. The latter methods are often termed internal consistency measures.

Repeated Administration

The logic of repeated administration as a method for determining the reliability of a measure is simple. If a test or observation is reliable, then if it is measured twice in the same individual without any change in the individual occurring, the value of the measurement should be the same. Test-retest reliability involves the administration of the same test or observation to a group of individuals at two points separated by a period of time. There is no simple guide to the ideal time period for test-retest reliability—essentially, it should be short enough to ensure that the sample has not changed in the aspect being measured but long enough to prevent individuals recalling their previous answers and using their recall as the basis for their responses on the second occasion. Periods of 2 to 4 weeks are typical. Some researchers advocate asking respondents to indicate whether they feel that they have changed in the construct under study between the two testing sessions, and then excluding those with a perceived change.

Interrater reliability refers to the consistency of measurement between two raters making independent observations of the same individuals. Interrater reliability is most commonly used in psychology where observational data are collected. Two individuals may observe either live behavior or a video recording of behavior and make ratings in terms of a standardized measurement. The independent ratings can then be observed. Simple measures of the percentage agreement and percentage disagreement can be calculated. The extent of agreement will depend to a large degree on how well the behaviors and the categories to be recorded are specified and the extent to which observers have been trained to use the scoring method. Extensive training and calibration in the measurement method prior to the research is an excellent way to ensure reliability of observational measurements.

In a large-scale study involving the observation of behavior, both interobserver and test-retest reliability measures may be taken. This is to avoid the potential for measurement error resulting from a change in the way raters make their observations over time. By reappraising data from earlier in the trial, it is possible to determine whether such measurement drift has occurred.

The statistical methods used to determine whether there is consistency across the two measurements for both test-retest reliability and inter-rater reliability depend on the nature of the data. For nominal data, Cohen's kappa statistic is calculated. This is the proportion of observations that agree across the two testing situations, corrected for chance levels of agreement. Values of Cohen's kappa range from 0 to 1.0, where 1.0 is perfect agreement. The following guide to the extent of agreement was produced by Douglas Altman:

0 to .6 poor agreement,

.6 to .8 satisfactory agreement,

.8 to 1.0 excellent agreement.

For ordinal data, the weighted kappa is used. This is an extension of Cohen's kappa but gives greater weight to disagreements far removed on the ordinal scale and smaller weight to disagreements falling on adjacent points. The values of weighted kappa are interpreted in the same manner as kappa.

Where the data tested for reliability are continuous, there are a number of statistical methods to determine the extent of consistency in the measurement. Some researchers have suggested the use of simple correlation statistics, but this is now considered inappropriate, since measurements could be perfectly correlated but differ in magnitude. To overcome this limitation, Bland and Altman suggested a simple method of plotting the data to explore the consistency of measurement. A Bland-Altman plot comprises a plot of the difference between two measurements on the same individual against the mean of the two measurements. Typically the overall mean and standard deviation of the two measurements are also placed on the graph. This allows the researcher to explore the range of magnitude of differences and, importantly, whether differences are larger at the extreme points of the measurement scale. This is important, since regression to the mean will affect extreme values most markedly. An alternative approach that is currently popular is to calculate the intraclass correlation (ICC) of the two sets of data. The ICC is a correlation coefficient where the intercept is forced to occur at the origin (0, 0) of the bivariate plot. The ICC is equivalent to a correlation coefficient and can be interpreted as such.

Single Administration

Single administration methods have the advantage that the consistency of measurement can be determined in a single assessment. They are therefore easier and more economic to undertake and especially useful where either the measurement changes the participant in some way, or there is a risk that the participant will change before a second observation can be arranged. These methods most commonly are used for questionnaires or observations with multiple related items measuring the same construct. The *split half* method works on the assumption that if all the items in a questionnaire are consistently measuring the same construct, then it should be possible to split the items into two halves that will correlate highly with each other. An obvious example would be to compare odd-numbered and even-numbered items. It is also possible to calculate all the possible split-half combinations of a questionnaire (given by the number of items − 1) and then calculate the average correlation between all the possible combinations. Generally, longer tests will show higher internal consistency, but using a split-half method means that the two forms of the scale are effectively half as long as the original. It is possible to correct for this in the calculation of the internal consistency statistic by using the Spearman-Brown formula.

Cronbach's alpha is a widely used measure of the internal consistency of scales. It is the average of the correlations of each item with the total score of the scale (excluding that item). The logic of Cronbach's alpha is that if all the items in a scale are reliably measuring the same construct, then they should all correlate highly with each other. Coefficient alpha will range from 0 (no consistency) to 1.0 (perfect consistency). For psychometric tests, an alpha above .7 is recommended, whereas for clinical tests, a value of alpha greater than .9 should be sought, according to Bland and Altman. Cronbach's alpha can be used where items have multiple response categories or in the situation where items have binary responses. In the latter case (binary response categories), Cronbach's alpha is equivalent to the Kuder-Richardson Formula-20, which has been used as a measure of internal consistency. However, since the two formulae are equivalent for the case where response categories are binary but, in addition, Cronbach's alpha deals with the wider case, alpha is generally the preferred statistic. Certain statistical packages will calculate Cronbach's alpha for a scale along with statistics for individual items within the scale (such as how well the scale performs when individual items are deleted). These statistics are often used to derive scales that are internally consistent by selectively removing items; this procedure can be an effective way of developing internally consistent scales, but some caveats should be noted: First, Cronbach's alpha is not suitable for very low numbers of items (three or two items); second, the scale derived by removing items may be internally consistent, but such a correction does not necessarily reflect the construct that the scale was originally devised to measure—measures of internal consistency give information on reliability, not validity.

The reliability of observations can generally be improved by adopting a range of methods. As mentioned previously, adding items to make a scale longer will improve reliability, provided that the items are conceptually similar. Ensuring that the meaning of all items is clear to participants will ensure that their answers are consistent. Item analysis—that is, exploring the psychometric properties of each item in a scale—will help identify "rogue" items that are lowering the reliability estimates. Item analysis includes exploring the correlation of the item to all the other items; those with an average interitem correlation less than .3 should be excluded.

It should also be noted that the reliability statistics calculated are related to the scores of a measure rather than the measure itself, and therefore will vary across different samples. Reliability estimates from one sample might differ from those of a second sample if the second sample is drawn from a different population. This is particularly true when samples are drawn from clinical and nonclinical samples. For example, a measure of eating disorder symptomatology may be extremely reliable in a sample of males without an eating disorder, since the entire sample will have very low scores on all items. However, in a clinical sample of women with eating disorders, there will be greater variation in scores that introduces greater possibility for measurement error and hence a nonreliable measure.

J. Tim Newton and Koula Asimakopoulou

See also Factor Analysis and Principal Components Analysis; Health Status Measurement, Construct Validity; Health Status Measurement, Face and Content Validity; Intraclass Correlation Coefficient

Further Readings

Altman, D. G. (1999). *Practical statistics for medical research* (2nd ed.). New York: Chapman & Hall.

Bland, J. M., & Altman, D. G. (1986). Statistical methods for assessing agreement between two methods of clinical measurement. *Lancet, 1,* 307–310.

Bland, J. M., & Altman, D. G. (1997). Statistics notes: Cronbach's alpha. *British Medical Journal, 314,* 572.

Cronbach, L. J. (1951). Coefficient alpha and the internal structure of tests. *Psychometrika, 16*(3), 297–334.

Shrout, P. E., & Fleiss, J. L. (1979). Intraclass correlations: Uses in assessing rater reliability. *Psychological Bulletin, 2,* 420–428.

HEALTH STATUS MEASUREMENT, RESPONSIVENESS AND SENSITIVITY TO CHANGE

For medical decision making, the purpose of measurement is often to measure change in health over time associated with treatment. With this in mind, there has been considerable attention paid to the ability of health status instruments to measure change, often called responsiveness or sensitivity to change. First, it should be noted that there is debate about whether or not to use change scores (the difference between scores at two points in time) at all, and although this discussion is beyond the scope of this entry, further readings have been provided as a starting point for those interested in delving more deeply into this topic. This entry defines responsiveness and sensitivity, provides context for the use of these terms, and explains the main approaches used in validation studies of health status measures.

Definitions

There is a significant body of literature about the appropriate methods to use when comparing measurement instruments over time in the absence of a gold standard. Unfortunately, there are several taxonomies in use, some with overlapping terms. Therefore, it is important to define key terms used in validation studies. Some have argued for using two terms, *sensitivity* and *responsiveness*, to describe the ability to measure change. Within this framework, *sensitivity* denotes the ability to detect any change at all and is assessed using calculations based on the variation within samples. These methods are often called *distribution-based*. *Responsiveness* refers to the ability to measure clinically important change and is calculated using external criteria, or *anchors*, to provide meaning for a specified magnitude of change in score; it is sometimes called an *anchor-based* approach. Another way of thinking about responsiveness is that it translates change on the new instrument into similar change on a familiar scale (the anchor), with the aim of enhancing the interpretability of results from the new measurement instrument. Commonly used external criteria or anchors

include clinical tests, performance tests, and ratings of status by providers, patients, and caretakers. For example, a responsiveness study may calculate how much change on New Scale X would be associated with patient-reported "mild improvement" or a one-level change in self-report of symptom level (e.g., from moderate to mild). In this way, various anchors may be used to calculate *minimal important difference* (MID), representing the amount of change in score that could be considered clinically meaningful. Implicit in the selection of the anchor is the perspective of interest for the external criterion.

There is continued dialogue about conceptual frameworks and optimal naming conventions. Some argue against the distinction made between validity and responsiveness, noting that responsiveness is the ability to measure "what is intended" as it changes and is, therefore, more appropriately named *longitudinal validity*. Using this framework, the terms *responsiveness* and *sensitivity* refer to aspects of construct validity. However, in practice, *responsiveness* and *sensitivity* are often used more generally to describe the ability to measure change. In this way, the terms are not meant to be distinguished from validity, or to distinguish between measuring meaningful change and measuring any change at all. In this entry, the term *responsiveness* is used to describe anchor-based aids to interpretability, to denote the ability to measure clinically meaningful change. The term *sensitivity* refers to distribution-based methods to characterize the ability to detect change. Both are framed within the realm of longitudinal construct validity studies.

Methods

A wide range of methods is available for appraising the responsiveness and sensitivity of measurement instruments, enabling researchers to choose the method that best suits their measurement purposes. However, this poses challenges for comparisons of validation studies and for facilitating the interpretation of changes in health-related quality of life (HRQOL) measurement instruments. A review conducted in 2002 reported 25 definitions of responsiveness and 31 different statistical measures. Studies comparing approaches report a range of agreement in results using different methods. While many debate the merits of various estimates, others call for consensus to minimize confusion and doubt about the validity of HRQOL measurement overall. Still others promote the benefits of the scope of information that comes from various approaches to validation studies.

Sensitivity to Change

Distribution-based methods for assessing sensitivity generally measure change relative to an estimate of variation expressed as the ratio of raw score change (Mean$_2$ – Mean$_1$) to measure of variance (standard deviation of the baseline score) and can vary depending on time points and patient groups selected. The types of variation considered can be generally categorized as reflecting one of three statistical characteristics. These are statistical significance (e.g., paired t test), sample variation (e.g., effect size and standardized response mean), and measurement precision (e.g., standard error of the measurement [SEM]). The effect size and standardized response mean (SRM) provide estimates of group change in terms of standard deviation units; so, for example, an effect size of 1.0 can be interpreted as change on the order of 1 standard deviation. The calculation for these statistics can be seen below. An effect size in the area of .2 is considered small, .5 is medium, and .8 is large. For the t test, effect size, and SRM, larger values indicate greater responsiveness. In contrast, SEM, as calculated below, estimates change for an individual, and smaller values represent better responsiveness.

$$\text{Effect size} = \frac{\text{Mean}_2 - \text{Mean}_1}{\text{Standard deviation}_{\text{baseline}}}.$$

$$SRM = \frac{\text{Mean}_2 - \text{Mean}_1}{\text{Standard deviation}_{\text{Change score}}}.$$

$$SEM = \text{Standard deviation}_{\text{baseline}} \sqrt{1 - \text{Reliability}_{\text{Test-Retest}}}.$$

Responsiveness

Various approaches have been developed to attach meaning to the magnitude of change in a measurement instrument. Characterization of MID requires comparison with an external criterion for health change. A common approach to MID is to calculate the mean change for the group within a study that fulfilled the criteria for important change. For example, in a validation study of health indexes, minimal important difference was defined as one level of change reported using a symptom satisfaction question and using a 10- to 19-point change in score using a disease-specific disability index. Approaches exist to elicit individual estimates of minimal important difference prospectively. Because MID estimates do not incorporate any information about the variability of the sample, methods have been developed to provide this information. For example, the responsiveness statistic (RS-MID) divides the MID by a measure of variation for those in the sample who were unchanged. The responsiveness statistic incorporates information about the distribution and judgment about meaningful change from an external criterion. It therefore is both distribution and anchor based. The criteria available for comparing MID estimates necessarily constrain the scope of interpretation of the responsiveness estimate. Therefore, the nature of the criterion—whether self-reported, performance based, clinician reported, or diagnosis based—must be considered when forming conclusions about the validity of the inferences that can be made from the instrument.

Interpretation

Differences between estimates of responsiveness and sensitivity using various approaches can be disconcerting. However, the interpretation of responsiveness and sensitivity estimates rests on the conceptual framework for the statistical procedures used. Below, a sample of the considerations related to a subset of measures is discussed.

The SRM uses a measure of variation in observed change of the sample in the denominator, while the effect size uses a measure of baseline variation of the sample at baseline. If the individuals all experience similar, large change, the SRM would be small relative to the effect size. Similarly, if there is little variation in the population at baseline, effect size will be relatively large. Some argue that statistics such as the SRM, using the standard deviation of change, characterize statistical significance rather than sample variation and should not be used in longitudinal validity studies. Theoretically, distribution-based statistics may capture change beyond measurement error that is not necessarily clinically meaningful.

Anchor-based approaches to estimating responsiveness provide information about the ability to capture change relative to a relevant, external criterion, or anchor, explicitly incorporating judgments about important change. MIDs do not incorporate sample variation or the variability inherent in the measurement system. Incorporating variability into MID may make interpretation of the measure more complex. MIDs are reported in the units of the system of interest and can be understood within the relevant context, while the dimensionless RS-MID is less familiar to most audiences than effect size, SRM and SEM, and MID in most circumstances and may be challenging to interpret. It may be that advantages of accounting for variability in the measurement system could be outweighed by the challenges of interpreting and communicating the meaning of this statistic.

Although it is distribution-based, the SEM is conceptually different from the effect size and the SRM. The SEM incorporates the standard deviation of the sample at baseline and the reliability of the measurement instrument and is used to interpret individual change. According to classical test theory, the SEM is a property of the measurement instrument and can be applied across populations. There is debate about the interpretation of the SEM relative to the magnitude and meaning of change. Various authors support the use of 1 to 2 SEM as an indication of change beyond measurement error. Furthermore, these thresholds are applied as thresholds for minimal important change. Investigations into the relationship between sensitivity and responsiveness measures have reported that MID estimates center on one half of a standard deviation, suggesting that 1 SEM is a reasonable threshold for important change.

From a practical standpoint, when planning a study, effect size or SRM would be useful to inform sample size calculation and system selection relative to distributional characteristics. If the treatment and study goals address a particular dimension, MIDs based on highly relevant anchors (e.g.,

symptom satisfaction) may add valuable information. To enhance interpretability, the SEM provides estimates of the threshold for significant change. The MID enhances the interpretability of change by estimating the threshold for important change on the group level from a specific perspective. MIDs from various perspectives may provide important information about the orientation of the measurement systems under consideration and therefore guide system choice.

Finally, responsiveness and sensitivity estimates make up a portion of a larger array of approaches available to study the validity of health status measurement instruments. By choosing statistical procedures based on their design to address specific hypotheses, and interpreting their results within this context, investigators contribute to the larger process of accumulating evidence about the level of confidence with which decision makers can make inferences based on scores from health status measurement instruments.

Christine M. McDonough

See also Health Outcomes Assessment; Health Status Measurement, Construct Validity; Health Status Measurement, Floor and Ceiling Effects; Health Status Measurement, Generic Versus Condition-Specific Measures; Health Status Measurement, Minimal Clinically Significant Differences, and Anchor Versus Distribution Methods; Health Status Measurement, Reliability and Internal Consistency; Health Status Measurement Standards

Further Readings

Beaton, D. E., Boers, M., & Wells, G. (2002). Many faces of the minimal clinically important difference (MCID): A literature review and directions for future research. *Current Opinion in Rheumatology, 14,* 109–114.

Cronbach, L. J., & Furby, L. (1970). How should we measure "change"—or should we? *Psychological Bulletin, 74*(1), 68–80.

Guyatt, G. H., Osoba, D., Wu, A. W., Wyrwich, K. W., & Norman, G. R. (2002, April). Methods to explain the clinical significance of health status measures. *Mayo Clinic Proceedings, 77,* 371–383.

Guyatt, G. H., Walters, S., & Norman, G. R. (1987). Measuring change over time: Assessing the usefulness of evaluative instruments. *Journal of Chronic Diseases, 40,* 171–178.

Liang, M. H. (2000, September). Longitudinal construct validity: Establishment of clinical meaning in patient evaluative instruments [See comment]. *Medical Care, 38*(9 Suppl.), II84–II90.

McDowell, I. (2006). *Measuring health: A guide to rating scales and questionnaires* (3rd ed.). New York: Oxford University Press.

Streiner, D. L., & Norman, G. R. (2003). *Health measurement scales.* New York: Oxford University Press.

Terwee, C., Dekker, F., Wiersinga, W., Prummel, M., & Bossuyt, P. (2003). On assessing responsiveness of health related quality of life instruments: Guidelines for instrument evaluation. *Quality of Life Research, 12,* 349–362.

HEALTH STATUS MEASUREMENT STANDARDS

Health status measurement is important in determining the health of a population. The definition of health represents one of the contemporary challenges in health services research, as defining health is complex and measures of health vary. Defining health status measurement is relative, as health is a multidimensional, multiconstruct concept for which users of any metric of health must provide appropriate context if they are to understand how the outcome applies to their research needs. Before further discussing health status measurement standards, one must have a clear definition of health.

What Is Health?

The most widely accepted definition of health was adopted in 1948 by the World Health Organization (WHO) for an individual anywhere in the world. WHO defines health as "a state of complete physical, mental and social well-being and not merely the absence of disease or infirmity." The global community did not adopt a definition of health to measure either presence or absence of disease. Health is multidimensional, involving the physical health of the body, mental/emotional health, and social well-being. This definition, as discussed by Donald Barr in his book *Health Disparities in the United States,* while all-encompassing in its appeal, has a limited perspective for health policy due to

the lofty, impractical expectation of health that few can truly achieve. By setting an unattainable standard of health, individuals are automatically positioned for failure to meet the expectation of health within this definition. WHO's widely accepted definition seems to provide a black-and-white view of health with few shades of gray—that is, one is either in good health or not. Thus, there is no way of tracking the degree to which health changes over time to determine improving or deteriorating health. Likewise, there are few mechanisms for comparison between individuals. The WHO definition provides an opportunity to understand the three approaches to health. These approaches address physical health, mental health, and social well-being. First, it is necessary to explore each approach and then discuss the potential for quantifying health.

Physical Health as the Absence of Disease: The Medical Approach

A definition of health provided by sociologist Andrew Twaddle in 1979 was used by the U.S. medical profession for much of the 20th century, according to Barr. Discussed in Twaddle's definition was the need for it to be understood that health first and foremost is a "biophysical state" and that illness is any state that has been diagnosed by a competent professional. These two components as identified by Twaddle according to the medical model include the following: (a) absence of symptoms (e.g., sensations noticed by the patient and interpreted as abnormal) and (b) absence of signs (e.g., objective criteria noted by a medical professional). This medical model approach tells us what health is *not*. If a person has abnormal signs or symptoms, according to this approach, the medical model does not define or discuss what health is. This is termed in medicine as a *rule-out* definition. Here, the health professional looks for the presence of abnormal signs or symptoms. And when both are absent, it is possible to rule out ill health. If one does not have ill health, then from this medical model perspective, the individual is healthy.

The medical approach in isolation creates problems. If the doctor and the patient disagree, which component takes precedence? Consider the scenario if a patient has the symptoms of a headache, yet the doctor, after running all available diagnostic tests, finds no signs of illness? Through ruling out ill health, the doctor can reassure the patient that he or she is healthy. However, the patient may still feel the headache and thus be unhealthy and expect to be treated as such. The converse is true, too. What if the patient has no abnormal symptoms? Consider a patient with high cholesterol. A person with high cholesterol develops symptoms over a period of time. Should we consider a person with elevated cholesterol to be unhealthy, if we also take into account that this individual's cholesterol may eventually lead to future health problems? Despite this person's feeling "fine," what might be the consequence of stigmatizing this person as "unhealthy"?

Within the medical approach, concerns exist about the reliability of objective testing measures creating abnormal illness signs due to variability of tests (e.g., EKGs, CAT scans, laboratory tests) both in individual interpretation (e.g., physician, test administrator) and due to differences in test specificity and sensitivity. Across the country, variations in the interpretations of findings by doctors have been documented, including variations in considering what comprises both a "normal" and an "abnormal" finding.

The Psychological Approach

The psychological state of the health of an individual, measured on a survey, is purely determined by the self-assessment of that individual and not by an independent evaluator. The question of how you would rate your overall feeling of well-being on a scale of 1 to 10 represents an example of such an assessment. Likert scales and a variety of other measures have been developed to measure self-perception of health. Often these measures are time sensitive, as time-specific individual circumstances are likely to influence answer choices and apt to cause change within these self-assessments of health. The mental health scores of an individual facing a particular stressor, such as an event or challenge (e.g., a test), may reflect a lower sense of well-being. However, after the stressor is resolved, that same individual may report substantially improved well-being. Additionally, issues with mental health reports by proxy have created a potential selection or interpretation bias. An example is if parents answer a questionnaire about their child's mental state and their subjectivity does not reflect their child's true mental health state.

Social Health and Functioning Approach

The level of functioning within one's social context was an approach to health taken by sociologist Talcott Parsons in 1972. This health approach applies less to the actual physiology of the individual and more to what the person is able to do with his or her body. This approach assesses the ability to function despite any limitations. Therefore, this concept removes the dichotomous view of health as defined by WHO and places emphasis on an individual's own social circumstances and social roles to define normal functioning.

Health comparisons between two individuals may be problematic again if this social health and functioning definition is considered in isolation. Differing states of health may be assessed when two people have different social roles and tasks but the same physical functioning. Consider the example of a concert pianist and a person who packs fish, both of whom are afflicted with carpal tunnel syndrome. The concert pianist may be seen as unhealthy because the condition affects the ability to play the piano and may be more likely to have a medical intervention. On the other hand, a fish packer on the assembly line with carpal tunnel syndrome may warrant little consideration despite the great discomfort and numbness of his hands. Inequalities in social economic status, including educational opportunities and attainment, may influence and lead to clearly dissimilar health experiences due to defined roles and tasks. Therefore, supporting this model of health in isolation may perpetuate these inequalities.

Functioning is important for defining health in people with disabilities and the elderly, as discussed by health services researcher Lisa Iezzoni. Iezzoni discusses "function status" as the end result of a person's health. Specifically for the evaluation of health for people with disabilities, function status measures have been typically grouped into activities of daily living (ADLs; e.g., eating, walking, bathing, dressing, toileting) and instrumental ADLs (IADLs; e.g., cooking, housework, shopping, using public transportation, managing personal finances, answering the phone). As described by Iezzoni in the book *Risk Adjustment for Measuring*

Healthcare Outcomes, measuring function status includes several challenges. Function status is not operationalized by demographics or clinical characteristics alone. Numerous studies have shown that demographics (e.g., age, sex, gender) and pathology explain only part of function status variation. Additionally, function status measures do not apply similarly across all conditions and patient populations, as there have been floor and ceiling effects with respect to function status measurement—that is, instruments have failed to detect improvement in functioning because those with poor health tend to remain constantly low (floor effect), and those with higher functioning remain unnoticed by instruments. Also, the mode of administration creates differences in functional status measurement, as face-to-face administration results in a more optimistic measure than self-administration. Moreover, disease-specific measures may be more appropriate than a generic universal measure of functioning. The use of condition-specific measurement scales (e.g., Arthritis Impact Measurement Scale, Visual Analogue Pain Scale, Gait Evaluation) are more sensitive to function changes for individuals with these conditions than a generic universal measure. Last, there exists conflict between single, composite, and summary measures of function versus multiple scales capturing different dimensions of function status. Single measures of health may well result in misrepresentation of function. In instruments like the 36-Item Short-Form Health Survey (SF-36), two summary measures of health are created, the Physical Component Summary (PCS) and the Mental Component Summary (MCS) scales. The implications of these composite measures are still being explored.

Health Is Multidimensional

Each approach to health described above implies something about individual health states; however, the overall state of health is more ambiguous. Health represents multiple dimensions. One health services researcher, Frederick Wollinsky, suggests dichotomizing health for each of the above three approaches (i.e., psychological, social, and absence of disease) into "well" and "ill" health, measuring health by ratio of "well" to "ill" dimensions of health. The SF-36 developed by John Ware and colleagues represents a multidimensional measure of health, except that, instead of the dichotomous measures suggested above, the SF-36 measures each dimension of health as a continuous measure of health.

The SF-36 uses different combinations of the 36 items in the instrument to create eight distinct scales, each measuring a different dimension of health. As discussed earlier, four of the eight scales create the PCS, which is a summary measure of physical health, and the remaining four create the MCS, which is a summary measure of mental health. The four scales to create the PCS are (1) physical functioning, (2) role limitations due to physical problems, (3) bodily pain, and (4) general health perceptions. The four scales that make up the MCS are (1) vitality, (2) social functioning, (3) role limitations due to emotional problems, and (4) general mental health.

Using a multidimensional instrument, such as the SF-36, allows providers and health service researchers to assess health across medical, social, and psychological constructs. These three constructs of health are causally linked to each other, as physical health changes create changes in social roles, which ultimately affect mental health. Each aspect of these dimensions is unique to the characteristics of both the individual and the environment in which that individual lives. These three dimensions are not the final outcome, but rather the intermediate factors that will ultimately affect health-related quality of life. Individual and environmental characteristics will buffer or enhance the health of an individual. For example, for an individual with strong social, psychological, and environmental support, a specific symptomatology may result in a smaller impact on functional status, whereas for another with similar symptomatology, weaker support may result in greater impact on function status, leading to poorer health. Quality-of-life measures are greatly affected by symptoms of illness and functional limitations; however, the presence of these symptoms alone will not result in reduced quality of life. For example, in a *BMC Public Health* 2008 article, "Age at Disability Onset and Self-Reported Health Status," Eric Jamoom and colleagues were able to show that the age at which one acquires symptoms or activity limitation is associated with health status differences. Health status measurement is tied intimately to context of health, and the jury is still out on a standard measure of health. Because health status is so complex, there is no single gold standard of health status measurement. Often a gold standard is considered a reference to determine whether a newer instrument adequately measures health as reflected in the older instrument. Therefore, an older survey is often used as a gold standard for a comparison to determine the criterion validity of a newer survey to ensure that the instrument still adequately represents the measures from the reference instrument. However, health status measures are subject to limitations with validity and reliability considerations, and definitions of health measurement are required to continue to understand the context for distinction.

Definitions of Health Status Measurement

A panel of 57 experts with backgrounds in medicine, biostatistics, psychology, and epidemiology participated in the COSMIN (COnsensus Standards for the selection of health Measurement INstruments) Delphi study to develop standards for selecting health measurement instruments. Definitions below are provided from the preliminary version of the COSMIN Checklist as designed in the protocol from Mokkink and colleagues in *BMC Medical Research Methodology*.

Reliability: The degree to which the measurement is free from measure error. The extent to which scores for patients who have not changed are the same for repeated measurement under several conditions: for example, using different sets of items from the same health-related patient-reported outcomes (HR-PRO) (internal consistency); over time (test-retest); by different persons on the same occasion (interrater); or by the same persons (i.e., raters or responders) on different occasions (intrarater).

Internal consistency: The degree of interrelatedness among the items.

Measurement error: The systematic and random error of a patient's score that is not attributed to the true changes in the construct to be measured.

Validity: The degree to which an instrument truly measures the construct it purports to measure.

Content validity: The degree to which the content of a HR-PRO instrument is an adequate reflection of the construct to be measured.

Construct validity: The degree to which the scores of a HR-PRO instrument are consistent with hypotheses based on the assumption that the HR-PRO instrument validity measures the construct to be measured.

Criterion validity: The degree to which scores of a HR-PRO instrument are an adequate reflection of a gold standard. A gold standard for HR-PRO instruments does not exist. When assessing criterion validity of a shortened questionnaire, the original long version may be considered as the gold standard.

Cross-cultural validity: The degree to which the performance of the items on a translated or culturally adapted HR-PRO instrument are an adequate reflection of the performance of the items of the original version of the HR-PRO instrument.

Face validity: The degree to which items of a HR-PRO indeed look as though they are an adequate reflection of the construct to be measured.

Eric W. Jamoom

See also Health Outcomes Assessment; Health Status Measurement, Construct Validity; Health Status Measurement, Face and Content Validity; Health Status Measurement, Reliability and Internal Consistency; SF-36 and SF-12 Health Surveys

Further Readings

Barr, D. A. (2008). *Health disparities in the United States: Social class, race, ethnicity, and health.* Baltimore: Johns Hopkins University Press.

Iezzoni, L. I. (1997). *Risk adjustment for measuring healthcare outcomes.* Chicago: Health Administration Press.

Jamoom, E. W., Horner-Johnson, W., Suzuki, R., et al. (2008). Age at disability onset and self-reported health status. *BMC Public Health, 8,* 10.

Kane, R. L. (2006). *Understanding health care outcomes research.* Sudbury, MA: Jones & Bartlett.

Mokkink, L. B., Terwee, C. B., Knol, D. L., Stratford, P. W., Alonso, J., Patrick, D. L., et al. (2006). Protocol of the COSMIN study: COnsensus-based Standards for the selection of health Measurement INstruments. *BMC Medical Research Methodology, 6,* 2. Retrieved January 20, 2009, from http://www.biomedcentral.com/1471-2288/6/2

National Quality Measures Clearinghouse: http://www.qualitymeasures.ahrq.gov

Research at the Research Rehabilitation and Training Center: Health & Wellness: http://www.ohsu.edu/oidd/rrtc/research/index.cfm

SF-36.org: A community for measuring health outcomes using SF tools: http://www.sf-36.org

World Health Organization. (2003). *WHO definition of health*. Retrieved January 20, 2009, from http://www.who.int/about/definition/en/print.html

Health Utilities Index Mark 2 and 3 (HUI2, HUI3)

The Health Utility Index Mark 2 and 3 (HUI2 and HUI3, collectively referred to as HUI2/3) are generic preference-based health status measures designed to provide utility scores for health outcomes evaluation. The HUI2/3 measure is generic, applicable to a wide range of conditions, treatments, and populations. Preference-based design provides a single-summary numerical score for each health state defined by the instrument. This form of presenting health outcomes is particularly useful in economic evaluation, where a single index of health-related quality of life that summarizes health status utilities is needed. The first version of the HUI was created in the 1970s to evaluate the outcomes of neonatal intensive care for very-low-birth-weight infants. Since then the HUI measures have continued under development, and there are now two versions available: HUI Mark 2 and HUI Mark 3. Nowadays, the HUI1 is rarely applied, while the HUI2/3 is continually used. Both of these measures have been employed in various clinical studies, in economic evaluations, and in population health surveys.

The HUI Mark 2/3 is a multi-attribute health status measure. In such a measure, the defined health is expressed in terms of key attributes of interest. In other words, the descriptive system, which is known as a classification system, comprises chosen attributes and reflects the health definition adopted by the instrument developers. The term *attribute* used here is the same as the term *domain* or *dimension* defined in other measures.

Development

The first version of the HUI was developed based on the pioneering work on the Quality of Well-Being (QWB) instrument by Fanshel and Bush in 1970. The conceptual framework of the QWB provided a template for developing the HUI instrument. To evaluate the outcomes of neonatal intensive care for very-low-birth-weight infants, Torrance and his colleagues in the 1980s expanded the QWB's descriptive system into the classification system of the HUI Mark 1, which consisted of four attributes: (1) physical function, (2) role function, (3) social-emotional function, and (4) health problems, with six, five, four, and eight levels per attitude, respectively, thus defining a total of 960 unique health states.

The HUI Mark 1 was further extended for pediatric application. Aiming to measure the long-term outcome of childhood cancer, Cadman and his colleagues reviewed the literature and created a list of potentially important attributes for health-related quality of life. They invited 84 parent-and-child pairs to select the most important attributes from the list and, as a result, a core set with six attributes was created. These six attributes are (1) sensory and communication ability, (2) happiness, (3) self-care, (4) pain or discomfort, (5) earning and school ability, and (6) physical activity ability. The six attributes identified by Cadman and his colleagues, plus an attribute of fertility, for capturing the impact of child cancer treatment on fertility, became the HUI Mark 2 classification system. Each attribute has three to five levels of function and, therefore, defined 24,000 unique health states. Although the development of the HUI2 is for measuring treatment outcomes of children with cancer, the HUI2 soon was used as a generic measure for adults, and it was applied to different populations and conditions due to its generic-like attributes. It is suggested that the HUI2 can be used as a generic measure for the child population after removing the attribute of fertility.

The HUI3 was developed to tackle some concerns of the HUI2, to be structurally independent, and to be applicable in both clinical and general population studies. There are several changes in the HUI3's multi-attribute system as compared with its predecessor version. The changes included removing the attribute of self-care and replacing it with dexterity to achieve structural independency, adding distinct components of sensation such as vision, hearing, and speech, and excluding the attribute of fertility. Therefore, there are eight attributes in the HUI3 system: (1) vision, (2) hearing,

(3) speech, (4) ambulation, (5) dexterity, (6) emotion, (7) cognition, and (8) pain. Each attribute has five to six response levels that are combined in such a way that the HUI3 defines in total 972,000 unique health states.

As described by the instrument's developers, the choice of attributes in the HUI2/3 was based on a "within the skin" approach, focusing on the attributes of physical and emotional health status that are fundamentally most important to health status measurement and excluding the aspect of participation in society, as in social activity or role performance. Furthermore, the design of the descriptive system of the HUI2/3 was aimed to record functional capacity rather than performance. The reason for this was that a measure of performance reflects the level of capacity of an individual on a chosen function. Thus, people with the same underlying functional capacity could have a different level of performance.

Utility

As a preference-based measure, each health state defined by the HUI2/3 descriptive system can be assigned a utility score. It is calibrated by applying a formula (a scoring algorithm) to a health state, which essentially attaches values (also called weights) to each of the levels in each attribute. The HUI2 scoring algorithm was developed from the valuation of a random sample of 293 parents of schoolchildren in Hamilton, Ontario, Canada. Both visual analog scale (VAS) and standard gamble (SG) methods were adopted to elicit preferences from the sample. Each participant was asked to value 7 single-attribute states and 14 multi-attribute states using a VAS. Participants were also asked to value 4 multi-attribute states that overlapped with those 14 states in the previous task, using the SG method. Based on the data, a power transformation was developed to convert the value of the health state measured by the VAS into a utility value as elicited by the SG. The scoring algorithm was developed based on the multi-attribute utility theory, where utility function for each attribute was estimated separately and a multiplicative function form was adopted in the final scoring formula.

Multi-attribute utility theory (MAUT) is a method to estimate a mathematical function, which allows for calibration values for a large number of health states defined by a multi-attribute classification system, based on values of a small, carefully selected set of those states. The basic approach is to measure the utility function for each single attribute and to identify an equation that expresses the overall utility as a function of these single-attribute utilities (details can be found in the paper by Torrance and his colleagues published in 1996, as listed in Further Readings, below). MAUT can reduce the number of health states required for valuation to develop a scoring formula by assuming a function form in advance. The choice of functional form imposes a restriction in terms of how each attribute in the classification system is related to the others. There are three typical function forms available—additive, multiplicative, and multilinear. The evidence obtained from the HUI2 studies by Torrance and his colleagues supported the choice of multiplicative functional form (multilinear form was not considered because it requires the measurement of a large amount of multi-attribute health states for calculation).

One of the unique features of the MAUT method is the corner state. The corner state is a multi-attribute state, where one attribute is set at one extreme (the worst level of functioning) and the rest are set at the other extreme (the best level of functioning), and participants are asked to value several corner states. However, the structural independence of the classification system is a prerequisite for evaluating such corner states. For instance, participants could not imagine and consequently had difficulty valuing a corner state where a person was unable to control or use arms and legs (mobility attribute) but had no problem with self-care attributes such as eating, bathing, dressing, and using the toilet. Therefore, it is necessary to have no correlation between attributes—these must be structurally independent in such a way that each corner state, combining the worst level in one attribute with others at the best level, is possible. This issue was first found in the valuation study of the HUI2, and it has now been taken into account in the redesign of the HUI3. That is to say, the HUI3 is structurally independent.

The scoring formula of the HUI3 used a similar approach based on the responses from a representative sample of 504 adults from Hamilton, Ontario. Each participant was asked to value three anchor and three marker states and 22 to 24 multi-attribute health states using a VAS, plus 5 states using the SG method. The study also examined the possibility of applying a simplified multilinear functional form, but it was concluded that the multiplicative form performed better in such a degree that the final scoring algorithm was based on multiplicative form.

Both the HUI2 and HUI3 offer a single numerical score for health states, anchored at 0 and 1, representing death and full health, respectively. A negative score indicating worse than dead is also allowed. The range of possible utility scores is from 1 to −.03 for the HUI2 and from 1 to −.36 for the HUI3.

There is extensive evidence supporting the reliability, validity, and responsiveness of the HUI2/3. The interested reader can refer to additional sources such as McDowell or Horsman and his colleagues, as listed in Further Readings, below. The minimal clinically important difference between HUI scores ranges from .02 to .04.

Current Versions

Currently, there are several versions of the HUI2/3 questionnaires available, depending on administration, whether they are self- or proxy assessed, and recall period. The HUI2/3 can be either self-completed or interviewer administered over the phone or in person. Both self- and proxy assessment are available. There are four different standard recall periods for each questionnaire available: 1 week, 2 weeks, 4 weeks, and "usual." The questionnaire with recall periods in weeks is usually applied in clinical studies or economics evaluation, while the questionnaire with the recall period, "usual," which does not specify the time, is mostly applied in population health surveys.

The HUI2 and HUI3 can be combined and applied together, which is known as the HUI. The HUI includes both classifications of the HUI2 and HUI3 and generates utility scores for both the HUI2 and HUI3. Further information on the HUI instruments can be found at the Health Utilities Inc. Web site.

Ling-Hsiang Chuang

See also Health Status Measurement, Generic Versus Condition-Specific Measures; Multi-Attribute Utility Theory

Further Readings

Feeny, D. H., Furlong, W. J., Boyle, M., & Torrance, G. W. (1995). Multi-attribute health status classification systems: Health Utility Index. *PharmacoEconomics, 7*, 490–502.

Feeny, D. H., Furlong, W. J., Torrance, G. W., Goldsmith, C. H., Zenglong, Z., & Depauw, S. (2002). Multiattribute and single-attribute utility function: The Health Utility Index Mark 3 system. *Medical Care, 40*, 113–128.

Health Utilities Inc.: http://www.healthutilities.com

Horsman, J., Furlong, W., Feeny, D., & Torrance, G. (2003). The Health Utilities Index (HUI): Concepts, measurement properties and applications. *Health and Quality of Life Outcome, 1*, 54–67.

McDowell, I. (2006). *Measuring health: A guide to rating scales and questionnaires* (3rd ed.). New York: Oxford University Press.

Torrance, G. W., Feeny, D. H., Furlong, W. J., Barr, R. D., Zhang, Y., & Wang, Q. (1996). A multi-attribute utility function for a comprehensive health status classification system: Health Utilities Mark 2. *Medical Care, 34*, 702–722.

Torrance, G. W., Furlong, W. J., Feeny, D., & Boyle, M. (1995). Multi-attribute preference functions: Health Utility Index. *PharmacoEconomics, 7*, 490–502.

HEALTHY YEARS EQUIVALENTS

The healthy years equivalent (HYE) provides a user-friendly metric that is needed for improved communication within and among researchers, decision makers, practitioners, and consumers. Unlike the quality-adjusted life year (QALY), which means different things to different people and often is not consistent with the underlying principles of cost-utility analysis (CUA), the HYE means only one thing—it is a utility-based concept, derived from the individual's utility function by measuring the number of years in full health, holding other arguments in the utility function constant, that produces the same level of utility to the individual as produced by the potential lifetime health profile following a given intervention. The measurement of HYE requires that individuals will be allowed to reveal their true preferences. This is because it seems reasonable, when asking the public to assist in the determination of healthcare priorities, to choose measurement techniques that allow the public to reveal their true preferences even if this requires the use of more complex techniques. If not, why do we bother asking them at all?

Concept

The underlying premise of cost utility/effectiveness analysis (CUA/CEA) is that for a given level of resources available, society or the decision maker wishes to maximize the total aggregate health benefits conferred by a proposed treatment. The principles underlying CUA/CEA are concerned with the simultaneous satisfaction of efficiency in both production (i.e., making sure that each level of outcome is produced with the minimum amount of resources) and product mix (i.e., making sure that the allocation of available resources between different "products" is optimal). In this way, CUA/CEA is consistent with the principles of welfare economics theory and a welfarist approach to economics. But to achieve the goal of maximizing health-related well-being (i.e., utility associated with health benefits) from available resources, the methods used to measure health-related well-being must be consistent with the theories on which the welfarist approach and principles of CUA are based. Under the welfarist approach, an individual's preferences are embodied in that individual's utility function. Thus, for a measure of outcome to be consistent with the welfarist approach, and hence CUA/CEA principles, it must be consistent with a theory of utility. Health (i.e., an expected profile of health over lifetime) is one argument in an individual's utility function.

From the perspective of the economist qua economist, "pure utility" is sufficient for comparing alternatives on the basis of individuals' preferences. Hence, for a von Neumann-Morgenstern (vNM)–type individual, for example, a single standard gamble (SG) question can provide the utility score (i.e., number of utils) for any potential lifetime health profile. But the utils measure, and the notion of cost per util, may not be very meaningful to individuals and organizations making choices among programs associated with different expected health profiles. Abraham Mehrez and Amiram Gafni, who were the first to introduce the approach, explained that the HYE responds to the need to improve communication within and among researchers, managers, practitioners, and consumers in a way that is consistent with the concept of utility and hence represents individuals' preferences. The HYE is *not* a direct measure of utility. It is an attempt to reflect individuals' preferences concerning uncertain

health profiles using one argument in their utility function (i.e., duration), holding health status constant (i.e., full health). The intuitive appeal of years in full health has been established by the QALY measure, which was designed to be thought of as an equivalent number of years in full health—a number of quality-adjusted life years (QALYs). A different name was chosen to distinguish the HYE, which is a utility-based concept, from the QALY. Furthermore, it has been argued that length of life in full health—that is, healthy-years equivalent—represents a much simpler concept to explain to decision makers than the variable quality of life health status annuity, which the QALY represents.

The need for distinguishing HYEs from QALYs stems from the observation that QALYs mean different things to different people. In the health services research literature, most proponents and users of the QALY approach do not subscribe to the notion of an underlying utility model. For them, QALY is simply an index (i.e., the QALY measures years of life adjusted for their quality) with intuitive meaning. It is a measure of the individual's health status as distinct from the utility associated with this health state. There are others who subscribe to the concept of QALY as a measure of utility and who identify the utility model for which this would be the case. Those who subscribe to this concept face the problem of communication (i.e., the QALY is intended to measure the number of utils generated by a health profile, not adjusted years of life). Finally, there are those who view the QALY as an index, but one in which the weights attached to durations in different health states are calculated using utility theory, typically, vNM utility theory. It has been argued that this unit of output is therefore the utility-adjusted life year, which may or may not be as intuitively appealing as the quality-adjusted life year.

In terms of the conceptual limitations of the HYE, it has been noted that the HYE definition imposes the same restrictions as the QALY in terms of the (implicit) underlying assumptions of utility independence between health and other commodities in the individual's utility function. It has also been noted that the current definition of HYE is equally as restrictive as the QALY approach in terms of the exclusion of externalities (i.e., one person's health status may affect another person's utility) from the individual's utility function. It has been suggested that the concept of external effects is much more applicable in the case of healthcare consumption than for most other commodities because of the special nature of the commodity, "health," that healthcare is expected to produce. Hence, such effects should be included when measuring outcomes. Finally, both the HYE and QALY use the same aggregation method to arrive at a social preference—an individual's health is measured in terms of QALYs or HYEs, and the community's health is measured as the sum of QALYs or HYEs (i.e., an additive model). This may not be consistent with the equity criteria adopted for the analysis.

Measurement

Can an algorithm be developed to measure HYEs that (a) does not require additional assumptions (i.e., in addition to the assumptions of the underlying utility theory) and (b) is feasible to use with the intended subjects (i.e., the number and complexity of questions asked is not too burdensome)? Proponents of the QALY as a direct measure of utility model have recognized that the additional assumptions of this model are restrictive but justify its use on the basis of measurement feasibility (i.e., price worth paying). While recognizing the importance of measurement feasibility issues, let's deal first with the question of a measurement algorithm and then the issue of whether the trade-off between feasibility and validity is necessary or appropriate.

The concept of HYE does not require that an individual subscribe to expected (i.e., vNM) utility theory. Any type of utility theory (i.e., non-vNM) can be used as a basis for generating algorithms to measure HYEs, and the choice of utility theory will determine the method of measurement. The only requirement is that preferences for health profiles are measured under conditions of uncertainty to reflect the nature of the commodity, health. For the case of a utility maximizer (i.e., vNM)–type individual and for the case of a decision tree (a typical case in medical decision making), HYEs are measured using the two-stage lottery-based method as follows: In Stage 1, SG is used to measure the utility of all potential lifetime health profiles. These are then used in association with the *ex ante* probabilities of each potential profile to calculate the expected

utility of each treatment option, measured in utils. Note that, as explained above, this is sufficient to determine which treatment is preferred by the subject, but the outcomes measured have limited intuitive appeal for users. In Stage 2, the expected utils of each treatment option are converted to HYEs (i.e., more intuitively appealing years in full health equivalents) using again the SG method.

Does the algorithm described above provide scores for health profiles that accurately reflect an expected utility maximizer preference ordering? It has been shown that in the case of uncertainty, *ex ante* HYEs always rank risky health profiles the same way as expected utility. The assumptions needed for the other measures are risk neutrality with respect to healthy time for expected HYEs; risk neutrality with respect to time in all health states and additive independence of quality in different periods for risk-neutral QALYs; and constant proportional risk posture with respect to time in all health states and additive independence of quality in different periods for risk-averse QALYs. In other words, it is possible to develop algorithms to measure HYEs in a way that either does not require additional assumptions to those required by the chosen utility theory or requires fewer and weaker assumptions as compared with those required by the QALY model. Thus, for those interested in a utility-based measure that has intuitive appeal to users while preserving the individual's preference ordering, the HYE concept provides a measure superior to the QALY.

In terms of the feasibility of the HYE measure, "the jury is still out." Measuring HYEs is likely to involve greater respondent burden, mainly in terms of the number of questions being asked. That it may be more complex and time-consuming does not imply that it should not or cannot be used at all. This has resulted in a debate between those who are willing to add assumptions (typically invalid assumptions such as additive independence) to ease the measurement burden and those who would like to relax as many assumptions as possible even at a price of a more complex technique. The need to simplify the assessment task (i.e., reduce the number of questions asked to generate HYE scores) is most evident in the case of large decision trees. This is because the number of different potential lifetime health profiles is likely to be large. However, there are many assumptions that researchers are making to populate large decision trees with numerical values. More empirical work is required to systematically test whether the use of more accurate measures of preference in the context of smaller and simpler decision trees provides more or less accurate ranking of societal preference as compared with the use of less accurate measures of preference in the context of large decision trees.

Finally, it has been suggested that, in principle, one can try to estimate the certainty equivalent number of HYEs that will always rank risky health profiles according to individual preferences using a time trade-off (TTO) question. In this case, the risky health profile to be assessed is framed as a probability distribution and is equated to the certainty equivalent number of healthy years. Note that this technique does not require that an individual be an expected utility maximizer. However, whether this could be done in practice is not known, as it is unclear whether that type of information can be processed in a meaningful way.

Amiram Gafni

See also Cost-Effectiveness Analysis; Cost-Utility Analysis; Expected Utility Theory; Quality-Adjusted Life Years (QALYs); Utility Assessment Techniques; Welfare, Welfarism, and Extrawelfarism

Further Readings

Ben Zion, U., & Gafni, A. (1983). Evaluation of public investment in health care: Is the risk irrelevant? *Journal of Health Economics, 2,* 161–165.

Bleichrodt, H. (1995). QALYs and HYEs: Under what conditions are they equivalent? *Journal of Health Economics, 14,* 17–37.

Gafni, A. (1994). The standard gamble method: What is being measured and how it is interpreted. *Health Services Research, 29,* 207–224.

Gafni, A., & Birch, S. (1995). Preferences for outcomes in economic evaluation: An economic approach in addressing economic problems. *Social Science and Medicine, 40,* 767–776.

Gafni, A., & Birch, S. (1997). QALYs and HYEs: Spotting the differences. *Journal of Health Economics, 16,* 601–608.

Gafni, A., & Birch, S. (2006). Incremental cost-effectiveness ratios (ICERs): The silence of the lambda. *Social Science and Medicine, 62,* 2091–2100.

Johannesson, M. (1995). The ranking properties of healthy years equivalents and quality adjusted life years under certainty and uncertainty. *International Journal of Health Technology Assessment in Health Care, 11,* 40–48.

Mehrez, A., & Gafni, A. (1989). Quality-adjusted life-years (QALYs), utility theory and Healthy Years Equivalent (HYE). *Medical Decision Making, 9,* 142–149.

Ried, W. (1998). QALYs versus HYEs: What's right and what's wrong. A review of the controversy. *Journal of Health Economics, 17,* 607–625.

HEDONIC PREDICTION AND RELATIVISM

Standard decision theory assumes that when choosing between options that have the same costs, decision makers evaluate which option will deliver the highest expected outcome utility and choose that option. This is known as a consequentialist utility analysis method. In reality, people rarely base their decisions strictly on this approach. In recent years, behavioral decision theorists have proposed that choices are often driven by decision makers' affect, or predicted experience, toward the choice options, and that such affect-driven decisions often lead to choices different from those that the standard utility analysis would prescribe. For example, before making a decision, they tend to think about the emotions that the outcomes of their choices are likely to trigger (i.e., decision makers predict their hedonic experiences). Evidence from behavioral decision research suggests that the emotions people expect to experience in the future are important determinants of their behavior. As a result of this development, decision theorists now make a distinction among three types of utilities—decision utility (as revealed by one's choice), experienced utility (feelings with the chosen option), and predicted utility (prediction of experienced utility). The last few decades have witnessed a large amount of research on the inconsistency between predicted and actual experience.

Hedonic Prediction

Hedonic prediction is a term denoting people's current judgments about what their emotions (e.g., happiness, distress, pain, fear) or preferences (e.g., for different health states or treatments) will be in the future. A substantial body of empirical research from a range of medical and nonmedical domains demonstrates that people typically exaggerate their emotional reactions (positive or negative) to future events. The emotions that have been investigated include pain, fear, and subjective well-being (happiness). For example, people tend to overpredict different types of acute pain (e.g., menstruation pain, headache, postoperative pain, dental pain) and chronic pain (e.g., arthritis pain and low back pain). Overprediction has also been observed when people forecast emotions such as fear and anxiety. For example, people overpredict their fear of dental treatments, confined spaces, snakes, and spiders.

Researchers have also investigated people's forecasts of the impact of specific positive and negative events that affect their well-being (such as significant life events, medical results, and treatments). In general, people overpredict the hedonic impact of negative events. For example, patients about to undergo surgically necessary amputations delay or opt out of the operations because they anticipate that their lives will be ruined without a limb. Similarly, women were found to overpredict their distress after receiving positive test results for unwanted pregnancies. There is also evidence that dieters overpredict their distress after being unable to achieve their weight-loss targets. One study demonstrated that people also overpredict the level of distress experienced by other people, for example, after positive HIV test results. People also tend to overpredict the impact of positive events. Existing evidence suggests that patients who decide to undergo cosmetic surgery are not necessarily happier after it. People are also found to overpredict the relief in distress that people with negative results experienced. Other studies have shown that people exaggerate the positive effect of a lottery win on their life, the pleasure that they will derive from a future holiday trip, and the happiness that they will experience if their favorite sports team wins.

Other related research suggests that people often have poor intuitions about the hedonic impact of gains and losses. For example, people overestimate how much hedonic benefit they will derive from small gains. People also believe that they will return to their hedonic baselines more quickly after a small loss than after a large loss even when the opposite is true. People also expect that the hedonic cost of a loss will be greater than the hedonic benefit of an equal-sized gain even when this is not so. People often think that they would be willing to pay the same amount to gain an item as to avoid losing it, while, in reality, they are willing to pay less.

In summary, the anticipation of unpleasant life events such as illnesses may be different from the actual experience of the event. In light of this difference, health economists have outlined a dual model for the evaluation of patients' preferences, which assesses patients' anticipation of an illness separately from their experience of it. Psychological accounts for the documented errors in hedonic prediction include the *projection bias*, according to which people underestimate or even completely ignore their ability to adapt to new circumstances and, as a result, tend to exaggerate the impact of positive and negative events on their well-being. Another psychological account is based on the *focusing illusion*, which states that people focus too much on the event in question (e.g., illness or treatment) and neglect other life events that will occur simultaneously with the event at the center of the attentional focus. As a result of this neglect of future events that will be competing for attention with the key event, people produce exaggerated predictions of the hedonic impact of the latter on their subjective well-being.

Relativism

When people make a choice, they tend to contemplate how they will feel if the alternative that they choose turns out not to be the best one. Such counterfactuals, between the expected outcome and those that would occur if a different choice was made, shape many decisions because they tend to trigger anticipated regret. According to regret-based models of decision making, the utility of a choice option (and, hence, the likelihood of selecting it) should depend on both anticipated regret and the subjective value of the option. Empirical research has documented that regret has a powerful effect on choice. For example, people feel regret after both action and inaction due to anticipated counterfactual regret (after receiving the outcomes arising from a choice, people experience emotions as a result of these outcomes and also as a result of the counterfactual comparisons of what the outcomes would have been, had they chosen differently). Some argue that all behavioral choices necessarily involve potential regret. This shows that the alternate option in a choice set influences the evaluation of each option, that is, that judgment and choices are relative, because the utility of an option is not independent of alternative options in a choice set. Such relativity has been demonstrated in studies showing that anticipated regret is exacerbated when people expect to receive feedback on the outcome of the foregone alternatives.

This relativistic paradigm is in line with behavioral evidence that people generate more accurate affective forecasts when they see an event within its context of other events. The explanation for this finding is that, by eliciting a context (i.e., the full set of outcomes), people realize that the specific event (or decision in question) is only one among many determinants of their well-being and often not the most important one. For example, some authors suggest that being exposed to other patients' posttreatment experience would allow patients to put a very unpleasant treatment within the context of the rest of their lives. The patients could then realize that what appears to be the focus of their lives at the time of the decision (i.e., the treatment and its consequences) may not be the focus of their lives later on.

Relativistic comparisons can also create certain biases. For example, when people miss a good bargain, they are less likely to take a subsequent one that is not as good. This phenomenon is termed *inaction inertia*, and according to regret-based explanations of it, people anticipate that buying the item will lead to regret, because it will remind them that they missed a better opportunity to buy it. This relativistic strategy is used when the difference between the previous and subsequent bargains is large. Studies have investigated the intensity of emotions caused by relativistic forecasts and have found poor accuracy in the prediction of the intensity of emotions. For example, in a negotiation task, subjects who made high offers overrated the regret that they would experience after they failed at a negotiation in which they had expected to succeed. Similar findings were obtained for disappointment. In another study, participants overrated the rejoicing that they would experience when they received marks for their coursework that were better than

what they had expected. Thus, this line of research demonstrates systematic prediction errors in both negative and positive decision-related hedonic forecasts. This evidence corroborates and complements previous work, in which accuracy was assessed by comparing judgments of forecasted with experienced emotions. One such study compared forecasted regret if a contest was lost with the experienced regret reported when respondents were led to believe that they had lost that contest. The forecasted predictions were overrated relative to the experienced regret. Similar findings emerged from two additional studies, in which commuters making only forecasting judgments overrated the regret that experiencing commuters reported after missing a train.

Note that some studies show the opposite effect of relativistic biases—that people underweight their expected emotional experiences. For example, if people are asked to analyze reasons before making a decision, then they are less likely to choose the option they will like later on (as compared with people not asked to analyze such reasons). Some researchers suggest that analyzing reasons focuses the decision maker's attention on more tangible attributes along which to compare the choice options (such as cost and benefits) and away from less perceptible feelings. Other research shows that if people are not explicitly asked to analyze reasons, they may still choose options that are rationalistic but inconsistent with predicted preferences; it suggests that people automatically seek rationalism in decision making (i.e., they spontaneously focus on rationalistic attributes such as economic values, quantitative specifications, and functions).

Shared Decision Making

Clinicians, healthcare experts, and policy makers have argued for shared decision making between patients and doctors regarding choice of medical and surgical treatments. According to this framework, the patient is a key medical decision maker in the care plan. At the center of such care plans are patient preferences, which are usually defined as positive or negative attitudes toward bundles of outcomes such as disease or treatment. However, since preferences can be predicted or experienced, a more precise definition should define them in terms of the experienced and predicted (positive or negative) feelings and emotions that patients associate with a disease and with the outcomes of its possible treatments. However, behavioral evidence suggests that people are poor at predicting the impact of an illness and its treatment on their subjective well-being, which suggests that they have little understanding of their own future feelings and preferences. Future research should aim to reveal how patients' self-forecasts affect their choice of treatments and whether such biased forecasts could be made more accurate.

Ivo Vlaev and Ray Dolan

See also Decision Making and Affect; Decisions Faced by Patients: Primary Care; Emotion and Choice; Experience and Evaluations; Health Outcomes Assessment; Models of Physician-Patient Relationship; Patient Decision Aids; Regret; Shared Decision Making; Utility Assessment Techniques

Further Readings

Dolan, P. (1999). Whose preferences count? *Medical Decision Making, 19,* 482–486.

Dolan, P., & Kahneman, D. (2008). Interpretations of utility and their implications for the valuation of health. *Economic Journal, 118,* 215–234.

Hsee, C. K., Zhang, J., Yu, F., & Xi, Y. (2003). Lay rationalism and inconsistency between predicted experience and decision. *Journal of Behavioral Decision Making, 16,* 257–272.

Sevdalis, N., & Harvey, N. (2006). Predicting preferences: A neglected aspect of shared decision-making. *Health Expectations, 9,* 245–251.

Sevdalis, N., & Harvey, N. (2007). Biased forecasting of post-decisional affect. *Psychological Science, 18,* 678–681.

Wilson, T. D., Wheatley, T., Meyers, J. M., Gilbert, D. T., & Axsom, D. (2000). Focalism: A source of durability bias in affective forecasting. *Journal of Personality and Social Psychology, 78,* 821–836.

Zeelenberg, M. (1999). Anticipated regret, expected feedback and behavioral decision-making. *Journal of Behavioral Decision Making, 12,* 93–106.

HEURISTICS

The term *heuristic* is of Greek origin and means serving to assist in finding out or discovering something. Imagine that you feel sick and decide to visit a doctor. He diagnoses heart disease and prescribes a new treatment. You might want to hear the opinion of a second expert before starting the treatment. You visit another doctor, who recommends a different medication. Now you must make up your mind rather quickly about which doctor you should trust. Inferential accuracy is also crucial: An error in judgment might lead to becoming more ill or even dying. How do doctors and patients solve the challenging task of making treatment decisions under time pressure and with limited information? One way to do it is to rely on heuristics.

There are two views on heuristics in the psychological literature. According to one line of thought, they are error-prone reasoning strategies that can lead to a number of cognitive illusions and biases. In another view, heuristics are cognitive shortcuts that can lead to as good or even better judgments than more complex decision strategies.

Error-Prone Reasoning Strategies

The first view of heuristics is the result of measuring human decision making against various normative standards, such as probability theory and logic. This research program was sparked by the seminal work of Daniel Kahneman and Amos Tversky in the 1970s. By comparing human reasoning and intuitive judgment with ideal standards of rationality, researchers within this program hoped to gain insight into the underlying psychological processes. Often, though, the program is charged with supporting the view that people are inherently faulty decision makers who use cognitive shortcuts that can lead to systematic errors.

Two of the more well-known heuristics studied in this program are *representativeness* and *availability*. Daniel Kahneman and Amos Tversky proposed that when using the representativeness heuristic, people judge the likelihood that an event belongs to a certain class, or is generated by a certain process, on the basis of its similarity to that class or process, neglecting its prior probability of occurrence. For example, most people will judge that the sequence of coin tosses head-tail-head-tail-tail-head is more likely than head-head-head-tail-tail-tail, because the former is perceived to be more representative of a random sample of coin tosses.

When people use the availability heuristic, they are estimating the likelihood of an event on the basis of how easily instances of the event come to mind. For example, people may overestimate the likelihood of certain causes of death, such as tornado or flood, because they are vivid and more likely to be talked about. In contrast, the likelihood of some more frequent but less "exciting" causes of death, such as heart attack or stroke, is underestimated.

This view of heuristics has spread to medical decision making. For instance, in a seminal study of how physicians process information about the results of mammography, David Eddy gave 100 physicians information about the prior probability that a patient has breast cancer, the hit rate or sensitivity of mammography, and the false-positive rate and asked them to estimate the probability that a patient with a positive mammogram actually has breast cancer. Eddy reported that most of the physicians had difficulties with probabilities and concluded that the physicians' judgments systematically deviated from statistical rules such as Bayes's rule, emphasizing cognitive illusions. Similar results were reported with physicians and students. From these studies, many researchers have concluded that the human mind does not appear to follow the calculus of chance or the statistical theory of prediction. If these conclusions are right, there is little hope for physicians and their patients.

Researchers tried to solve this problem by training the physicians to use decision-support tools, which weight and combine the relevant information by using regression, instead of relying on their intuitive judgment. For instance, physicians at the University of Michigan Hospital are trained to use the Heart Disease Predictive Instrument, which consists of a chart listing approximately 50 probabilities. The physicians have to check for the presence or absence of seven symptoms (evidence of which is routinely obtained during the patient's admission process) and can then find the probability that the patient has heart disease. The probability scores are generated from a logistic regression formula that combines and weights the dichotomous information on the seven symptoms. When using the Heart Disease Predictive Instrument, physicians achieve more accurate decisions than when they rely on their intuitive judgment. Many

doctors, however, are not happy using this and similar systems, typically because they do not understand logistic regression. Even though this understanding is not necessary to use the prediction systems, the lack of transparency and the dependence on probability charts leaves them uncomfortable.

There is, however, an alternative: Another view of heuristics is that they are cognitive strategies that can provide good solutions to complex problems under restrictions of time and cognitive capacity.

Cognitive Shortcuts

The concept of cognitive shortcuts providing good solutions is the opposite of the traditional view that human decision making should be evaluated in comparison with models of unbounded rationality, such as Bayesian or subjective expected utility models or logistic regression. These models must often assume—unrealistically—that people can predict all consequences of their choices, are able to assign them a joint probability distribution, and can order them using a single utility function. But in real life, people rarely have the time or cognitive capacity to think of all the possible scenarios for the future, their likelihood, and their subjective utilities. Real life often involves so many possible choices and so many possible outcomes that the optimal solution to a problem rarely exists, or if it does, the solution requires prohibitively long and complex computations. Instead of trying to find the best solution, people may *satisfice*—that is, look for solutions that are good enough for their current purposes. The father of this *bounded rationality* view, Herbert Simon, argued that people rely on simple strategies that can successfully deal with situations of sparse resources.

A recent representative of the bounded rationality approach is the simple heuristics research program. This approach, championed by Gerd Gigerenzer, Peter M. Todd, and the ABC Research Group, proposes that heuristics may be the only available approach to decision making for the many problems for which optimal solutions do not exist. Moreover, even when exact solutions do exist, domain-specific decision heuristics may be more effective than domain-general approaches, which are often computationally unfeasible. This research program focuses on precisely specified computational models of fast and frugal heuristics and how they are matched to the ecological structure of particular decision environments. It also explores the ways that evolution may have achieved this match in human behavior.

In line with this approach, Lee Green and David R. Mehr constructed a simple heuristic for the patient admission process in a coronary unit. This heuristic, a fast and frugal decision tree, relies on simple building blocks for searching for information, stopping the information search, and finally making a decision. Specifically, it first ranks the predictors according to a simple criterion (the predictor with the highest sensitivity first, the predictor with the highest specificity second, and so on), and information search follows this order. Second, the search can stop after each predictor; the rest are ignored. Third, the strategy does not combine—weight and add—the predictors. Only one predictor determines each decision. This decision rule is an example of one-reason decision making.

The fast and frugal decision tree proposed by Green and Mehr works as follows: If a patient has a certain anomaly in his electrocardiogram, he is immediately admitted to the coronary care unit. No other information is searched for. If this is not the case, a second variable is considered: whether the patient's primary complaint is chest pain. If this is not the case, he is immediately classified as low risk and assigned to a regular nursing bed. No further information is considered. If the answer is yes, then a third and final question is asked: whether he has had a heart attack before. The fast and frugal decision tree thus ignores all 50 probabilities of the original Heart Disease Predictive Instrument and asks only a few yes-or-no questions.

The fast and frugal tree, just like the Heart Disease Predictive Instrument, can be evaluated on multiple performance criteria. Accuracy is one criterion, and it turns out that the tree is more accurate in classifying heart attack patients than both physicians' intuition and the Heart Disease Predictive Instrument. Specifically, it assigned correctly the largest proportion of patients who subsequently had a myocardial infarction to the coronary care unit. At the same time, it had a comparatively low false alarm rate. Being able to make a decision fast with only limited information is a second criterion, which is essential in situations where slow decision making can cost a life. The fast and frugal decision tree uses less information than the expert system and uses less sophisticated statistical calculations. A third criterion is the transparency of a decision system. Unlike logistic regression, the steps of the fast and frugal tree are transparent and easy to teach. Therefore, in complex situations such as the patient admission process in a coronary unit, less is more. Simplicity can pay off.

Another well-studied cognitive strategy within the simple heuristics program is take-the-best, which is a domain-specific rather than a general problem-solving strategy, meaning that it is useful in some environments and for some problems but not for all. When using this heuristic, people infer which of two objects has a higher value on some criterion based on just one reason, or cue. An example would be inferring which of the two cities has a higher mortality rate based on the average January temperature, the relative pollution potential, or the average percentage of relative humidity. Like the fast and frugal decision tree of Green and Mehr, this heuristic considers cues sequentially in the order of how indicative they are of the objects' values and makes a decision based on the first cue that discriminates between objects. This heuristic is particularly successful when one cue is much more important than other cues, but it has been shown to be as good as computationally more demanding procedures in other environments, as well.

Empirical evidence suggests that take-the-best is a plausible behavioral model, especially when searching for information in the environment is costly or when decisions have to be made under time pressure. By "betting on one good reason" and disregarding the surplus information, this fast and frugal heuristic may be particularly useful for patient populations whose computational resources are limited due to aging or illness.

Future Research

Medical situations promote the use of heuristics because decisions in such contexts often need to be made under pressure and with limited information. Fast and frugal heuristics for medical decision making have the potential to be powerful alternatives to the prescriptions of classical decision theory for patient care. A strategy that ignores information and forgoes computation can be not only faster, more frugal, and transparent but also more accurate. Simple tools for making accurate decisions under time pressure in the medical arena should be a major research topic for future investigation.

Rocio Garcia-Retamero and Mirta Galesic

See also Bias; Bounded Rationality and Emotions; Decision Making and Affect; Motivation; Trust in Healthcare

Further Readings

Garcia-Retamero, R., Hoffrage, U., & Dieckmann, A. (2007). When one cue is not enough: Combining fast and frugal heuristics with compound cue processing. *Quarterly Journal of Experimental Psychology, 60,* 1197–1215.

Garcia Retamero, R., Hoffrage, U., Dieckmann, A., & Ramos, M. (2007). Compound cue processing within the fast and frugal heuristic approach in non-linearly separable environments. *Learning & Motivation, 38,* 16–34.

Gigerenzer, G., & Goldstein, D. G. (1996). Reasoning the fast and frugal way: Models of bounded rationality. *Psychological Review, 103,* 650–669.

Gigerenzer, G., & Kurzenhäuser, S. (2005). Fast and frugal heuristics in medical decision making. In R. Bibace, J. D. Laird, K. L. Noller, & J. Valsiner (Eds.), *Science and medicine in dialogue: Thinking through particulars and universals* (pp. 3–15). Westport, CT: Praeger.

Gigerenzer, G., Todd, P. M., & the ABC Research Group. (1999). *Simple heuristics that make us smart.* New York: Oxford University Press.

Green, L., & Mehr, D. R. (1997). What alters physicians' decisions to admit to the coronary care unit? *Journal of Family Practice, 45,* 219–226.

Kahneman, D., Slovic, P., & Tversky, A. (1982). *Judgment under uncertainty: Heuristics and biases.* Cambridge, UK: Cambridge University Press.

Kahneman, D., & Tversky, A. (1973). On the psychology of prediction. *Psychological Review, 80,* 237–251.

Pozen, M. W., D'Agostino, R. B., Selker, H. P., Sytkowski, P. A., & Hood, W. B. (1984). A predictive instrument to improve coronary-care-unit admission practices in acute ischemic heart disease. *New England Journal of Medicine, 310,* 1273–1278.

Simon, H. A. (1983). Alternative visions of rationality. In H. A. Simon (Ed.), *Reason in human affairs* (pp. 7–35). Stanford, CA: Stanford University Press.

Tversky, A., & Kahneman, D. (1974). Judgment under uncertainty: Heuristics and biases. *Science, 185,* 1124–1131.

HOLISTIC MEASUREMENT

Holistic measurement is an approach to the measurement of preferences for health states or treatments in which a rater assigns values to each possible health state or treatment, where a state or treatment represents a combination of many attributes. During the assessment, the rater thus considers all the relevant attributes simultaneously.

Valuing Health States or Treatments

Basically, there are two different approaches to measuring preferences for health states, services, or treatments: the holistic and the decomposed. The decomposed approach expresses the overall value as a decomposed function of the attributes. It enables the investigator to obtain values for all health states or treatments without requiring the rater to assign values to every state or treatment; the rater is asked to value the attributes only. Holistic measurement is mostly used for health state valuation, but in some instances, it is used for the valuation of treatments or services as well, for example, in the willingness-to-pay method and the treatment trade-off method.

Holistic valuations of health states encompass valuations of the quality of life of those states, and the valuations are therefore sometimes called preference-based measures of quality of life, as distinct from descriptive measures of quality of life. Descriptive measures of quality of life generally generate quality-of-life profiles, that is, a combination of scores on different dimensions of quality of life, such as physical functioning, emotional functioning, and social functioning. A well-known example of such a descriptive instrument is the Medical Outcomes Study SF-36. These descriptive approaches to quality-of-life evaluation are not suitable for the purpose of decision making. In decision making, different attributes of treatment outcomes have to be weighed. On the one hand, different aspects of quality of life may have to be balanced against each other. Does, for example, the better pain relief from a new neuralgia medication outweigh the side effects, such as sedation and confusion? On the other hand, quality of life and length of life may have to be weighed against each other. Does the increased survival from chemotherapy outweigh the side effects, or, on the contrary, are patients willing to trade off survival for improved quality of life? For such decisional purposes, a valuation of the health outcome is needed.

Holistic Methods

Several holistic methods exist to assess preference-based measures of quality of life. The standard gamble and the time trade-off measure the utility of a health state, a cardinal measure of the strength of an individual's preference for particular outcomes when faced with uncertainty.

Standard Gamble

In the standard gamble method, a subject is offered the hypothetical choice between the sure outcome A (living his remaining life expectancy in the health state to be valued) and the gamble B. The gamble has a probability p of the best possible outcome (usually optimal health, defined as 1) and a probability $(1 - p)$ of the worst possible outcome (usually immediate death, defined as 0). By varying p, the value at which the subject is indifferent to the choice between the sure outcome and the gamble is obtained. The utility for the sure outcome, the state to be valued, is equal to the value of p at the point of indifference ($U = p \times 1 + (1 - p) \times 0 = p$).

Time Trade-Off

In the time trade-off method, a subject is asked to choose between his remaining life expectancy in the state to be valued and a shorter life span in normal health. In other words, he is asked whether he would be willing to trade years of his remaining life expectancy to avoid the state to be valued. As an example, a 65-year-old man is asked how many years x in a state of optimal health he considers equivalent to a period of 15 years (his remaining life expectancy) in a disability state. By varying the

duration of x, the point is found where he is indifferent to the choice between the two options. The simplest and most common way to transform this optimal health equivalent x into a utility (ranging from 0 to 1) is to divide x by 15.

Visual Analog Scale

A visual analog scale is a rating scale, a simple method that can be self-administered and, therefore, is often used to obtain evaluations of health states. Subjects are asked to rate the state by placing a mark on a 100-mm horizontal or vertical line, anchored by optimal health and death (or sometimes best possible health and worst possible health). The score is the number of millimeters from the "death" anchor to the mark, divided by 100.

The visual analog scale does not reflect any trade-off that a subject may be willing to make in order to obtain better health, either in terms of risk or in years of life. It can therefore not be considered a preference-based method, and transformations have been proposed to approximate standard gamble or time trade-off utilities. The choice of the method is still a matter of an ongoing debate. All three methods have been shown to be subject to biases in the elicitation process, but many of these biases can be explained by prospect theory.

Magnitude Estimation

Magnitude estimation is a scaling method that was developed by psychophysicists to overcome the limitations of the rating scales, that is, the lack of ratio-level measurement and the tendency of respondents to use categories equally often (verbal scale) or not to use the upper and lower ends of the scale (visual analog scale). The respondent is given a standard health state and asked to provide a number or ratio indicating how much better or worse each of the other states is as compared with the standard. For example, the research participants are instructed to assign the number 10 to the first case, the standard. Then a case that is half as desirable receives the number 5, and a case that is regarded as twice as desirable is given the number 20. Magnitude estimation is seldom used, since it is not based on any theory of measurement and since the scores have no obvious meaning in the context of decision making. They do not reflect utility and as such cannot be used in decision analyses.

Person Trade-Off

A different variant called the person trade-off has gained popularity among health economists and policy makers. It was formerly known as the equivalence method, and the task is to determine how many people in health state X are equivalent to a specified number of people in health state Y. From a policy perspective, the person trade-off seeks information similar to that required by policy makers. It has been used in the elicitation of disability weights for the DALYs (disability-adjusted life years), a measure used by the World Health Organization as a summary measure of population health.

Willingness-to-Pay

The willingness to pay is a method used primarily by health economists. To value health states, it asks the respondents what amount, or what percentage of their household income, they would be willing to pay to move from a less desirable state to a state of optimal health. More frequently, it is used to assess respondents' willingness to pay for treatments and services. It is most commonly used in cost-benefit analyses, in which all outcomes are expressed in monetary terms, in contrast to cost-effectiveness analyses, in which health outcomes are expressed in (quality-adjusted) life years. As is the case for magnitude estimation and the person trade-off method, this method does not result in a utility.

Probability Trade-Off

The probability trade-off or treatment trade-off method assesses, in a holistic manner, respondents' strength of preference for a treatment (relative to another treatment). In these methods, preferences for combined process and outcome paths are elicited in the following way. The patient is presented with two clinical options, for example, Treatments A and B, which are described with respect to (chances of) benefits and side effects, and is asked to state a preference for a treatment. If Treatment A is preferred, the interviewer systematically either increases the probability of benefit from Treatment B, or reduces the probability of benefit from Treatment A (and vice versa if Treatment B is preferred). The particular aspects of the treatments that are altered in this way, and the direction in which they are changed, are decided on beforehand, according to the clinical characteristics of the problem and the nature of the research question. For example, these may include the probability of side effects of treatment, risk of recurrence, or chance of survival. The relative strength of preference for a treatment is assessed by determining the patient's willingness to accept side effects of that treatment or forego benefits of the alternative treatment. This general approach has been adapted specifically to a variety of treatment decisions. Examples are decisions about adjuvant chemotherapy in breast cancer, benign prostatic hypertrophy, treatment of lupus nephritis, and radiotherapy for breast cancer.

The resulting preference scores are idiosyncratic to the original decision problem, and only the strength of preference for Treatment A relative to Treatment B is obtained, not a utility. For formal decision analysis they are therefore not suitable. However, for decision support they seem appropriate as they are tailored to the clinical problem at hand and will reflect the real-life situation more than does utility assessment. These methods have indeed been used "at the bedside," using decision boards as visual aids. They seem a promising way to help patients who wish to engage in decision making to clarify and communicate their values.

Anne M. Stiggelbout

See also Contingent Valuation; Decomposed Measurement; Person Trade-Off; Prospect Theory; Utility Assessment Techniques; Willingness to Pay

Further Readings

Bleichrodt, H. (2002). A new explanation for the difference between time trade-off utilities and standard gamble utilities. *Health Economics, 11,* 447–456.

Llewellyn-Thomas, H. A. (1997). Investigating patients' preferences for different treatment options. *Canadian Journal of Nursing Research, 29,* 45–64.

Stiggelbout, A. M., & De Haes, J. C. J. M. (2001). Patient preference for cancer therapy: An overview of measurement approaches. *Journal of Clinical Oncology, 19,* 220–230.

HUMAN CAPITAL APPROACH

The human capital approach to economic evaluation places a monetary value on loss of health as the lost value of economic productivity due to ill health, disability, or premature mortality. More specifically, the human capital approach uses the present value of expected future earnings, often adjusted for nonmarket productivity, to estimate the potential loss to society if an individual dies or becomes permanently disabled. It is commonly employed in cost-of-illness (COI) analyses that distinguish between direct costs, chiefly medical care, and the indirect costs of lost productivity. It is also employed in certain cost-effectiveness and cost-benefit analyses, particularly in older publications.

The idea that a human life can be valued by capitalizing the value of future earnings goes back to Sir William Petty in England in the late 1600s. The application of human capital to economic evaluation of health interventions can be traced to Burton Weisbrod in the 1960s. Under this approach, productivity is calculated as the present value of the sum of expected labor market earnings in future years, adjusted for life table survival probabilities and discounting. It is standard practice to take the current pattern of average earnings stratified by age and sex and assume that an individual's earnings trajectory will trace the same pattern, adjusted for expected increases in future labor productivity and inflation-adjusted earnings. For example, in the United States, it is conventional to assume that future labor productivity will increase at 1% per year. If one combines this with a 3% discount rate as is recommended in the United States, one gets estimates roughly equivalent to use of a 2% discount rate without assuming future productivity increases.

It is standard in health economic evaluations to include the imputed value of household production as well as paid earnings in human capital estimates, although cost-benefit analyses in environmental policy typically do not do so. The inclusion of household productivity is particularly important for older people and women, who tend to have high values of household productivity relative to paid compensation. Time spent in household production can be valued using either the individual's own wage or imputed wage (opportunity cost method) or the average wage paid to workers performing similar services (replacement cost method); the latter is more commonly employed. The original justification for the inclusion of household services was to reduce the lower valuation placed on women's lives because of lower labor force participation. Although in principle one could put a monetary value on other uses of time, such as volunteer service and leisure, this is rarely done.

Earnings are typically calculated as gross earnings, including payroll taxes and employee benefits, and are intended to capture the full cost of employee compensation. The rationale for the human capital approach is that the marginal productivity of labor is equal to the compensation paid to the average employee and that the withdrawal of that individual's labor due to premature death or permanent disability would result in a loss to society of that individual's future production. In most applications, average earnings are estimated for everyone within a given age-group, stratified only by gender. This avoids the ethical problems that can result from using different earnings for individuals of different socioeconomic or ethnic groups, which can have the effect of causing diseases affecting disadvantaged groups to appear less costly. The same argument can be applied to the use of sex-specific earnings estimates, given that in almost all countries average earnings are lower for women than for men, even after taking household services into account.

The chief alternative to the human capital approach is the friction cost approach developed by Dutch economists in the 1990s who objected that the presence of unemployed labor made human capital estimates of productivity losses too high. This approach presumes that replacement workers are readily available and that the only loss in productivity due to a worker's death or disability is the short-term cost of recruiting and training a replacement worker. Human capital estimates of productivity losses are many times higher than those calculated using the friction cost method.

Older cost-benefit analyses typically used the human capital approach to put a monetary value on lost life. In recent decades, it has become standard to use estimates of willingness-to-pay (WTP) to value health, particularly in environmental and transportation policy analyses. WTP estimates of the value of a statistical life based on occupational mortality and compensating wage differentials are typically several times higher than human capital estimates. Unlike WTP estimates, human capital estimates do not place a monetary value on pain and suffering or the grief experienced by family members and friends at the loss of a loved one. Because of the difficulty in putting a monetary value on such intangible costs, cost-benefit analyses published in medical journals often use the human capital approach for monetary valuations of health, which results in relatively conservative estimates of benefits as compared with cost-benefit analyses using WTP estimates.

Older cost-effectiveness analyses also often included productivity costs. However, the U.S. Panel on Cost-Effectiveness in Health and Medicine in 1996 recommended that reference case cost-effectiveness analyses conducted from the societal perspective only include direct costs of care and exclude productivity costs, a term that was suggested to supplant the term *indirect costs*. The rationale offered was that quality-adjusted life-years, or QALYs, recommended as a measure of health outcomes could entail double counting with economic productivity. The National Institute of Health and Clinical Excellence (NICE) in the United Kingdom likewise recommends that only direct costs be included in cost-effectiveness analyses.

The leading use of human capital estimates is in COI studies used to call the attention of stakeholders to the economic impact of diseases or injuries and the potential gains from allocating funds to research and prevention, but they can also be used in the economic evaluation of programs or interventions. For example, the economic benefit of folic acid fortification policies for the prevention of certain types of birth defects, spina bifida and anencephaly, has been calculated as the present value of lifetime earnings for averted cases of anencephaly, which is uniformly fatal in the neonatal period, and the present value of averted medical and educational costs and gains in economic productivity from the prevention of lifelong disability and early mortality resulting from averted cases of spina bifida.

Scott D. Grosse

Disclaimer: The findings and conclusions in this report are those of the author and do not necessarily represent the official position of the Centers for Disease Control and Prevention.

See also Cost-Benefit Analysis; Costs, Direct Versus Indirect

Further Readings

Grosse, S. D., Waitzman, N. J., Romano, P. S., & Mulinare, J. (2005). Reevaluating the benefits of folic acid fortification in the United States: Economic analysis, regulation, and public health. *American Journal of Public Health, 95,* 1917–1922.
Luce, B. R., Manning, W. G., Siegel, J. E., & Lipscomb, J. (1996). Estimating costs in cost-effectiveness analysis. In M. R. Gold, J. E. Siegel, L. B. Russell, & M. C. Weinstein (Eds.), *Cost-effectiveness in health and medicine* (pp. 176–213). New York: Oxford University Press.
Max, W., Rice, D. P., & MacKenzie, E. J. (1990). The lifetime cost of injury. *Inquiry, 27,* 332–343.
Verstappen, S. M., Boonen, A., Verkleij, H., Bijlsma, J. W., Buskens, E., & Jacobs, J. W. (2005). Productivity costs among patients with rheumatoid arthritis: The influence of methods and sources to value loss of productivity. *Annals of the Rheumatic Diseases, 64,* 1754–1760.
Waitzman, N. J., Scheffler, R. M., & Romano, P. S. (1996). *The cost of birth defects.* Lanham, MD: University Press of America.

HUMAN COGNITIVE SYSTEMS

Human cognitive systems are the systems in the human mind that involve the conscious processing of information of various types and that help individuals deal with self, others, and the world. Human cognitive systems as they reside in the human mind are typically described as being mental processes that are typically accessible by only the individual. As the individual behaves in the world and as that individual communicates with others, the individual can share to some degree (but does not have to) what is going on in his or her own mind.

The processes underlying human cognitive systems, such as thinking and deciding, for the most part, are not held in consciousness but remain as unconscious or subconscious processes.

Referent of the Term *Cognition*

The term *cognition* can be used to refer to the *processes* of thought, the process of thinking, the applying of rules, the development of plans in humans, the weighing of risk and benefit, or the performances of operations such as mathematical operations, or to the *results of such processes* in humans, animals, and machines. The term can apply to the processes of thinking, deciding, and perceiving, or to the results of such cognitive activity. The term *cognition* can apply to beliefs of as well as knowledge of individuals, groups, or populations.

The term may also apply to some views of perceiving (perception) but not necessarily to certain views of sensing (sensation). The construction of sensations into perceptions may be considered by some to be a cognitive process even though such construction or processing can occur unconsciously or subconsciously. And these perceptions often occur instantaneously, as when we see a tree and we see (perceive) this tree as having a back side, even though we do not see that back side in our perception. Yet if we walk around that tree, the argument continues, we would be surprised to find that it did not have a back side and was just, for example, an elaborately constructed stage prop and not a tree at all.

Preferences and Decision Making

Cognitive science in the late 1970s to early 2000s focused on the notion of mind and intelligence in terms of representation and computational procedures of human intelligence versus machine intelligence (artificial intelligence), with cognitive research on medical artificial intelligence, artificial intelligence in choice and explanation, artificial neural networks, prediction of medical conditions and disease processes such as community-acquired pneumonia, and computer-based explanations of decision theoretic advice, among others. Yet cognitive science of the late 1970s to early 2000s also needs to be recast in terms of its definition and needs and seen as taking on different dimensions than the cognitive science of the 1950s. Yet both domains still share crucial similarities.

Today, the concept of cognitive science goes beyond this notion. The cognitive sciences today, particularly as they apply to medical decision making, also explore the notions of patient preferences, how patients make decisions on their own (descriptive decision making), and how this descriptive

decision making compares with other models of how decisions should be made (normative decision making). In terms of normative decision making, human preference in medical choice situations is compared with normative models of decision making, such as expected value theory. Today, it can be argued that emotion (and emotive theory) also has a role to play in the cognitive sciences.

However, today, the ways in which humans think, problem solve, and weigh decisions in terms of output of human mental processes (human intelligence) are not compared with machine intelligence (artificial intelligence) but rather are contrasted to the outputs of alternative approaches of how decisions should be made (normative theory, such as expected value theory) or alternative theories regarding how decisions are actually made by humans (psychological theory, such as prospect theory).

In such later comparisons a different form of cognitive science arises, one that—in essential qualities of comparison—is not that dissimilar in terms of methodology from the attempt of the earlier view of cognitive science to capture human mental output and problem-solving skills in terms of representations and computational procedures and then compare how human intelligence compares and contrasts with artificial intelligence.

Framing and Choice

Amos Tversky and Daniel Kahneman describe their work in choice and decision making in relation to the basic model of mind given above. When the authors talk about decision making, they use the term *decision frame* to refer to the decision maker's conception of what he or she considers—consciously, unconsciously, or subconsciously—as the acts, outcomes, and contingencies associated with a particular choice. They further note that this frame adopted by the decision maker is influenced by the way the problem is formulated and partly by the decision maker's own norms, habits, and personal characteristics.

Tversky and Kahneman compare their perspective on alternative frames for a decision problem to perception, particularly, the alternative perspectives on a visual scene. The term *veridical* means coinciding with reality. Tversky and Kahneman note that veridical perception requires that the "perceived relative heights" of two neighboring mountains should not reverse with any change of vantage point of an observer. In a similar vein, the authors argue that rational choice requires that the preference between options should not reverse with changes of frame or perspective. They then link the imperfections of perception in the human being with the imperfections of human decision making. For the authors, changes of perspective, in fact, often reverse (or at least in some way influence) the relative apparent size of objects, and changes of perspective, in fact, often reverse (or at least influence in some way) the relative desirability of options.

Tversky and Kahneman thus characterize their own research in framing as an attempt to describe and thus represent the human cognitive system in terms of the systematic reversals of preferences. Their own research discovered that by varying the framing of acts, their contingencies, and their outcomes, human cognitive systems of study volunteers respond to such changes (descriptive decision making) in ways that are not predicted by normative models of decision making, such as expected utility theory.

Language Learning and Problem Solving

Just as Tversky and Kahneman consider their framing effects as almost akin to human perceptual effects, there are many basic questions raised by the application of framing effects into medical decision making that raise issues in other areas of human cognitive systems: namely, the capacity for language and problem solving.

Tversky and Kahneman's research, based on their concept of framing, focused on one type of study design methodology: choices between "a simple gamble" or "a sure thing," each with an objectively specified probability and at most two nonzero outcomes. Typical choice situations were based on monetary gains and losses or survival (health-related) gains and losses.

Tversky and Kahneman were interested in "gain" and "loss" situations. In a gain situation, a typical monetary choice given by Tversky and Kahneman to study participants was a sure gain of $250 versus a 25% chance to gain $1,000 and a 75% chance of gaining nothing. A typical monetary choice in a loss situation involved consideration of a sure loss of $250 versus a 25% chance of losing $1,000 and a 75% chance of losing nothing.

A typical survival-mortality choice situation given by Tversky and Kahneman to study participants for consideration involved a disease outbreak where the overall baseline situation is a disease outbreak with an overall expectation of 600 people being killed, but there is a gain scenario and a loss scenario. The gain scenario is illustrated by the choice given between two programs, Vaccine Program A, which if adopted would allow 200 people to be saved (+200 being saved), versus Vaccine Program B, which if adopted would result in a one-third chance of 600 people being saved (+200 being saved) and a two-thirds chance of no one being saved. In terms of loss, a typical survival-mortality choice situation that could have been given by Tversky and Kahneman to study participants for consideration could have involved a new vaccine first to be used in a human population that has an as yet unknown defect. This flawed vaccine—instead of saving lives—will cause more people to be killed until the fact that the vaccine is flawed is identified. The choice given is between two programs using the flawed vaccine, Flawed Vaccine Program C, which if adopted would allow 200 additional people to be killed of an at-risk group that the vaccine was intended to save (200 individuals being killed), versus Flawed Vaccine Program D, which if adopted would result in a one-third chance of 600 at-risk people being killed (200 individuals being killed) and a two-thirds chance of no one being killed.

Part of the challenges faced by the study volunteers in each of the above thought experiments is the extent to which the study participants could imagine the gains and losses to be real considerations in their own lives while answering the questionnaires in a study setting. This challenge also related to Tversky and Kahneman's methodology, specifically relating to the fact that it may be difficult to invent choice scenarios in survival-mortality contexts that involve gains and losses, as in the flawed vaccine example, to make the scenario believable enough that the study participants can place themselves in the scenario as the individual targeted to make the decision.

In general, it is also important for study investigators to recognize that some study participants are unwilling to agree to participation in questionnaire studies that require them to consider gambles in relation to human life. Such individuals hold personal beliefs that will not allow them to participate in such studies, and thus, these individuals' opinions will not be reflected in the study results of such research endeavors in decision making.

The internal constraints—study of one type of choice between "a simple gamble" or "a sure thing," each with an objectively specified probability and at most two nonzero outcomes—explicitly placed by these two psychologists on their rigorous study methodology (with the aim of understanding what types of choices humans make in specifically defined choice situations involving gains and losses and considerations of gambles vs. sure things) allowed them to construct a Nobel prize–winning theory that was highly dependent on at least two capacities of human cognitive systems in addition to perception: language learning and problem solving.

Literacy and Numeracy

Here, language learning has two components: the ability to work with words (*literacy*) and the ability to work with numbers (*numeracy*). The problem that arises for Tversky and Kahneman is what happens when the citizens of a population have difficulties with literacy, numeracy, or both. An additional problem arises when the citizens of a population prefer to discuss issues such as are found in medical decision making in terms of quality expressions of chance (probability), that is, in terms of words and not in terms of numbers. David H. Hickam and Dennis Mazur have found that in discussion of risk in medicine, patients prefer to discuss risk with their physicians in terms of qualitative expressions of chance (probability), such as "rare," "possible," and "probable," and not in terms of numerical expressions of chance (probability), such as "percents."

The very understanding of medical decision making has been argued to require a high propensity for verbal and numerical abilities for those patients and consumers interested in participating in considering scientific evidence derived from research studies as part of their own decision making in relation to shared decision making between patients and their providers, or in terms

of physician-based decision making where the patient may not want to make a decision on care but does want to track those decisions.

Yet there are many reasons to believe that solutions to these basic issues of literacy and numeracy in a population are not easy to move in positive directions beyond the research finding that a majority of patients do not want to discuss risk with their physicians in terms of numbers (quantitative expressions of probability) and prefer to discuss risk in terms of words (qualitative expressions of probability). This entry now considers an alternative to simple numbers: graphical data displays, for example, pie charts.

To date, graphs have been forbidden in the United States by federal regulation in direct-to-consumer advertisements used to sell medical products (prescription medicine and medical devices) to consumers through broadcast advertising over television because of the ways data can be unfairly manipulated in graphic data displays.

Jessica S. Ancker and colleagues note both the positive and negative impacts of graphs used to display data in medical and public health decision making. First, an example of a positive aspect of a graph is that it may allow patients and consumers to understand more clearly through a visual graphical display part-to-whole relationships. In helping patients understand data and scientific evidence in medicine, graphical data displays can help patients visually attend to key components of chance (probability) that can be expressed as a ratio of two numbers (e.g., a fraction with a numerator over a denominator). This fraction can also be expressed by a graph visually expressing the relationship between a numerator (the number of people sustaining adverse outcomes) and the denominator (the entire population studied), for example, in a pie diagram.

Second, graphs may be used to manipulate the very same numbers, for example, when the developer of the graph elects to display only the numerator in a graph used in a direct-to-consumer advertisement. A graph that displays only the numerator can be intentionally used to appear to inflate the perceived risk and, thus, induce risk-averse behavior on the part of the consumer. The *U.S. Code of Federal Regulations* attempts to guard against such manipulation by product manufacturers and their advertisers in the federal regulation of direct-to-consumer advertising of prescription medicines.

Challenges facing direct-to-consumer advertising of prescription medicines and medical devices in cases where consumers and patients are not attending to numbers or graphs include the attention paid by (and the weight given to information by) consumers and patients to nonnumerical and nongraphical information such as *who* is endorsing the medical product. Directing consumers away from a full understanding of the numbers and scientific evidence that surrounds a medical product is often a key goal of a financially successful direct-to-consumer advertising program.

Dennis J. Mazur

See also Decision Psychology; Prospect Theory; Unreliability of Memory

Further Readings

Ancker, J. S., Senathirajah, Y., Kukafka, R., & Starren, J. B. (2006). Design features of graphs in health risk communication: A systematic review. *Journal of the American Medical Informatics Association, 13,* 608–618.

Baron, J. (2000). *Thinking and deciding.* New York: Cambridge University Press.

Fagerlin, A., Zikmund-Fisher, B. J., Ubel, P. A., Jankovic, A., Derry, H. A., & Smith, D. M. (2007). Measuring numeracy without a math test: Development of the subjective numeracy scale. *Medical Decision Making, 27,* 672–680.

Føllesdal, D. (1969). Husserl's notion of noema. *Journal of Philosophy, 66,* 680–687.

Lipkus, I. M., Samsa, G., & Rimer, B. K. (2001). General performance on a numeracy scale among highly educated samples. *Medical Decision Making, 21,* 37–44.

Mazur, D. J., & Hickam, D. H. (1997). Patients' preferences for risk disclosure and role in decision making for invasive medical procedures. *Journal of General Internal Medicine, 12,* 114–117.

Seebohm, T. M., Føllesdal, D., & Mohanty, J. N. (Eds.). (1991). *Phenomenology and the formal sciences.* Dordrecht, The Netherlands: Kluwer Academic.

Smith, D. W., & McIntyre, R. (1982). *Husserl and intentionality: A study of mind, meaning and language.* Dordrecht, the Netherlands: D. Reidel.

Tversky, A., & Kahneman, D. (1981). The framing of decisions and the psychology of choice. *Science, 211,* 453–458.

Woloshin, S., Schwartz, L. M., Moncur, M., Gabriel, S., & Tosteson, A. N. A. (2001). Assessing values for health: Numeracy matters. *Medical Decision Making, 21,* 380–388.

HYPOTHESIS TESTING

A scientific hypothesis is tested by evaluating the logical consistency of its implications and/or the accuracy of its predictions. Other grounds for assessing hypotheses include breadth of prediction, scientific fertility, simplicity, and aesthetic appeal; however, the term *hypothesis testing* refers only to accuracy. Statistical hypothesis testing, a form of inductive inference, is used extensively in medical research and described here as a form of proof by contradiction.

A hypothesis is rejected by a test if the hypothesis logically implies something false or strongly predicts something contradicted by data. The 2,500-year-old proof by Hippasus of Metapontum that $\sqrt{2}$ is not a ratio of whole numbers exemplifies the former. Hypothesizing the opposite, that $\sqrt{2} = a/b$ for whole numbers a and b, Hippasus deduced the impossible: that both numerator and denominator must remain divisible by 2, even after all possible cancellations of 2 from both a and b. Unable to deny the logic of this contradiction, a rational mind instead rejects the hypothesis, concluding that $\sqrt{2}$ *cannot be* such a ratio. This is proof by contradiction or, from the Latin, *reductio ad absurdum*.

Data may also contradict hypotheses. In deterministic settings, that is, when predictions are made with certainty because all relevant influences are presumed known, one valid incompatible datum overturns a hypothesis. The hypothesis "Elixir A cures all cancer" is overturned by a single treatment failure, demonstrating conclusively that other treatment is sometimes required. This is an empirical analog of proof by contradiction.

In medical sciences, though, knowledge is incomplete and biological variability the rule. Hence, determinism is rare. Medical hypotheses describe tendencies that are exhibited variably, in complex systems governed by probabilities rather than individually predictable fates. The hypothesis "Elixir A increases the fraction of cases alive two months postdiagnosis" does not imply that a particular individual will live for 2 months. Unless 2-month survival is already extremely high, this hypothesis cannot be overturned by one or even several early deaths.

But suppose, in a trial of Elixir A, that all 10 clinically similar but otherwise unrelated patients who receive it die before 2 months postdiagnosis. If extensive data show that only half of similar untreated cases die this quickly, most would reconsider further use of Elixir A. Although 10 patients on any new treatment may all be unlucky, the chance of this happening in a specified study is below $2^{-10} = .098\%$ if Elixir A is beneficial. Logically, either luck has been extraordinarily poor, or Elixir A doesn't work as hypothesized. A longer consecutive run of deaths would be even less likely, for example, $2^{-15} = .003\%$ for 15 deaths, and hence more difficult to attribute to bad luck. With "enough" accumulated evidence, most persons bow to its weight and reject the initial hypothesis, because the hypothesis made a strong prediction that failed. Specifically, the hypothesis had predicted strongly, that is, with very high probability, that data would show a 2-month case fatality more similar to what the hypothesis describes (< 50%) than to what was actually seen (100%).

Such probabilistic proof by contradiction exemplifies statistical hypothesis testing, the focus of this entry. Statistical hypothesis tests influence most research on which medical decisions are based. Their general use is to select, from among statistical associations in data, those hardest to explain by play of chance in a particular data sample. The selected associations, unless explicable by study design problems, receive preferential evaluation for causal involvement in disease initiation, promotion, progression to disability, and therapeutic benefit.

Statistical Hypotheses, Distributions, and Evidentiary Standards

Statistical hypothesis testing presupposes a scientific hypothesis of interest, H, and a source of relevant data, for example, clinical or laboratory experiment, observational epidemiological study,

or clinical database. The notation H_C is used for the complement, or negation, of H. Testing constitutes a formal confrontation of a prediction from either H or H_C with the data. This involves several steps, starting with a choice to test either H or H_C and selection of a basic probability model for the data-generating process. The probability model consists of a collection of probability laws assumed to include one which accurately portrays this process. These laws are usually constructed from component probability distribution functions, for example, binomial, Poisson, normal (Gaussian), or lognormal distributions, thought to describe the origins of individual observations or sets of observations from a patient. This class is then partitioned into two subsets of probability laws, respectively, consistent with H and with H_C. From this partition follows a *statistical hypothesis* H_0, postulating that the data arise from a member of the subset associated with whichever scientific hypothesis, H or H_C, was chosen for testing.

Predictions about data can then be based, when the scientific hypothesis selected for testing is correct, on one or more probability laws from the subset associated with H_0. Along the lines of "the enemy of my enemy is my friend," data discrepant with predictions from H_0 contradict the scientific hypothesis H or H_C on which H_0 is based, supporting the other. Note that the sometimes important distinction between testing a scientific hypothesis H using predictions from H_0, and testing whether H_0 contains an accurate probability model for the data, is often dropped in application. For simplicity and brevity, we must also sometimes drop it below.

In the 10-patient trial above, one hypothesized H, that a cancer patient treated rapidly with Elixir A stood more than a 50% chance of surviving at least 2 months after diagnosis, rather than H_C, a 50% chance or less. Based on the clinical similarity and presumably independent results of otherwise unrelated patients, the probability model consists of all binomial distributions Bin(10, π), with π the chance a patient survives 2 months, and Bin(n, π) the mathematically proven probability law describing a count of accumulated events from n independent tries of the same process, each with chance π of producing the event. These distributions with $\pi > 50\%$ reflect H and with $\pi \leq 50\%$ reflect H_C. H_0, based on H, hypothesizes that the data arise from one of the former group. H_0 is said to be a "composite" versus "simple" hypothesis because it contains more than one distribution. Any Bin(10, π) in H_0 predicts some 2-month survivors with probability exceeding 99.9%. Total absence of survivors disconfirms this strong prediction based on H and supports H_C, that Elixir A is ineffective or even harmful.

Scientifically, one usually hopes to demonstrate presence rather than absence of a relationship. Thus, when H posits a relationship, H_0 is usually based on H_C, hypothesizing its absence or opposite. H_0 is then called the *statistical null hypothesis,* motivating the conventional subscripted 0. The researcher wishes to assemble enough data to contradict H_0, discredit H_C, and hence confirm H.

Suppose H_0 has been chosen based on some scientific hypothesis H. A method is then selected for locating the observed data on a scale of discrepancy from H toward H_C, in relation to other possible study results that might have but did not occur. The scale is defined by the value of a summary statistic, for example, a count (as above), proportion, mean, difference, or ratio of these or the maximum probability of the observed data for a probability law from H_0. Any such scale defines a possible hypothesis test. The scale ordinarily incorporates whether testing is "one sided" or "two sided." For instance, in the one-sided example above, 2/10 = 20% early deaths are less discrepant from H_0 ($\pi > 50\%$ for survival) than are 6/10 = 60% early deaths, but would be more discrepant on a reasonable scale for two-sided testing of H_0^*: Elixir A has no effect (H_0: $\pi = 50\%$).

Research results sufficiently discrepant to reject H_0 are determined, using the selected discrepancy scale, by designating a maximum allowable chance of erroneous rejections when H_0 applies. This probability, symbolized by α, is called the *significance level* or simply *level* of the test. The collection of results discrepant enough to reject is then formed by successively including possible results, from most discrepant toward less discrepant from H, as ordered by the summary statistic. The process stops when rejections based on the next value of the summary statistic would raise the accumulated rejection probability above α for some distribution in H_0.

The level α serves as a probabilistic standard for strength of evidence required to reject H_0. For tests

based on continuous probability distributions, α is the chance that a true hypothesis will be erroneously rejected and otherwise is an upper bound. In practice, α is often chosen from among 10%, 5%, 1%, and 0.1%; lower values require stronger evidence to reject H_0. The Neyman-Pearson approach to statistical hypothesis testing, invoked explicitly by considerations of statistical power, also requires the specification of an *alternative hypothesis H_A* that comprises probability laws possibly applying when H_0 is false.

The steps above prescribe how to test H_0 using any data that occurs. The summary statistic and its location on the discrepancy scale are determined. This location indicates whether the evidentiary standard for rejection has been met and hence whether the test is passed or failed. If the latter, H_0 is rejected, and the effect, trend, or "signal" in the data is labeled "statistically significant." If the former, some say H_0 is accepted, others that it is retained, that the test fails to reject, or that the signal is not statistically significant. *Accepted* is a technical term in this context; literal acceptance is rarely if ever justified in medical hypothesis testing.

Technical Aspects and Examples

Most generally, a statistical hypothesis test may be viewed as partitioning the universe U of possible data sets that might be observed in a study into a *rejection region U_R* and its complement U_C. U_R is chosen so that, when H_0 is true, the maximum probability of observing data within U_R, called the *size* of the test, equals or is minimally below α. Among possible such choices of U_R, a region is selected with high chance of containing data likely to occur from the type of relationship one expects, and hopes to detect, if H_0 is false.

Implementation involves rejecting H_0, or not, based on the location of a summary *test statistic* within a reference probability distribution. The test of a genuinely null hypothesis, that is, one representing no difference between quantities such as averages or proportions over time or between groups, is then analogous to a clinical diagnostic test. In diagnosis, the detection target is disease in a patient; in statistical hypothesis testing, the target is a systematic statistical relationship in the population generating the data. The hypothesis test may mistakenly reject H_0 when true, a Type I error, or mistakenly retain H_0 when false, a Type II error. These errors are respectively analogous to false-positive and false-negative diagnoses. The Type I error probability is the size of the test, which for simplicity we now assume equals the stipulated level α. Its complement, the chance $1 - \alpha$ that H_0 passes the test when true, is analogous to diagnostic specificity. Type II error probability is represented by β. Its complement $1 - \beta$, the chance of rejecting a false H_0, is the test's *power*, analogous to diagnostic sensitivity. Power and β are functions of the extent to which reality departs from H_0. Tables 1 and 2 show the analogy. In diagnosis, one desires highest possible sensitivity for given false-positive rate. In hypothesis testing, one desires highest possible power for given test level α.

Suppose one conducts a parallel group randomized trial comparing a new drug with placebo and wishes to demonstrate differences in mean diastolic blood pressures (DBP) and proportions of patients who experienced a myocardial infarction (MI) after 1 year. For DBP, blood pressures might be assumed normally distributed, and H_0 might state that DBPs within each group have identical distributions. The ubiquitous Student's t statistic is the ratio of the difference between mean DBPs among patients receiving the new drug and receiving placebo (essentially, the signal in the data), to its estimated standard error, a measure of sensitivity to random variation among patients, that is, statistical noise. U_R contains data sets for which this ratio differs from 0 more than would occur $100(1 - (\alpha/2))\%$ of the time if H_0 were true, as calculated from a Student's t distribution, the relevant reference probability law.

For MI, H_0 states that probability of MI within a year is unaffected by drug. An equivalent version of the well-known Pearson chi-square test uses the ratio of the difference between proportions of

Table 1   Diagnostic test probabilities

Disease	Test Result	
	Negative	Positive
Absent	Specificity	False-positive rate
Present	False-negative rate	Sensitivity

Table 2   Hypothesis test probabilities

Null Hypothesis	Test Result	
	Retain	Reject
True	$1 - \alpha$	Type I error: α
False	Type II error: β	Power: $1 - \beta$

patients who experienced an MI to its estimated standard error when H_0 is true. U_R is determined as above, but using a different reference distribution.

Use of unsigned differences and $\alpha/2$, as above, pertain to two-sided tests. In one-sided testing, U_R contains only data sets reflecting the anticipated direction, up to accumulated probability $100(1 - \alpha)\%$. In the examples, only differences of prespecified sign would justify rejection. Since rejection in one direction is precluded, a one-sided test allows easier rejection of H_0 in the other, anticipated direction, than does a two-sided test if both are at level α.

Extensive theory guides selection of a hypothesis test to use information in data from a given scientific setting most efficiently, stemming from work of J. Neyman and E. S. Pearson on testing with stipulated or optimum power against a specified alternative hypothesis H_A. Many methods for constructing U_R have been developed. Likelihood ratio testing orders data sets for placement into U_R by the ratio, lowest to highest, of the highest probability of the data under a distribution in H_0 to their highest probability under a stipulated broader class of distributions (e.g., H_0 or H_A, if an H_A has been specified). Other methods, such as score and Wald tests, also use test statistics calculated from assumed or approximated underlying probability laws. Reference probability distributions are also derived from a priori mathematical models for data generation processes or from theoretical approximations to the random behavior of summary statistics from large samples.

Sometimes a reference distribution may be developed based on a verifiable property of the data collection process or on symmetry considerations in a related "thought experiment." Thus, when treatment assignments are randomized, a reference distribution may be obtained by considering how a test statistic would vary across all possible randomized assignments. Such randomization tests have high credibility due to conceptual simplicity and freedom from mathematical assumptions.

Information is lost when tests are reported as statistically significant, or not, at a fixed level. If statistical significance is reported at 5%, researchers with a more stringent evidentiary standard, say 1%, are left ignorant as to whether their standard has been achieved. If nonsignificance at 5% is reported, other researchers with a less stringent evidentiary standard, say 10%, are left similarly ignorant. Most researchers therefore report the p value of a test, defined as the lowest level for which the test is statistically significant, allowing each reader to assess statistical significance relative to an individual standard. Modern software automates reporting of p values.

Some take this further, by omitting prespecification of α and U_R altogether and using the p value as an index of compatibility of the data with H_0, on the discrepancy scale that underlies the hypothesis test. Values close to 0 reflect discrepancy; values above 0.1 reflect compatibility, increasingly with the value. Such use reasonably accords with the views of founders of biometrics, including K. Pearson, W. S. Gosset, and R. A. Fisher, but is in some respects incompatible with the Neyman-Pearson theory that followed. Thus, somewhat different testing philosophies coexist in general scientific practice.

This discussion has focused on the frequentist-based hypothesis tests that dominate the current biomedical literature. A Bayesian inferential perspective offers useful alternatives by treating both data and hypotheses as subject to probability distributions and incorporating a priori probabilities of hypotheses. Due to their subjectivity, Bayesian hypothesis tests have not been widely accepted in scientific practice. The increasing capabilities of "objective Bayes" methods, emphasizing prior distributions that limit effects of subjectivity, may overcome resistance.

Peter B. Imrey

See also Bayesian Analysis; Coincidence; Confidence Intervals; Effect Size; Frequentist Approach; Likelihood Ratio; Managing Variability and Uncertainty; Probability; Sample Size and Power; Statistical Testing: Overview

Further Readings

Barnett, V. (1999). *Comparative statistical inference* (3rd ed.). New York: Wiley.

Carlin, B. P., & Louis, T. A. (2008). *Bayesian methods for data analysis* (3rd ed.). New York: Chapman & Hall.

Cox, D. R. (1977). The role of significance tests. *Scandinavian Journal of Statistics, 4*, 49–70.

Edgington, E. S. (1995). *Randomization tests* (3rd ed.). New York: Dekker.

Fisher, R. A. (1959). *Statistical methods and scientific inference*. Edinburgh, UK: Oliver & Boyd.

Fisher, R. A. (1970). *Statistical methods for research workers* (14th ed.). New York: Hafner.

Lehmann, E. L., & Romano, J. P. (2008). *Testing statistical hypotheses*. New York: Springer.

Mayo, D. G., & Cox, D. R. (2006). Frequentist statistics as a theory of inductive inference. In J. Rojo (Ed.), *Optimality: The second Erich L. Lehman symposium* (pp. 77–97), May 19–22, 2004, Rice University, Houston, TX; Beachwood, OH: Institute of Mathematical Statistics.

Neyman, J., & Pearson, E. S. (1966). *Joint statistical papers of J. Neyman and E. S. Pearson*. Berkeley: University of California Press.

Pearson, K. (1948). On a criterion that a given system of deviations from the probable in the case of a correlated system of variables is such that it can reasonably be supposed to have arisen from random sampling. In E. S. Pearson (Ed.), *Karl Pearson's early papers*. Cambridge, UK: Cambridge University Press. (Reprinted from *Philosophical Magazine, Series 5, 50*, 157–175, 1900)

Wald, A. (1955). *Selected papers in probability and statistics*. New York: McGraw-Hill.